THE ARCHAEOLOGY OF DISEASE

THE ARCHAEOLOGY OF DISEASE

FOURTH EDITION

Charlotte A. Roberts, Mary E. Lewis,
Jacalyn Duffin, and Keith Manchester

The History Press

First published in the USA by Cornell University Press, 2026
First published in the UK by The History Press, 2026

The History Press
97 St George's Place, Cheltenham,
Gloucestershire, GL50 3QB
www.thehistorypress.co.uk

British Library Cataloguing in Publication Data.
A catalogue record for this book is available from the British Library.

ISBN 978 1 83705 206 6

Typesetting and origination by Cornell University Press
Printed and bound in Great Britain by TJ Books, Padstow, Cornwall

FSC www.fsc.org MIX Paper | Supporting responsible forestry FSC® C013056

The History Press proudly supports

Trees for Life

www.treesforlife.org.uk

EU Authorised Representative: Easy Access System Europe
Mustamäe tee 50, 10621 Tallinn, Estonia
gpsr.requests@easproject.com

Dedicated to Ann Manchester and Ann Hunter

Contents

Foreword

Anne L. Grauer

I remember it clearly. He sat cross-legged on his living room floor scrutinizing images of paleopathological conditions. Were more needed? Could any be discarded without compromising the message? Would they be more effective for readers as half or full-page plates? This was my introduction, in 1982, to Keith Manchester's soon-to-be-published book, *The Archaeology of Disease.* I hadn't read the text. I had no idea of the extraordinary impact the book would have on the fields of bioarchaeology and paleopathology. That soon would change.

Exploration into ancient diseases has been an interest of medical practitioners for almost a century. By the 1970s, with a growing inclusion of archaeologists and anthropologists, scientists made great headway into both the diagnosis of disease and placing health and disease into larger contexts. Journal articles and books emphasizing the importance of careful diagnosis based on clinical and archaeological or historical knowledge and taking geographic and populational approaches informed professionals and students alike. Missing, however, was a resource that synthesized a myriad of information and perspectives bound within a single cover. Cue *The Archaeology of Disease.*

From the very first page, it was evident that Keith Manchester's book was unique. It began with Part 1, Diseases and Mankind, followed by Part 2, Diseases *of* Mankind. The distinction between these sections, while subtle, was significant. First, prior to discussing specific diseases, foundational archaeological/anthropological concepts were tackled. These included the importance of taking an evolutionary approach toward understanding disease and recognizing that human behavior, which included changes to subsistence strategies and human/environmental interaction, were essential variables to consider when exploring past diseases. The need to recognize and contend with biases inherent to the assessment of mummified and skeletal remains was also emphasized. Readers were warned that we only get a glimpse of the presence and impact of diseases in the past, and that great care was needed when formulating conclusions.

Unequivocally, this fourth edition builds on the scaffolding assembled by Keith Manchester and later strongly reinforced by Charlotte Roberts, coauthor of the following two editions. For one, each chapter in this new edition deftly incorporates biases and issues inherent to both the diagnosis of diseases (or conditions) and to their interpretation. This is germane to the field of bioarchaeology and paleopathology, as the paths to offering conclusions are seldom straight. Each chapter emphasizes the need for diagnostic rigor and transparency. Amidst discussion of the many new accomplishments in molecular techniques, such as DNA and isotopic analyses, readers are encouraged to embrace uncertainty; to become comfortable with complex differential diagnoses and indefinite conclusions. They are warned about the great potential and unfortunate pitfalls of using modern clinical data as a basis for diagnoses and about simplistically interpreting the impact of a disease on the lives of an individual or a population in the past.

Readers are also informed of the importance of understanding the history of anatomical collections and archaeological excavation and current conversations involving the ethical treatment of human remains. We aren't studying the history of disease in a vacuum. Decisions and actions based on entitlement have led to the creation of collections and our opportunity to study human remains—remains of those who did not consent to their bodies being used as a curiosity, a "treasure," a teaching tool, or object of scientific inquiry. As emphasized by the authors, this recognition is not tangential to the study of disease in the past. It is integral.

Much like the first edition, but moving well beyond, this edition also emphasizes the need to incorporate multiple lines of evidence into analyses. Yes, the title of the book highlights the role that archaeology plays in understanding the past, but the content clearly recognizes the need to incorporate new medical and biological knowledge, new diagnostic techniques, as well as new historical and archaeological data, leading to a far richer understanding of all disease categories. For instance, great strides have been made in understanding the pathogenesis and detection of infectious diseases, as well as cancer. These data, alongside historical documents and archaeological analysis, provide a greater foundation upon which we can explore the evolution of disease, the spatial and chronological distributions, and ways in which individuals and populations biologically and culturally adapted.

Appreciating individual and population-level approaches also resonates throughout this book. In each edition, and especially in this new fourth edition, discussion of multiscale research is introduced, regardless of the disease or condition under investigation. Disease does not solely affect individuals, but rather develops, spreads, waxes, and wanes within groups defined and influenced, in part, by geographic area, genetic ancestry, environmental interactions, and human sociocultural behavior, to name a few. The authors recognize this and deftly communicate the complexities of diagnosing the presence of disease on one hand and interpreting its significance on the other. Discussion of recent advances in mathematical modeling and statistical analyses further allows readers to appreciate the presence and potential impact of diseases on population-level scales.

The emphasis on modern contexts of diseases in earlier editions of this book truly set the books apart from others. Manchester and Roberts wisely communicated that diseases of the past did not disappear but, rather, played significant roles in the lives of individuals and within populations today. This edition of the book further emphasizes this point. Discussion of each condition, each disease category, is firmly established in today's world. The result of this perspective is twofold. First, it provides a context for comparing current trends with those of the past. Second, and perhaps more importantly, it allows us to appreciate and, hopefully, scientifically test the roles that multiple variables play in the presence and progression of disease. Readers are introduced to the many ways in which understanding the past, alongside the present, can inform our future. What role did environmental change play in contributing to or reducing the presence of disease in the past? How might it inform us about the effects of climate change today? How can our understanding of maternal and generational health help us predict diseases and potentially ameliorate them?

Arguably, one of the greatest influences within bioarchaeology and paleopathology has been the incorporation of social theory into the interpretation of disease. We've moved far past the trope of "high status versus low status" as the key social variables influencing health and disease—especially since the terms were rarely, if ever, defined. Many factors influence the presence and interpretation of health and disease, including complex social interactions between individuals and groups, changing roles one takes throughout life, and individual and group perceptions of "disease" itself. Much to the credit of the authors of this edition, human identities (created and/or perceived by oneself or others), human agency, and concepts of "disability" are folded into the evaluation of disease in the past. So, too, is the recognition that social roles and identity might or might not be linked to physiological development. Hence, socially constructed categories of "subadult," or "infant," or "juvenile," or "adult" are neither universal classifications nor absolute predictors of disease. Rather, exploring the complex interactions between human development within social contexts is essential. The authors also carefully dissect the concept of "disability." They inform readers that the presumption that having a condition or a disease left one unable to fully contribute to their group or in need of help inexcusably simplifies the varied ways individuals operate within groups. It ignores the fact that humans must rely on one another throughout their lives, even if they are deemed "healthy."

Finally, it is interesting to note the parallels between the ever-increasing complexity of bioarchaeological and paleopathological analysis and the inclusion of two new authors of this edition. The widening scope of the topic the "archaeology of disease," now propelled by hypothesis-driven inquiry, requires the incorporation of many experts from many fields—a transdisciplinary approach. Scholars trained in medicine, biology, history, imaging, veterinary medicine, ecology, statistics, and anthropology/archaeology, to name a few, provide both a breadth and depth of understanding that a single individual (or single discipline) rarely can achieve. Hence, our field, as well as this edition, is strengthened immeasurably by inclusion. With the four authors—Keith Manchester, a practicing physician, Charlotte

Roberts, trained first in nursing and later as a paleopathologist, Mary Lewis, a bioarchaeologist whose work has focused on health and disease of children and adolescents, and Jacalyn Duffin, a hematologist and medical historian—this edition offers a broad and synthetic view. The message to the reader is clear: Regardless of whether you are a scholar, a student, or simply interested in the subject, recognizing the social and evolutionary complexities of health and disease, alongside issues surrounding scientific analysis itself, are as important to address as successfully diagnosing the presence of disease in the past.

Preface

On the publication of the fourth edition of *The Archaeology of Disease*, it seems fitting to consider the book's history. In 1978, Keith Manchester had been invited to join the then University of Bradford's School of Archaeological Sciences as a part-time lecturer. Alongside his general practitioner commitments, Keith's undergraduate teaching and linked research became the foundation of a one-year master's degree in human osteology, paleopathology, and funerary archaeology. Charlotte Roberts came on board to help develop, run, and teach on that course in 1989, having previously served as Keith's research assistant from 1983 to 1989. The course was launched in 1990. Paleopathology and bioarchaeology have continued to thrive at Bradford to the present day. The early 1980s saw the publication of the first edition of this book, Manchester (1983), with the second edition published twelve years later, Roberts and Manchester (1995), followed ten years after that by the third edition, Roberts and Manchester (2005). When Keith wrote the first edition, more than four decades ago, the University of Bradford generously and enthusiastically agreed to publish his book; without this support, this book would not exist. Thank you, University of Bradford! This book is now used by scientists around the globe. The third edition was translated by Grace Hua Zhang into Chinese and published in 2010 by Shandong Huabao Publisher; at that time Grace was a PhD student at Simon Fraser University in Canada.

When Charlotte suggested that perhaps the 1983 book should be revised, Keith was enthusiastic that his work would continue and, so it was, the second edition appeared in 1995, courtesy of Alan Sutton Publishing and Cornell University Press, this time with the cover bearing a color image. Ten years later, Charlotte had moved to Durham University, but her collaboration with Keith continued and the third edition was published by Sutton Publishing Limited (2005; by then taken over by The History Press), first in hardcover and then in paperback.

When thinking about a fourth edition, Charlotte and Keith decided that they needed another paleopathologist, particularly someone who could add much-needed consideration of the health and well-being of children and adolescents. Mary Lewis (University of Reading, England), a 1993 graduate of the Bradford MSc course, has spent her career researching and publishing on the health of non-adults, and it seemed only fitting that they ask Mary to join them in early 2021. They were also aware that previous editions contained a lot of medical historical facts and figures. Neither Charlotte nor Keith are medical historians (i.e., those who study historical sources and iconography for evidence of disease), although they had tried to utilize relevant information alongside paleopathological evidence. So, Charlotte, Keith, and Mary began a search for a medical historian who might be interested in being part of this new volume. They found just who they were looking for in Jacalyn Duffin (Queens University, Kingston, Canada) in early 2022. During her long career, Jacalyn has served as president of the American Association for the History of Medicine and the Canadian Society for the History of Medicine, and has published many books and articles in this area. Charlotte and Keith are eternally grateful to Mary and Jacalyn for agreeing to join the team and for all the insights they have made to this new edition. Finally, with everything in place, this author team submitted the proposal to Cornell University Press in June 2022, received very positive reviewers' comments and helpful suggestions (thank you!), and began work in October 2022.

The reader may be surprised to learn that the chapters of *The Archaeology of Disease* have not changed much since 1983, although in this fourth edition we decided to abandon Chapter 2, incorporating relevant sections into the introductory and concluding chapters, and pointing the reader to excellent texts that will give them a good grounding in human osteology. While we recognize that paleopathology has moved on considerably as a discipline in the past forty years, especially in the development of thematic and theoretical approaches, the same chapter format still allows us to emphasize the importance of past disease to the understanding of, for example, urbanization, identity, subsistence, migration, and climate change. In addition, we discuss the relevance of paleopathology to the present and future: We refer to the United Nations Sustainable Development Goals and the World Health Organization (and vice versa); and we insist that public engagement should be at the forefront of our minds as we do our work.

The astounding rise of paleopathological study, methods, and interpretation around the globe since our first edition is described in Chapter 1 and in each following chapter. Using macroscopic and other evidence, paleopathologists in the academic and heritage sectors (and beyond) are now working with other disciplines and practitioners to answer ever more complex questions about past health and disease. This is because many more methods are at our disposal since the previous edition of this book.

Along with many changes to the contents of each chapter, the range of images used in the current edition has also changed. While the previous editions primarily contained photographs of pathology affecting skeletons derived from sites in the UK, we have made a considerable effort to include photographs that represent the paleopathological evidence more globally. We have striven not to include images of bones from Indigenous peoples in the USA, but where this is the case we thank the communities of these individuals for consenting to the use of images of their ancestor's skeletal remains for illustration and education purposes. Linked to this change, we have addressed the important issue of ethics in relation to archaeological human remains in relevant chapters.

The covers of our successive editions have evolved too. The first edition was in a large hardbound format, almost twice the size of the later editions, and had a black-and-white image of a skull with cranial trauma on the cover. The second edition had a color image of a skull with a head wound. Both formats of the third edition retained color on the cover, but this time it was a compilation of images—hardbound (three photos): a rather garish green radiograph of porotic hyperostosis, a red scanning electron microscopic image of a rib showing osteoporosis, and a blue thin section of a bone. The paperback edition cover featured four images: a green photograph of a burial; a yellowy skull with treponemal disease evident; the scanning electron microscopy image from the hardbound edition, this time in blue; and a red skull with evidence of leprosy. Our fourth edition has no images of real bones or teeth on its front cover. This was a conscious decision because we accept the argument that human remains should not be used to "advertise" books or confront a casual browser in a bookstore. However, inside the book itself, we have used photographs of actual human remains to instruct the reader on the types of lesions that they may encounter during their teaching and research. Ethical practices are, of course, the *primary* consideration for any study of human remains from anywhere in the world, and from any time.

Finally, we hope that readers of this volume enjoy it and gain useful information that will be applicable to their day-to-day work, research, and leisure reading. Our aim is, as it always was, to inspire new research and encourage researchers into this wonderful discipline. We are deeply grateful to our global community of colleagues who have so generously provided photographs for this new volume and provided valuable feedback on individual chapters. It has been an absolute pleasure to work as a team of four. Please note that any errors contained within are, of course, ours.

THE ARCHAEOLOGY OF DISEASE

1

The Study of Paleopathology

The field of paleopathology, like many scientific disciplines, has changed profoundly over the past decades. Technological advances, new theoretical approaches, and the inclusion of diverse voices in the creation and discourse surrounding data collection and analysis have influenced all aspects of our understanding of health and disease in the past.

—A. L. Grauer, *The Routledge Handbook of Paleopathology*

What Is Paleopathology?

Disease and injury have affected human populations since time immemorial, and paleopathology has been documenting the evidence for hundreds of years. But what is paleopathology? Let us start with pathology. *Pathology* stems from the Greek word *pathología* ("the study of suffering"). It is a branch of medical science concerned with the cause, development, structural or functional changes, and natural history associated with disease (Funkhauser 2018, 217). The study of pathology is central to the practice of evidence-based medicine (Reid and Harrison 2008, 4) and has various specialisms: cellular pathology, morbid anatomy (postmortem dissection), forensic pathology (crime scene investigations), microbiology (infectious diseases), hematology (blood diseases), clinical biochemistry (body chemistry), immunology (a person's defenses against external threats, such as infections and allergens), and genetics (inheritance of genes that cause or predispose to diseases).

Paleopathology is the study of ancient (paleo-) suffering using human remains from archaeological sites. It examines the origin, evolution, progress, and history of disease from a deep-time perspective. By so doing, it explores how humans and other animals have adapted to changes in their environments. Relevant to evolutionary medicine (Nesse and Williams 1994; Plomp et al. 2022b), paleopathology provides primary evidence for the state of health of our ancestors, and it combines paleopathological information with methods and data from many disciplines: from archaeology, medicine, medical anthropology, medical geography, and history to genetics, chemistry, and biology. It is a wide-ranging holistic multi- and transdisciplinary field of study (Buikstra et al. 2023), and is a subdiscipline of biological anthropology and bioarchaeology. Since our third edition, bioarchaeology has developed rapidly into a highly scientific area of study that is posing and answering ever more important and complex questions about our ancestors' lives (Roberts 2023a). Current developments and the future of paleopathology are exciting and are discussed further in the final chapter of this book.

Today, good health and well-being on local, regional, national, and global scales are goals that many people and organizations strive for (WHO 2018; United Nations 2023; *Nature* 2023). Indeed in 2015, the United Nations (UN) set up a Sustainable Development Group with seventeen global goals that they aimed to achieve by 2030; many are relevant to paleopathology (e.g., health and well-being, hunger, inequality, poor sanitation, and the health effects of industry, innovation, and infrastructure). Issues surrounding poverty, health, and climate are of increasing concern (Kickbusch and Alakija 2023). The editors of *Nature* (2023, 229) commented that they "strongly support efforts to learn from the past and to take heed of evidence." We would argue that this should include evidence from the distant past. As the World Health Organization (WHO 2018, 5) stated "good health is a precious thing, and when we are healthy we can learn, work, and support ourselves and our families. When we are sick, we struggle, and our families and communities fall behind. After all, and as we know, being unwell affects mental and physical abilities to live well and take advantage of the joys of being alive."

Organizations like the WHO and the UN were not around in the distant past to help communities attain and maintain healthy bodies. Even so, we should remember that humans are good at adapting to changing circumstances and being resilient against all odds, something that our ancestors, such as hunter-gatherers, would have had to learn (Temple and Stojanowski 2019) and that we are currently learning as we confront climate change (Berrang-Ford et al. 2021; Brooks et al. 2019).

One of the most common questions asked of paleopathologists, especially by the media, is about the relevance of our field to helping people with disease today. This can be a tricky question to answer, but increasingly we are making our research more relevant to the here and now, and we are learning from the past to inform challenges of contemporary significance (Roberts 2024; Buikstra et al. 2022; Buikstra 2019b). More frequently, paleopathology uses thematic approaches to address themes relevant to both the past and the present (e.g., see Grauer and Buikstra 2019a). These themes include migration; climate; subsistence and diet; the lived environment, such as urbanization or industrialization; occupation; trade and contact; and care and treatment. Different themes are increasingly brought together through evidence for disease or injury—for example, climate change and violence (Harrod and Martin 2014); urbanization, industrialization, occupation, and respiratory disease (Roberts et al. 2016); and migration, colonization, and infectious disease (Guzmán-Solís et al. 2021).

A key development since the 2005 edition has been the adoption of an evolutionary medicine paradigm, an "elephant in the room" that had been waiting to be taken forward by paleopathologists since it became prominent in the 1990s (e.g., Nesse and Williams 1994). Paleopathology and evolutionary medicine are obvious "bedfellows," and the latter has impacted clinical studies in many fields, from understanding drug resistance to curing infections. Indeed, we now recognize a mismatch between the relatively slow evolution of humans over thousands of years and the rapid development and change in our environment that has taken less than one generation (Gluckman and Hanson 2006, 7). As they say, we need to understand better the interaction of genes, environment, and development. This mismatch has set the scene for lifestyle-related diseases such as diabetes, dental decay, mental health conditions, dementia, cancer, cardiovascular disease (e.g., stroke, heart attack), and chronic respiratory disease such as obstructive pulmonary disease. However, developing an environment that prevents these diseases and promotes healthy populations in the future cannot be achieved by working in the present alone; detailed insights from the past are fundamental to our understanding of conditions today (Plomp et al. 2022b, 2). To make our data matter, we must continue to take a holistic approach, combining medical, scientific, archaeological, and historical data to interpret our evidence.

Paleopathology concentrates on the primary evidence for disease—the people themselves—derived from skeletons, cremated remains, and preserved bodies, such as mummified remains from Egypt or bog bodies from northern Europe (Aufderheide 2000). This evidence is the only reliable indication that a once-living person had a health problem; but whether a specific diagnosis can be made, a cause of death assigned, or hard evidence produced to indicate that a person had a specific affliction is challenging. Since our third edition, one particular gap in our knowledge of paleopathology is now being filled: an increasing focus on babies, young children, and teenagers from the past is giving them a voice to tell stories about their health (e.g., Halcrow and Gowland 2019; Lewis 2018).

Secondary forms of evidence for disease and injury experienced in the past include historical sources (documents) and iconography (artwork) produced during the time period under investigation. This goes alongside exploring contextual factors that influenced what diseases were present in specific places and time periods. Unfortunately, observations left by writers, physicians, and historians are relatively recent in terms of human existence; medical and pharmaceutical texts can rarely be dated prior to 2000 BCE, with Egypt, India, Iran, and China vying for recognition as holding the earliest documents. Furthermore, the traces that can be read now are often fragmentary and imbued with the priorities and scientific concepts of their own time; therefore, retrospective diagnosis is fraught with difficulty (Grmek 1991; Karenberg 2009). All literary works must be studied carefully within the traditional framework in which their facts are presented (Mitchell 2017). In addition, those aspects of an illness that we now consider to be of vital importance in identifying a disease may have been considered of no consequence to observers in the past. There are also circumstances where a disease description does not correspond with any known disease in the modern world. This may be because it cannot be recognized through its historical representation, or perhaps because it no longer exists. Nevertheless, they lure armchair explorers to retrospective diagnosis: examples abound, such as the Plague of Athens described only by Thucydides in the fifth century BCE, or the sweating sickness of early modern Europe (Duffin 2021; Bridson 2001). Long before physicians embraced anatomy, biochemistry, and the microscope to identify diseases, diagnostic clues came only

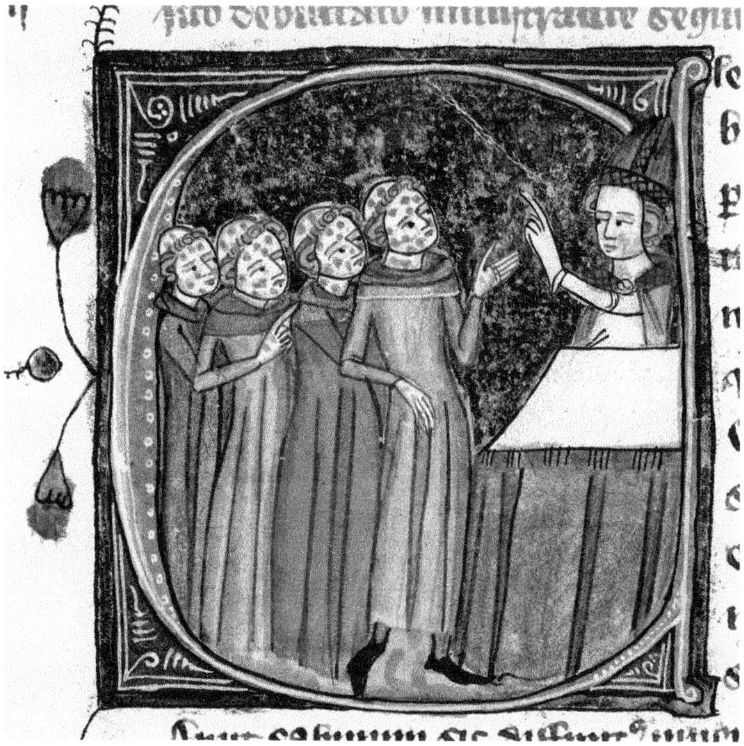

Figure 1.1. Clerics with leprosy receiving instruction from a bishop, 1360–1375 CE. https://commons.wikimedia.org/wiki/.

from the observation of signs of diseases and the patient's account of feelings (symptoms). How does one differentiate between types of pain experienced, or the skin rashes of chickenpox, leprosy, plague, and measles (Fig. 1.1)?

Specific areas of the body may be affected by different conditions, and the nature of the "lesion" (abnormality) may differ. Another example is the clinical picture associated with respiratory disease: cancer, chronic bronchitis, and tuberculosis can all result in coughing up blood (hemoptysis) and shortness of breath (dyspnea), but how can (or should) we distinguish them from one another in the written record if only hemoptysis and dyspnea are described? To be able to determine what disease is being displayed in writing or art necessitates a detailed representation and great faith in the reliability of the source (Mitchell 2017).

Another consideration about using secondary evidence is that artists and authors in the past may have tended to illustrate and describe the more visual and dramatic diseases, and ignored those that were more commonplace. The mundane, common illnesses and injuries are lost to the paleopathologist if this type of evidence is considered alone. For example, the mutilating deformities of leprosy, the devastating effects of the bubonic plague, and the curiosity factor regarding people of short stature have led to abundant representations of these conditions in art; but coughs, colds, influenza, and gastrointestinal upsets, along with cuts, bruises, burns, and sprains, may have been so common that they did not merit recording. In antiquity, diseases with the greatest impact in terms of mortality (death), personal disfigurement, or social and economic disruption may have evoked the greatest response from society (and its authors and artists). In other words, the records may not have been lost; they may never have existed. Secondary sources are also unreliable for establishing statistical inferences about epidemiology or "pathocoenosis," a term Grmek (1991) used to describe the constellation of diseases at a certain time and in a specific place (Arrizabalaga 2018; Dutour 2013; Sabbatini and Fiorini 2008–9).

Secondary sources are especially valuable in establishing evidence about diseases that are not displayed in the skeletal record: those affecting only the soft tissue, such as malaria; childhood diseases such as whooping cough and mumps; cholera and typhoid. Their traces may be recorded only in art and documentary sources. Paleopathologists recognize that solely considering skeletal remains for the evidence of disease allows us to deal with only a small percentage of the disease load in a population, notwithstanding that biomolecular analysis or DNA, for example, has detected some soft tissue diseases (see later in the chapter). As Horden (2000, 208) stated: "The greater the number and variety of perspectives on the pathological past with which we can engage, the greater the chance that our analysis will not be completely disabled by problems of retrospective diagnosis."

History and Development of Paleopathology

Anne Grauer (2012, 2) once noted that "when chronicling the development of paleopathology . . . individual perspectives shape the scope, direction and intent of the discourse, resulting in many crafted explanations." Indeed, there have been numerous accounts of the development of our discipline, and what follows is no different in its individual perspective. More extensive histories can be found by Buikstra (2023), Grauer (2018; 2023, 1–2), and Buikstra and Roberts (2012), especially with regard to the colonial influence on paleopathological study. For a brief history of the development of child paleopathology, see Lewis (2018, 1–2).

Interest in ancient pathological bones began with the study of nonhuman fossils—with the first publication credited to Johann Frederik Esper (1732–1781), who in 1774 published a report of bony lesions on the femur of a cave bear. Esper considered the lesions to be the result of a fracture callus—while Roy Moodie (1880–1934) later suggested that Esper had diagnosed an osteosarcoma (tumor), and this diagnosis has since dominated the history books (Waldron 2015). The first human paleopathology "manual" was published in the United States in 1886 by William Whitney (Armelagos et al. 1971), although the term *paleopathology* seems to have been coined later by Robert Wilson Schufeldt (1893), who used it while describing pathology in fossil bird bones (Waldron 2015). The honor of being the first "official" paleopathologist perhaps goes to Roy Moodie, who was employed under this title by Henry Wellcome in 1929, following his books on nonhuman fossil pathology: *Paleopathology* and *The Antiquity of Disease*, both published in 1923. For an amusing account of the life and influence of Moodie, see Waldron (2015).

The focus on human remains really began with Marc Armand Ruffer (1859–1917) who, while chair of bacteriology in Cairo, met Grafton Elliot-Smith and Frederic Wood Jones, and began histological examinations of mummified tissues (Waldron 2015). The first woman to publish on paleopathology in the *American Journal of Physical Anthropology* was Sheilagh Brookes in 1963, on an individual with cleft palate from California (2000–4000 BCE). From these early beginnings paleopathology evolved into a more biomedical-focused discipline, creating diagnostic criteria for specific diseases and using archaeological evidence to understand their evolution and epidemiology (Ortner 1979). Great advances were made in our understanding of leprosy (Andersen 1969; Manchester 1984; Møller-Christensen 1961, 1978); the treponemal diseases (Hudson 1965; Hackett 1976; Baker and Armelagos 1988); and tuberculosis (Buikstra 1981)—often making use of contemporaneous developments in radiography. Paleopathology was a subject of interest not only in North America and the UK, but also around the globe (see chapters in Buikstra and Roberts 2012). In addition, a series of International Congresses (ICEPID) brought scholars from different disciplines to discuss specific diseases (e.g., syphilis, Toulon, 1993; tuberculosis, Szeged-Budapest, 1997; leprosy, University of Bradford, UK, 1999: Fig. 1.2). The Paleopathology Association, formerly the Paleopathology Club (1973), held its first meeting in 1974 (and the first European meeting a year later in London). This still thriving association of several hundred members worldwide brings together people interested in, and studying, paleopathology from a wide range of disciplines including anthropology, archaeology, medical history, pathology, genetics, veterinary medicine, biology, and many more (www.paleopathology.org). Its publication, the *International Journal of Paleopathology* was launched in 2011. Additionally, the World Committee on Mummy Studies, formed in 1992 after the first World Mummy Congress, represents the interests of people researching mummified remains.

In the 1980s and 1990s, the concept of stress and the complexity of disease stimulated new interest in "nonspecific indicators of stress" such as enamel hypoplasia, cribra orbitalia, and Harris lines, which speak to the general health (or ill health) of a population. The focus centered mostly on the adaptation of groups of people transitioning to agriculture in North America (Huss-Ashmore 1982; Goodman et al. 1984), and because many of these indicators form during childhood, there was an

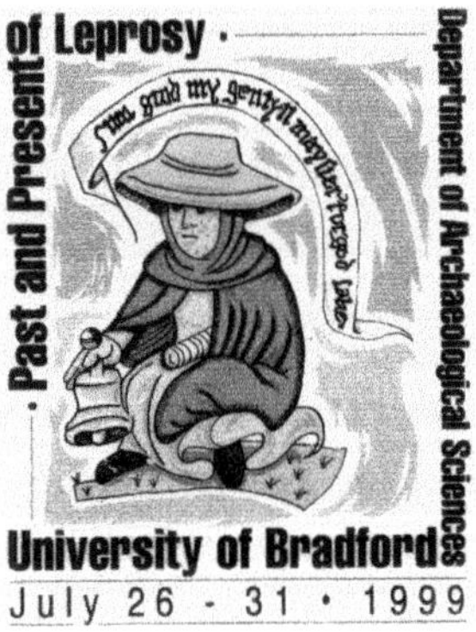

Figure 1.2. Cover of the program for the International Leprosy Congress, University of Bradford, England. Drawn by Mary Lewis.

increasing interest in the paleopathology of children (e.g., Lewis and Roberts 1997). The emphasis on diagnostic rigor and intricate investigation into the causes and clinical expression of many of these conditions is an approach that persists today (see Baker et al. 2020 on treponemal disease). This is most recently illustrated by research into the cause of porous lesions, including cribra orbitalia (Brickley 2018). The health of ancient children has also now come into sharper focus, with themes relating to trauma and metabolic disease advancing our understanding of how pediatric bone reacts to trauma, infection, and dietary deficiencies during growth (Lewis 2018; Brickley et al. 2020). While the 1980s may have seen a move away from focusing on single skeletons and mummied remains in favor of "population-based" studies on large groups to aid a statistical approach, we now recognize the value of both perspectives. Big data projects have also collated a mass of evidence by focusing on the prevalence of disease through time—for example, Steckel et al. (2002) on the Western Hemisphere, Roberts and Cox (2003) on the UK, and Steckel et al. (2019) on Europe. There has also been a rise in detailed osteobiographies (e.g., Hosek and Robb 2019), while the bioarchaeology of personhood has become a key focus, and there are many narratives from the viewpoint of the person who had the diseases and injuries (e.g., Boutin 2016).

Some of the most recent developments in paleopathology have been brought about by technological advances that allow us to ask ever more detailed questions about people's experience of disease, using stable isotopes to reconstruct their diet, ancient DNA (aDNA) to identify infections before they affect the skeleton, or to explore the etiology (cause) of specific lesions (Müller et al. 2014). Similarly, increasingly sophisticated imaging techniques such as microcomputed tomography (CT), 3D reconstructions, and geometric morphometrics allow us to explore and display lesions in amazing detail (e.g., Colombo et al. 2015). A recognition that humans, the natural world, and other animals have an impact on the spread of disease has resulted in the One Health/Paleopathology Initiative, where in the latter, zooarchaeologists and paleopathologists work together to understand disease dynamics in the past, and help inform disease patterns of the present and for the future (MacKenzie and Jeggo 2019; Buikstra et al. 2025).

Notably, and prior to the twenty-first century, paleopathology was Eurocentric and focused on a narrow subset of populations who colonized the globe over time (i.e., white Europeans and European descendants in the Americas). A concerted effort to "decolonize" our field places a greater focus on the health of nonwhite populations (e.g., see Buikstra et al. 2022; de la Cova 2023). This work is coupled with an understanding of how our collections of human remains in museums were collated, who these people were, and what sociostructural factors of the past are embedded in their bones. This move to a more global appreciation of past health is helped by an increase in scholars working in other areas of the world as well as more people entering the field of paleopathology, thanks to training that is available at different levels around the world—for example, undergraduate and postgraduate courses in higher education.

Arguably, the other most important paleopathological development of the twenty-first century is the adoption of social theory and generational health approaches that help us make sense of these scientific data from a human perspective. While social theory has been applied to the understanding of disease since the 1980s (at least in North America; Grauer 2023, 4), theoretical models adopted from the social and medical sciences now permeate our work, such as disability studies (Roberts 2000), the bioarchaeology of care (Tilley 2015; Tilley and Schrenk 2017; Roberts 2022), and measures of frailty (Marklein et al. 2016; Zedda et al. 2021). Research into the mother-infant nexus has been inspired by life history theory and the developmental origins of health and disease hypothesis (DOHaD), which posits that the diseases we experience as adults have their roots in the health of our mothers and grandmothers (Gowland 2022). Attention is now being given to intersectionality theory and health disparities (Mant et al. 2021; Yaussy 2022), and to syndemics (Perry and Gowland 2019), that is the presence of two or more diseases that already interact with each other, negatively affecting the mutual course of each disease (Lancet 2017). This enhances vulnerability and is made worse by inequality. Intersectionality, although challenging to study due to many hidden variables, considers how a person's multiple identities coincide to shape their experience of life and access to resources, depending on the time period or location in which they lived. As an example, contrast a wealthy, Black young male migrant with a poor, white, old, local female. Migrants may be considered "outsiders" in one society and treated in a way that may be reflected in the greater burden of ill health seen on their skeletons (for example, denied jobs and kept in poverty). These theoretical approaches and expansion into wider geographical areas of study will ultimately provide a more informed paleopathology, a wider worldview of the long history of disease, and the effects of social interactions, genetics, and ancestry on population health.

Limitations of Paleopathology

In any discipline there are limitations; some may eventually be overcome, may take years to address, or may never be solved. It is important to emphasize that the individuals and populations being studied in paleopathology are long dead and unlikely to fully represent the living population that resulted in the skeletons in a funerary context. The human remains that bioarchaeologists study range from preserved bodies to inhumed skeletons and cremated burials, and they come from many different contexts that represent varying funerary rituals. These can range from large urban and small rural cemeteries, prehistoric contexts that may hold very small numbers of individuals, and more unusual burials, for example, in peat bogs, caves, and glaciers. Excavations are often in advance of modern developments, such as the building of new hospitals, supermarkets, and housing, and are usually carried out by commercial archaeology companies. Less common are research-led and grant-funded excavations, which are often organized by universities. As an example of commercial excavation in the UK, since the establishment of Policy Planning Guidance (Department of the Environment 1990), which was replaced by Planning Policy Statement 5 (Department for Communities and Local Government 2010), there is a legal requirement to survey areas proposed for development. If archaeological evidence is found, then it has to be excavated prior to that development (e.g., excavation in advance of the building of the new high-speed rail line (HS2) from London to Birmingham, which has included a number of large cemeteries). These "planning" developments have created a more professional and managed approach to excavation and post-excavation work that is now developer-funded; more employment opportunities for archaeologists, including bioarchaeologists; and more money available to pay good salaries and support detailed post-excavation work (e.g., human skeletal reports).

With the above in mind, however, bioarchaeologists are usually dealing with a sample of a sample of a sample . . . of the original living population. Total excavation of a whole cemetery is unusual, meaning that often only a portion of the original buried population will be examined (Fig. 1.3). Skeletal remains can be fragmentary and poorly preserved, and the integrity of older adult skeletons may be particularly affected by postmortem processes before, during, and after burial because their bones have a lower density (Stodder 2018). The different burial patterns of adult males, adult females, and children may bias the data, while some members of the population may have been buried in other places—for example, children and people with impairments or specific diseases, such as leprosy. In some cultures, children were not buried in the cemetery serving the general population; in Roman period England, many babies were buried in domestic spaces (Millett and Gowland 2015). While there is a common misapprehension that child skeletons do not survive well in the ground, cemeteries have yielded hundreds of perinatal and child remains from all periods, and where adult skeletons survive, child skeletons do too (Lewis 2019a). Children are, however, more often buried in shallow graves that can be easily disturbed by later activity, and their bones are small and may be missed during excavation, or misidentified as faunal remains. So, unless the burial environment is not conducive to their preservation, it is more likely that cultural practices dictate their discovery.

Even if a complete cemetery were to be excavated, we cannot assume that everybody buried there lived in the area; some of the people could have been migrants from another area, or even people who just wanted to be buried there but had not lived in the village or town, as we might see today. Neither do we know *how many* people had migrated from elsewhere, near or far. Nevertheless, the increasing use of

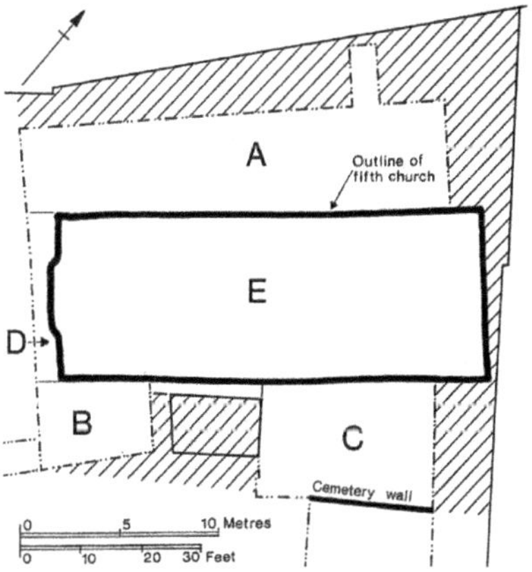

Figure 1.3. Plan of the excavation of the late medieval church (E) cemetery (twelfth to sixteenth centuries CE) of St. Helen-on-the-Walls, York, England. The hatched areas are those not excavated that may contain age- and biological sex-specific groups of people that could change the demographic profile of the populations, if excavated. Dawes and Magilton 1980, 8, with kind permission from York Archaeology.

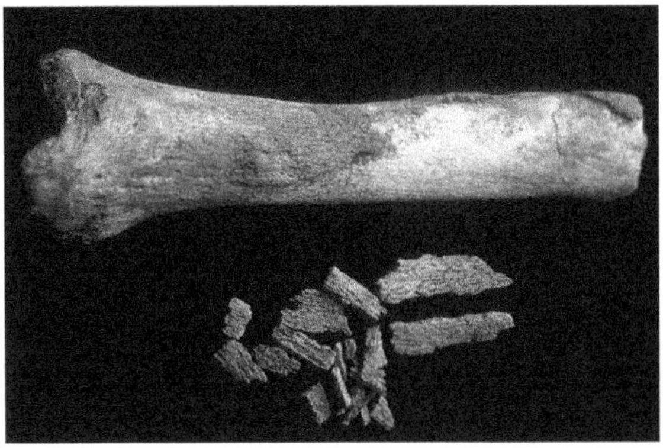

Figure 1.4. Detachment of new bone from the original cortex. Photograph courtesy of Anwen Caffell.

stable isotope analysis to study the origins and migration of people is now helping to identify nonlocal individuals in cemeteries (see Biomolecular Analysis later in the chapter). This may at least provide some indication of the proportion of people buried in a cemetery who were born and raised nonlocally.

Pathological bones and teeth are inherently fragile and may be damaged while buried and not survive to be excavated; thus, disease frequency will be an underrepresentation of real frequency. Skeletons (and pathological bones and teeth) can also be damaged during analysis and handling (e.g., Caffell et al. 2001), and evidence may be destroyed because of environmental conditions that affect the integrity of the lesions themselves—for example, detachment of periosteal new bone (Fig. 1.4). Acute infections likely killed people quickly in antiquity, as they can do today. In these cases, no pathological lesions would be visible (or expected) because the person died before the bone had time to react. Many diseases affect only the soft tissues (e.g., some tumors, influenza), even though aDNA analysis may detect some of them. We might find other evidence of soft tissue diseases if we know what we are looking for, both in the grave and with the skeleton. For example, bladder, kidney, and gall stones may be found in burial contexts, perhaps located where these organs were anatomically positioned in the buried body. Similarly, calcified tissues, such as blood vessels, indicating cardiovascular disease (Binder and Roberts 2014; Binder et al. 2023), and calcified pleura, suggesting lung disease (e.g., Roberts et al. 1998), have also been identified. In addition, postmortem damage on bones and teeth may be misread as a pathological lesion, known as a pseudopathology (Fig. 1.5). We should also remember that several different diseases may induce similar lesions on bone. Deciding which came first and last is usually difficult if not impossible, but it may be important when considering life expectancy (Owen et al. 2023). Finally, we should be careful of ascribing disease where none existed on the basis of normal variation in the skeleton, that is, a nonmetric trait (Fig. 1.6; e.g., see Scott and Turner 1997: teeth; Saunders and Rainey 2008: bone).

In most circumstances, we are unable to ascribe a cause of death to an individual. Rare exceptions include a weapon embedded in the skeleton in its grave, an unhealed perimortem injury, or evidence for other fatal trauma, such as decapitation or trauma to the hyoid bone or ossified neck cartilages, which occurs in

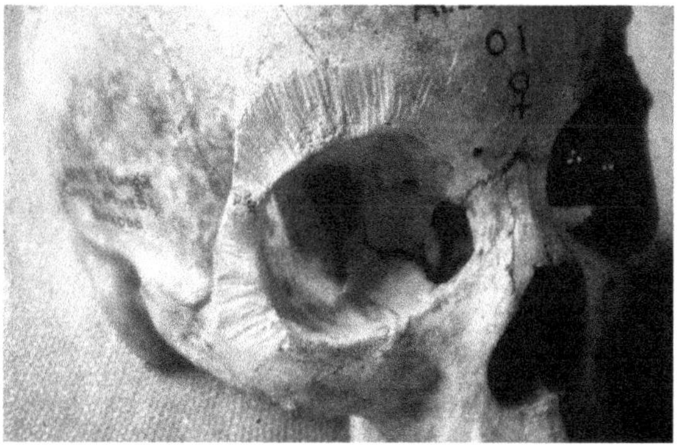

Figure 1.5. Postmortem (pseudopathological) lesions around the right eye socket due to gnawing from a rodent in the grave. With kind permission from Jo Buckberry, Calvin Wells Collection, University of Bradford.

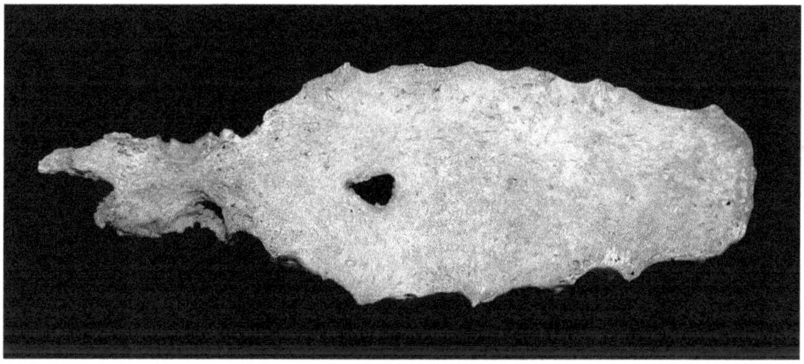

Figure 1.6. Sternal foramen, a nonmetric trait that may be confused with sharp force trauma to the chest. The proximal end is on the right. Photograph by Charlotte Roberts.

strangulation. Preserved bodies, such as those from northwest European bogs (Giles 2020), can provide a more obvious cause of death (e.g., cut to the throat) because the soft tissue survived. We can, however, deduce the diseases that an individual may have experienced in life, and whether the disease was active or not at the time of death. Therefore, we should not dwell too much on our inability to assign a specific cause of death to skeletal remains; there is also ample evidence from clinical research and historical data that assigning the correct cause of death is not, and was not, easy (e.g., McGivern et al. 2017; Gamage et al. 2021).

Limitations also affect our interpretations of past population health. Selective mortality and the nonstationary nature of populations were highlighted as major problems for inferring health by Wood et al. (1992) in their paper "The Osteological Paradox." Within any cemetery population, we are dealing with an unknown mix of people with different susceptibilities to contracting a disease, displaying a lesion, and/or dying, and this hidden frailty may mean certain diseases are overrepresented. The development of analytical methods in recent years is helping interpretations; for example, aDNA analysis is providing information about susceptibility to infectious diseases, such as by looking at changes in DNA sequences of genes that make a person more likely to acquire a disease (mutations). Stable isotope analysis is also enabling us to explore the movement of people over their lifetime, journeys that may have predisposed them to poor health. Essentially, we have a better toolkit than we had in the early 1990s, and it is more sensitive to the problems originally outlined by Wood et al. (1992). We have developed ways to measure frailty in skeletal remains too, and to explore lesion specificity, which is the likelihood that a lesion represents the disease that we think it does (Boldsen and Milner 2012). We have also begun to develop strategies to account for hidden susceptibility to diseases that may be influencing selective mortality in our populations, with an approach that emphasizes cultural factors, testing ideas about risk using cemeteries from defined periods and contexts, and examining the "nonsurvivors" in that group, that is, the children (DeWitte and Stojanowski 2015).

Identifying disease is not straightforward. First, the "classic" appearance or distribution of lesions in the skeleton described in clinical or paleopathological texts, which often emphasize the late chronic stages, may not always fit what we see in an archaeological skeleton. Some features may be the same, but others may differ. Indeed, often we do not know what the early stages of a disease look like. Second, we cannot assume that the bone changes now used to identify a specific disease have not altered over time. Skeletal changes associated with a disease in the past may not be described clinically because they were not deemed important, or because they are not seen on a radiograph in a living person, such as the new bone formation on the internal aspects of ribs that may form with lung infections. Some diseases common today are thought to have been rare in the past too: for example, rheumatoid arthritis (WHO 2024h); often, its identification is prefaced as "possible" or "probable," reflecting challenges in diagnosis and potential confusion with other joint diseases (Mant et al. 2024). Absence of evidence may reflect nondiagnosis due to nonrecognition, confusion with another joint disease, or that it really was rare in the past. Finally, as mentioned earlier, it is also possible that some diseases today may not have been present in the past and, conversely, we may be observing lesions of a disease that no longer exists today.

As paleopathologists, we cannot talk to our skeletons, but clinicians gain detailed knowledge of a patient's experience of a disease, its progress (pathogenesis), and the underlying reasons for its appearance. However, their knowledge may be confined to a few weeks, months, or years. By considering longer periods of time and many skeletons, paleopathologists can explore major alterations in disease patterning and its evolution over hundreds and thousands of years. While the importance of documented (identified) skeletons is recognized (Santos 2020), we often observe natural expressions of disease without the influence of drug therapy or other treatment intervention; therefore, we can explore the cumulative effects of disease or injury over a person's lifetime. Interpretation of the evidence is very challenging, though. We can read clinical texts to infer how a disease affects a person's body, but we cannot know how an individual experienced the disease: What their symptoms were and how disabling. We also cannot "note the progression of any changes" (Waldron 2021, 345), but sometimes we may be confident in thinking that a particular disease or injury seen in a skeleton would have caused suffering: for example, a dental abscess, bone cancer, or a poorly healed fracture of a lower limb bone would have caused pain and problems with mobility.

Having reviewed many of the limitations of studying disease in the skeleton, one might begin to wonder what we can *actually* say about the experience of disease in the past. That is what this book aims to do.

Diagnosis and Description in Paleopathology

Before paleopathologists consider how to describe and interpret lesions, a record of each skeleton is created. This involves using established osteological methods to estimate the person's biological sex, age at death, stature, and ancestry. These data help us build a demographic profile for the cemetery sample under study, and in the case of a single skeleton, a detailed osteobiography that can aid in any diagnosis. Collecting these data is important because some diseases are more common in particular age groups or a particular sex. Without knowledge about these key variables, it is not possible to make meaningful interpretations and conclusions about individual skeletons showing disease, or about a population's health status.

Paleopathology naturally starts with having a detailed anatomical knowledge of the bones and teeth of the skeleton, including characteristics of normal structure, function, and development—it is only by understanding "the normal" that diseases can be identified, recorded, and interpreted (Lynnerup and Klaus 2019; Klaus and Lynnerup 2019). The bones of each skeleton differ slightly from those of the next, and the skeletons (and bodies) of everyone who has ever lived are unique. For information on skeletal anatomy and how to apply methods for biological sex estimation, age at death, and other osteological techniques we refer you to key texts such as White et al. (2012), Efthymia (2017), and for children, Cunningham et al. (2016). Understanding patterns of disease or injury in the group under study is vital for exploring biological differences in susceptibility to disease, as well as the sociostructural factors such as unequal access to resources and/or culturally sanctioned maltreatment that may have provoked that pattern in males, females, religious groups, or people of different ages and ancestries (Halcrow and Schug 2022; Zuckerman et al. 2023).

The strength or weakness of a person's immune system will influence whether or not they contract the disease to which they were exposed, and differences in immunity between the sexes and with aging are a major area of current clinical research (e.g., Gubbels Bupp et al. 2018). The immune system depends on the properties and products (antibodies) of specific cells in the blood, marrow, and lymph nodes. Immunity to a disease may be natural/innate (i.e., inherited and independent of any previous exposure to specific pathogenic microorganisms), or it may be acquired—stimulated by exposure and adaptation to foreign proteins of invading pathogenic microorganisms. The integrity of both forms of immunity relies on the individual's general health and nutritional status. Adaptive/acquired immunity is characterized by the retention of a specific memory for the invading pathogen so that a "tailor-made" defense mechanism is in place for future invasion by that pathogen. A child's ability to rally against invading organisms alters as they grow. In the newborn, antibodies are acquired passively through their mother's breastmilk until they can create their own short term/passive immunity (Palmeira and Carneiro-Sampaio 2016). The move from passive to acquired immunity through the exposure of an increasing range of environmental pathogens means the mortality rate of 2–5-year-olds from infectious disease is often the highest.

Adolescence sees a divergence of male and female immunity patterns, with females developing more autoimmune conditions (where the body attacks itself) and males more prone to inflammation and infections (Bupp 2015; and see Lewis 2018, 5–7). Unfortunately, the levels of natural and acquired immunity in past human groups cannot be ascertained; however, evidence for chronic disease indicates that a person's immunity was effective enough to prevent death in the acute phase. Conversely, a child who died with no bone changes of disease may indicate that their immune status was not developed enough for them to overcome and recover from it. Nevertheless, not only can aDNA analysis identify the presence of pathogens in the past, but it has also recently begun to be used to explore human susceptibility to infection and resistance genes (e.g., Kerner et al. 2023).

Macroscopic Descriptions

Paleopathologists have a variety of methods at their disposal to study skeletons for evidence of disease. Primarily this relies on macroscopic (or visual) observation. A description of abnormal changes in bones and teeth and their distribution in the skeleton are prerequisites to attempting a diagnosis of the disease. Mays (2023, 20–21) defines macroscopy as "gross examination of remains with the naked eye, perhaps augmented with low power magnification . . . or with basic measurements." It is the mainstay of teaching and research in paleopathology.

Unambiguous terminology is of utmost importance so that readers and future researchers who wish to use these data understand its meaning, which may lead to a different diagnosis, especially if they are to use the data for comparison or reinterpretation. Unfortunately, the clinical and paleopathological literature abounds with different terms describing various changes in disease. Without a common, agreed-upon set of terms, there can be little hope of comparative studies of paleopathological data on a global perspective. The authors recommend the use of Manchester et al. (2016) for prefixes, suffixes, and terms to use in describing pathological lesions. Manchester et al.'s "Nomenclature in Palaeopathology" is published online and accessible through the Paleopathology Association website (www.paleopathology.org). Buikstra and Ubelaker (1994, chap. 10) addressed methodological standardization in paleopathology. Along these lines, the British Association for Biological Anthropology and Osteoarchaeology (BABAO) has produced two shorter documents for use on British-derived skeletal remains (Brickley and McKinley 2004; Mitchell and Brickley 2017). Furthermore, the Global History of Health Project's European module developed a standardized recording system that was applied to over 15,000 European skeletons so that comparative analysis could be undertaken (Steckel et al. 2005, 2019). Other recording systems do of course exist. As we stated, the bone changes seen on the skeleton represent chronicity, but a person may have lived throughout life with more than one disease and bear the scars of all these conditions, making for tricky interpretations. We emphasize that creating careful descriptions of all findings, as opposed to providing a specific diagnosis, is key.

The bone changes of disease may be either proliferative—initiated by the bone forming cells: osteoblasts ("blastic"), or destructive—initiated by the bone destroying cells: osteoclasts ("clastic/lytic"). A mixture of both bone forming and bone destroying activities may be evident on a single bone. Destructive activity can be seen in the teeth and jaw bones too (e.g., dental caries and periodontal disease, respectively). In the normal physiological state, a balance exists between osteoblastic and osteoclastic activity, which allows for continuous change in the structure and form of the bone (i.e., remodeling) throughout life. As a person ages, however, bone loss overtakes bone formation and leads to a decline in bone density, called osteopenia, and eventually osteoporosis. Pathological stimuli provoke an imbalance in osteoblast/osteoclast activity, producing changes of atrophy, hypertrophy, hyperplasia, dysplasia, or metaplasia. The cellular changes in bone are stimulated by an alteration in oxygen supply to the tissues: high blood oxygen tension stimulates osteoclast activity, and low blood oxygen tension stimulates osteoblasts. Hypertrophy involves an increase in cell size and may be induced physiologically—for example, in people with heavy manual occupations whose muscles become increased in size. Atrophy occurs with a decrease in cell size—for instance, in paralysis when limbs are not used. Hyperplasia indicates cell division and an increase in the number of cells and the cellular content of the tissue, such as with abnormal levels of hormones. Dysplasia denotes problems with the development of the bones, joints, or cartilage. Metaplasia involves the change in differentiation of cell type, for example, in tumors when, under pathological stimulus, cells assume the morphological and functional characteristics of other cells.

The bone formed in a disease process may be woven (or fiber) bone, also called immature or primary bone, which is porous and disorganized in structure (Fig. 1.7), or more mature, older, better organized, lamellar bone (Fig. 1.8). The former indicates that the disease process was active at the time of death, and the latter indicates that the process was quiescent or had been overcome and/or become chronic. The presence of active lesions does not necessarily indicate that the pathological process was the cause of death; rather that it may have contributed to it, along with other factors. It is also of importance to study whether a pathological lesion is healed (smooth bone with rounded edges) or unhealed (sharp, unremodeled edges) because this gives an indication of the disease state at the time of death. Nevertheless, determining the ante-, peri-, or postmortem nature of lesions can prove challenging. In addition, bone can react to a pathological stimulus in only a limited number of ways. For example, new bone formation on the lower leg bones (tibia and fibula) may represent the inflammation inherent in the specific infectious diseases of leprosy or treponemal disease, but it can also occur with trauma, nonspecific infection, cancer and scurvy. These conditions would not be diagnosed solely on the basis of this change, because the fuller picture (distribution pattern) of all the pathological lesions would also be considered. Some paleopathologists also attach a degree of severity to lesions observed, but their appearance may not necessarily reflect a gradation in the actual disease process. If grades for disease are to be included, a clear

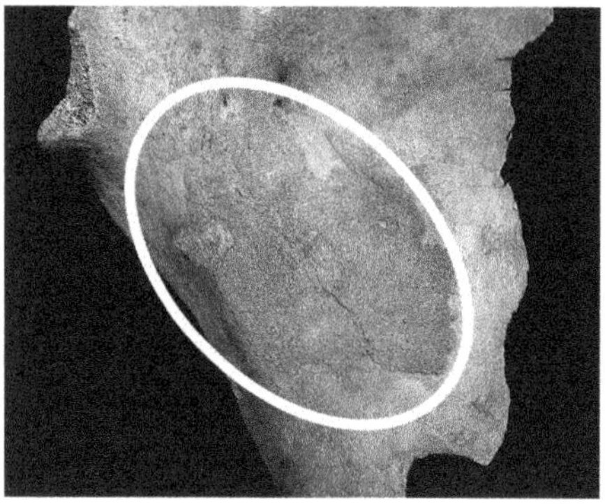

Figure 1.7. Scapula bone with woven new bone formation on top of the original cortex indicative of an active lesion. With kind permission from York Osteoarchaeology.

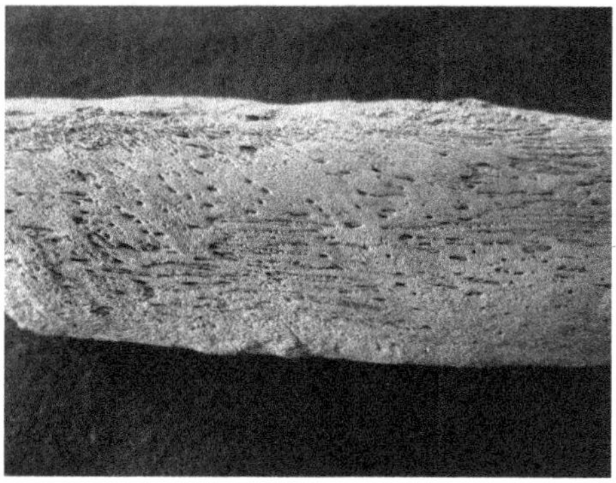

Figure 1.8. Long bone with lamellar new bone formation indicative of a healed lesion. Photograph by Charlotte Roberts.

definition of the grades (including photographs) should be provided so that future researchers understand their meaning (e.g., Davies et al. 2021a: maxillary sinusitis).

It is beneficial to study complete skeletons, since observation of the distribution pattern of lesions is necessary in attempting a diagnosis based on modern clinical criteria, although these criteria may not always be applicable to an ancient skeleton. Clinical data also provide signs and symptoms for diseases that help in interpretation of the impact of lesions. Just as different diseases may produce similar signs and symptoms, people with the same diseases may experience the same, different, or similar signs or symptoms, and disease progression will vary on an individual basis (e.g., see Roberts 2017 on the application of the Index of Care to a medieval skeleton with evidence of leprosy).

Inferring symptoms is a particular challenge, and pain is a good example. Levels of pain and their relationship to bone changes of disease can be difficult to assess, as demonstrated by studies of living populations. Fillingim (2023) noted a greater prevalence of chronic pain in females compared to males, indicating that biological and psychosocial factors contribute to these sex differences, as too, it seems, do genes. In their genetic metastudy, Toikumo et al. (2024) identified 126 genes that were associated with pain in over half a million people of diverse ancestry in the United States. They also found that intensity was genetically correlated with other pain phenotypes (expression of the genetic code, or genotype), and with substance use and related disorders, psychiatric traits, education level, and cognition.

Once the distribution pattern of lesions has been established, consideration of all possible differential diagnoses for the abnormalities described is essential (Appleby 2023; Lawler 2017). Producing a list of possible (differential) diagnoses may be the closest we can get to deciding what disease(s) affected the once-living person, rather than producing a specific diagnosis. The aforementioned lack of certainty in diagnosis, or lack of engagement with hypothesis testing, has resulted in an abundance of "probable" and "possible" diagnoses in paleopathology (Zuckerman et al. 2016, 375), which has inspired more recent developments in "weighted diagnostic

Table 1.1 Appleby's adapted diagnostic terminology framework

Certainty level	Description
Undefined	Currently undefined, but with possible lesion involvement
Not consistent with	Not consistent with the condition
Consistent with (pathophysiologically)	Consistent with the pathophysiology of the condition, but unreported in the clinical literature
Consistent with	Can be associated with the condition
Highly consistent with	The lesions can be associated with the condition, and there are few other possible causes
Typical of	The lesions are usually associated with the condition
Diagnostic of	Pathognomonic (specific) lesion, not associated with any other condition

Source: Adapted from Appleby 2023, 53.

criteria." Appleby et al. (2015) recommended a system for diagnosis widely used in forensic medicine for the identification of torture and argued that application of this slightly modified terminological framework would encourage consistency between paleopathologists and make data more comparable (Table 1.1). As we will see, similar diagnostic threshold criteria have been developed for rickets, scurvy, and the treponemal diseases. Vlok (2023) discussed the pros and cons of such systems, suggesting they could be improved if lesion severity was also included—and if other lesions led to the "exclusion" of a particular disease being considered likely. We too recommend the use of diagnostic threshold criteria to help assess the importance of pathological lesions in the diagnosis of specific conditions.

Even in modern clinical settings, with an array of tests at hand, diagnosis is often challenging; it may also change as more tests are carried out and a specific and accurate diagnosis may never be achieved (Waldron 2021, 61). This ambiguity provides paleopathologists with a bit of comfort when they are trying to diagnose disease, even in a well-preserved skeleton. Paleopathologists have increasingly turned to documented skeletal collections to inform observations and interpretation of disease. These collections usually date from the late nineteenth and early twentieth centuries when skeletons were often collected for medical research (Santos 2020 for a list; Hunt and Albanese 2005: USA; Eliopoulos et al. 2006: Greece; Cunha and Wasterlain 2007: Portugal; Dayal et al. 2009: South Africa; and Chi-Keb et al. 2013: Mexico). Skeletons in these collections have various information linked to them—for example, age at death, biological sex, stature, ancestry, medical history, and aspects of their lifestyle (e.g., their occupation). While not without their ethical problems (Henderson and Cardoso 2018), they provide an unrivaled opportunity for paleopathologists to test hypotheses in research and for teaching. However, many of these individuals may have had the advantage of modern medical interventions that could have altered the natural progress and appearance of a disease or injury.

Mays (2018) has argued that diagnosis in paleopathology is a two-part process: type 1, intuitive—paleopathologists often compare the lesions they see with those reported for a particular disease in the clinical literature or with reference to bone changes already related to that disease in other skeletal remains; and type 2, analytical—a process that is "slower, reflective and effortful [and] the application of specific procedural approaches in order to arrive at conclusions based on evidence" (Mays 2023, 25). This type 2 process involves careful and detailed observations on the location and characteristics of the bone changes in relation to information derived from the biomedical literature, and in relation to hard and soft tissue changes and anatomical structures. It is also important to seek negative evidence—lesions or biological changes that argue against the favored diagnosis (Mays 2018). Along with Mays, we consider such approaches to be essential when making paleopathological diagnoses.

Some attempts at developing new methods of diagnosis in paleopathology have been explored, including probabilistic approaches to leprosy and tuberculosis (Boldsen 2001; Pedersen et al. 2019; Yaussy 2023). Yes, as a first step, diagnosis primarily relies on appreciating the known skeletal patterning of the different diseases under consideration in modern clinical circumstances. A probable diagnosis may be made, but it may not be possible to be more specific. Good-quality, detailed photographs and other types of imaging—for example, radiographs—are also essential when reporting pathological lesions and may help future researchers assess the conclusions in light of future information. Such reporting can result in a considerable amount of data. Since our third edition, numerous advances in the storage of both visual and textual data have appeared (e.g., Wrobel et al. 2019), and journal papers routinely include supplementary data accessible online. However, the ubiquity of present-day image sharing has raised increasing concerns about the use of human remains in publications, online, and via social media (e.g., see Ericksen and Thompson 2019; Smith and Hirst 2019).

Methods of Analysis Beyond Macroscopic Recording

Radiography and Computed Tomography

Imaging plays a large part in the diagnosis of disease and trauma, and this is especially the case for unwrapped mummified bodies (e.g., see Ryan and Milner 2006; Taylor and Antoine 2014; Chiara et al. 2019). Plain film radiography and micro- and macro-CT scanning comprise the main methods used in paleopathology; it is possible to look inside bones and teeth using these techniques, all of which are nondestructive (Fig. 1.9). Radiographs produce a 2D image of a 3D bone or tooth, and therefore their different layers are superimposed on each other. This limitation makes a CT scan, which focuses on layers in slices, much more valuable for detailed information of pathological lesions (Fig. 1.10); however, its cost can be considerable. Databases containing digital radiographs have not only enhanced understanding of observed lesions but also enabled sharing among scholars—making them globally accessible while protecting the often delicate pathological bones from being damaged through handling (Villa and Jørkov 2023; Digitised Diseases 2024).

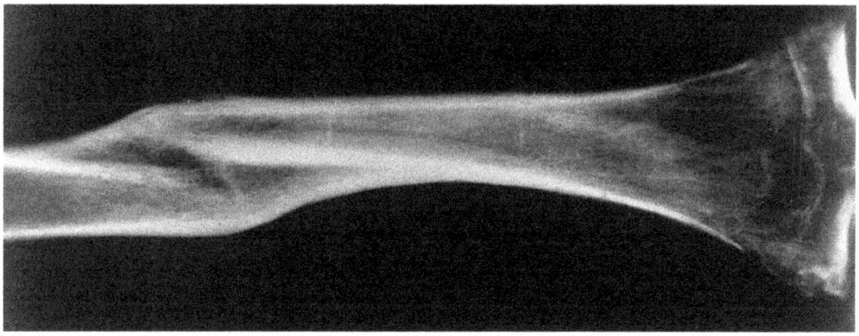

Figure 1.9. Radiograph of a tibia showing a healed fracture. Photograph by and courtesy of Jean Brown. Right is the proximal end.

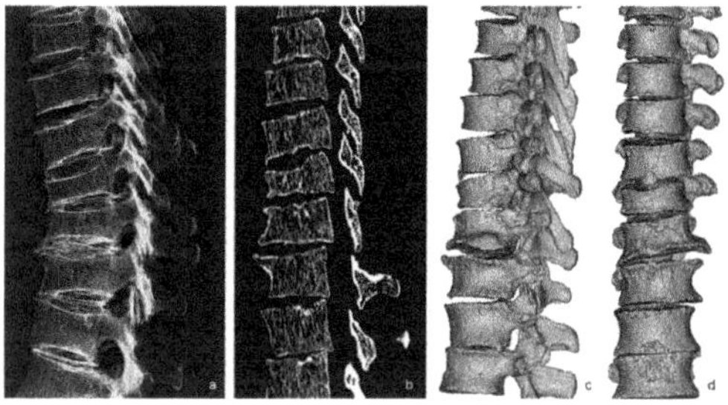

Figure 1.10. Degenerative changes on thoracic vertebrae: (a) plain film radiograph; (b) sagittal CT scan; (c) CT 3D visualization, left lateral view; (d) CT 3D visualization, anterior view. Photograph courtesy of Chiara Villa.

Microscopy

Microscopy also features in some paleopathologists' repertoire of methods, but it is perhaps the least used (Assis and De Boer 2023). One reason is that it is destructive, and consequently it is not always possible to take samples of bones or teeth, especially from museum collections. Another reason is that, relative to other analytical methods, little training is available. Nevertheless, microscopy has proved advantageous for many studies; has helped in diagnosis, especially for the metabolic diseases (Stout et al. 2019); and is also useful for identifying pseudopathological changes (Assis et al. 2015). Transmitted light electron microscopy (TEM) and scanning electron microscopy (SEM) have been used in paleopathology for diagnosing disease and trauma (Fig. 1.11), although only a few diseases have specific histomorphological changes, for example, osteitis deformans (Aaron et al. 1992) and osteomalacia (Welsh et al. 2020; see De Boer et al. 2013 for a review of paleomicroscopy).

Biomolecular Analysis

Several other destructive (biomolecular) methods have seen a sharp increase in use since our third edition. These primarily include stable isotope and aDNA analyses, but also analysis of ancient proteins and the amino acids, such as peptides, that constitute them (Hendy 2023). From an ethical standpoint, taking samples for destructive

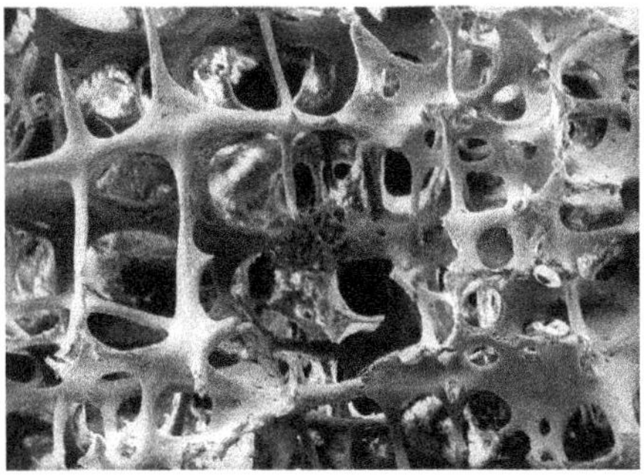

Figure 1.11. Scanning electron microscopy image of a section from a third lumbar vertebra showing a healed microfracture in its center (early medieval, eighth–tenth centuries CE, Raunds Furnells, Northamptonshire). Photograph by and courtesy of Jean Brown.

analysis requires various steps to be taken (see Ethics below). As an example, in England guidelines have been published by the Advisory Panel on the Archaeology of Burial in England (2023). The decision should take into account the rarity of a particular set of human remains, documentation of the bones or teeth pre- and postsampling, and permissions to do the work (Sabin and Stone 2023, 138–141). Laboratory protocols should also be in place to facilitate the production of authentic data, and data management should be conducted ethically following the project's end. We should emphasize that the biomolecular methods do not provide answers to all questions we might like to ask about the past. It requires macroscopically recorded biographical information to form the basis for interpretation of data. Therefore, macroscopic analysis should not be omitted in paleopathological research, although it is absent from many biomolecular publications. Indeed, Mays (2023, 19) addressed the reasons why macroscopy is often overlooked and commented that it has "formed the foundation of study since the dawn of the discipline." Perhaps bioarchaeologists, and biomolecular scientists who are not bioarchaeologists, are pushing back against each other's practices to promote and protect their respective fields of enquiry for the future. Scholars applying stable isotope analysis, aDNA, and protein analysis to paleopathology should also be engaging with the literature beyond archaeology and into other sciences, such as ecology, agriculture, physiology, and nutrition (O'Connell 2023). Having a broader awareness of other disciplines essentially grounds our data.

Stable isotope analysis is used to answer many questions about our ancestors' lives. Isotopes are chemical elements that can be found embedded in teeth and bones of skeletons. Two areas of interest that can be explored using this type of analysis relate to diet and mobility histories. Diet can be reconstructed using stable isotopes of carbon (^{13}C, extracted from bone collagen, indicating the type of plant foods eaten), nitrogen (^{15}N, extracted from both bone collagen and dental enamel, reflecting levels of dietary protein), and of oxygen ($\delta^{18}O$) in tooth enamel to indicate the oxygen levels in the groundwater water these plants and animals utilized (see Chapter 6; see also Afshar et al. 2019). Like diet, mobility histories have also become increasingly of interest to bioarchaeologists. Migration can take diseases to people in new places and at the same time expose people on the move to diseases they have not previously encountered (e.g., see reviews: Katzenberg and Waters-Rist 2018; Gregoricka 2021; Stantis and Kendall 2023). Generally speaking, stable isotopes are used to explore the origin and mobility of people during their lives. In the teeth, strontium ($^{87}Sr/^{86}Sr$ ratio) reflects local geology and oxygen ($\delta^{18}O$) the local water supply and climate (Lugli et al. 2019; Filipek et al. 2022). While reflecting diet and subsistence, ratios of ^{13}C, ^{15}N and ^{34}S (sulfur) have also been used together to identify people whose origin differed from their place of burial, that is, when the traditional isotopes of strontium and oxygen cannot be analyzed (Wißing et al. 2019). In addition, new procedures involving multiple sequential sampling of the dentine of teeth are used to explore changes in an individual's diet during tooth formation, with the data linked to pathological lesions (see Goude et al. 2020). Scholars are also starting to, directly explore the impact of mobility on disease transmission (e.g., Richards and Montgomery 2012; Kendall et al. 2013; Inskip et al. 2015; Toyne and Turner 2020). However, some studies suggest that the biological effect of disease on the skeleton can alter stable isotope values in bone (Katzenberg and Lovell 1999; Plomp et al. 2020b; Stantis and Kendall 2023).

Like stable isotope and aDNA analyses, the study of proteins in archaeology has seen a rise in interest over the past 20 years; this has included interrogating the ancient proteome, which is a complete set of proteins in an organism, and the metaproteome, which is all the protein samples recovered from environmental sources (Hendy 2021; 2023). Proteins are among the oldest biomolecules that have been identified. At times aDNA may not survive in the archaeological record, leaving proteins to tell the story, which may include diseases experienced. Proteins can be found in viruses and bacteria and they have been found in bones, teeth, preserved bodies, and dental calculus. Although their study in paleopathology is not yet as advanced as aDNA analysis, proteins are providing surprising information about the past, including about diet and subsistence (e.g., Hendy et al. 2018), dairy consumption (Bleasdale et al. 2021), dental health (Jersie-Christensen et al. 2018), biological sex (Stewart et al. 2017), and diseases, such as infections, and immune and physiological responses (e.g., Barbieri et al. 2017; Corthals et al. 2012). We should also emphasize the revolution in analyzing dental calculus and the preservation of a huge range of biomolecular inclusions (see Chapter 3).

Finally, we come to human and pathogen aDNA analysis (mitochondrial and nuclear, respectively). In the 1980s researchers discovered that the soft tissues of mummified remains (Pääbo 1985) and dry bones (Hagelberg et al. 1989) could preserve DNA. Since then, its analysis, like that of stable isotopes, has become almost routine; for overviews, see Stone and Ozaga (2019), Sabin and Stone (2023), and Brown (2023). Ancient DNA analysis started with a rocky road of criticisms, especially regarding questionable laboratory protocols and reproducibility of results (e.g., Barnes and Thomas 2005; Roberts and Ingham 2008), and even whether it was truly preserved DNA or the result of contamination. Cooper and Poinar (2000) made recommendations. Methods developed initially from polymerase chain reaction (PCR) sequencing to next-generation sequencing (NGS) in the early 2000s. NGS enabled ultrahigh throughput of samples on a broader scale and increased the speed of analysis. It has more power and sensitivity to detect genetic material. It can also sequence hundreds and thousands of genes, or even a whole genome, in a shorter period of time, and it overcame a key limitation of PCR-based techniques that could not distinguish ancient from modern microbial DNA contamination (Dalal et al. 2023). In paleopathology, the study of aDNA of infectious pathogens has produced the most research since the first discoveries in the early 1990s—for example, with the work of Salo et al. (1994) on tuberculosis. In the early years of aDNA analysis, the genus and species of pathogens were identified, most notably the animal and human species of tuberculosis. More recently, a closer look at the origin and evolution of infectious diseases is enabled by phylogenetic characterizations of pathogen DNA, that is, ancient strains of infectious organisms seen in particular geographic locations today, together with data from modern DNA. This technique, together with stable isotope and mitochondrial DNA data has been extremely useful for exploring the movement of people with their infections in the past, as well as the comorbidity of different diseases (Bonczarowska et al. 2022; Fernandez-Dominguez 2023). Ancient pathogen genomes have also been published in recent years. Excellent overviews are provided by Duchêne et al. (2020); for plague: Bos et al. (2011); leprosy: Schuenemann et al. (2013); tuberculosis: Bos et al. (2014); and treponemal infection: Giffin et al. (2020).

Other Measures of Poor Health

While the identification of tangible bone changes associated with disease and injury form the main components of the paleopathologist's endeavor, other, possibly more subtle health measures are important to consider. An example is exploring growth estimations for children, where a dental age at death (a more reliable age indicator) is compared to long bone lengths as a proxy for the child's height (see Chapter 7). These are then compared to other groups of archaeological children—for example, in urban and suburban populations (Vilumets et al. 2024), or with modern standards of healthy children—often by creating z-scores (Fig. 1.12; and see Spake and Cardoso 2021). If the growth of the child or group falls below what is expected, it suggests that disease or dietary insufficiency was involved; this was the case when Roberts et al. (2016) identified multiple diseases in an eighteenth- and nineteenth-century boy who displayed short bones for his dental age. In life, children may "catch up" their growth should conditions improve (Cooke et al. 2023), or continue to fall behind the expected growth attainment if they do not. However, paleopathologists can only judge the growth of that individual child at one point in time: death (as we rely on cross-sectional data). Instead, if growth faltering occurs within a specific age cohort of a group (e.g., 2–3 years), it might indicate what factors are responsible, such as weaning or insufficient food. If these adverse conditions persist for the group, adult skeletons will have a shorter than expected stature too.

Measures of variation in attained height reflect many factors: genetic, environmental (e.g., living conditions), subsistence and diet, hormonal, and socioeconomic. Stature also varies between geographic locations, in different climates, and between ethnic groups (Davies et al. 2023). While stature displays a strong inherited genetic component (Mittal et al. 2021), Cox et al. (2024) concluded that height was more driven by culture in their study. They used aDNA, bone measurements, diet, and evidence for disease from over 1,500 Early Neolithic individuals in north-central and south-central Europe, the Mediterranean, and Balkan regions

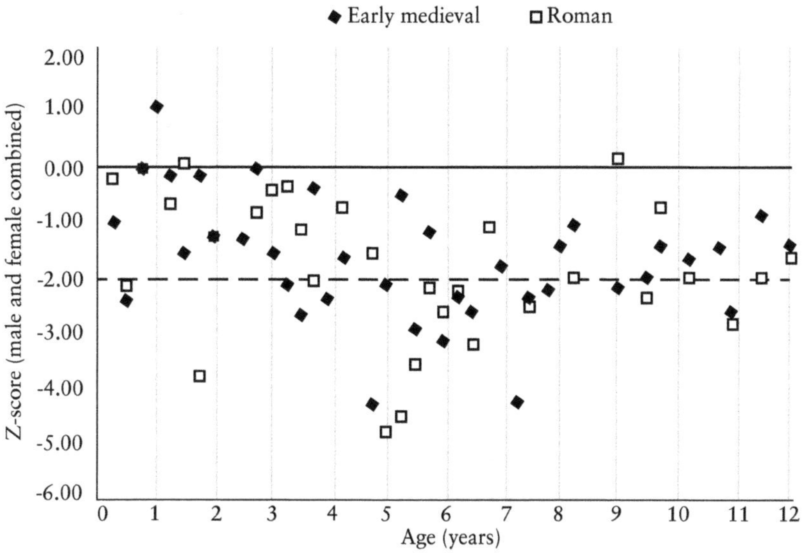

Figure 1.12. Hypothetical example of a z-score used to estimate average growth attainment in non-adult skeletal remains. Any individuals (represented by a point) falling two standard deviations below 0 are considered to be faltering. Figure by Mary Lewis.

(8000–6000 BCE). Genetic predictions of height were statistically identical in skeletons from all regions and for both males and females, but they found a large difference in actual height between the sexes, suggested to be caused by cultural and environmental drivers.

Height has been used by many paleopathologists to assess inequality, and to explore nutritional deprivation and level of income, particularly in the twentieth and twenty-first centuries (e.g., Orr et al. 2021: England). This work has revealed, not surprisingly, that deprived children are more likely to have relatively shorter stature than those who are not deprived (Orr et al. 2021), and that higher-status people are taller, thus reflecting inequality in the biological standard of living (Steckel 1995). Perhaps the most dramatic declines in stature have been seen in studies of populations making the transition to farming (e.g., Cohen and Armelagos 1984). Consideration of stature is therefore advisable because it provides potential evidence for the reasons behind shorter than expected height. Long bone lengths alone, rather than lengths being used in regression equations, are increasingly being employed (e.g., see Steckel et al. 2019).

Paleodemography considers the size, structure, and dynamics of a dead (not living) population derived from the biological sex and age estimates for that group. It provides a window into life expectancy, fertility rates, and risk of dying in past populations (Boldsen et al. 2022: 115). Population figures and their patterns are of immense value to the paleopathologist because population size and growth can be explained in terms of socioeconomic development, and in the case of rapid population expansion through changing birth and death rates, the spread of disease and famines. Furthermore, the changing population pattern may have a bearing on modern disease and its possible causation. While many diseases can be seen on

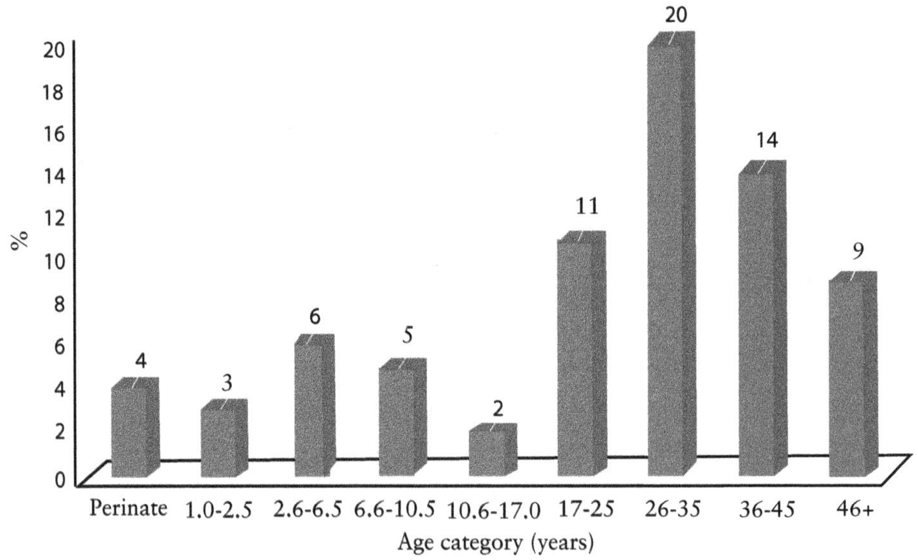

Figure 1.13. Example of a mortality profile chart, showing the percentage of people dying within specific age groups. Figure by Mary Lewis.

archaeological skeletal remains, many cannot, and rapidly fatal (acute) or soft tissue diseases will not leave their mark. A demographic profile may be the only way to explore the impact of acute diseases on a population—for example, the plague pandemics in sixth- through sixteenth-century Europe (Castex and Kacki 2016), or the impact of the 1440–1730 CE Little Ice Age in Japan (Nagaoka et al. 2019).

Demographic profiles may incorporate a mortality profile, a survivorship curve, and a life table. Mortality is the relative frequency of deaths in relation to population numbers, and the mortality profile shows at what age people were dying and whether there are any differences between male and female adults (Fig. 1.13). Death affects all age groups but in differing frequencies depending on time period, geographic location, and intrinsic and extrinsic factors referred to earlier. A survivorship curve is another way of presenting the data and shows the proportion of people in each age group, starting at 100% for the youngest age group represented. The juvenile ratio is used to calculate the fertility or birth rate.

The study of paleodemography has a long history, but it has been fraught with problems. These pertain to the accuracy of biological sex and age data, selective mortality, burial exclusion, the presence of inherent (and hidden) frailty, unknown immigration and emigration patterns, and underrepresentation of the very young and the very old. For example, fertility rates will be affected if not all the children from a site are recovered, or if not all babies who died were buried in the general cemetery. Hoppa and Saunders (1998) and Paine and Harpending (1998) warned that underrepresentation of the oldest in the population might inflate crude birth rates by up to 20%. Also, cemetery samples are often made up of people buried over many generations and hundreds of years, and it is unlikely they all experienced the same advantages and disadvantages in life, even within the same social group (Boldsen et al. 2022). The integration of demographic profiles with data on health and disease for archaeologically derived populations is essential to understand the impact of disease on our ancestors. A paleodemographic profile should not be based on the skeletal data alone. In addition to paleopathological, archaeological, and historical data, a picture of the population under study is helped by radiocarbon dating of the site and cemetery, archaeological evidence for buildings and settlement size, burial registers (for historic populations), and aDNA data to help understand genetic diversity (French et al. 2021; McFadden 2021). Fortunately, most scholars are optimistic about the future of paleodemography as more researchers adopt a multiproxy and multidisciplinary approach to address its limitations (McFadden 2021).

Estimating Disease Frequency

Individual skeletons and large population groups may be studied in paleopathology; each has strengths and weaknesses. The former tells us much about that individual, but not the wider picture of diseases that affected the population in which that person lived—who was affected and what determined that disease distribution (paleoepidemiology), which provides insight to when diseases rose and declined and what contextual factors were important. In clinical medicine, frequency of disease is expressed in two ways—incidence and prevalence (Waldron 2021, 326):

- Incidence = number of new cases in the *population* at risk ÷ the total number in the population at risk
- Prevalence = number of cases in the *study group* ÷ the total number in the study group

To estimate disease incidence, a disease is recorded in a specific group of people; it is then followed by counting new people with the disease after a specified period of time. The time period selected depends on the disease, whether it is rare or not, and its nature. Prevalence is estimated as the number of cases expressed as a proportion of an identified group of people (or cohort). Essentially, paleopathologists can only use the prevalence estimate, and it is "a point prevalence at that" (Waldron 2021, 329). There are three ways that disease frequency may be presented using archaeological data. They are determined by the number of individuals in the study group, and the number of specific bones and teeth that are represented. Taking tuberculosis (TB) of the spine as an example, we may calculate:

1. The frequency of skeletons affected by spinal TB regardless of how many of the skeletons had a preserved spine to observe for this disease (not recommended)
2. The frequency of skeletons affected by spinal TB according to the number that had a preserved spine to observe (crude prevalence rate, or CPR)
3. The number of preserved vertebrae affected by TB overall for the population (true prevalence rate)

Two more examples address these definitions. First, if the prevalence of left hip joint osteoarthritis, for example, is to be studied, then the observer needs to know how many left femora and acetabulae are preserved for observation in order to estimate the prevalence of left hip joint disease. Second, if five out of ten people are reported to have evidence for leprosy, the assumption must be that all bones that are commonly affected in leprosy were preserved for observation (facial, hand, foot, and lower legs). Therefore, it is important to not only include the number of bones and teeth observed for any group, but also what bones and teeth relevant to diagnosis of specific diseases were present to observe. Naturally, the number of skeletons used for calculating frequency rates for disease depends on how many are excavated and analyzed from a site, and their relationship to the original living population. This will be determined by who was buried where, how they were buried, whether their remains were preserved to be excavated, and how much of the cemetery was uncovered; all these processes determine the final number, and it is inevitable that this number will be only a fraction of the original.

When calculating the frequency of disease throughout the time period of a cemetery, the calculation becomes even more difficult. Some cemeteries span several hundred years, and stratification detail is usually not available to allow the division of burials into subperiods, although exceptions exist (e.g., Stroud and Kemp 1993; Connell et al. 2012). As Waldron (1994, 22) suggested, if there are no temporal subunits within a cemetery for the population being analyzed, then only a mean prevalence rate for specific diseases can be produced. This is all well and good, but it does not pick out the peaks in disease prevalence that may have occurred throughout the time span of the cemetery. Additionally, experimental studies have shown that marked discrepancies can occur in how data are recorded in paleopathology, especially if a severity grading system is used (Waldron and Rogers 1991; Miller et al. 1996). Therefore, incorporating inter and intra error tests to ensure consistency in pathological recording is advised (see Mays 2023, 32–35). A recent study by Biehler-Gomez et al. (2020) shows how challenging description can be. Ten participants (five forensic pathologists and five anthropologists) were invited to describe thirty bone lesions on dry bones and photographs. The contradictions and inaccuracies, especially in describing lesion characteristics and new bone formation, indicate potential consequences for the frequency of diseases that were diagnosed. To be able to compare prevalence rates between different cemetery groups, methods of recording and the data generated must be consistently collected using the same methods and observations to make them comparable among scholars worldwide.

Interpretation: Context Is Everything

Understanding the context for the occurrence of human disease in the past and the present is therefore essential for paleopathology; without that knowledge it is not possible to usefully interpret the information about disease we find in human remains. While data about context are readily available for the present, we also have detailed information about the past through archaeological and environmental evidence, and historical documentation, albeit inevitably with less detail and gaps in information. To contextualize our data, bioarchaeologists interrogate this evidence to learn about people's lives, what diet they ate, what type of housing they lived in, what social-structural situations they were exposed to, what work they did, and how mobile they were, in order to interpret how healthy they were and what risk factors for disease were present in their environments. Understanding the time period of individuals with particular diseases is also vital. For example, the precise dating of skeletons with bone changes consistent with venereal (acquired) syphilis is important for the discussion of the pre- or post-Columbian nature and origin for this disease (Baker et al. 2020; see also Chapter 6). Since humans evolved, the health challenges that human populations have faced, as well as those that we face today, are very much part of our identity, like our age, gender, ancestry, social class, and faith (e.g., Knudson and Stowjanowski 2020). Intersectionality theory is providing a more nuanced approach to understanding how people experienced the world in which they lived, how the individual aspects of identities may not necessarily be mutually exclusive, and that they may change across the life course and even work together to create disadvantage (Collins and Bilge 2020).

Taking some of these aspects of identification, we do not know how important it was in the past to assign an age to a person (Gowland 2006). It is probable that progression through life was related to specific events, and when the person reached a particular developmental stage, such as crawling or walking, then their status within the group changed. These achievements may also have affected their health. For example, walking increases the risk of having more accidents, and weaning may lead to diarrhea, which could lead to death. People who lived into later age may have lost their social network of family to support them and, depending on time and place, they may have acquired increased risks for particular diseases (Appleby 2024); such frailty may or may not have been tolerated by their society.

Ethnic identity is also an important factor in the occurrence and type of disease that people are exposed to. First, in a racist society, social inequality can generate impoverished childhoods and greater exposure to malnutrition and disease that impact later life and the next generation, according to the DOHaD hypothesis. Second, as we will see throughout the following chapters, some conditions, such as genetic anemia, evolved almost exclusively in African and southern Mediterranean populations and climates (tropical or temperate). Important too is consideration of health beliefs in different groups, which will, in turn, affect whether and how a disease might be treated. For example, Roberts and Buikstra (2003) discussed differing approaches to tuberculosis in a variety of living populations around the world. We should be aware, however, that many of the so-called documented collections that have been used to develop osteological techniques (biological sex, age, ancestry) and to explore pathological change are biased toward selected groups of individuals whose remains were collected, sometimes using exploitive practices and associated with limited documentation. Many individuals would have experienced health inequality as the result of structural racism, leading to higher levels of violent trauma, for example; therefore, we should be cautious in how we interpret the findings (de la Cova 2011, 2017; Razai et al. 2021).

Knowing the time and place from which the skeletons under study came is essential for understanding the evolution of disease. "Epidemiological transitions" describe changes that occurred at different periods of time and geographic locations and affected the lives of humans, other animals, and their environments around the globe (Barrett et al. 1998). The first transition occurred around 10,000 years ago and documents the development of farming of plants and animals, creation of permanent settlements, a movement away from a hunting-and-foraging way of life (Cohen and Armelagos 1984; Temple and Stojanowski 2019) and, later, the formation of urban centers (Rawcliffe 2013; Betsinger and DeWitte 2020). The second transition (industrialization) includes four phases (Armelagos 1990; Groumpos 2021); three had been transitioned by the end of the twentieth century: (1) mechanization, (2) technological (e.g., electrification), and (3) automation, or the digital revolution, enabling development of the information and communication superhighway. The fourth transition (digitization) since 2000 has encompassed "the application of information and communication technologies mainly to industry but also to the rest of societies' activities" (Groumpos 2021, 466). We now live in a globalized world, which enables easy and rapid movement, mirrored by the easy and rapid spread of new diseases.

Health has been affected in all the transitions. Until the advent of agriculture, many people lived in reasonable harmony with their environment, but this equilibrium was destroyed with the development of farming; it still remains a challenge for many, as Garrett et al. (2021) have shown for the Amazon region. Ploughing, crop rearing, and tending domesticated animals increased exposure to new organisms. In association with environmental change, be it deforestation, land cultivation, or urbanization, people also came to live closer to a variety of animals and their diseases. Paleopathologists have often documented a decline in health with farming in the Americas (Steckel et al. 2002), Europe (Steckel et al. 2019), and more globally (Cohen and Armelagos 1984; Cohen and Crane-Kramer 2007). The development of farming supported higher population sizes, and consequently urban communities were established in towns and cities. Greater numbers of people living in close contact, often in poorly ventilated, unhygienic houses, put pressure on scarce resources and enabled transmission of infectious diseases (for historical examples see Dyer 1989; Clark 2007; Smith et al. 2012; Rosen 2015; and Galor 2022). In the early stages of village and town development, little thought was given to waste disposal, and the health hazards of poor water quality or open sewers were not understood. Within this framework, waterborne infections, such as cholera, flourished and still do (Amicizia et al. 2019). With industrialization also came problems of increased health inequality, but by the early twentieth century, antibiotics and vaccinations reduced the impact of many infections. Increased wealth improved health through better standards of living and nutrition, which according to McKeown (1988, 79, 198) made a greater contribution to the decline of tuberculosis than medicine. Nevertheless, new infections and reemerging (old) infections (e.g., tuberculosis), alongside antibiotic resistance, became challenges by the end of that century (Hall et al. 2018; Ayorinde et al. 2023). In addition, the chronic degenerative noncommunicable diseases of old age (NCDs) rapidly increased due to lifestyle changes and longer life expectancy, at least in the Western world.

The movement of people across long distances is not only a pattern of modern life. In the past, the movement of people, either as individuals or conquering nations, aided the spread of disease. Soldiers on active service were and are notorious for spreading infectious disease, crossing frontiers and seas on campaigns to distant lands (e.g., Kaushik and Sougat 2018). They were often crowded together, poorly nourished, and usually exhausted by the stress of battle. Explorers from the Old World who reached the Americas introduced new diseases to which Indigenous populations had no resistance (Nunn and Qian 2010). In more recent centuries, activities related to colonization, including enslavement, compromised the health of those colonizing and the colonized; indeed, Indigenous communities still experience poor health (Wispelwey et al. 2023). Now many people travel much more rapidly and frequently than ever, and infections continue to go and return with them.

Coastal or inland, island or mainland, highland or lowland, rivers, lakes, or estuaries, hot, cold, dry, or humid; all these environments affect the range of diseases experienced. For example, metals leaching from naturally occurring sulphate soils in both coastal and inland settings can damage the brain or peripheral nervous system, and in Finland it has been suggested they have been associated with multiple sclerosis (MS; Åström and Roos 2022). However, the precise cause of MS remains unclear. Copper mining has health risks too, particularly via the food chain because of soil pollution: headaches, liver cirrhosis, renal failure, cancer, and respiratory disease have been recorded in residents living near copper-mining areas (Chen et al. 2022). The causal relationship between the development of goiter—a swelling of the neck caused by an enlarged thyroid gland—and nutritional deficiency of iodine is well known. It is due to low iodine levels in water and food of inland mountainous areas—for example, the Alps, Andes, and Himalaya (Zimmerman 2009; see Chapter 7). The combination of latitude and its associated climate and weather patterns can also have a profound effect on the incidence of certain diseases today, as it did in the past. Vitamin D deficiency in northern latitudes, especially in winter, is also attested (e.g., Mendes et al. 2020; Cui et al. 2023; Oskarsson et al. 2022).

The health hazards of the work that people have done and do are also clear. A hunter-forager may live in a healthy environment with a good, well-balanced diet; however, the dangers of injury from hunting wild animals may compromise health and well-being (e.g., Scott et al. 2019, Vietnam). Work in pottery, textile, and mining industries generates particles in the environment that, when inhaled, can induce inflammation and infection in the respiratory tract (e.g., Liu and Liu 2020). Spending long hours cooking over smoky fires may also lead to respiratory tract diseases (Bălă et al. 2021). The modern trades that today create environments conducive to injuries and zoonoses include tanning (Alam et al. 2020), farming (e.g., Johnson et al. 2021), and butchery (Espinosa et al. 2020), although Milstein et al. (2020) have also described mitigating risks of wild meat preparation.

Ethics

In the previous editions of this book, we did not discuss ethical considerations for human remains, which was a terrible oversight, especially considering the developments and reflections over the past 20 years (e.g. see Squires et al. 2019b). We agree with de la Cova (2023, 382), who said paleopathologists have had a strong tendency to skirt around the "deep ethical issues" that surround the study of human remains. This is probably because it was convenient not to act, and no one was preventing us from excavating and analyzing skeletons and preserved bodies.

First, we should remember that human remains represent people who had identities and lived experiences. They represent once-living and breathing human beings like everyone reading this book. They are not pottery sherds, plant remains, animal bones, or gold artifacts, and we need to remember this when we are excavating and recording them, taking samples for scientific analysis, curating them for future teaching and research, and displaying them in museums. That is why we recommend that we use words to describe skeletons or mummified remains that do not lead to objectification. Commonly used terms applied to human remains include: *case, specimen, subject, sample, material,* and *object*. *Case*, *specimen*, and *subject* reflect the medical influence on paleopathology, and one could argue may have originated from the processes and outcomes of colonization. *Sample* is increasingly used because of the rise in biomolecular analysis where they are taken from human remains; *material* is used perhaps because journal paper structure includes a section called "materials and methods"; and *object* is used in curation where everything in a museum's care may be called an object.

Moving away from objectification of human remains is recommended for the future, as de la Cova (2023) also suggested. In fact, when discussing people with disease in the past, it is worth noting the old adage often attributed to Hippocrates (fifth century BCE), emphasizing that it is more important to know about the person with the disease than what disease they have had. Care includes "compassion and dignity, advocacy and common sense" (Sullivan 2010, 24), and this definition should apply to caring for human remains, from excavation, through analysis, to curation. Inappropriate treatment of human remains and mentioning specific words or cultural practices (e.g., cannibalism), interpersonal violence, or even particular diseases (e.g., syphilis, leprosy) can lead to stigma, which can be particularly distressing to living Indigenous communities and for their histories (e.g., Lambert 2012). Diseases that have been stigmatized in the past leave their legacies for living populations; for example, in medieval times the word *leper* equated the sufferer with the disease, and during the recent pandemic some people with COVID-19 were labeled "lepers." In the early history of paleopathology individual skeletons, bones and mummified remains were the focus, before we developed more population-focused studies. More recently, we have seen a return to the individual, where now the complex identity of the individual and their life is reconstructed (an osteobiography). This, together with the application of the Index of Care (Tilley and Cameron 2014), which focuses on the individual's experience of disease or injury and the possible reaction of their family and community, is a long way from "objectification."

Consideration of ethics in relation to archaeological human remains has increased enormously over the past 20 years. First, ethical considerations increasingly pervade, and have pervaded, all aspects of our world including medicine (Varkey 2021).

While paleopathologists often describe the most severe symptoms and outcomes of a disease in our communications about people in the past, we need to be sensitive toward individuals who may have the same diseases today. Care should be taken about how we discuss these signs and symptoms so as not to sensationalize that condition or a person's experience of it. Research into conditions is particularly fraught with ethical challenges. As Titelbaum et al. (2022, 250) explained, the words we use to describe these conditions are loaded with negative connotations. For example, "malformation" comes from the Latin for "evil" (*malus*), and "defect" from the Latin for "fail" (*deficere*), and it is clear how terms such as "abnormal" and "abnormality" may impact the well-being of people with developmental conditions today who may read our articles and books. Additionally, there is a move away from the use of eponyms in medical science, especially where the condition is named after a physician whose practices are deemed unethical today, or where the name has racial connotations; for example, Reiter's syndrome is named after a doctor involved in Nazi atrocities, and Down syndrome is linked to Langston Down, who originally referred to the condition as "mongolism" (Castillo Aleman 2021). Alternatively, there is a call for leprosy to be once again referred to as Hansen's disease after the physician who discovered it, to shield people with the disease from its stigma (Souza et al. 2024; and see Chapter 6).

While true collaborations in research can be mutually beneficial, Butlin and Peters (2022) have noted that some researchers take advantage of regions of the world that are less well regulated in terms of ethics. Paleopathologists must be aware of this failing when working in places where ethical policies and practices may not be established, or where colonization once took place that led to scientifically focused collection of skeletons that were taken far from their origin. In addition, considering culturally embedded beliefs about the proper treatment of the dead should be an essential part of a paleopathologist's toolkit, and these beliefs must be respected, even if it means not having access to the human remains that they wish to study.

It can be argued that the impetus for bioarchaeologists to practice their work more ethically was precipitated in North America toward the end of the twentieth century. Indigenous peoples became concerned about the excavation of their ancestors' remains, and they objected to the housing of remains for teaching and research in museums, universities, and other institutions. Their efforts resulted in the passing of the National Museum of the American Indian Act in 1989 (National Museum of the American Indian 2024) and the Native American Graves Protection and Repatriation Act in 1990 (National Park Service 2024). Further regulations followed in 1995 and 2023 on the research and stewardship of these remains. These legislative measures recognized that Indigenous communities feel spiritually linked to their ancestors, and that the spirits of their ancestors were being mistreated in museums (Lambert and Walker 2018). Importantly, in 1989 the Vermillion Accord on human remains was adopted at the World Archaeological Congress (WAC 2024), paving the way for inclusion of Indigenous voices in discussions about human remains within codes of conduct in the archaeological and museum fields.

As a reaction to these developments, professional organizations, such as the American Association of Physical (now Biological) Anthropologists (AABA), published their own ethical guidelines. BABAO first published its ethics and practice guidelines in 2010, updated in 2019. New guidance was also established for digital imaging and photography of human remains (BABAO 2024), emphasizing that taking and sharing images can compromise the dignity and respect that should be afforded to human remains. The requirements for a specific focus on ethics when researching diseases in the past led the Paleopathology Association in 2023 to introduce a Statement of Ethical Principles that recognized "decision-making and relationships with other researchers and communities may be complex and challenging" and urged researchers to be mindful of "the impact of their research on the lives of people living with diseases today." De la Cova (2023) reported new calls for ethical reform, including an African American Graves Protection and Repatriation Act (Dunnavant et al. 2021; see https://www.congress.gov/bill/117th-congress/house-bill/6805/text). However, as she wrote: "regardless of how noble our intentions are, these actions do not change past behaviors and violence perpetrated by our anthropological founding fathers, which continue to resonate into the present" (2023, 381). If we do not proactively deal with these issues, then our actions will become empty gestures. Definitions of dignity and respect will also vary among different cultures (past and present). As de la Cova stated, we must confront histories that put bioarchaeologists in the past to shame, and "include perspectives of scholars who come from marginalized and oppressed groups, deconstructing colonial stereotypes, and allowing descendant communities to take active roles in creation, production, and control of knowledge about their ancestors" (2023, 385). It is clear from the many publications on this subject that paleopathologists feel a duty of care for human remains that should extend to encouraging dialogue with all parties of interest, including descendant communities, regardless of whether all opinions are welcomed (e.g., see Buikstra 2016; Lambert and Walker 2018; Roberts 2018, chap. 2; Turner et al. 2018; Roberts 2019a). These considerations have extended to recommendations for teaching, developer-led archaeology, museums, display, social media, 3D data, sampling for destructive analyses, and more, recently publishing in bioarchaeology (e.g., see Squires et al. 2019a, 2022; Cassman et al. 2007; Giesen 2013).

There has also been a focus on ethics and aDNA analysis. For example, Wagner et al. (2020, 190) provided advice on questions that should be addressed before starting any projects, along with suggestions for community engagement strategies and example data and storage agreements. As they wrote, "globally, researchers need to understand the politics and local laws (including Indigenous community regulations) of the country in which they are working. Every member of the research team is responsible for fostering ethical aDNA work" (see also Márquez-Grant and Fibiger 2011). Alpaslan-Roodenberg et al. (2021) made five recommendations for aDNA research: (1) ensure all regulations are followed according to the geographic location of the research; (2) prepare a detailed plan prior to any study; (3) minimize damage to human remains; (4) make the data available following publication; and (5) engage with other stakeholders to ensure respect and sensitivity to stakeholder perspectives. This paper has been criticized more recently for insufficiently addressing community engagement (Kowal et al. 2023). Squires et al. (2019a) also provided detailed guidance for sampling and analysis, but it is clear that much more work is needed to define the ethical issues surrounding aDNA analysis in any human remains, whether Indigenous or not, as has occurred with living population DNA studies (e.g., Takashima et al. 2018; Eman and Mahsa 2019; Moodley et al. 2022). Indeed, disparities have been identified between the protocols for modern and ancient studies (e.g., Gibbon 2020).

Paleopathologists strive to give voices to the individuals that they study across their life courses, and to provide these people with identities. If the reader of this book takes anything away from it, we hope it will include as a priority the important ethical dimension to human remains from archaeological sites. We would also advocate the guidelines of de la Cova (2023, 387–393) moving forward:

1. Challenge our past by engaging with it and deconstructing it
2. Acknowledge that we need to break free from our enlightenment chains
3. Restore the social and the biological through multidimensional analyses
4. Remember your privilege and positionality
5. Clearly communicate with the public and descendant communities
6. Stop the perpetual cycle of structural violence
7. Be aware of our own ethical biases

In studying disease and injury in human remains from archaeological sites we should always remember that we do not have a right to do this; it is a huge privilege and one we should respect.

Public Engagement

In the third edition of this book, we wrote little about the need to engage with people beyond academia about our research: politicians, policy makers, and the general public. As seen in the previous section, we have an ethical responsibility to communicate with the public and other interested parties. That this area has relatively recently come to the fore may be explained by increased scrutiny of our work in terms of value not only to our own discipline, but to others for whom there can be pushback. First, we need to ask ourselves why we are paleopathologists and what our aims are in doing the work we do. Some scholars appear to be content to do their work and make a difference to understanding the past, but others are increasingly keen to address contemporary challenges, as many recent publications indicate (e.g., Buikstra 2019a; Buikstra et al. 2022, section 2.2; Cheung et al. 2019; de la Cova 2023, 390–392; DeWitte 2016; Martin et al. 2013, chap. 10; Roberts 2020ab; Schug et al. 2023; Schug and Halcrow 2022). Outreach activities are an important avenue for us to connect to the public and beyond academia. Indeed, we are fortunate that the public are generally fascinated with ancient bodies and what they can tell us, probably because everyone has a skeleton and is interested to learn more about it. As the bestselling author Bryson has said, we spend our whole lives in one body and yet most of us have practically no idea how it works and what goes on inside it (Bryson 2019; see also Black 2020). Paleopathologists have at their fingertips much knowledge about the skeleton, its associated soft tissues, and how the body works, and they have lots of stories to tell the public about the human remains they study. They also work with researchers in evolutionary medicine to document the origin, evolution, and history of disease, which also fascinates the public (Zuckerman et al. 2012; Plomp et al. 2022b).

In the UK, there is much emphasis on how archaeology can have an impact beyond academia, influencing a range of people, practices, and organizations, and we imagine it is similar elsewhere. Our knowledge has had an influence on the heritage sector, practicing archaeologists, planning authorities, agriculture, forestry, nature conservation, policy advisers and makers, the tourism sector, developers, creative art industries, education across all levels, the socially disadvantaged, mentally ill citizens, citizen scientists, journalists, the media, and artists (Roberts 2024, table 15.2; Mattingley and Foster 2023). These effects were presented most recently in the sixty-one impact case studies in archaeology submitted in 2021 for the periodic Research Excellence Framework (REF 2022), an exercise that considers quality of research in UK universities. REF defines impact as "an effect on, change or benefit to the economy, society, culture, public policy or services, health, the environment or quality of life, beyond academia." Some of these REF impact case studies give a flavor of the value of our research: *Healing Heritage: Facilitating and Evaluating the Impact of Museums and Museum Encounters on Health and Wellbeing; Let the Dead Teach the Living: The Applications of Palaeopathological Research to Industry; The Identification of King Richard III: The Economic and Social Impact; and Continuing Bonds: The Long Dead Change Understanding of Death and Bereavement in the Present.* Despite its long history of engagement with people beyond academia, bioarchaeology still has work to do to impact policy advisers and makers, particularly in governments, perhaps using guidance on the dos and don'ts provided by Oliver and Cairney (2019), Sasse and Haddon (2019), and Sanderson (2023). The will is there, and paleopathologists have the necessary skills and knowledge. More generally, paleopathology has many communication methods at hand and much to offer the modern world in addressing global challenges. Kintigh et al. (2014), Barker et al. (2015), and Schofield (2024) illustrate the value of archaeological research generally, but paleopathology is integral to understanding the lives of past communities and how poor health could impact the very functioning of societies. Paleopathology feeds into all of Kintigh et al.'s (2014) "grand challenges in archaeology" focused on the dynamic cultural practices that operate within human and natural systems.

The Archaeology of Disease: Its Scope

Paleopathology was defined in 1910 by Marc Armand Ruffer as the science of diseases whose existence can be demonstrated on the basis of human and animal remains from ancient times. Diseases in animal bones are generally not discussed in this book, not because we do not think they are important, but because they are an increasing focus of zooarchaeological study, and because we simply do not have the space. Animal diseases are relevant to the One Health concept; as starting points, the reader is directed to Thomas (2012, 2019), Bartosiewicz and Mansouri (2023), and a special issue of the *International Journal of Osteoarchaeology* (2022;32(3)). We hope that zooarchaeologists will expand their studies of disease in animal bones from archaeological sites in the future. At the very least, paleopathologists studying human remains need that perspective because many diseases originated in animals and the information is important for reconstructing the origin, evolution, and history of disease. The study of mummified remains is also not generally dealt with here, although we recognize that preserved bodies potentially provide more extensive information about people's lives than skeletons. They survive in certain parts of the world only where environmental conditions in the burial context are conducive to preservation; therefore, there are many fewer preserved bodies than skeletons. Furthermore, none of the authors work with mummified remains. For overviews of research on preserved bodies, see Aufderheide (2003), Lynnerup (2019), Nystrom et al. (2023), and Wilson et al. (2023). Finally, while the majority of individuals studied by paleopathologists are represented by skeletons (inhumations) and fewer are cremated remains, exceptional work has been done on cremains from many parts of the world (e.g., Thompson 2015; Schmit and Symes 2008; McKinley 1994, 2000). Nevertheless, cremains do not usually provide as much pathological information compared to bones, and therefore, for the purposes of this volume, we made the decision to exclude them.

Care has been given to the terminology we have used throughout the book, although we may not always get it right. For example, bioarchaeologists estimate a biological sex (male or female) from skeletal remains, rather than gender. Sex is a biological characteristic whereas gender is socially constructed. Biological sex and gender are not necessarily binary values in the living or the dead. It is well known that estimating the biological sex of an individual is more of an art than a science, and skeletons can often demonstrate a mixture of male and female morphological traits. In bioarchaeology, we have long estimated biological sex along a spectrum, placing skeletons into those that appear very male, very female, or who we cannot assign a definite sex due to their mix of characteristics (Kaufman et al. 2023). With a grounding in medical science, paleopathologists use "male" and "female" to understand patterns of disease susceptibility because this is how the clinicians present these data, and hence, these binary terms are used throughout the book. Forementioned concerns about the use of unethical language or eponyms have also been considered throughout, most notably, but not exclusively, in Chapter 2 (e.g., "Down syndrome" is replaced by "trisomy 21," and "defect" is replaced with "anomaly").

In a book such as this, it is not possible to consider all the bone and dental diseases that may occur in ancient human remains. Many diseases are rare in modern populations and were likely rare in the past—as discussed by Gresky et al. (2021). Instead, it is our intention here to focus on diseases that are more commonly seen and, crucially, what they can tell us about life in the past. Throughout we provide guidance for scholars in the discipline and other interested readers about the advantages and limitations of a paleopathological approach to the interpretation of the past human experience within a cultural (archaeological) context.

In the following chapters the most common diseases that affect bones and teeth are discussed. Each chapter outlines a series of conditions and lesions associated with a defined disease classification as follows:

- **Congenital and developmental conditions:** encompassing conditions present at birth or that occur during the birth process
- **Dental disease:** those diseases or conditions affecting the teeth and associated tissues
- **Trauma:** fractures and other lesions that result from injury or deliberate modification of the skeleton
- **Joint disease and skeletal indicators of activity:** those that affect the joints of the body and associated soft tissues
- **Infectious disease:** diseases caused by invading living organisms such as bacteria and parasites
- **Metabolic and endocrine disorders:** ailments caused by a disturbance in the normal processes of cell metabolism (metabolic) or an over- or underactivity of the endocrine glands, which secrete hormones (endocrine)
- **Neoplastic disease:** "new growths," which may be benign (localized to the site of growth) or malignant (progressive growth, which invades and destroys surrounding tissues and spreads to more distant sites in the body)

2

Congenital and Developmental Conditions

> Detecting developmental [anomalies] within a prehistoric skeletal population permits interpretive projections for the occurrence of major [disorders], biological affinities, and both cultural and environmental influences.
>
> —E. Barnes, *Developmental Defects of the Axial Skeleton in Paleopathology*

Developmental conditions include a wide range of structural and functional changes to both the soft tissue and skeleton that occur during embryonic and fetal development (Moore et al. 2019). They can be identified before or at birth, or become manifest later in life (WHO 2023b). These conditions vary in their severity, from the most minor anomaly of development, which may never produce signs or symptoms in the individual, to a severe condition that is incompatible with life. Today, 94% of congenital conditions occur in low- and middle-income countries, with the incidence increasing as other causes of infant mortality, such as infectious disease, decline (WHO 2023b). An estimated 240,000 newborns currently die within 28 days after birth due to congenital conditions worldwide, with a further 170,000 dying between the ages of 1 month and 5 years (WHO 2023b). Children born with skeletal anomalies are more likely to survive than those born with problems in the development of soft tissue systems (Pearce and Goldblatt 2001). In archaeological terms, it is mainly children who survived birth that are recognized, whereas the number of children with developmental conditions represented by intrauterine deaths is unknown. It is likely that in antiquity, the actual percentage of infants and children who died directly as the result of a developmental condition was low. Many more would have died as a result of common infections of gastroenteritis and pneumonia, diseases that can affect any child. In the modern antibiotic era, where control of infantile infection is usually successful and commonplace (particularly in Western countries), the proportion of deaths due to developmental conditions has hence increased (WHO 2023b). Numerically, though, the deaths attributable to the problem may have remained fairly stable; it is their significance relative to other infantile diseases that has changed. While, as we shall discuss, many developmental conditions are of unknown etiology, viewed through the lens of the United Nations Sustainable Development Goals, information on the frequency of congenital anomalies in different environments in the past are relevant to our understanding of poverty (1), nutrition (2), environmental pollution (6, 11, 12), and social inequality (10).

Many terms used to describe developmental conditions in the literature are used interchangeably (e.g., "variation," "anomaly"), but they all occur as the result of four different processes (Moore et al. 2019):

1. A problem with the shape of an organ or bone during initial development
2. Where the shape of the already formed organ or bone is changed due to mechanical pressure
3. Disruption in the initial development of the organ or bone due to an external factor such as a toxin, trauma, or infection
4. The abnormal development of a part of the body, which in terms of the skeleton means affecting one or more of the bones

Because they result from problems of formation, developmental conditions are classified as the total failure of development (aplasia), partial failure of development (hypoplasia), overdevelopment (hyperplasia), or problems with normal cell development or function (dysplasia). Like most medical classifications, this is perhaps too simple, but it is nevertheless practical and convenient for the paleopathologist. The full extent of disorders of fetal development is not and may never be known, as many end in a spontaneous abortion of the fetus early in development. Modern data are fraught with problems; even with the most sophisticated diagnostic methods used today, 10% of all miscarriages have an unknown cause (Papas and Kutteh 2020) and the lack of standardized terminology, and the different levels of reporting in different countries, means that the true frequency of these conditions across the globe is difficult to assess (Modell et al. 2018). From an archaeological perspective, faults in soft tissue development may be recognizable in preserved bodies, but these represent only a very small proportion of the remains recovered, and so it is mainly the skeletal anomalies that are identified and recorded.

It is worth noting that an individual possessing one anomaly is likely to possess a second and different anomaly (Garne et al. 2011), as if nature deals a double blow. For example, an infant with a cleft palate or a club foot is more likely also to have an anomaly of the nervous system (Hall et al. 2020), and 50% of individuals with trisomy 21 (previously Down syndrome) have a heart defect (Dimopoulos et al. 2023). The occurrence of such different and seemingly unrelated problems in a single individual is due, in fact, to a disruption of fetal development at a specific age (called organogenesis), at a time when several organ systems are developing independently and concurrently from hitherto undifferentiated cells within the fetal body, and adverse environmental (teratogenic) influences can co-occur with ultimate gross anatomical or physiological consequences. The occurrence of any disturbing factor during the different trimesters of pregnancy predicts which areas of the body's development are affected and, as many of the body's systems develop at the same time, may result in multiple anomalies (Fig. 2.1). In many cases, the association is between the skeleton and soft tissue. In archaeology, as the latter is often undetectable, such associations may be impossible to record.

The difficulty of identifying such changes in tiny perinates (where the most severe changes are likely to be evident) and a paucity of population-based skeletal research

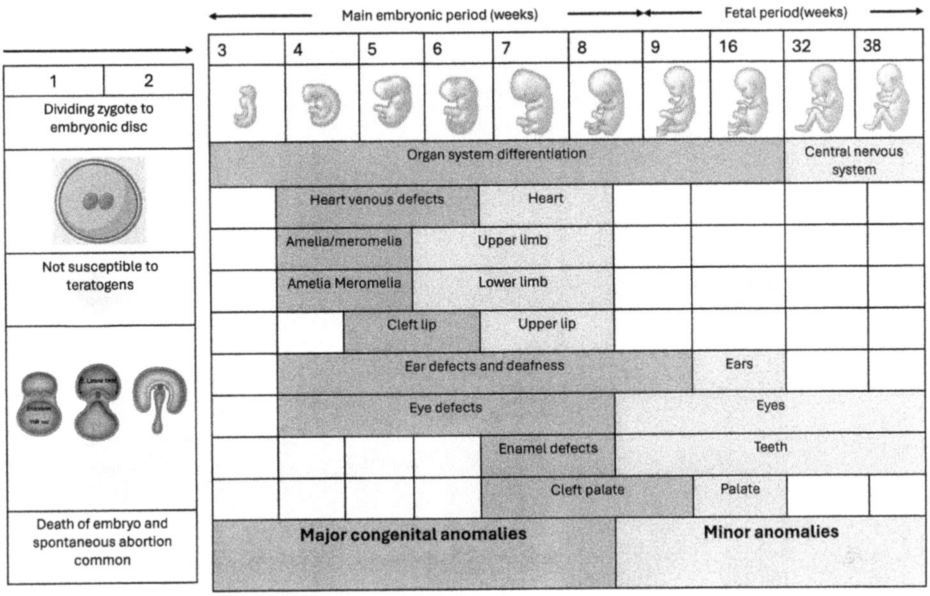

Figure 2.1. Critical periods in human prenatal development. Maternal exposure to toxins and infections during particular embryonic or fetal weeks will have the most effect on the organs and body systems undergoing major development during that period. Adapted from Moore and Persaud 2007, 473.

has limited our understanding of these conditions in the past. Nevertheless, studies of developmental variation in archaeological populations from North America (e.g., Barnes 1994; Titelbaum 2020), medieval and early modern Europe (e.g., Sture 2002; Masnicová and Beňus 2003; Tancock 2014), and South America (e.g., Fabra and Salega 2016: Argentina) have been carried out, commonly finding a concentration of anomalies in the spine. Greater familiarization and training in analyzing and interpreting perinatal skeletal remains has resulted in an increase in evidence for developmental conditions in their remains since the third edition of this book (Pedersen and Anton 1998; Case et al. 2006; Dudar 2010; Irurita et al. 2015; Lewis 2018, 32; Titelbaum 2020). In order to identify an anomaly that may point to a congenital condition, scholars must first be versed in the normal skeletal anatomy of a perinate. We should also consider that children with congenital impairments may have been subject to infanticide, stigmatized when they were alive, and/or buried away from the main community when they died. This will affect whether they are visible within the archaeological record, and hence whether they are available to be studied.

Various conditions, some more common than others, have appeared in the literature throughout the history of paleopathology, and along with neoplastic disease, reports of congenital conditions are dominated by individual skeletons or mummified bodies. What is most apparent is that they are fairly rare compared to other pathological conditions such as trauma or infectious disease. Furthermore, many of the skeletal anomalies that we record would have been asymptomatic in life and would have had no significance to the person concerned.

Causes of Developmental Variation

Just as with other diseases, faults in normal development can rarely be ascribed to a single cause. Instead, potential causes are many and can be grouped in more simple terms as either intrinsic or extrinsic. Intrinsic factors (hereditary/genetic) affect the constitution of the fetus, resulting from a single gene alteration, a combination of recessive genes in the parents, or a chromosomal disorder (Waldron 2021). Evidence for a genetic influence in many congenital diseases rests upon the recording of the repetition of the anomaly in siblings and other close blood relatives. Such evidence can usually only be seen in contemporary and closely documented families. For example, Waters-Rist and Hoogland (2013) reported on a remarkable Dutch family with short-limbed dwarfism from nineteenth-century Middenbeemster, suggesting a familial transference of the condition.

Barnes (1994) noted that similarities in patterns of developmental anomalies indicates a homogeneous population, and that different patterns suggest separate populations or varied gene pools. The likelihood of congenital complications is increased if parents are themselves close blood relatives (consanguinity). For example, marriage between first cousins is commonplace within certain religious groups today, where higher rates of congenital conditions have been noted (Sharkia et al. 2023). Indeed, the legality of consanguineous marriages fell in and out of fashion in Roman, early medieval, and later medieval Europe (Archibald 2001). Procreation between closely related males and females in the small isolated groups of antiquity may, of necessity, have been common and, if so, will have had a similar influence upon the rate of developmental anomalies. A high prevalence of clefts to the atlas neural arch and retained deciduous canines in Neanderthal individuals from El Sidrón in northern Spain led Ríos and coworkers (2015) to suggested these groups experienced an ever-decreasing gene pool in small and isolated groups, resulting in this increase in congenital anomalies.

Extrinsic, or environmental, factors (known as teratogens) include viral and bacterial infections of the mother (e.g., rubella, measles, mumps, chickenpox, and shingles), the effects of drugs and alcohol, and exposure to chemicals and radiation (Moore et al. 2019). For example, during pregnancy drugs can pass across the placenta to the unborn child, and the first trimester of pregnancy (between 2 weeks and 3 months of intrauterine development) is when very serious fetal anomalies can occur (Benjamin et al. 2002, 964). Phenytoin, used to treat epilepsy, can cause cleft lip and palate, and tetracycline, an antibiotic, can lead to damaged bones and teeth (Benjamin et al. 2002, 965). In the 1950s, the therapeutic administration of thalidomide to treat morning sickness during organogenesis in the first trimester resulted in severe anomalies in the development of the limbs and cranium. It is likely that people in distant antiquity sought to remedy their physical ills with herbal remedies, just as they do today. These unrefined agents may have helped to relieve symptoms, but it is also possible that they contributed to congenital conditions in their unborn children. Exposure of the mother to radiation may also lead to skeletal anomalies developing in the fetus. For example in 2003–2004 in Iraq, US weapons firing depleted uranium projectiles were believed by many to be behind the increases in birth anomalies in the population (Allen 2003). The projectiles disintegrate into fine particles and contaminate the soil, water, air, and ultimately people. Furthermore, in Vietnam, some 30 years after the war, there were still many people suffering birth anomalies and other conditions such as cancer, probably because of contamination of the land by Agent Orange, a herbicide used to decimate the jungle, which contains one of the most virulent poisons known to humans (Scott-Clark and Levy 2003).

The majority of anomalies (up to 60%), however, are of unknown etiology and occur because of a complex mixture of intrinsic and extrinsic factors influencing the mother (Moore et al. 2019). The varying importance of these factors will of course differ in populations spread geographically and through time. These conditions occur when there is disturbance of development at a "threshold level." This level is genetically determined, and variant genes and nongenetic factors can upset normal development, usually in the form of a delay in timing of a threshold event as the embryo develops. Identifying exactly what caused a particular condition in the past is difficult because there are often very few specific archaeological data to provide clues. It is not an easy task today, with clinicians stressing the importance of records that link developmental anomalies and birth rates in order to help us fully understand the risk factors (Botting and Abrahams 2000). We can hypothesize that indoor and outdoor pollution as a result of poorly ventilated smoky housing, or even volcanic eruptions, and people being exposed to poor air quality through the mining, metalworking, and pottery industries, both in prehistory and history, may have exposed parts of the population to chemicals and other contaminants (Trumble and Finch 2019). With the advances in aDNA analysis for identifying family relatedness, infectious diseases, and population movements, it was only a matter of time before genes related to specific congenital conditions were isolated (Maxiner et al. 2021; Boer et al. 2017; Cassidy et al. 2020).

Understanding how congenital conditions may have affected the individual, and the way in which their community treated them, is an exciting departure in paleopathology and reflects a growing field of disability history (Rembis et al. 2018). Such approaches add a new dimension to these reports of single affected individuals. For example, clinical data, assessment of joint mobility through bone measurements, and musculoskeletal stress markers (MSMs) were used to assess the limited movement an older adult male must have experienced with chronic arthritis and subsequent joint fusion, and who lived in New Mexico, USA (1550–1672 CE). His progressive mobility issues led Hawkey (1998, 337–8) to conclude that "although severely impaired, the individual . . . was well cared for, permitting him to survive to middle age" (Fig. 2.2). Similarly, the skeleton of a 16-year-old female with probable osteogenesis imperfecta, who survived despite the fact they may never have walked or eaten regular foods, was found in the Hind Site (c. 3000 BCE) of present-day Ontario, Canada (Vairamuthu and Pfeiffer 2018).

Such interpretive approaches have evolved into an Index of Care (Tilley 2012; Tilley and Schrenk 2017) that takes a staged approach to map detailed information about an individual's physical constraints and appearance, combined with information about the resources that would have been required to support that person within that specific community. Being physically impaired does not necessarily

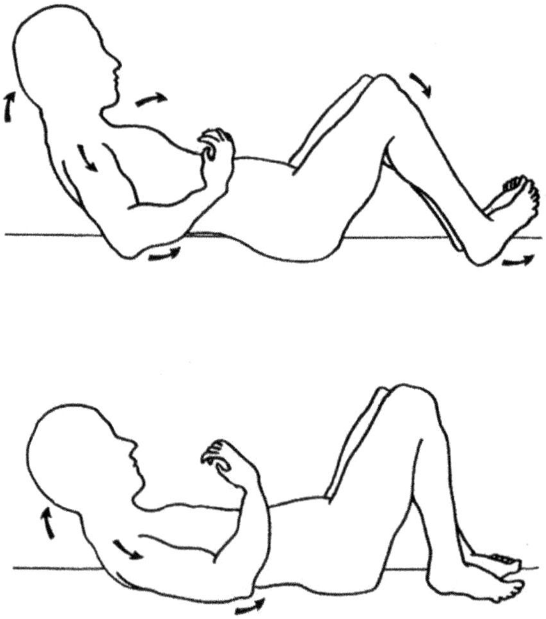

Figure 2.2. Estimated physical movement (arrows) possible for a male with juvenile-onset chronic arthritis as a non-adult (top) and from early adulthood (bottom). Gran Quivira Pueblo, New Mexico, USA, reproduced with kind permission from Diane Hawkey.

imply the individual was considered disabled within their community, nor does that person's survival mean that a whole community cared for them. For example, a person's experience of the same physical impairment may differ because of the nature of their personality or spiritual beliefs (King et al. 1999; Rembis et al. 2018), and those will impact how they view their condition, what pain they may experience, and how those factors impact their ability to function within their community. Humans have an incredible ability to adapt. Hippocrates referred to an impaired but not "disabled" child with a congenitally dislocated hip, crawling and using their hands to pull themselves around, allowing them to remain mobile (Laes 2008). Individuals with the same physical impairment may also be differentially stigmatized across time, cultures, and in contrasting economic contexts. For example, a hunter-forager population almost continuously on the move would have more challenges supporting a physically impaired person than a settled agricultural community. Murphy (2000), while studying developmental anomalies in two Iron Age seminomadic Siberian populations, concluded that they were accepted by their peers and supported in life, because they were treated the same in death as the other members of their community (i.e., buried in the same cemetery and in the same manner). It is important that due consideration of the burial context of an individual affected by a major developmental anomaly in the past is always made, such as where the grave is located and whether it differs in structure from the rest of the cemetery graves. This can tell us much about how they were considered and cared for (or not) by their community.

Age and social status may also have had an impact on whether an individual with a congenital condition was accepted within a community, as well as the role that person would have been expected to play. A survey of 260 child skeletons from archaeological contexts with developmental anomalies worldwide revealed 49 individuals who would have been born "physically distinctive" (e.g., variously with evidence for polydactyly, a short neck, cleft palate, deafness, a club foot, trisomy 21, and restricted movement). Some of these conditions would have become evident only when the child was expected to walk and talk. The fact that 47% of these children survived into adolescence indicates that they were accepted, at least by their immediate family, and at least while they were perhaps still classed as children (Lewis 2016). Being deaf-mute may have been of no consequence to a society if an individual was of lower status and could still perform manual work, while a high-status individual may have experienced stigma if their role in life was to be a leader or orator (Laes et al. 2013).

The following discussion considers some of the developmental conditions that have been observed in the archaeological record. Many of the examples have been identified in adults, but as research into the paleopathology of non-adult remains increases, the extent of conditions reported in children is also rising. There are some caveats to the diagnosis of developmental conditions in children. Although the difficulty of identifying anomalies in the multiple and tiny remains of babies has been mentioned, for older children it is important to also be aware of the time at which the skeleton would normally develop. Spina bifida occulta, for example, is difficult to identify until the sacrum is fully developed, around 15 years of age (Merbs 2004), and irregularities of the axis of the second cervical vertebra associated with torticollis should be diagnosed with caution until the terminal epiphysis of the dens has fused, around the age of 12 years (see Lewis 2018 for examples of how to identify anomalies in younger individuals).

First, we will focus on conditions affecting the skull and vertebrae (the axial skeleton), second on the lower limb bones (the appendicular skeleton), and finally on conditions where both axial and appendicular skeleton can be affected. Being unable to consider all conditions that have been identified in past populations, we will instead consider those anomalies that are more commonly reported in archaeological skeletal remains, those that would have made the person physically distinctive, and conditions that may have led to disability or stigma.

Axial Skeleton

Anencephaly

Perhaps the most severe congenital anomaly that has been noted in paleopathological contexts is anencephaly. The condition has a modern incidence of 5.1 in every 10,000 births worldwide (Salari et al. 2022a). The anomaly is incompatible with independent life after birth; only 25% of affected babies are born live and, tragically, die within days. The etiology of this neural tube defect has genetic links, in particular rare variants in genes associated with chromatin modification (Zou et al. 2020), but it has also been strongly linked to folic acid deficiency in the mother, particularly during the first trimester (Kalter 2003), exposure to toxins, and maternal fever. Anencephaly has a higher frequency in females of low social-economic status (Munteanu et al. 2020) and is more common in twin births (Mastroiacovo et al. 1999). Folic acid is found naturally in green leafy vegetables, shellfish, liver, and meat, but can be destroyed by boiling. Quite possibly the causes of anencephaly operated with the same frequency in antiquity, but the failure of postnatal survival of afflicted infants accounts for the extreme rarity of direct evidence from the past. The thin, fragile bones of neonates do not readily survive to allow for the recognition of skull vault anomaly. Nevertheless, detailed descriptions of the shape individual cranial elements may take on, using anatomical examples, have been provided by Irurita and colleagues (2015) (Fig. 2.3) and Berezina and Buzhilova (2021). The basic defect consists of the lack of development of the cranial vault and the associated failure of brain development, and it is often associated with other midline neural tube anomalies such as spina bifida cystica and cleft palate (Zou et al. 2020).

Anencephaly has a long history, with accounts of "headless" infants dating to 426 BCE and the first archaeological example, of a mummified child from Thebes, in ancient Egypt dated to the first century BCE (Charon 2004). The child was recovered from the Catacombs of Hermopolis, built to house sacred monkeys and birds (ibises), and it is thought the child was included as "an animal born of a woman" (Charon 2004). The failure of postnatal survival of the anencephalic child is a problem of equal significance today as it must have been in antiquity. Because of the very nature of the condition, medical management is powerless, although today early detection is highly possible. The personal grief of the new mother in ancient Egypt was probably as great as that of a mother living in the twenty-first century. Notwithstanding the resigned acceptance of infant death in antiquity, pregnancy, then as now, held an expectation of success. The delivery of an anencephalic baby must have been psychologically very traumatic.

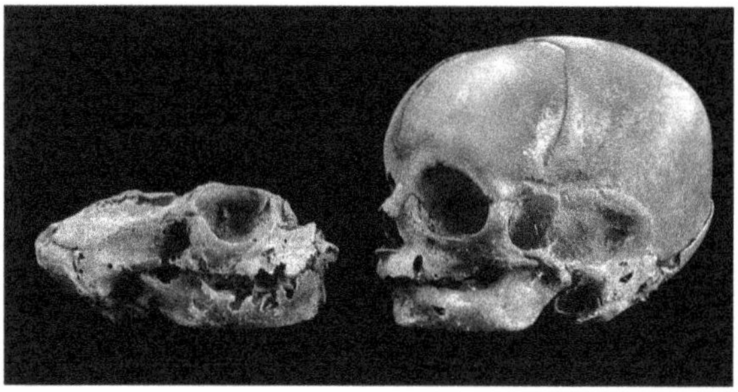

Figure 2.3. Anencephaly (left) in a newborn compared to an unaffected cranium of a child of similar age (right). From the identified collection of non-adult skeletons from San José Granada University, Spain. Photograph courtesy of Javier Irurita.

Microcephaly

A less severe congenital condition, but one which is of profound significance in the social interpretation of antiquity, is microcephaly. This anomaly has a variety of causes including an autosomal recessive gene, fetal alcohol syndrome, radiation exposure, pre- and postnatal iodine deficiency (Sampson et al. 1997; Hollowell and Hannon 1997), and infection, including in more recent times congenital Zika virus infection (de Araújo et al. 2018). Microcephaly is characterized by a statistically significantly small skull circumference (Aufderheide and Rodríguez-Martín 1998, 56) and general severe cognitive impairment (the brain weight is considerably reduced). The frontal and parietal bones recede, the occipital bone is flattened, and the cranial capacity is reduced to less than 1000 cc (as opposed to the usual 1200–1850 cc), with a circumference of less than 46 cm. In addition, the cranial sutures fuse earlier than normal and the face is larger compared to the rest of the head (Aufderheide and Rodríguez-Martín 1998, 56). When using measurements to identify microcephaly, it is recommended that these measurements be compared to a suitable reference sample that is controlled for biological sex (Mank et al. 2023). Frequencies for microcephaly may be up to 1 in 2,000 births in populations with a restricted genetic pool (Barnes 1994, 158). It is a rarity in archaeology, and since Richard's review in 1985, limited new evidence for microcephaly has been identified, with the exception of the study by Mank et al. (2023), who identified microcephaly in three adult females from the nineteenth-century Meerenberg psychiatric hospital, in the Netherlands.

Cleft Palate

Cleft palate results from a failure of bone union of the two halves of the palate during fetal development and may be associated with a defect of the upper lip and bone beneath, called the cleft lip (Fig. 2.4a and b). Cleft lip and palate are among the most common birth anomalies resulting from environmental factors (Oner and Tastan 2020). The modern incidence of the two conditions combined is 0.45 in 1,000 live births, but of the cleft palate alone it is 0.33 per 1,000 live births globally (Salari et al. 2022b). The two problems of cleft palate/lip and of cleft palate alone are in fact somewhat distinct entities with different causative factors. Cleft palate, more common in females, has multifactorial causes but a strong family history suggests that it is predominantly genetic in origin (Barnes 1994, 175). The problem was probably as common in the past as it is today. Cleft lip frequency does not vary as much as cleft palate among populations (Barnes 1994, 174) and may be more related to environmental influences, such as exposure to tobacco smoke, rubella, or a lack of folic acid (Orkar et al. 2002). The severity of the defect in the palate will vary from a minor cleft, to a U-shaped deformity. Around 50% of children born with cleft palate are asymptomatic (Oner and Tastan 2020), but for a child with a severe defect, in which there is an open connection between the mouth and nasal cavities, sucking, and hence breastfeeding, is impossible. In the past, breastfeeding must surely have been the norm (Stuart-Macadam and Dettwyler 1995), and the mother would need to find an alternative way to feed her baby if it was to survive.

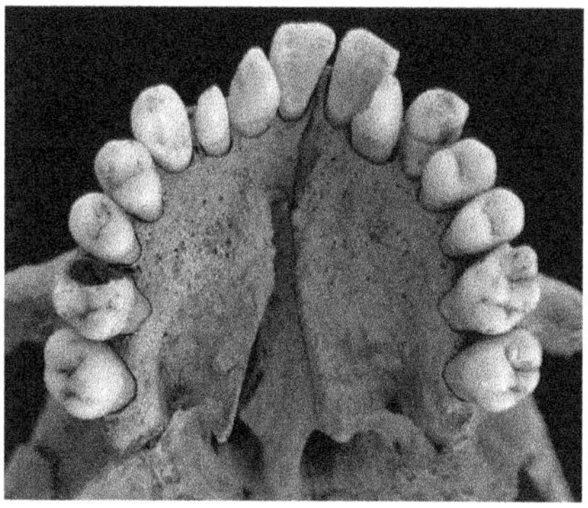

Figure 2.4a. Unilateral cleft palate in a male adolescent (16–18 years) from Dunajská Streda, Slovakia (postmedieval, seventeenth–eighteenth centuries CE). Photograph courtesy of Silva Bodoriková.

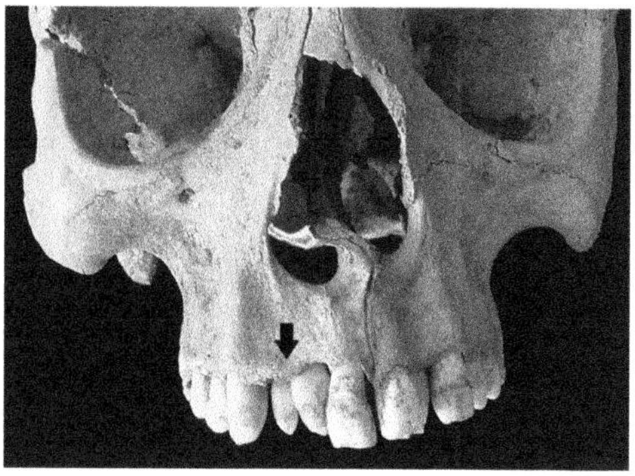

Figure 2.4b. Unilateral cleft lip in the same adolescent (16–18 years) from Dunajská Streda, Slovakia (postmedieval, seventeenth–eighteenth centuries CE). Photograph courtesy of Silva Bodoriková.

Today, neonates with severe cleft palate require very time-consuming and laborious spoon-feeding of maternally expressed milk or specialized artificial teat adaptation, and evidence for feeding bottles, which may have helped in this endeavor, have been found in the archaeological record (Drinkall and Foreman, 1998). Such care is accepted and can be provided today, but may have been unacceptable or impossible for earlier people, for example, in hunter-forager populations. Neonatal death of babies with cleft palate may therefore have been common in the distant past. In fact, in many developing societies (with a relatively low level of economic and technological development) today and in the past, affected neonates, including those with manifest cleft palate and cleft lip, may have been subject to infanticide (or at least, no effort was made to ensure their survival). Liston and Rotroff (2013) identified cleft palate in a number of infants found within a well at the Athenian Agora, suggesting that their poor prospects for survival, whether due to problems with feeding or the associated stigma, singled them out for this treatment. People with cleft lip can appear outwardly disfigured, even with modern treatment, and have difficulties in the clarity of speech as a result of the open communication between the oral and nasal cavities, which prevents the normal pronunciation of consonants; this may have meant people were stigmatized or ostracized. There are also instances, such as those recorded in early medieval England and ancient China, where surgical correction of a cleft lip was undertaken to help these individuals (Kesling 2020 and Ma 2000, respectively).

Poor preservation of the fragile bones of the maxilla can make the diagnosis of cleft palate challenging, and in some cases minor anomalies can go unnoticed unless accompanied by dental anomalies or other skeletal anomalies such as cleft vertebrae. Despite such difficulties, several examples of cleft palate/lip in children have been identified in the archaeological record, within normal burial contexts (Lewis 2018:38; Bodoriková et al. 2022). Significantly, severe defects have been identified in adults—demonstrating the desire and ability of communities to feed them as babies. Individuals with crania exhibiting both cleft palate and cleft lip have been excavated in California and dated to 2000–4000 BCE (Brooks and Hohenthal 1963). These

Native American individuals were between the ages of 25 and 35 years at death. Another example of both palatal and lip deformities comes from England in an eleventh- to twelfth-century 40–50-year-old male (Anderson 1994). The cleft lip made his face asymmetrical, but his survival into adulthood indicates he may have been accepted within his social group and was not differentially treated after death. Spinek et al. (2023) reported bilateral cleft palate in a 50-plus-year-old male from eighteenth-century Krakow, Poland, who had been fitted with a palatal prosthesis, shaped to fit the opening. These examples show that, perhaps contrary to certain influential theories (Ariès 1962), parental devotion to infant rearing is not a phenomenon of modern times; this was also an ethic of the past.

Hydrocephalus

Of all the anomalies of development affecting people, few are more dramatic in their presentation than hydrocephalus. Literally, *hydrocephalus* means "water on the brain," but in strict terms, it is applied to the condition where there is an enlargement of the normal fluid-containing spaces within the brain substance associated with increased pressure due to accumulation of cerebrospinal fluid (Johanson et al. 2008). Cerebrospinal fluid formation and resorption in the brain is a dynamic continuum. If this function is disrupted and the fluid is produced but not resorbed, then pressure-induced atrophy of the cerebral cortex occurs, with consequent motor and sensory loss causing blindness and paralysis. This may be an acutely developing and life-threatening change. In the infant, the buildup of fluid results in cranial enlargement with characteristic skeletal manifestations. In the twenty-first century, the sequence of hydrocephalic development may be arrested or prevented by surgical intervention and drainage of cerebrospinal fluid into the jugular vein. Such a facility was clearly not available to the hydrocephalic child of antiquity, the majority of whom would not have survived, and the paleopathological evidence has been lost.

The usual clinical presentation is of a rapidly enlarging head in infancy or childhood, and this can be recognized in archaeological skeletons. The condition can arise as a congenital anomaly, in which case the unborn fetus itself has a large head (0.48–0.81 per 1,000 live births), and may be caused by inflammation as the result of rubella or mumps, or the presence of spina bifida, a tumor, or trauma (McAllister 2012). Because of the enlargement of the unborn child's head, congenital hydrocephalus was probably not compatible with fetal or maternal survival in antiquity. This would likely have resulted in obstructed labor, which was a fatal problem of past childbirth. Notwithstanding varied evidence for Caesarean sections dating as far back as 1795 BCE (Lurie and Glezerman 2003), safe Caesarean section is a relatively modern concept. Today, hydrocephalus is normally the result of an acquired viral infection that occurs in the first six months of life (Persson et al. 2005). Bacterial infections, today cured using antibiotics, may still result in hydrocephalus, but in antiquity, they were probably fatal before hydrocephalus developed. In rare cases, a slowly growing tumor within the skull can provoke it.

The diagnosis of hydrocephalus in archaeological contexts rests upon the recognition of skull enlargement (Fig. 2.5a–c), with subsequent widening of the cranial sutures, numerous sutural bones, and a flattened cranial base (Murphy 1996), and upon the anatomical configuration of the facial and cranial skeleton (Richards and Anton 1991). Hydrocephalus developing in later childhood may not result in appreciable enlargement of the head once the fontanelles and frontal sutures have fused, making it unlikely to be identified (Kinsman and Johnson 2016). Therefore, examples of paleopathological interest probably had their origin within the first six months of life. Survival of such children, many of whom must surely have had physical impairments, possibly indicates a caring community in the society of antiquity. In addition, if the child was mentally impaired, the care and attention demanded of the parent or social group might have been considerable. In these same individuals, the disease progression may have been arrested and not ended in death. In a study published just as surgical shunts were becoming available, Laurence (1958) noted that the condition becomes arrested in 46% of individuals, usually when they are between the ages of 9 months and 2 years; a similar situation may have existed in antiquity.

In paleopathological records hydrocephalus is rare, but Richards and Anton (1991) indicated that about thirty possible examples had been identified, mainly from Europe and dating from 10,000 BCE to 1670 CE (Richards and Anton 1991; Murphy 1996). Eleven of these are found in children (Lewis 2018, 27). The earliest individual recorded in Britain is of Romano-British date, and is of an adult with a cranial capacity of 2,600 cm^3 compared with the normal capacity of about 1,500 cm^3 (Trevor 1950). The condition in both an English early medieval adolescent of the sixth century CE, aged 14–16 years (Manchester, 1980), and a medieval adolescent of 16–18 years from Westerhus, Sweden (Gejvall 1960), was probably caused by an intracranial tumor. A young adult Egyptian male from the Roman period had asymmetry of the limbs suggestive of paralysis associated with his hydrocephalus (Derry 1913). More recent examples include a 4–5-year-old child from Iron Age Aymyrlyg, southern Siberia (Murphy 2000), a fourteenth–eighteenth-century 1–2-year-old from Žumberak, Croatia (Bedić et al. 2019), and a 3-year-old child from Middle Paleolithic Qafzeh, Israel (Tillier et al. 2001).

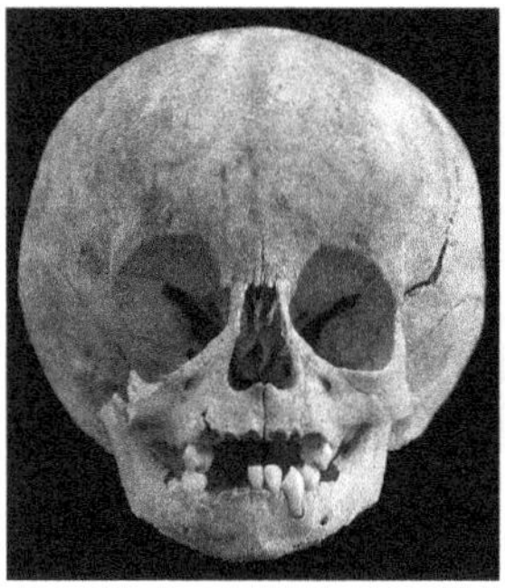

Figure 2.5a. Hydrocephalus in a 1.5–2.0-year-old from early modern Žumberek, Croatia, showing the frontal aspect. Photograph courtesy of Mario Šlaus.

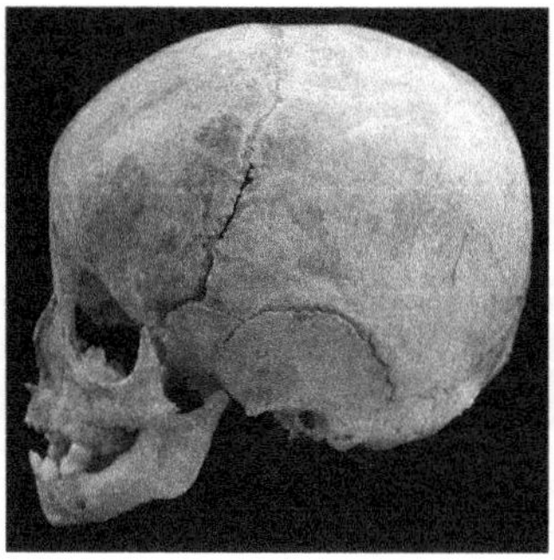

Figure 2.5b. Hydrocephalus in a 1.5–2.0-year-old from early modern Žumberek, Croatia, showing left lateral aspect. Photograph courtesy of Mario Šlaus.

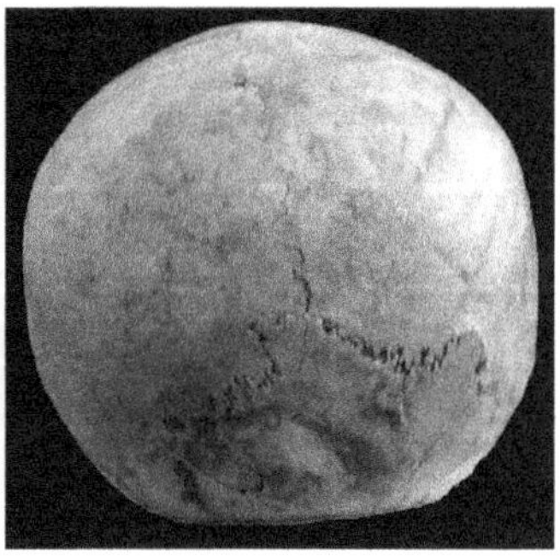

Figure 2.5c. Hydrocephalus in a 1.5–2.0-year-old from early modern Žumberek, Croatia, showing the posterior aspect. Photograph courtesy of Mario Šlaus.

Anomalies in Cranial Suture Development

The cranial sutures may also be subject to problems in normal development; this might include lack of a suture or premature closure of sutures (Fig. 2.6a and b). The former is usually termed sutural agenesis, and a genetic basis for its occurrence is under study (Stanton et al. 2022; Yapijakis et al. 2023). Premature suture fusion, or craniosynostosis, can cause an abnormal cranial shape, or craniostenosis (Cohen 2005). The changes may impact cerebral morphology resulting in cognitive, visual, and other neurological problems (Dalmas et al. 2020). While around 259 genetic conditions and syndromes have been associated with premature suture fusion (Oostra et al. 2005), in a third of individuals with premature suture closure the etiology is known, and may occur as the result of hyperthyroidism, vitamin D deficiency, birth trauma, intrauterine infection, Hurler's skeletal dysplasia, genetic anemia, and infant head binding (Khanna et al. 2011). Early fusion, most often of the sagittal suture, leads to changes in the shape of the skull, with the resulting shape depending on which sutures are affected and the age at which fusion occurs (Cohen 2005). Despite normally fusing between the ages of 20–30 years, Bolk (1915) noted that premature fusion of the sagittal suture after the age of 6 years did not cause a change in cranial morphology. A number of reports of people with agenesis and premature fusion of sutures have appeared in the paleopathological literature, several of which are summarized in Barnes 1994.

Spina Bifida

Spina bifida is probably the most common developmental defect to be reported during pregnancy, and it is estimated to have occurred in 5.05 per 10,000 births in the European Union between 2005 and 2022 (European Commission 2024). This "neural tube defect" varies in frequency worldwide, and is highest in low- and middle-income countries, with mandatory folic acid for some pregnant women changing global distribution patterns. Males are more frequently affected than females generally, and genetic and environmental factors are potential causes—for example, deficiencies in maternal folic acid, vitamin B_{12}, zinc, and selenium while the fetus

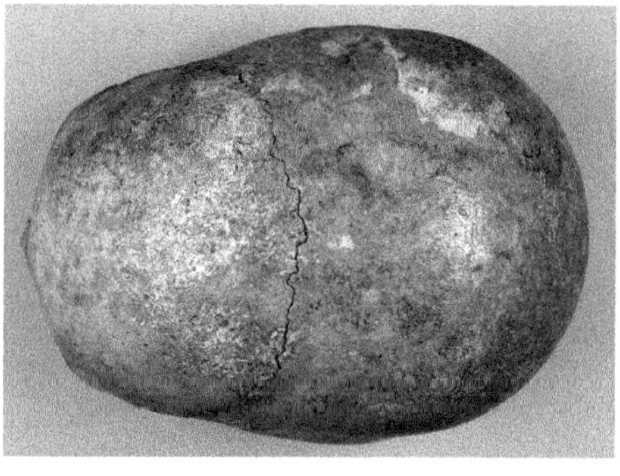

Figure 2.6a. Superior view of a cranium with premature closure of the sagittal suture. Photograph by and with kind permission from Jeff Veitch.

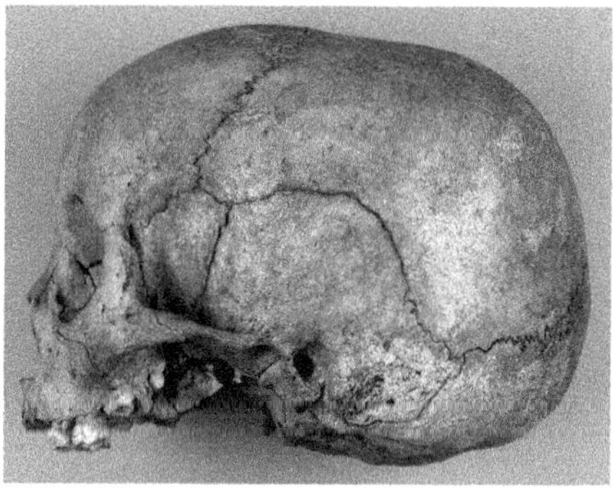

Figure 2.6b. Lateral view of the same cranium. Photograph by and with kind permission from Jeff Veitch.

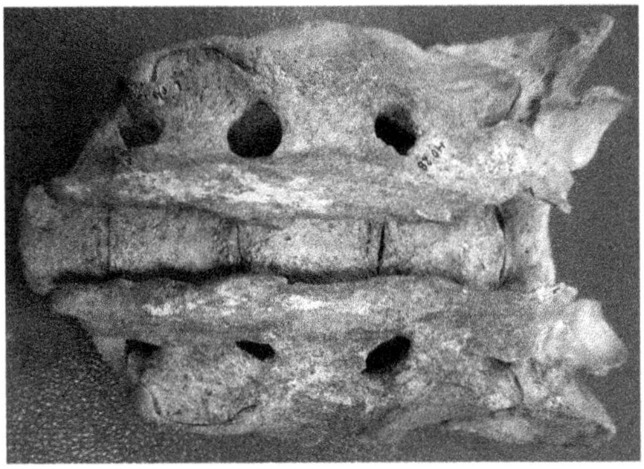

Figure 2.7. Spina bifida occulta showing open posterior sacrum in an adult from early medieval Addingham (sixth–eighth century CE, England, UK). Right is the proximal end. Photograph by and courtesy of Jean Brown.

is developing. Although global distribution patterns are changing, low consumption of fortified foods, poverty, and exposure to chemicals such as arsenic have limited folic acid's protective effect (Koch et al. 2024). In the archaeological record, it is the occulta, rather than cystica, type that is described most frequently. Spina bifida occulta refers to the incomplete fusion of the posterior neural arches of the vertebral column, mainly in the sacral segments and/or lumbar vertebrae (Fig. 2.7). No structures such as the central nervous system, meninges, spinal nerves, or cerebrospinal fluid protrude out through the space and, thus, no complications such as infection of spinal canal structures or peripheral motor or sensory function loss occur. *Occulta* means hidden, and this condition is usually not detected in a living person because of the lack of external signs or symptoms, although it may be identified on a radiograph of the spine. Absent or underdeveloped neural arches of the first, fourth, and fifth sacral vertebrae may be normal for a particular person or population, and this finding must not be confused with pathologically induced spina bifida affecting the whole sacrum. To be able to compare population frequencies, an accepted standardized recording system should be used.

The more severe form is spina bifida cystica, which is often fatal in early life. Aufderheide and Rodríguez-Martín (1998, 61) describe three forms of severity: meningocele, myelomeningocele, and myelocele. The first involves protrusion of the nerve roots and meninges through the osseous defect, with the spinal cord and issuing spinal nerves remaining in the vertebral canal, but the osseous deficiency is covered by skin. The second (in 60% of individuals) involves the added protrusion of the spinal cord through the defect without a normal skin covering. In the third (and most severe) the skin and meninges fail to close at the defect; subsequent infection leads to death. Evidence of spina bifida cystica with meningomyeocele is likely only to be identified through careful examination of the unfused neural arches of perinatal and infant skeletons, which may be widened and curved outward due to pressure from the fluid-filled sac (Barnes 1994, 49). In older children, paralysis, an underdeveloped pelvis, hydrocephalus, or scoliosis may be evident as secondary complications (Ortner 2003). Dickel and Doran (1989) described a 14–16-year-old individual with spina bifida cystica buried in early archaic (6000–5000 BCE) Florida, having open neural arches from the third lumbar vertebra to the second sacral vertebra, and subsequent disuse atrophy of the long bones, which may represent resulting paralysis. Another example from Peru is of a 6-year-old child, also with spina bifida affecting the lumbar and sacral vertebrae, whose spine included an extra sixth lumbar vertebra (Castro de la Mata and

Bonevia 1980). More data are available for spina bifida occulta. For example, reports from three sites in early medieval Britain described absolute but variable frequencies of spina bifida occulta (percentage of sacra affected) ranging from 2.7% to 8.7% (Brothwell and Powers 1968; Roberts and Cox 2003).

Lumbarization and Sacralization

Lumbarization and sacralization occur in the spine as a result of what is termed upward or downward "border shifting" due to an error in genetic signaling (Barnes 2012). The affected vertebra takes on the features of the adjacent vertebra in the neighboring region. If the shift is upward, then it is called a cranial shift, or sacralization, and the fifth lumbar vertebra takes on the morphology of the first sacral vertebra. If the shift is downward, it is caudal, or lumbarization, and the first sacral vertebra looks like a fifth lumbar vertebra. Identifying these conditions can be difficult if the complete spine is not preserved (often the case in an archaeological context), or if the sacrum is still unfused (i.e., before around 12 years of age). In 1995, López-Durán reported that 3–5% of the population were affected by shifting at the lumbosacral border and that two-thirds were sacralizations (Fig. 2.8). Both conditions have been reported in the paleopathological literature (Roberts and Cox 2003; Barnes 2012). It is unlikely that these anatomical skeletal shifts had any symptomatic sequalae.

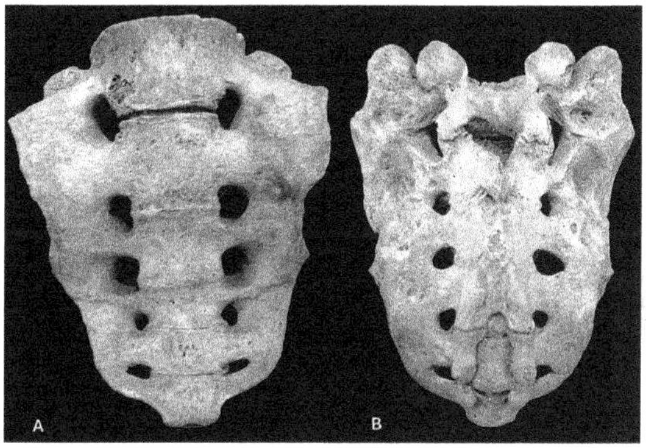

Figure 2.8. Sacralization of the fifth lumbar vertebra in an adult male from early medieval Oxford, England, seen from the anterior (A) and posterior (B) aspect. Photograph courtesy of Ceri Falys and Thames Valley Archaeological Services.

Spondylolysis

The lower parts of the spine are also the site of another, possibly developmentally related, anomaly, spondylolysis. This defect to some extent bridges the gap between congenital and acquired anomalies. In the bony union of parts of a vertebra early in life, bone development may be dysplastic, and the pars interarticularis of the posterior vertebral arch may fracture due to the continual stresses and strains of an upright posture. Spondylolysis is recognized in skeletal remains as a separate and seemingly ununited posterior part of a vertebra. In most instances the defect does not create symptoms. Occasionally, however, it creates sufficient instability of the spine to allow one vertebra to move anteriorly in anatomical alignment upon its neighbor, compressing the spinal cord and the nerves issuing from it, with resultant neuropathic symptoms of the lower limbs, as well as bladder and bowel impairment.

This dislocation, known as spondylolisthesis, is sometimes recognized in skeletal remains (see Chapter 4 for further discussion on spondylolysis).

Appendicular Skeleton

Congenital Dislocation of the Hip and Congenital Hip Dysplasia

In modern medical practice the congenital diseases of anencephaly and spina bifida cystica are readily apparent. In the former, the lesion is totally untreatable, and in the latter the lesion is sometimes treatable, allowing survival of the affected infant. In past societies, both lesions would have been obvious at birth. There is also a developmental condition with genetic risk factors that, with modern knowledge, is both diagnosable and curable shortly after birth. The problem is that of congenital acetabular dysplasia, indicating that the problem occurs in the womb, during the development of the acetabulum of the hip joint (Resnick et al. 2024, 1135). Congenital dislocation of the hip (CDH) may occur at birth, either as a result of this anomaly or due to trauma incurred during the birth process (Davidson et al. 2008). In past societies these problems became apparent only when the child started to walk, by which time treatment, had it been available, would have been ineffective. The recurrent dislocation of the joint during weight-bearing provokes a characteristic swaying gait and predisposes those with the condition to the early development of degenerative arthritis in the hip joint. In the archaeological record, the condition is recognized usually when a falst joint (or pseudoarthrosis) has been created to accommodate the misplaced femoral head, while the original socket (acetabulum) becomes very shallow and triangular in shape. The femoral head can also be flattened. Figure 2.9 shows the same condition in a developing child—where subtle changes above the articular surface and to the shape of the femoral head are also evident. The dysplastic form of the condition has a genetic predisposition, with a modern incidence in 10–20 of 1,000 live births; it is more common in females. The condition can affect both hips or a single side in equal measure (Eng et al. 2009; Tao et al. 2023). There is marked geographical variation in incidence today, perhaps indicating both genetic and environmental factors are responsible. Dislocation during the birth process is associated with 30% of breech delivered babies (Resnick et al.

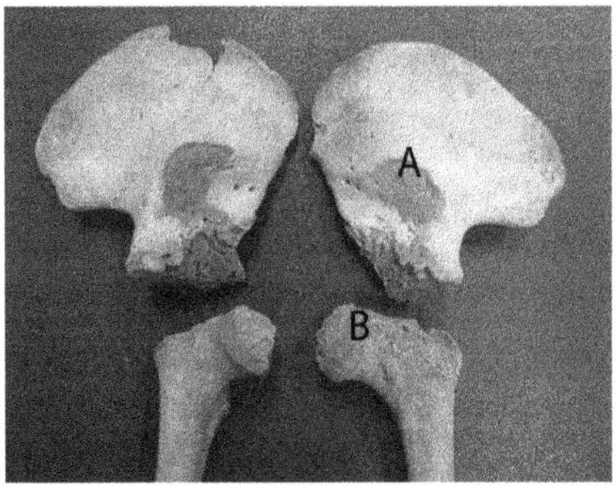

Figure 2.9. Congenital dislocation of the hip in a 6–7-year-old from Fishergate House, York, England (1120–1360 CE). Note the enlargement of the left femoral head (B) and development of false joints (pseudarthroses) on the ilia (A) above the original acetabulae that have not developed normally. Photograph by Charlotte Roberts.

2024, 1135). Today, immediate postpartum checks of the neonate normally identify and rectify the problem without further problems for the child.

Clearly with such an unusual gait, and with such severe arthritis, an individual may have been unable to efficiently do any activity that involved walking, and may also have had constant incapacitating pain. Their role in society in the past, particularly in those societies dependent for their existence on hunting and foraging, may have been restricted. There is, however, an example of bilateral CDH, with severe osteoarthritis of the hip joints, in the skeleton of an adult male who was a member of the Royalist Garrison in seventeenth-century Sandal Castle, Wakefield, England. His condition was compatible with an active military role, but whether it was combatant or supportive is not known (Manchester 1978). The condition has been recognized in skeletons from many periods from both the Old and New Worlds (Roberts and Cox 2003; Aufderheide and Rodríguez-Martín 1998). Mitchell and Redfern (2008) have provided a classification system for recognizing the condition. The youngest individual with possible hip dysplasia is a six-month-old from medieval rural Wharram Percy, England, where an abnormally shallow acetabulum on the unfused ilium suggests dislocation would have occurred when the child began to crawl (Mays 2007a,186).

Club Foot

A less common condition in paleopathology is club foot, or *talipes equinovarus*. The most numerous and perhaps visually convincing evidence for this condition in the past is in pictorial sources from Egypt, in which the classically inverted feet of this condition are admirably demonstrated in drawings (Dasen 1988). The modern incidence is 1 in 1,000 live births, and it is more common in males. Nearly 25% of individuals affected have a blood relative with a club foot, while a higher percentage occurs in identical twins. This suggests a strong genetic component, although the exact genetic factors behind this pattern are still unknown (Dobbs and Gurnett 2009). In 43–50% of occurrences, club foot occurs with additional congenital anomalies, and other nongenetic etiologies range from vascular or muscular deficiencies to unusual fetal foot placing (Dobbs and Gurnett 2009). Brothwell (1967a) detailed the skeletal changes that may be expected, by reconstructing the bones of the affected foot and ankle in comparison with the unaffected side, and highlighting the consequences of such a condition (e.g., lack of use of the leg and disuse atrophy, and even the use of crutches to move around). Club foot is a progressive deformity, and changes are the result of years of walking on affected feet, perhaps explaining why all the evidence reported in the paleopathological literature is in adults (Mann and Owsley 1989; Owsley and Mann 1990; Curto and Fernandes 2022). The earliest dated examples of (bilateral) club foot are in individuals from the ancient Maya city of Tikal, Guatemala (Wright 2011), and Bronze Age Thailand (Domett et al. 2022). In Britain, the earliest individuals with club foot have only one foot affected and are from Neolithic Nether Swell (Brothwell 1967a) and fourth-century CE Kingsholm, Gloucester (Roberts et al. 2004). The latter revealed atrophy (wasting) of the left leg bones and disruption to the articular facets of the talus indicative of limited use of the limb and a misplaced foot. The changes to this individual were reassessed in 2017

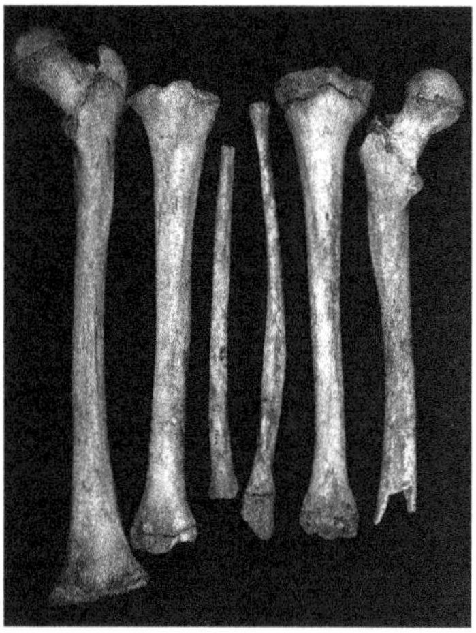

Figure 2.10a. Club foot evident in an adolescent individual from Kingsholm, Gloucester, England (Romano-British fourth century CE). Affected left lower leg bones (right) compared to normal right side (left), showing a mediolaterally flattened fibula and more slender femur. Photograph by and courtesy of Jean Brown.

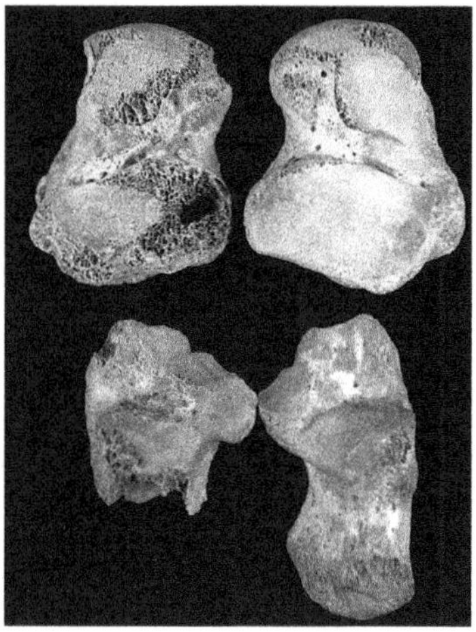

Figure 2.10b. Club foot evident in an adolescent individual from Kingsholm, Gloucester, England (Romano-British fourth century CE). Comparison of the normal right side with affected left talus (top) and calcaneus (bottom) showing changes to the articular surfaces. Photograph by and courtesy of Jean Brown.

by Castells Navarro et al., who argued that this was a case of acquired (rather than congenital) club foot as the result of post-polio syndrome, which caused the leg to be permanently paralyzed (Fig. 2.10a and b). Just as with congenital dislocation of the hip, the main problem of having a club foot is its effect on the ability to walk, and no doubt the same restriction of activity would have applied.

Other, more rare developmental problems of the appendicular skeleton have also been reported in the paleopathological literature—for example, polydactyly, or the congenital duplication of one or more toes or fingers (Murphy 1999; Case et al. 2006), congenital absence of the patella (Patrick and Waldron 2003), radio-ulnar synostosis (Lorrio 2010), Madelung's deformity of the radius (Anderson and Carter 1995), and arthrogryposis multiplex, where muscles are stiff and weak, causing joint contractures (Anderson and Thomas 1997).

Syndromes

Achondroplasia

Skeletons representing people of shorter stature than the norm for their population are generally rare in the paleopathological record, although there are many types of dwarfism (to use the accepted medical term) described in the clinical literature. In Britain, for example, from the prehistoric to postmedieval periods only five such skeletons were identified (Roberts and Cox 2003). These individuals had either proportionate dwarfism, where the body is short but the limbs are in proportion, or disproportionate dwarfism, where only some parts of the body experience restricted growth.

The most common form of clinically short stature, achondroplasia, is genetically based and follows simple dominant inheritance, but it most commonly develops as the result of a gene aberration, with 80% occurring from a de novo germ cell mutation linked to advanced paternal age. The worldwide pooled prevalence of the condition is 4.6 in 1,000,000 live births, making it a rare condition today (Foreman et al. 2020). The problem arises in the process of ossification, or bone formation, in the skeletal precursors of the fetus. Ossification takes place by two different methods: *intramembranous ossification* governing the formation of the bones of the skull vault, the face, and the clavicle; the remaining bones of the skeleton develop by *intracartilaginous ossification*. In achondroplasia, the first method progresses normally whereas the second is faulty. Hence the skull vault, face, and clavicle develop as usual, although the nasal area is depressed. The remainder of the skeleton—that is, the limbs—are shortened, with achieved adult stature usually less than 140 cm (Aufderheide and Rodríguez-Martín 1998, 360). Consequently, the characteristic small stature and short-limbed appearance of a person with achondroplasia is recognizable even from artwork of antiquity (Enderle et al. 1994). More than any other developmental anomaly of the past, achondroplasia is portrayed in statuettes and tomb illustrations. The role of the achondroplastic individual in society seems to have achieved prominence. For example, the Egyptian gods Phtha and probably Bes, are depicted with the short limbs of dwarfism. The Roman emperors Tiberius and Alexander Severus (and also Mark Antony) retained individuals with achondroplasia as counselors (Johnston 1963), and the little figure named in the Bayeux tapestry as Turold, clearly held a position of importance in the entourage of Duke William of Normandy (Lewis et al. 2011). Their role as "objects of interest" in the medieval period is shown by the record of a gift of nine "dwarfs" to Charles IX of France from the king of Poland. Precisely why honors and roles such as Egyptian deification, Roman Imperial advisers, or medieval court entertainers should be bestowed upon those with this condition is difficult to understand and is an object of historical inquiry (Findlen 1996; Fleming 2011; Spinks 2015).

There is skeletal evidence of dwarfism from both the Old and New Worlds. The earliest recorded skeletal example is an adolescent from Romito, Italy, and of late Upper Paleolithic date (Frayer et al. 1987). What social role the individual played can only be wondered at, because they were buried in a seeming embrace with an adult female. Typical shortened limb bones and characteristic skull shapes have been described in remains from Predynastic Egypt and from the Dynastic tombs of King Zer and King Mersekha (Brothwell and Powers 1968), as well as in North America and medieval Poland (Gladykowska-Rzeczycka 1980; Snow 1943). Other examples are described by Ortner (2003) and include a child from Belle Glade, Florida, United States, dating from 1000 BCE. The youngest individual identified with achondroplasia is an 18–24-month-old from early medieval Wales, United Kingdom (Sables 2010). An example of particular note is from a known wealthy Dutch family from nineteenth-century Middenbeemster. The mother, and possibly her adult son and 10-year-old daughter, displayed different expressions of achondroplasia-like dwarfism (Waters-Rist and Hoogland 2013). In 2017, Boer and colleagues advanced our potential to use paleogenetics to understand rare diseases when they extracted aDNA from an individual with achondroplasia (180 years old) curated at a museum in Amsterdam, and identified the G1138A mutation of the fibroblast growth receptor gene (*FGFR3*) believed to occur in 97% of people with the condition. Such advances may make it possible in the future to confirm less clear examples of these conditions in the archaeological record.

Osteogenesis Imperfecta

A similarly generalized, genetically determined anomaly of connective tissue is osteogenesis imperfecta, or "brittle bone disease." It is a condition of great rarity today, and the evidence from the past consists of four archaeological skeletons. As its name suggests, the disease is the result of the inadequate formation of bone collagen (protein), but it also affects the dentine of the teeth, skin, and ligaments (Resnick et al. 2024, 1157–1161; and see Figure 2.11). The bones are, in consequence, brittle and distorted. Their fragility leads to frequent and multiple fractures sometimes occurring during the birth process. There are four main types of the disease recognized today (and many subtypes within these). In the mild form (type I), people will be unaware of it until they break a bone (Glorieux et al. 2002; Basal and Steiner 2009). Type I is the most common form, seen in between 1:15,000 to 1:20,000 births today. Type II is a lethal form causing death of the perinate, while types III and IV are the severe but nonlethal and moderately severe forms, respectively (Chhabra et al. 2023). Although today the afflicted individual can be nurtured into adulthood, this may have been rare in the past. Death from fractures

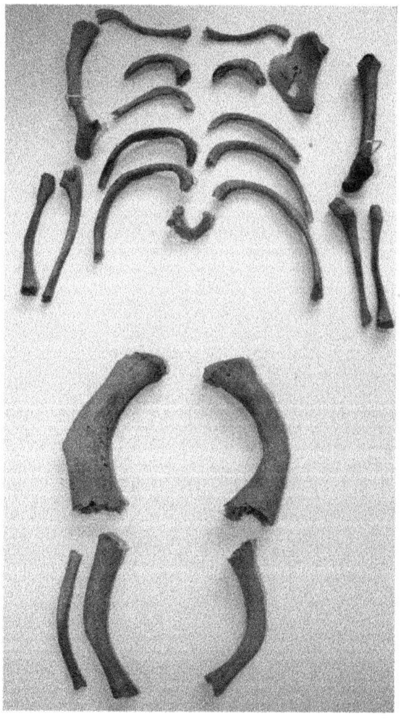

Figure 2.11. Possible osteogenesis imperfecta in a 2-year-old from Speos Artemidos, Beni Hassan, Egypt (1000 BCE). The left distal humerus displays a healed fracture while the femora are bowed and osteopenic. Photographs taken with kind permission from Daniel Antoine and the Trustees of the British Museum.

and their complications must have been the pattern in early childhood, as is indicated by the Egyptian 2-year-old suggested to have the condition in the XXI Dynasty, around 1000 BCE (Gray 1969). The skeletal preservation of this child is remarkable, displaying an occipital bone made up almost entirely of a complex series of cranial ossicles (Fig. 2.12), marked anterolateral bowing of the long bones, with disproportionately thickened femora and osteopenia. Fractures are evident in the ribs, spine, and humeri (Lewis 2018, 61). A younger and more recent example of osteogenesis imperfecta in a perinate was identified by Cope and Dupras (2011) from the Roman Dakhleh Oasis, while a single bone from early medieval England (seventh century CE) has been described—although the evidence rests only on the fractured and distorted femur of an older individual (Wells 1965). The relationship between osteogenesis imperfecta and an inherited autosomal recessive gene in the offspring of consanguineous marriages (Stephen et al. 2015) makes it tempting to hypothesize that the affected children from Egypt (high status and Roman) were the result of such practices, which were sanctioned at the time.

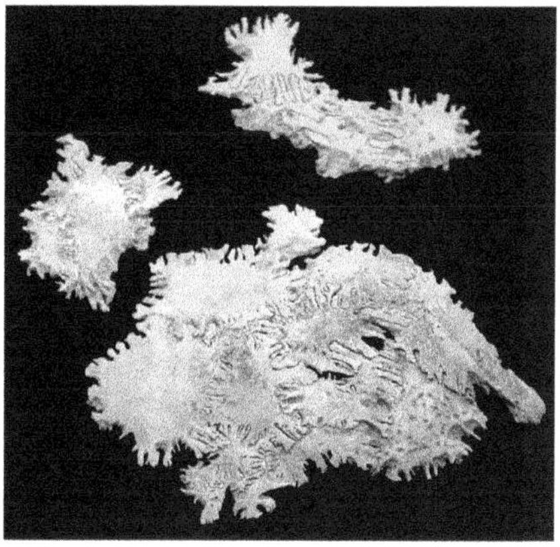
Figure 2.12. Possible osteogenesis imperfecta in a 2-year-old from Speos Artemidos, Beni Hassan, Egypt (1000 BCE). The occipital comprises multiple small ossicles. Photographs taken with kind permission from Daniel Antoine and the Trustees of the British Museum.

Trisomy 21

Trisomy 21, first named after Langston Down, who studied the condition, falls under the trisomy group of congenital conditions, in which a person has three chromosomes rather than the usual pair, or an additional chromosome 21. Trisomy 21 is one of the most common congenital conditions today, present in 1 in every 800 live births (Patton 2008), although this frequency is not reflected in the archaeological record. The condition is characterized by a spectrum of cognitive and physical changes, including short stature and distinctive facial features. The skeletal features are principally of the skull and consist of a relative shortening of skull length associated with some flattening at the back of the cranium and of the nose. These features, together with a deficient growth of the base of the cranium and the facial skeleton, give rise to an overall reduction in the capacity of the skull. Growth rates are slowed in adolescence, and the distal segments of long bones have growth deficiency. The individual may experience delay in walking and talking, as well as cognitive impairment (Cronk 1993, 685). Individuals affected may also suffer infections, congenital heart anomalies, and acute leukemia. Skeletally, they are of short stature and can have hip dislocation. There may also be a variety of dental anomalies, including dental fusion and, more commonly, agenesis of the lateral incisors (Reuland-Bosma and van Dijk 1986).

Trisomy 21 has been described in at least four individuals from archaeological contexts, and all but one of these are children. The earliest to be described is from tenth–eleventh century CE Breedon-on-the-Hill in Leicestershire, England. This child was about 9 years of age, and may have been cared for by members of the monastery connected to the site (Brothwell 1960). An adult from the late Hallstatt period (350 BCE) Taubischofscheim, Germany, has skeletal changes similar to the child from Breedon-on-the-Hill (Czarnetski 1980). Charlier (2008) suggested trisomy 21 as a diagnosis for a 13–14-year-old adolescent from late Bronze Age Rome (1200–850 BCE), and Rivolatt et al. (2014) described the features of trisomy 21 in a 5–7-year-old from fifth–sixth century France. Most recently, almost by accident, Cassidy et al. (2020) identified trisomy 21 through genetic analysis of a male infant from Neolithic Ireland, the oldest known evidence to date. The child had been breastfed, hinting at their level of acceptance into the community, or at least by their mother. Although a child with trisomy 21 may be born to any mother, it is much more common in women who give birth when they are over the age of 40—a frequency of up to 1 in 25 births (Patton 2008). Starbuck (2011) identified eight possible depictions of children with trisomy 21 in paintings dating from 1455 CE, and also described it in ancient figurines and pottery dating from 1500 BCE to 1500 CE. The general paucity of evidence for this condition in the archaeological record has been caused by the difficulty in diagnosing such a myriad of skeletal and dental changes, and it is possible that older women were less likely to survive childbearing in the past. However, things might be about to change. A remarkable study that, for the first time, used aDNA analysis to screen for trisomy 21 in 9,855 individuals from prehistoric and historic sites across the world, identified six individuals with the condition—all in infants and perinates—and one with trisomy 18 (Edwards syndrome). Although the presence of this congenital condition in perinates may suggest such children were "disposed of" at birth, their careful burial suggests that, just as with the other cases of trisomy 21 in the archaeological record, these children were cared for in death as they were in life and accepted as members of the community (Rohrlach et al. 2024). This study provided an opportunity to assess osteological markers for trisomy 21 in these tiny remains, but no clear skeletal signatures were found. The results confirmed the presence of trisomy 21 from fifth–sixth century France and that the prevalence of the condition in the past was similar to that of today.

Epilogue

In this outline of the paleopathology of congenital and developmental conditions, only the most common or dramatic and significant anomalies have been discussed. The less significant anomalies and the variety of skeletal features, which may be counted as normal variations, have been omitted. The conditions discussed were doubtless of grave significance to those affected and to their communities, but they perhaps illustrate the care and tolerance shown by communities to those less fortunate living in the past. The recognition of developmental anomalies in skeletal remains can be challenging—especially in non-adult remains where unfused elements can hide morphological changes—but population-based studies and advances in aDNA analysis have the potential to inform modern discourses on the role of social inequality, poor nutrition, and environmental pollution on their causes and prevention.

3

Dental Disease

> No structures of the human body are more likely to disintegrate during life than teeth, yet after death none have greater tenacity against decay.
>
> —C. Wells, *Bones, Bodies, and Disease*

The mouth, or oral cavity, forms part of the digestive tract and contains the tongue, teeth, and gums (gingiva). The teeth, gums, and underlying jaw bones may all be separately or concurrently affected by dental disease. Teeth are the hardest and most chemically stable tissues in the body because they are mainly composed of mineral; they are much stronger than bone and can sometimes be the only part of the body that survives the burial environment. Their use in documenting human evolution over thousands of years testifies to their long-term preservation (Jheon et al. 2013). This is very fortunate for bioarchaeology as, "despite their small size, they [teeth] are a densely packed record of our lives" (Ullinger and Loewen 2023, 36). Not only do they have the potential to provide information about diet, dental health, oral hygiene, and dentistry, but they also may reveal evidence for childhood growth disruption or physiological stress (enamel hypoplasia), a person's occupation (using the teeth as a tool), culturally related behaviors such as tooth ablation or pipe smoking, and subsistence economy (e.g., dental disease in relation to farming domesticated cereal crops). The mouth functions primarily as a food processor, taking in food to be chewed, mixed with saliva to moisten and lubricate it, and moved around the mouth prior to swallowing it (Wilson 1995, 171–172). Food type determines the microorganisms present in the mouth (the oral microbiome), and the condition of a person's teeth can reflect the types and composition of the food to which they have been exposed. The oral cavity also produces sound and is important in respiration and heat and fluid regulation, among other functions.

In recent years, the medical profession and bioarchaeologists have come to better appreciate the diverse communities of microorganisms that live within the mouth and make up the oral microbiome (Warinner et al. 2014; Deo and Deshmukh 2019). This array of organisms was first noted by Dutch microbiologist Anthonie van Leeuwenhoek when observing dental plaque in the seventeenth century (He and Shi 2009), although their role in the cause of disease and caries was not yet established.

Bioarchaeologists and others have embraced this knowledge and applied it to the analysis of dental calculus (calcified plaque) from ancient skeletons and mummies, which has led to astounding discoveries (e.g., see Gancz et al. 2023: diversity in pre-industrialized microbiomes that helps us appreciate the origins of chronic noncommunicable disease today).

The composition of a person's oral microbiome has implications for oral and overall health. For example, periodontal disease, caries, lung and cardiovascular diseases, diabetes, and systemic inflammation can all be linked to organisms within the oral microbiome (Sharma et al. 2018; Sheikh 2020). In a meta-analysis of studies that have linked oral diseases with systemic noncommunicable diseases, twenty-eight were found to be associated with poor oral health, either as a result of the condition limiting oral self-care, or as a direct consequence of dental disease on a person's immune system (Botelho et al. 2022). These observations have endorsed the importance of incorporating dental care within general health care systems (Carstairs 2022, 150–153; Quiñonez et al. 2011). The paleopathological study of dental diseases is beginning to benefit from appreciating this link, even if many of the associated diseases are not readily identifiable in human remains. For example, dental pulp calcification/stones, identified using radiographs in the living, are associated with cardiovascular disease; they have also been found in the teeth of people from archaeological contexts (Tomczyk et al. 2014).

Dental disease is a common affliction of human and nonhuman populations today, in spite of the availability of dentists and, for humans, health education promoting more effective oral care to prevent dental problems. Nonetheless, this is not a global picture, and dental disease is more frequent in people who are disadvantaged. Not only is dental disease potentially life-threatening, but it can also provoke excruciating pain; dentists were among the first to promote the use of general anesthetics (Barnett 2017, 160–163; Bause 2009). In 2022, the World Health Organization (2022a) published the first report on the state of global oral health, finding that nearly half of the World's population was affected (3.5 billion), making it the most common noncommunicable disease today. Indeed, a number of the United Nations Sustainable Development Goals are particularly relevant to dental disease: (1) no poverty; (2) good health and well-being; and (10) reduced inequalities. In paleopathology, dental diseases and anomalies such as impacted "wisdom" teeth are, along with joint diseases, the most commonly occurring afflictions reported in ancient human remains. When integrated with other forms of evidence from an archaeological site, they provide valuable sources of information about both the lives of individuals and of wider populations (e.g., Seiler et al. 2013 and Klaus 2010, respectively). In this chapter we do not consider dental anomalies, notwithstanding that some anomalies, such as impacted wisdom teeth, may cause pain and could lead to suffering and even premature death. Research on dental diseases may involve evidence from macroscopic, microscopic, radiographic, and biomolecular analyses of teeth, as well as the use of supplementary information from art, historical documents, archaeology, and ethnography. Normal variations in dental morphology have also been used to explore relationships between populations (e.g., Scott and Pilloud 2019; Manabe et al. 2011), and ancient DNA (aDNA) analysis of teeth has been used to explore genetic ancestry (e.g., Silva et al. 2021), while isotope analysis of dental enamel has documented mobility histories of people in the past (e.g., Depaermentier et al. 2020) and helped to reconstruct past diet (Petersone-Gordina et al. 2020).

Dental disease is normally classified as either infectious (e.g., caries), degenerative (periodontal disease, calculus, tooth loss), or developmental (e.g., enamel hypoplasia, and lack of, or more than the expected, number of teeth). Caries are one of the most common diseases reported in past populations, and thanks to ever more sophisticated analytical techniques available to paleopathologists, dental calculus is becoming one of the most valuable sources of information that can be found in skeletons and mummified bodies, providing a range of evidence from dietary constituents to microorganisms and more. Of course, dental diseases rarely form in isolation and often have a complex relationship with other tissues. For example, a person could develop plaque deposits on their teeth, which can irritate the surrounding soft tissues (gingivitis) and underlying bone (periodontal disease), which, in turn, may lead to loss of alveolar bone and antemortem tooth loss.

Today, great emphasis is placed on taking care of our teeth; the use of toothpaste and dental floss and visiting a dentist are regular and consistent parts of many people's lives throughout their life course, but this varies globally. In the past, access to dental surgery and dental cleaning implements and substances, although evidently available to some individuals in some populations, was also not consistent across all populations and through time. Absence of evidence, however, is not proof of absence; methods used for dental care may result from no trace being left for a paleopathologist to find, or from the fact that these practices were never part of the people's culture. Essentially, a paleopathologist is recording a true reflection of the dental problems experienced by individuals, not dental problems that have been shaped by the practice of significant modern oral hygiene or dentistry interventions. What is observed is more a reflection of dietary components, a lack of care of the teeth, and the use of the teeth as tools.

Although teeth survive well in archaeological contexts, great care is needed when cleaning them and the jaws that contain them, once excavated. The mandible, or lower jaw, is more robust than the maxilla, or upper jaw, as the latter tends to suffer fragmentation during burial and/or excavation. Soil can become impacted in the nasal aperture, and the integrity of this part of the facial skeleton may be damaged. The single-rooted anterior teeth can become separated from the jaws during burial, excavation, or cleaning, although the multirooted teeth (e.g., the molars) are more stable in the jaws. Vigorous brushing of the teeth and jaws to clean them is not advised in an archaeological context; calcified plaque (calculus) can be dislodged and the fragile alveolar bone surrounding the teeth can become damaged.

Hillson (2023) provided details on tooth structure and the number and types of teeth expected in the deciduous (milk/primary) and permanent dentitions. As the dentition develops, a mixture of the two types of teeth appears until all the deciduous teeth are lost and replaced by the permanent teeth. The following sections discuss the types of dental diseases that occur most commonly in adults and children from archaeological contexts. We consider their etiology (cause), appearance, methods of recording, and examples of research. Some diseases affect both the bones and teeth (e.g., congenital syphilis), and dental signatures specific to these conditions will be outlined both here and in the relevant chapters. In some respects, the use of modern clinical observations as a base for interpretation is more appropriate for dental diseases than bone diseases. Dentists today can observe the tooth surfaces (just as in an archaeological situation), but can only indirectly visualize the surrounding bone through the use of imaging (radiography) or during surgery.

Dental Caries

Dental caries (Latin: *caries*, or rottenness) is one of the more frequently reported dental diseases in archaeological populations (Fig. 3.1). Caries first appears as opaque spots on the enamel surface, and it may progress to become an obvious cavity on the root or crown (Hillson 1986, 287). Now considered an infectious disease, caries results from fermentation of dietary sugars, especially sucrose, by bacteria in plaque, such as *Lactobacillus acidophilus* and *Streptococcus mutans* (see J.S. Zhang et al. 2022a on the dental microbiome and caries). Starches in the diet may also cause caries, but less frequently (Hancock et al. 2020). Progressive destruction of the tooth structure is initiated by microbial action on the tooth surface. If the correct combination of plaque bacteria and sucrose occurs, the resulting low pH acids (a by-product of fermentation) demineralize the teeth and leave cavities in their wake.

Caries can develop on any part of the tooth where food debris can accumulate. Most frequently, this is the tooth crowns of the premolars and molars, and between the teeth along the cemento-enamel junction. Factors contributing to caries development can include environmental (e.g., trace elements in food and water), exogenous (diet, poor oral hygiene, dental modification), endogenous (shape and structure of teeth, genetics), and pathogenic agents (caries-causing bacteria). For example, the cultural practice of dental modification predisposed fifteenth- to seventeenth-century African enslaved individuals from Portugal to caries in the modified surface because of exposure of the pulp cavity, just as it had affected the sixteenth-century people of African ancestry buried in Panama (Wasterlain 2019 and Smith-Guzmán et al. 2020, respectively). The use of night bottles or sugared rags to console nursing or teething infants has also been linked to rampant childhood caries, today (Chandra and Adlakha 2015; Castilho and Rocha 2009) and in antiquity

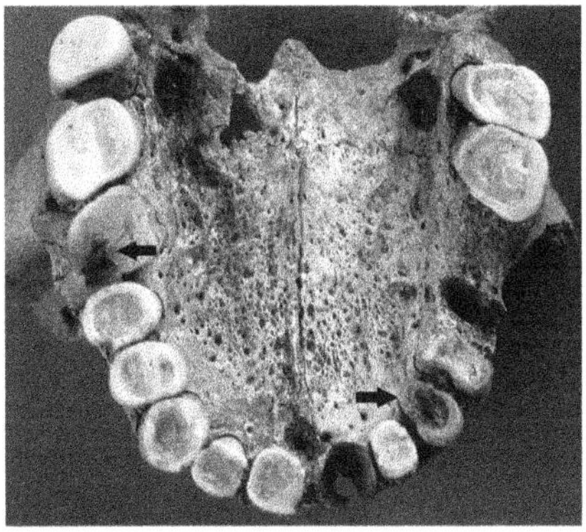

Figure 3.1. Dental caries affecting the left maxillary first molar and right canine tooth (black arrows); also note wear on the teeth and antemortem tooth loss of the right first molar. First century BCE–first century CE, Late Iron Age/early Roman, Hereford and Worcester, England. Photograph by and courtesy of Jean Brown.

(Bonsall et al. 2016). Various studies of saliva proteins and bacterial genetics, along with research on human twins and animals, have revealed specific genes related to low and high caries susceptibility (Cogulu and Saglam 2022). For example, the tuftelen gene along with the presence of the *Streptococcus mutans* bacteria can increase susceptibility. Caries may also occur with other oral pathologies, such as periodontal disease. In a study of the dentitions of skeletons excavated from a fourteenth- to sixteenth-century cemetery in London, UK (medieval St. Mary Graces), people with both periodontitis and dental caries died at an earlier age than those who were unaffected (DeWitte and Bekvalac 2010).

These potential etiological factors should all be considered in any bioarchaeological study of caries. As no one factor alone can necessarily be attributed to their development, taking into account contextual factors for the time and place is essential. As an example, a study of the dentitions of Mexican forager-farmers dated to the early Agricultural period (1660 BCE–200 CE) concluded that high rates of caries and antemortem tooth loss were caused by consumption of locally sourced cariogenic cacti and legumes (Watson 2008). Some trace elements in food and water may also prevent or predispose a person to caries. Fluoride in water can protect a person's teeth, but levels that are too high may cause fluorosis, which affects the strength of the teeth and bones (Whelton et al. 2019); some parts of the world (e.g., China, India, and Pakistan) have naturally high levels of fluoride in the water (e.g., Rasool et al. 2018; Wang et al. 2021; Nizam et al. 2022). This is a consideration for paleopathologists who may be working with skeletons excavated from these regions. Other dental problems may also weaken the normal structure of the teeth, making them more susceptible to carious attack. For example, deciduous teeth with enamel hypoplasia from the Libben population (Late Woodland, Ohio, United States; 800–1100 CE) were found to have a moderate increase in caries when compared to unaffected deciduous teeth (Duray 1990). Severe wear on the surfaces of the teeth can also weaken the tooth structure. This allows the entry of bacteria into an exposed pulp cavity, with consequent abscess development at the root of the tooth—another infectious lesion (see later in the chapter). As an infectious disease, caries can spread from a mother or sibling to a child through kisses or the sharing of cups and spoons (Wan et al. 2003). Nield et al. (2008) also provided a review of this issue, while Li et al. (2023) confirmed Wan et al.'s findings, and Riggs et al. (2019) suggested improving maternal dental care to reduce the incidence of caries in infants.

Recording of caries should include the number of teeth observed, tooth affected (incisor, canine, premolar, molar), tooth location (anterior, posterior), and the location of the lesion on the tooth, although documenting the size of lesions is more subjective. These variables help to explain underlying etiological factors. For example, the areas between teeth and the occlusal surfaces of molar teeth are places where plaque can accumulate if it is not removed. Care should be taken not to record caries when it does not exist: discolored, darkened areas on the enamel caused by taphonomic processes, as well as soil in the occlusal surface fissures, may both be mistaken for caries (e.g., see Garot et al. 2023). Hillson (2001, 2019) produced a more detailed scoring system for caries, and Lewis (2018, 76) documented a reporting system for nonadults that takes into account the presence of mixed dentitions and unerupted teeth. Some scholars have presented frequency rates for caries as a percentage of the individuals studied (known as a crude prevalence rate, or CPR), but this assumes that all teeth are preserved in all of the individuals and/or that the teeth lost postmortem were not affected by caries. Others present caries according to the number of teeth present and those affected (known as a true prevalence rate, or TPR), and still others include both sets of data. Whichever method is used, it should be clearly explained so that any comparative work between populations can be reliably conducted. We must also remember that some carious lesions may not be detected without the use of radiography (Smith and Warinner 2022).

The estimation of dental disease frequency according to biological sex has a number of implications for males and females; females today and in the past tend to have higher rates (Lukacs 2011). This was the case for a study of skeletons from two medieval London cemeteries (twelfth–sixteenth centuries CE), a time when famines were a regular event. Reproductive age-related biological factors, dietary differences for males and females, or different access to dietary resources during famine years were suggested to have been responsible for this difference (Walter et al. 2016). Lukacs and Largaespada (2006) in their study of Guanche mummified remains from Tenerife, Canary Islands, Spain, have also emphasized the importance of hormonal fluctuations in females, which can have a considerable impact on their oral health. In children, girls appear to have higher rates of caries than boys perhaps because teeth erupt earlier in females, meaning that they have a longer time in the mouth to develop them. In children aged from birth to five years, key causal factors are poor feeding and oral hygiene practices, poverty, and lack of parental education (Anil and Anand 2017; see also Lewis 2018, 68–70).

While both biological sex- and age-at-death-related rates for caries are usually provided in paleopathological studies, the interpretation of age and caries occurrence is complex. For example, a person with caries aged 40–50 years at death may have developed a number of carious lesions throughout their life—and the risk factors for caries may vary during different stages of their life course. The different teeth of both the deciduous and permanent dentitions erupt into the gums at various ages and at that point become vulnerable to caries; as age increases there is more chance that caries will develop. The gradual eruption of teeth and exposure of each tooth to caries may provide a more detailed timeline for the predisposing factors underlying caries. If appropriate archaeological contextual information is available, it may also be possible to provide a more nuanced understanding of the etiological factors.

The socioeconomic status of an individual adds another factor to our understanding of caries etiology. We often find differences in caries rates between the rich and people living in poverty, but not always in the same direction (e.g., for a modern example, see Foley and Akers 2018; and for a nineteenth-century example, see Geber and Murphy 2018). Boyce et al. (2010) studied decayed, missing, and filled teeth of living children from different socioeconomic backgrounds in the San Francisco Bay Area of California. They suggested that psychosocial, infectious, and stress-related biological processes were all at play in the development of caries in the disadvantaged children. It might be hypothesized that affluent people in the more distant past had easier access to cariogenic foods, including exotic products with high levels of sucrose, as seen in a study of a Classic period (250–900 CE) Mayan population from Mexico (Cucina and Tiesler 2003). Results showed that the highest antemortem tooth loss rates occurred in elite males, that is, those who would have more likely had access to a softer, more refined diet, demonstrating the intersection of biological sex and/or gender and status in poor oral health. Alternative interpretations could also have emerged: that the elite would have had access to more protein, which resulted in healthier teeth due to a more alkaline oral environment—but not in this case (Larsen 2015; Giacaman 2018). At Trakai, a sixteenth- to seventeenth-century site in Lithuania, poverty and poor-quality carbohydrates are thought to account for the high rates of caries and tooth wear found in laypeople buried in the churchyard. In contrast, people buried inside the church had lower caries rates, which could be attributed to a higher-quality and less cariogenic diet for the elite people buried there (Miliauskienė and Jankauskas 2015).

Globally, there are many studies of caries in past human populations, with the data interpreted in terms of risk factors operating within their environment, particularly their subsistence base. At the transition to agriculture from hunting and foraging, fermentable carbohydrates became available and initiated an increase in caries, although there are exceptions. In their study of the dentitions of infants and children from prehistoric sites in Thailand and Cambodia (ca. 4000–1500 BCE), Halcrow et al. (2013) found that dental health did not worsen over time and attributed this to a diet including (noncariogenic) rice. Moving east to Japan, Yao period farmers (ca. 2500 BCE–300 CE) showed no significant differences in caries rates when compared to the foragers from the earlier Jomon period (Temple and Larsen 2007). However, in a study of three populations from northern China with different subsistence patterns (intensified agriculture, hunting-foraging-fishing with some agriculture, and pastoralism), intensive farmers had the poorest oral health—including the highest rate of caries (Zhang et al. 2016).

Moving to the United States, the dentitions of pre-agricultural (1000 BCE–1150 CE) and agricultural (1150–1550 CE) populations on the Georgia coast were studied (Larsen 1984). Caries increased by around 10% for both sexes and all tooth types, with females showing the greatest rise. The increase was attributed to the adoption of maize agriculture. However, this is a rather simplistic interpretation. For example, Cucina et al. (2011, 560) studied caries rates in a maize-consuming pre-Hispanic Mayan coastal population from north Yucatan, Mexico, and stressed the limitations imposed by understanding carious lesions solely in terms of single dietary components, such as maize consumption, without taking into account broader aspects of cultural and socioeconomic relevance. Other studies confirmed this finding, illustrating the complexity of interpretation of caries rates. Hodges (1987) examined skeletons from the Formative (1400 BCE), Classic, and Postclassic (950 CE) periods in the Oaxaca Valley, Mexico, a time of agricultural intensification. She divided the fourteen archaeological sites studied into intensive and nonintensive farming groups. Here, a decline in caries was observed, from 17.9% in the Formative to 16.9% in the Classic to 11.1% in the Postclassic. Only males experienced an increase in caries, but this was confined to their molars. Overall, this suggested that a similar level of carbohydrate ingestion occurred across the periods, and there was no difference between the two groups.

Other research focuses on skeletons from the European continent. A "big data" multiperiod study of health in 103 sites from across Europe (second–nineteenth century CE) included rates of dental disease (Witwer-Backofen and Engel 2019). Here, dental caries increased with age, females were more affected than males, and caries showed an increasing trend from 500 CE (early medieval period) to 1800–1900 CE (Industrial period). Lower caries rates were reported at coastal sites, perhaps due to high levels of fluoride in marine resources; this compared to higher rates in urban sites. While this research covered a long time period, many sites and a wide geographic location, most studies are focused on far fewer sites, and often one site or region. An example of a site-specific study comes from Karsten et al. (2015), who studied skeletons of farmers from the Tripolye culture, Ukraine (approximately 5500 to 2750 BCE). Researchers found almost 10% of farmers' teeth had caries, while hunter-fisher-foragers had none. A comparative regional example comes from the Andes, South America, where a review and interpretation of published evidence for dental disease, including caries, concluded that these farming populations likely maintained a mixed subsistence pattern over a long period of time, and that Spanish colonialism rather than Inca imperialism affected these populations more (Gagnon 2020). Other big-picture studies include Bennike's (1985) research exploring Danish dental health. There were no caries in Mesolithic (hunter-forager) teeth, whereas 160 of the 7,062 (2.3%) Neolithic teeth were affected. Collated data for British populations from the Mesolithic to the postmedieval period (ca. 8000 BCE–1850 CE) suggest a link between increased dental caries across time, with the exception of the early medieval period (fifth–eleventh century CE) where frequencies declined (Roberts and Cox 2003, table 8.2). Prior to the sixteenth century CE in England, the main sweetening agents were likely honey and fructose from fruit, and at times luxury imports such as figs and dates, with bread being the main source of carbohydrate. The widespread availability of cane sugar and relaxation of import duties in northern Europe together with the rise in tobacco use saw a massive increase in caries rates (Moore and Corbett 1975; Jones 2014, 9, 113). By the end of the nineteenth century, sugar consumption was estimated at 20 pounds (9 kg) per person per year. By 1900 CE, it was 90 pounds (approximately 40 kg) and included large amounts of chocolate, treacle, and jam. The mean rate of caries in postmedieval sites in Britain was 11.2% of 12,993 teeth observed (Roberts and Cox 2003) but, as for the other periods, these were pooled data that included high and low rates, which varied depending on the site studied; in a study of two postmedieval populations in the UK (1712-1849 CE), the frequency of teeth affected in the high-status individuals buried at Chelsea Old Church, London was 21.5%, compared to 26.5% in the poorer people buried at St. Brides Church (Mant and Roberts 2015).

Clearly, the recording, analysis, and interpretation of dental caries is complex, and their multifactorial etiology warrants serious consideration when assessing results of studies. For example, dental caries and periapical lesions such as abscesses may lead to antemortem tooth loss (see Lukacs 1995, who developed a "caries correction factor" method to compensate for antemortem tooth loss due to caries). In paleopathology, for valid comparisons to be made between groups, agreement on methods of assessing and recording primary data is as paramount as it is for any other pathological condition.

Periapical Lesions

Dental caries can predispose an individual to the development of inflammatory-induced periapical lesions in the alveolar bone of the mandible and maxilla. In addition, dental wear, trauma, and dental modification such as filing can expose the pulp cavity and allow infiltration of bacteria, leading to lesions in the jaw (e.g., see Rufino et al. 2017). When microorganisms accumulate in the pulp cavity, inflammation occurs and a body of pus collects (dead cells and bacteria); this is called an abscess and it can track to the apex, or base, of the tooth root and into the surrounding tissues (Hillson 1986, 316). Abscess formation can also occur if an individual develops periodontal disease and a periodontal pocket. This is initiated by the accumulation of plaque between the soft tissue of the gum and the teeth. As the pus in the periapical region accumulates, pressure builds, and eventually a hole (sinus), or fistula, develops on the surface of the jaw to allow the pus to escape into the skin or mucous membranes of the mouth (Fig. 3.2). The pain may be severe before this occurs. It is at this stage in the process that the presence of a periapical abscess can be identified archaeologically as a hole on the alveolar bone. Prior to this, identification is not possible unless radiography is undertaken and shows a translucent destructive area at the tooth's apex. Potentially the tooth can die and eventually be lost antemortem.

Following the publication of the third edition of this book, other important contributions on this subject were published (e.g., Dias et al. 2007; Ogden 2008). Prior to 1997, paleopathologists tended to call all periapical lesions "abscesses," even though Dias and Tayles (1997) had emphasized that a cavity in the bone around a tooth root may not necessarily be an abscess (i.e., be pus forming) and could be a more benign condition, such as a cyst. The most common response to an infection is a granuloma, which may become a periapical cyst in time (Dias and Tayles 1997).

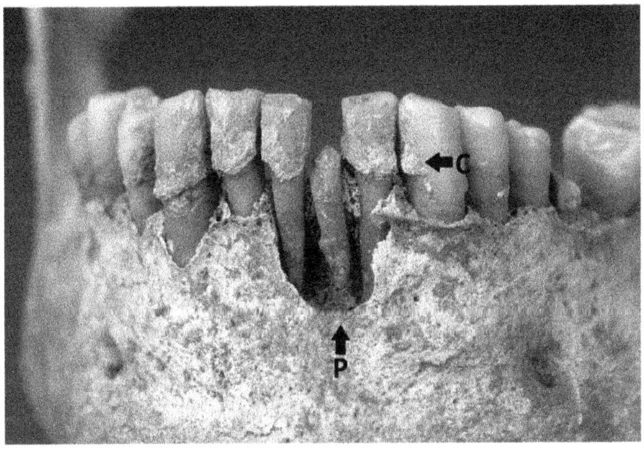

Figure 3.2. Periapical lesion (P) at the roots of the mandibular incisors (late medieval, twelfth–sixteenth centuries CE, France); note the extensive calculus deposits on the majority of the teeth (C). Photograph by and courtesy of Jean Brown.

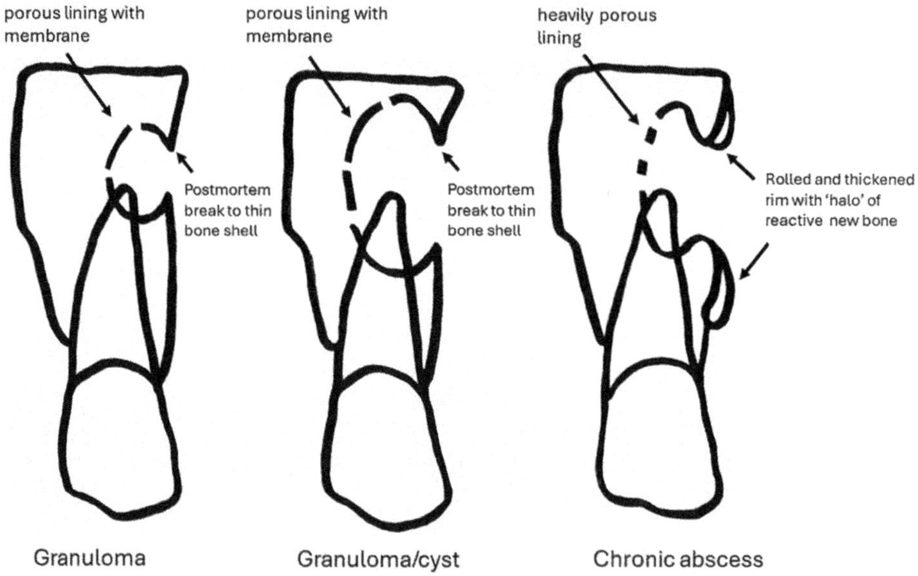

Figure 3.3. Types of periapical lesions. Adapted and redrawn from Ogden 2008 by Mary Lewis, with kind permission from the Ogden family.

An abscess can also develop from a granuloma or cyst. While abscesses have roughened irregular edges, granulomas are described as 2–3 mm in diameter with smooth walls, and cysts are larger (3-plus mm); radiography may be needed to identify some lesions. Even so, distinguishing granulomas from cysts is not always possible, and Ogden (2008, 297) provided a useful illustration to show the morphological differences (Fig. 3.3).

Because of the problems of identification, including the need for radiography, it is likely that periapical lesion frequency in the past is an underestimation. Further, abscess sinuses on the surface of alveolar bone may be mistaken for holes caused by postmortem damage. The roots of the teeth, especially in the anterior area of the upper jaw, are very close to the surface of the bone, and postmortem damage can occur over those roots. Dental abscess frequency in skeletal remains from Britain are low, ranging over 12,000 years from 1.0% of tooth sockets in the Bronze Age to 3.9% for the Roman period (Roberts and Cox 2003, table 4.2). By contrast, Pietrusewsky and Douglas (2002, 58) found at Ban Chiang in northeast Thailand that 6.4% of total adult tooth sockets revealed abscesses, with a significant difference between male (7.6%) and female (4.9%) frequencies. This latter finding is concordant with the differences in rates for caries and antemortem tooth loss at the site.

Dental Calculus (Calcified Plaque)

Another commonly observed dental condition is dental calculus. Dental plaque found on the teeth of the living (a biofilm) consists of microorganisms embedded in a matrix partly created by the organisms themselves, and partly derived from proteins in the saliva (Lieverse 1999). It accumulates on the teeth faster when there is a high-protein and/or carbohydrate diet that favors an alkaline oral environment. Apart from diet, a lack of oral hygiene and excessive mouth breathing (e.g., see Mummolo et al. 2020) are risk factors. Notably, diseases that lead to congestion of the nose—for example, leprosy—can cause mouth breathing (Reichart et al. 1976). While studies of dental calculus in children from archaeological contexts are rare, the consumption of soft weaning foods may contribute to a buildup of dental plaque, and erupting teeth are particularly susceptible during teething (Prowse et al. 2008). If plaque becomes long standing and chronic, it can become mineralized into calculus (Fig. 3.4) where crystallites of minerals in saliva—mainly calcium and phosphorus—are deposited in the plaque. Organic components make up a smaller but very important proportion of the calculus, containing a range of different remains of microparticles (e.g., from plants) and biomolecules (e.g., DNA and microorganisms).

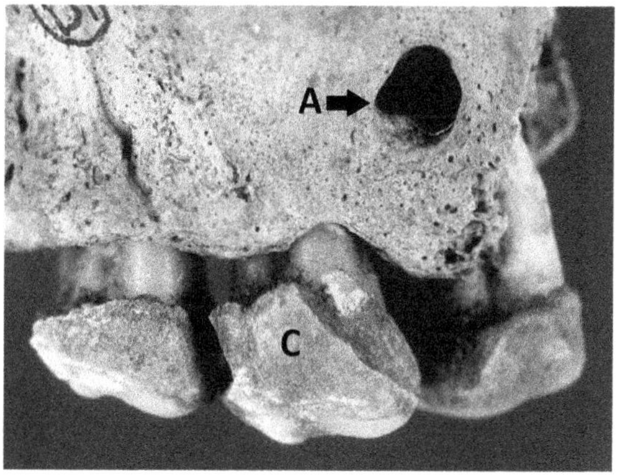

Figure 3.4. Dental calculus (C) on upper teeth (late medieval, twelfth–sixteenth centuries CE, France); also note the sinus of a dental abscess (A). Photograph by and courtesy of Jean Brown.

Two types of calculus are seen: supragingival calculus (above the gum) is more common and is usually thicker and gray or brown, while the subgingival type (below the gum) can be seen on exposed tooth roots and is associated with periodontal disease; it is harder and green or black in color. Calculus develops most commonly on the teeth nearest the salivary glands (tongue side of the lower incisors and cheek side of the upper molars) and is a common finding on archaeological teeth, which perhaps reflects a lack of attention to removing plaque (and thus calculus) from the teeth. Of interest is that although the microbes in historic and modern dental calculus have been found to be similar, there are several differences related to biofilm physiology. Velsko et al. (2019) noted that these differences are important when producing and interpreting datasets that are comparing dental plaque and calculus. Today, people have less diverse microbes in the mouth but are more at risk from dental diseases (Adler et al. 2013).

Methods of recording calculus, albeit subjective, have developed and vary from slight, medium, and considerable (Brothwell 1981, 155) to more detailed descriptions, where thickness and extent of deposit are considered (Dobney and Brothwell 1987). Ancient calculus has been variously analyzed to assess what makes up its composition. A large range of inclusions have been revealed in the past 20 years and include plant remains such as phytoliths, diatoms, starch, pollen, spores, and macro plant remains from cereals, tubers, and legumes. This goes alongside insect parts, animal hairs, microorganism DNA, charcoal, proteins, and even medicinal plants and human DNA (Ozga et al. 2016). Multiple pathways through which plaque can entrap inclusions have also been described (Radini et al. 2017). Furthermore, stable isotope analysis of calculus is now being explored (e.g., using $\delta^{13}C$ and $\delta^{15}N$ as a proxy for diet: see Price et al. 2018; and Salazar Garcia et al. 2023 for a review).

Several studies of dental calculus are enabling paleopathologists to reveal more nuanced pictures of our ancestors' lives. For example, a study of skeletons from England, Germany, and Poland found that the transition to farming changed the microbes of the mouth and that during the Industrial Revolution, bacteria causing dental caries became common (Adler et al. 2013). In a study of the skeletons of seventeenth-century soldiers who had survived the Battle of Dunbar, Scotland, and were eventually buried in Durham, England, Millard et al. (2020) reported evidence of food proteins, human proteins linked to the immune system, and bacterial DNA indicating gum and respiratory disease. They even identified soot in the dental calculus. Another interesting find has come from a prehistoric Sudanese burial site where a low frequency of caries was noted. Buckley et al. (2014) hypothesized that these people were likely consuming a particular tuber that inhibits an organism that causes dental caries, *Streptococcus mutans*. Some discoveries in calculus are really surprising: hunter-foragers in the Mesolithic Balkans were found to have consumed not only meat but also domesticated plants (Cristiani et al. 2016); respiratory irritants were a problem in Lower Paleolithic Israel (Hardy et al. 2016); and different sources of drinking water were consumed by people in the sixteenth–eighteenth centuries on Easter Island, Polynesia (Dudgeon and Trump 2014). Information about Neanderthal behavior, diet, and disease 48,000 years ago has also been interpreted from calculus studies, including self-medication in an individual with a dental abscess and a gastrointestinal pathogen (Weyrich et al. 2017). Fiorin et al. (2019) reported a specific fern used as a medicine in medieval Spain; Tromp et al. (2020) documented the importance of forests and arboriculture during the settlement of Remote Oceania; Tang et al. (2023) used protein in calculus as evidence of dairying in prehistoric pastoralists in Tibet; and Ventresca Miller (2023) identified yak dairy consumption by elite individuals of thirteenth-century Mongolia. Finally, Mackenzie et al. (2023) found plant material (cotton), fungal and yeast spores, wood particles, wool fibers, microcharcoal, and imported plants (e.g., New World maize) in the calculus of nineteenth-century people living in Manchester, northwest England. These examples of research display the enormous potential for future studies of calculus.

Studies of archaeological human populations indicate that, in general, calculus is common across time and space. Comparisons of frequency rates between different populations are challenging because most authors report calculus on the basis of individuals affected (CPR), often regardless of whether a complete dentition was preserved for recording or not, rather than basing prevalence on the total teeth observed (TPR). That calculus survives well in the archaeological record, and potentially holds much information about the individual and the population within which they lived, means that it has become a common target for sampling. For this reason, curators of skeletal collections need to be sure that photographs and casts of the teeth are taken before sampling. While this advancement provides an opportunity to use an often overlooked lesion to enhance our understanding of the past, not every individual had calculus, and so samples need to be reserved for the most rigorous research. We should not forget that the biographical information derived from the bones of the individual is as important as that emanating from the calculus, and the two should be integrated for the final interpretation (Radini and Nikita 2023).

Periodontal Disease and Antemortem Tooth Loss

The periodontium surrounds and supports the teeth, and comprises the periodontal ligament, the alveolar bone, cementum, and the gingival tissues (i.e., gums). Periodontal disease first affects the periodontium (periodontitis), and subsequently (but not inevitably) the bone. Resorption of the bone occurs, initially creating periodontal pockets, along with loss of the periodontal ligament holding the tooth. The distance between the bone and the cementoenamel junction (CEJ) increases, and eventually loss of teeth occurs (Fig. 3.5). Details of the development of periodontal disease have been described by Hillson (2019).

Calculus accumulates in crevices between the tooth and the soft tissue and jaw bone, forming periodontal pockets; this is a major predisposing factor in the development of periodontal disease. Because calculus was very common in the past, we would expect periodontal disease to also have been common, and this appears to be the case. As a degenerative condition, however, periodontal disease is less common in children when compared to adults (Lewis 2018, 77). Periodontal disease affects 1 in 10 people today and is a major cause of tooth loss (Janakiram and Dye 2020). It has been linked to other diseases, such as those affecting the heart, nervous system, and immune system (Hajishengallis 2022), something to bear in mind when periodontal disease is identified archaeologically. Specific bacteria have been associated with it in clinical studies: *Porphyromonas gingivalis*, *Treponema denticola*, and *Tannerella forsythia* (Visentin et al. 2023). These same organisms have been found preserved in the dental calculus of ancient skeletons (e.g., Mackenzie et al. 2018).

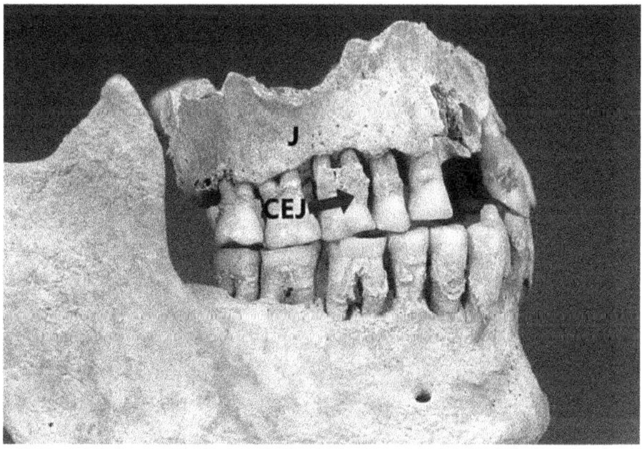

Figure 3.5. Periodontal disease and extensive calculus, with exposure of the tooth roots (late medieval, twelfth–sixteenth centuries CE, France). Note distance between the cementoenamel junction (CEJ) and the bone of the upper jaw (J). Photograph by and courtesy of Jean Brown.

Identification of this dental disease in archaeological skeletons is challenging. The distance between the CEJ and the crest of the alveolar bone may increase, and remodeling of the alveolar bone may be present (Clarke and Hirsch 1991). This may not necessarily be due to periodontal disease. Periodontal disease may be overdiagnosed in skeletal remains, if the distance between the alveolar and CEJ is increased due to continuing eruption of the teeth (through the deposition of secondary cementum on the roots), and/or as a response to severe wear. It is important to check whether wear is present on the occlusal surfaces of the teeth. Signs of inflammatory pitting and new bone formation on the jaw bones around the teeth, and/or periodontal pockets around the teeth in association with exposure of tooth roots, are more likely to secure a positive diagnosis for this dental disorder. Bone may be lost horizontally affecting the whole of the alveolus, or vertically around a few teeth, and increasing age, poor oral hygiene, and diets rich in sucrose are key predisposing factors. There is also a general lack of standardized recording, knowledge, and agreement as to what actually constitutes periodontal disease. Davies et al. (1969), Brothwell (1981, 155), Levers and Darling (1983), Kerr (1988), Karn et al. (1984), Lukacs (1989), Hillson (2019), and many others all describe and illustrate different methods to record and classify this dental disease. Whiting et al. (2019) emphasized that many factors contribute to the development of periodontal disease, its progression, and ultimately the prevalences reported, and concluded that Kerr (1988) offered the most useful recording method. Apart from the problems already outlined, the postmortem damage that occurs to the jaws often mimics loss of bone around the roots of the teeth.

Periodontal disease leads ultimately to tooth loss, and it was probably a major risk factor in the past as it is today, although caries and apical lesions can lead to loss too, and a combination of factors can be at play. Antemortem tooth loss (AMTL) can usually be recognized only if there has been some healing of the edges and bases of the tooth sockets or infilling of the affected sockets with new bone (Fig. 3.6). Unfortunately, no systematic surveys of periodontal disease in paleopathology using identical methods have been accomplished; therefore, reliably collected and standardized data are lacking and comparisons are impossible. Alongside a general decline in health with escalating social complexity, increases in caries and tooth loss at the transition to agriculture (perhaps due to periodontal disease) were noted for many of the studies in Cohen and Armelagos (1984), in the Western Hemisphere Health Project (Steckel et al., 2002), and in the European Health Project (Witwer-Backofen and Engel 2019).

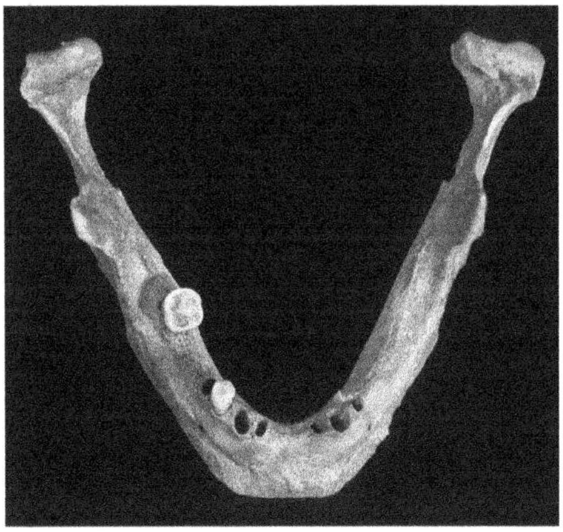

Figure 3.6. Antemortem tooth loss of most of the teeth of this mandible. Photograph by Charlotte Roberts.

Notwithstanding problems with recording and data interpretation, interesting studies have been published, many deploying the simple scale from Brothwell (1981, 155): slight, medium, and considerable. Two contrasting studies using different methodological approaches illustrate the periodontal disease challenge, particularly the question of how data can be compared if different methods are used to generate the data. The first used extant data collected by different scholars from the Museum of London's Wellcome Osteological Research Database, but using Brothwell's (1981) method. DeWitte (2012) reported frequencies in male and female Londoners buried in the fourteenth-century East Smithfield Black Death catastrophic cemetery (ca. 1349–1350 CE) and in the post–Black Death attritional cemetery of St. Mary Graces (ca. 1350–1538 CE). No differences between males and females were noted for the former, but males were more affected in the latter. A link between periodontal disease and subperiosteal lesions on the tibiae of individuals in the post–Black Death cemetery was also found, suggesting a number of possible etiological factors, such as immune incompetence and susceptibility to pathogens (DeWitte and Bekvalac 2011). The authors suggested that this finding may have resulted from the differential impacts of diet on each sex during the Great Bovine Pestilence (ca. 1319–1320 CE), prior to the Black Death. The second study used Kerr's (1988) recording method, which includes five categories that describe architectural form and textual appearance of interdental alveolar bone. Wasterlain et al. (2011) found a 73.8% frequency of periodontal disease in nineteenth- to twentieth-century documented skeletons of Portuguese individuals (University of Coimbra); males were more affected, and frequency increased with age. The findings were suggested to be similar to modern epidemiological studies.

Enamel Hypoplasia

Teeth can also retain a record of other events in a person's life, particularly during their growing years. There are many risk factors that may disrupt the development of dental enamel (see Smith and Warinner 2022, table 6.1), but they can be categorized broadly into systemic disruptions, such as nutritional deficiencies and disease (e.g., rickets, congenital syphilis, fluorosis); dental trauma; and inherited conditions (e.g., amelogenesis of osteogenesis imperfecta). These are generally known as dental enamel hypoplasia. Enamel hypoplasia have attracted the attention of many researchers in studies of both living and ancient populations. These aberrations in enamel development (amelogenesis) can be visualized macroscopically as well as microscopically as Wilson's bands (Antoine et al. 2009). Wilson's bands represent accentuated brown striae of Retzius, or incremental growth lines that run parallel to the normal striae in the enamel. They include the "neonatal line" that indicates a live birth (although it can take several days after birth for it to appear; Whittaker and White 1989). Wilson's bands are caused by short periods of stress (hours/days), while enamel hypoplasia, visual to the naked eye, result from longer periods of stress (weeks/months) (Larsen 2015, 49).

Essentially, an event in the person's life causes enamel-forming cells—ameloblasts—to stop working; as a consequence, flaws are left on the enamel

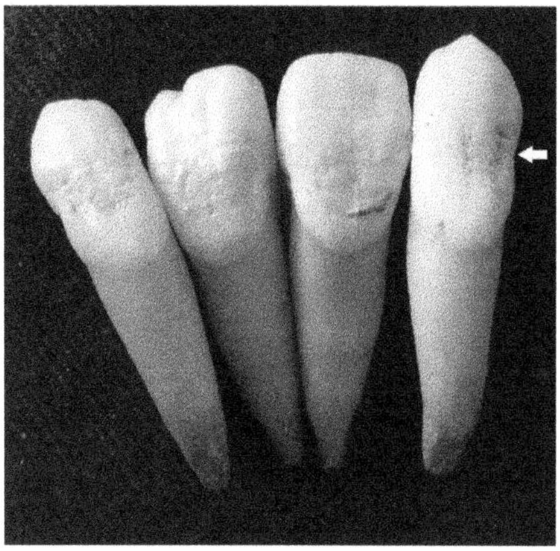

Figure 3.7. Dental enamel hypoplasia on the buccal surfaces of mandibular teeth of a child, eighteenth–nineteenth century CE, Coach Lane, North Shields, Tyne and Wear. Photograph by Charlotte Roberts.

surfaces or internally (Smith and Warinner 2022). The specific teeth developing at the time of the event are affected. For example, anomalies in the deciduous teeth indicate a disruption any time from the third trimester in utero to one year of age, and may provide information on maternal stress. These deficiencies in enamel matrix composition are often termed a nonspecific "indicator of stress" in bioarchaeology. They are one of many physiological stress-related indicators described in the bioarchaeological literature (also see Chapter 8). The word *stress*, however, has a very broad definition. Stress affects people biologically and psychologically (O'Connor et al. 2021), and specifically identifying a cause for a particular stress indicator such as enamel hypoplasia in bioarchaeology is very challenging.

Enamel hypoplasias are observed in several forms: as pits, furrows or grooves (also termed linear enamel hypoplasia), or plane form hypoplasia, and occur as the tooth crowns are developing in childhood (Ogden et al. 2007). Hypoplasia are situated circumferentially around the crown and are usually more easily seen on the labial surfaces of the incisor and canine teeth (Fig. 3.7). Despite being a permanent dental record of "stress" (enamel does not remodel), severe dental wear can obliterate these lesions, and calculus can obscure them.

Some studies have explored the age at which enamel hypoplasia developed in a person's life. This has been achieved by comparing the position of the lesion on a tooth with known enamel formation time sequences for tooth crowns in both deciduous and permanent dentitions of relatively modern populations. While the overall chronology of tooth formation is known, such work has been criticized for "formidable problems of diagnosis" (Hillson 2019, 298). This is, not least, because earlier enamel layers with defects may be hidden by subsequent enamel layers as the tooth develops. Research using histological (microscopic) analyses of enamel may well resolve these issues (e.g., Reid and Dean 2000, 2006), alongside dental development research (e.g., Alquatani et al. 2010). Studies on the age at formation of enamel hypoplasia have to presume that the relatively recent study populations on which crown formation ages are based (often those of Massler et al. 1941 and Sarnat and Schour 1942) were the same in the past as they are today, and that there was no variation between and within populations of different time periods, geographic areas or archaeological contexts.

Most recording of dental hypoplasia is undertaken macroscopically. The number and type of teeth affected, number of lesions, their appearance, and their severity are all standard data that should be recorded. Hillson (2019), among others, advocated for histological analysis using higher-power magnification to gain better accuracy (although see a more traditional study by Hassett 2014). Interestingly, Propst et al. (1994) showed that recording the lesions on dental casts rather than on the teeth themselves was easier, more productive, and more accurate. Whatever the method, as they reflect systemic physiological stress, enamel hypoplasia should occur on multiple teeth (with the exception of stress in later childhood, which may be evident only on the third molar), in a position that corresponds to the relative formation of each tooth crown at the time the stress occurred.

A range of thematic approaches has been applied to the study of enamel hypoplasia, especially for exploring subsistence economy. For example, Goodman et al.'s 1984 study at Dickson Mounds, Illinois (950–1300 CE), encompassed skeletons from three different groups (hunting-forager, mixed hunter-forager/agriculture, and agriculture). Enamel hypoplasia increased through time from hunting and foraging to farming. Many similar studies have come to the same conclusions. Further agricultural intensification does not always increase their frequency. Hodges (1987) did not find an increase in enamel hypoplasia with intensification in a study of skeletons from fourteen archaeological sites in Oaxaca, Mexico (nonintensive agricultural group—1400–500 BCE, and an intensive agricultural group—500 BCE–1400 CE). The Western Hemisphere and European Health Projects also found an overall rise in enamel hypoplasia over time with the development of increasingly larger and more complex societies that relied on agriculture (Steckel et al. 2002 and Bereczki et al. 2019, respectively). The latter study of 6,813 European individuals from premedieval to the Industrial period found some interesting trends: people living in the pre- and early medieval periods did not see a decline in health based on enamel hypoplasia, but rates of hypoplasia rose in urban environments, with some variance in their frequency in rural settings, and rates were higher in "transport-isolated landlocked areas" (Bereczki et al. 2019, 192).

Ethnographic studies have much to offer paleopathologists when interpreting what is seen in the archaeological record. For example, Ungar and Crittenden (2017) studied a living group of Hadza in Tanzania who spent their infancy and early childhood in three different environments: (1) in the bush, where they consumed wild foods; (2) in the village, where the weaning diet was dominated by domesticated cereals; and (3) transitioning between the village and the bush. A higher linear enamel hypoplasia rate was found in the village group, likely due to malnutrition. Turning back to bioarchaeological evidence, in China, Merrett et al. (2016) found that 72.7% of people buried at a site on the Dongbei plain, northeast China (2250–2050 BP), had enamel hypoplasia; in this case they practiced mixed hunting–foraging–fishing with some limited millet cultivation. Other thematic approaches have included their link to climate change. Lukacs and Walimbe (1998) studied individuals living in Inamgaon, India, between 1100 and 700 BCE, showing that health improved with a climatic shift to aridity and a change to nomadism and hunting and foraging. Socioeconomic status has also been explored using different funerary contexts, reflecting low-, middle-, and higher-status individuals, showing the higher-status burials experienced lower levels of enamel hypoplasia (Nakayama 2015).

As paleopathology now increasingly focuses on multiple morbidities expressed in the skeletal record, and their associations, many studies have explored enamel hypoplasia and their association with other "indicators of nonspecific stress." Watts (2015) compared their correlation with reduced vertebral neural canal (VNC) diameters to examine the impact of growth disruptions during infancy, childhood, and early adolescence in later medieval and postmedieval London, England. The aim was to assess whether, like reduced VNC, hypoplasia were linked to an increased risk of early adult mortality, but no association between the presence of enamel hypoplasia and age at death was seen. Conversely, an earlier age at death for Libben population individuals with enamel hypoplasia was found (Ottawa County, Ohio). Duray (1996) suggested that damage to the immune system during pre- or postnatal development may have resulted in the lesions. In a study of long bone length (reflecting height), cribra orbitalia and porotic hyperostosis (reflecting a range of conditions, such as an iron-deficient diet), and enamel hypoplasia were recorded for 9,021 individuals to explore potential links between early life growth disruption and age at death (Roberts and Steckel 2019). In this case, hypoplasia were positively associated with earlier mortality.

For many years, age at formation of enamel hypoplasia has been used to study weaning (Corruccini et al. 1985; Blakey et al. 1994), and more recent work relies on stable isotope data (e.g., De Armas 2022). However, Hillson and Bond (1997) showed nearly all age-at-formation studies using macroscopically identified hypoplasia reveal defects occurring between 2 and 4 years, and Smith and Warinner (2022, 99) remind us that, despite many enamel hypoplasia studies suggesting a potential weaning age of between 1 and 4 years in many societies, "this association does not prove a causal relationship" between hypoplasia and when mothers cease breastfeeding.

Dental Problems Associated with Specific Diseases

Several dental problems may be associated with specific disease processes. While any person who develops a health problem during the development of their teeth may have enamel hypoplasia, there are specific patterns of dental changes in certain diseases. For example, the more severe form of leprosy (lepromatous leprosy—see Chapter 6) has been suggested to induce constriction and shortening of the dental roots, especially in the central upper incisors. The change is hypothesized to be the result of direct action of the *M. leprae* causative organism, but more research needs to be done because it has not been reported in living people with leprosy, to our knowledge. In any case, this finding has been reported in some medieval skeletons from the Naestved leprosy hospital cemetery in Denmark (Danielsen 1970), and by Matos and Santos (2013), again from a Danish leprosarium (Odense). Likewise, the treponematoses (especially congenital syphilis) can affect the normal development of the teeth, producing Moon's molars and Hutchinson's incisors. Moon's molars are normal in appearance, but the tips of the cusps are very close together (Hillson et al. 1998; and see Chapter 6). Hutchinson's incisors occur because one of the three cusplets on the incisor edge is poorly developed and therefore a notch occurs. A number of sites have recorded the occurrence of these dental anomalies. For example, Iouannou and Henneberg (2017) reported them in individuals from the early twentieth century in the Hamann-Todd documented skeletal collection curated in Cleveland, Ohio, and Tomzcyk et al. (2015a) described an affected eighteenth- to nineteenth-century child from Radom, Poland. Notably, care should be exercised in the diagnosis of treponemal disease-related dental lesions, especially in the case of molar malformations, when severe enamel hypoplasia unrelated to the infection should be considered in the differential diagnosis. In the past, mercury was used for the treatment of syphilis and other diseases, such as leprosy, and its effects on the dentition have also been used to identify congenital syphilis in both infants and children (e.g., Ioannou and Henneberg 2017). While enamel hypoplasia and vitamin D deficiency are regularly reported together in paleopathology (e.g., see Ogden et al. 2007), recent work also documents interglobular dentine—an area of poorly mineralized dentine matrix—associated with vitamin D deficiency in clinical and archaeological contexts (Reed et al. 2017; D'Ortenzio et al. 2018a; see Chapter 7).

Dental Wear: Attrition, Abrasion, and Erosion

The predisposition of teeth to dental caries from dental attrition has already been discussed. Although not a dental disease per se, dental attrition results from tooth-on-tooth contact between the upper and lower teeth and between neighboring teeth and includes tooth grinding, or bruxism (Hillson 2019; Foley 2020). As the teeth wear down, secondary dentine is produced under the worn enamel to protect the pulp cavity (Fig. 3.8). Another form of wear is erosion of the tooth enamel. This may be caused by acid reflux from the stomach, which can be linked to eating disorders and consumption of acidic drinks or foods. Abrasion is defined as wear from contact with objects other than the teeth (Hillson 2019) and may be the result of cultural activities—e.g., for example, brushing the teeth with an abrasive substance or holding the stem of a pipe in the teeth while smoking it. One major factor causing wear on the teeth in past populations was the processing of foods, for example, grinding grain on a stone mortar, with the resulting flour containing stone particles from the mortar (Fig. 3.9). Modern Westernized diets tend to be much softer and easier to chew and digest than those in the past; therefore, wear on the teeth, certainly in the West, is not as significant today.

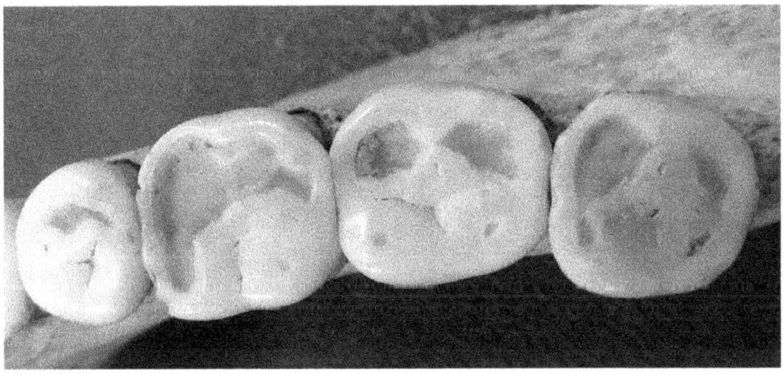

Figure 3.8. Exposure of dentine as a result of dental wear on canine and molar teeth.

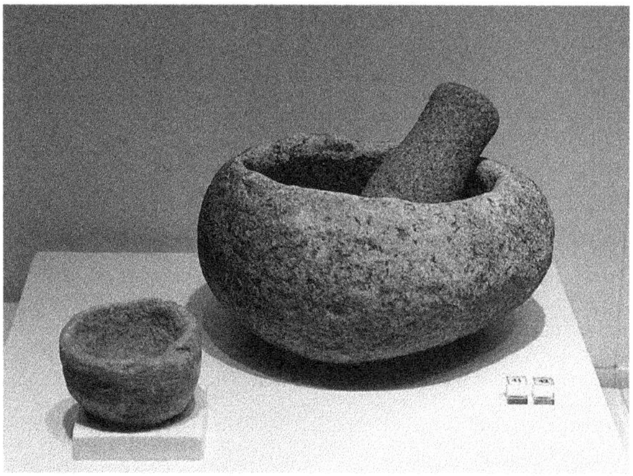

Figure 3.9. Mortar and pestle with a limestone bowl (Kissonerga-Mosfilia, Late Chalcolithic period, 2800–2500 BCE). Collection Archaeological Museum of Paphos, https://commons.wikimedia.org/wiki/.

Many methods of recording attrition to explore age at death have been developed for archaeological human groups, that is, observation of the patterning and rate of dentine exposure (e.g., Brothwell 1981, 72; also see Mays et al. 2022), although attrition, as we have seen, also reflects sociocultural risk factors. Clearly, attrition will vary between groups, time periods, and geographic areas; therefore, one method of recording developed on a particular group for age estimation may not be applicable to another population. Teeth also compensate for wear and maintain their height by "continually erupting" (Glass 1991), thus complicating the recording and interpretation of periodontal disease described earlier. While most scholars record macroscopic evidence for dental wear, it can also be seen microscopically (see Burnett and Irish 2017). Microscopic analysis of tooth wear can provide us with data on diet, use of the teeth as tools, and the mechanisms of chewing (e.g., see Mahoney 2006). For example, scanning electron microscopy enables the analysis of the intricacies of tooth wear in the form of pits and scratches. Summaries of research on microwear in various populations of human and nonhuman groups are described by Larsen (2015, 292–297; see also Fig. 3.10). Differences in food textures and abrasiveness, methods used for processing foods, and types of diet have all been explored. For example, the adoption of pottery and its use in cooking created softer diets with subsequent declines in scratches and pits on the tooth surface.

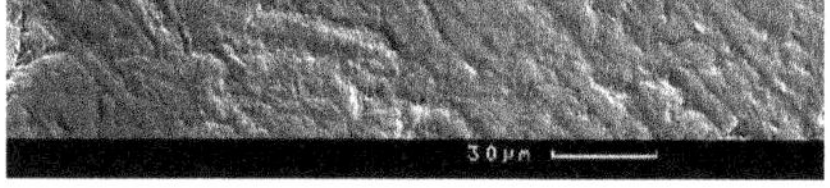

Figure 3.10. Microwear (grinding facet) evident on occlusal surface of the lower third molar of the Ohallo II skeleton (H1) Levant, 23,000 years BP (scanning electron microscopic image of a high-resolution cast, magnification 500 x; SEM operating in secondary electron emission mode; spot size of 3.0; accelerating voltage of 15 kV). Photograph courtesy of Patrick Mahoney.

The impact of severe attrition may be reflected in two other areas of the oral cavity. Degeneration of the temporomandibular joint (TMJ) may occur and has been observed in association with attrition in some archaeological populations (e.g., Pechenkina and Benfer 2002: Neolithic China; Stone et al. 2020: prehistoric Palau, western Micronesia). Hodges (1991) found TMJ disease and attrition co-occurring in British archaeological populations. Furthermore, Merbs' 1983 study of an Inuit population identified a link between the two conditions, especially in females; this, he suggested, reflected the use of the jaws and teeth as tools for culturally related activities, such as stretching and softening animal skins to make into clothing. Another condition seen in the oral cavity that may be present alongside heavy dental wear and TMJ disease, are the mandibular, maxillary, and palatine tori, which, it is believed, reflect high levels of masticatory stress that produce a bony reaction (Fig. 3.11). New bone forms along the lingual aspects of the mandible and maxilla, usually around the molar region, and along the midline of the palatal bones.

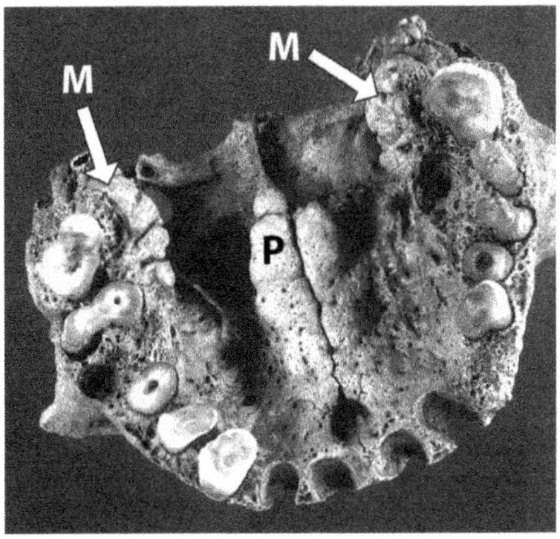

Figure 3.11. Maxillary (M) and palatine (P) tori (arrowed) and severe attrition on many teeth (early medieval, eighth–tenth centuries CE, Raunds Furnells, England). Photograph by and courtesy of Jean Brown.

Culturally Induced Dental Alteration

As previously discussed, dental diseases can be closely associated with sociocultural behavior. The final area of study in this chapter focuses on evidence of the effects of cultural behavior on the dentition. A large literature exists both on living and dead (archaeological) populations on how people use (and might have used) their teeth for various culturally related activities, for example, in farming, hunting and foraging, and various industries.

Macroscopic alteration of teeth may be intentional, related to (1) trauma (violence); (2) oral surgery; or (3) ritual purposes, to express group identity or beautification (Fig. 3.12). Intentional alteration of tooth shape or avulsion (removal) of teeth may be evidenced (Barnett 2017, 32–33; Durband et al. 2014: Roonka, Australia). Extraction of teeth and inlaying teeth with precious stones may also be part of the behavior of specific populations, linked to the appearance of an individual, their perceived status, and personal identity

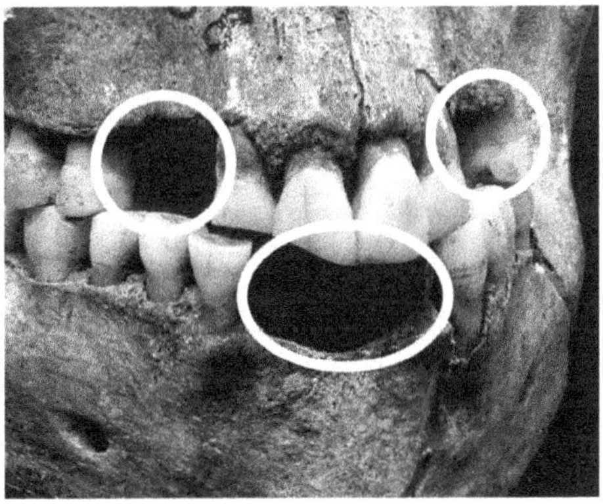

Figure 3.12. Dental modification: bilateral ablation of maxillary canines and first premolars, as well as all mandibular incisors (Yoshigo, Kyoto, Japan; Jomon period: 3500–2300 BCE—end of the Late Jomon/Final Jomon period). Photograph by Scott E. Burnett, courtesy of Kyoto University.

(De Groote and Humphrey 2016: tooth ablation/evulsion in prehistoric northwest Africa). Schroeder et al. (2014) documented both dental modification and an African origin (based on strontium isotope analysis) for three individuals buried in the Dutch part of St. Martin Island in the Caribbean. In the New World, the Maya developed the art of inlaying (mainly) incisor and canine teeth using stones such as jade (Tiesler 2024). Lower-lip plugs (labrets) are also known archaeologically and ethnographically as a body modification in North America, Europe, and Asia (Frayer et al. 2020). Dental modifications may thus represent a specific time or event in a person's life where this procedure took place, or that it was used purely for decorative purposes.

Macroscopic unintentional alteration of teeth relates to the use of the jaws and dentition as tools, but also as masticators of foodstuffs. While fractures and chipping of the enamel occur, probably the most common alteration to teeth is that caused by activities related to work. Patterns of tooth wear and alteration from normal shape may be induced by activities such as habitually pulling flexible materials through and over the teeth (e.g., plant fibers for basketry work), or holding materials static between the teeth to allow manipulation (Fig. 3.13). These actions may also be associated with loss of teeth and TMJ disease (e.g., Merbs 1983, 154). Differences in tooth wear between groups with different subsistence economies may be striking, allowing differentiation of hunter-foraging groups from farming groups, but dental changes are induced not only by activities essential for survival, but also by activities related to leisure (e.g., see Molnar 2008). In a unique study of skeletons from a prehistoric cemetery in Italy, Sperduti et al. (2018) found notches, grooves, and microstriations on teeth, suggesting an activity involving plant fibers, possibly basketry, and there was evidence of preserved hemp fibers in their dental calculus. Only by comparing patterns of tooth alteration seen in living populations with observations of dentitions of past populations can we make suggestions for their modification through cultural behavior; in some instances, however, no comparative data are available.

Evidence for oral surgery in archaeological populations is relatively rare, although it may have originated in Europe up to 14,000 years ago (Atiyeh et al. 2023). For example, Zias and Numeroff (1987) described an individual from Israel, dated to 200 BCE, with a 2.5 mm-long bronze wire implanted in a tooth. Bennike and Fredebo (1986) reported on a skeleton dated to between 3200 and 1800 BCE from a passage grave in Denmark (Middle Neolithic). The individual had drilled cavities between roots of the upper second permanent molar and between the first and second molars; these teeth had caries, suggesting that this action comprised a specific treatment. Other examples of tooth drilling come from 1300–1700 CE

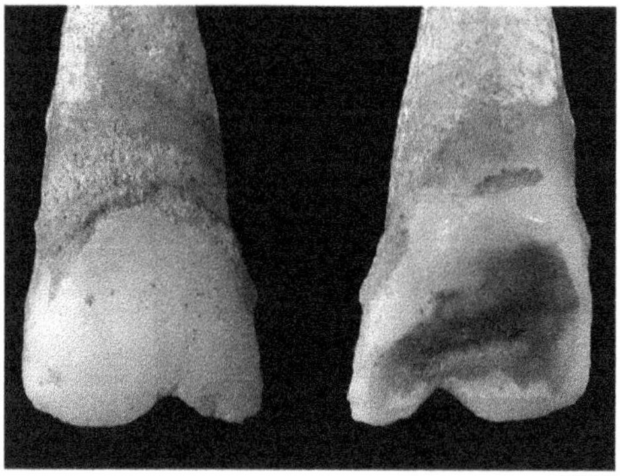

Figure 3.13. Notches in teeth in a 16–20-year-old male, from Palace Green Library, Durham (seventeenth century). Photograph courtesy of Anwen Caffell.

Alaska (Schwartz et al. 1995), where the alveolar bone around a central incisor contained a hole that appeared to have been drilled deliberately to treat an abscessed tooth, and from 1025 CE Colorado, where an occlusally drilled canine tooth was associated with a dental abscess (White et al. 1997). Of interest too are three prehistoric individuals from the US state of Maryland with evidence of tool marks in both the enamel and dentine borders of carious lesions, again suggesting deliberate intervention (Nase et al. 2022). Although rare, fillings in diseased teeth also have been reported. A mature adult from Denmark (fifteenth century CE) was found to have a carious mandibular tooth filled with a bone rosary bead (Møller-Christensen 1969a; Fig. 3.15), and Bernardini et al. (2021) reported beeswax as a filling 6500 years ago in Slovenia (Neolithic). Furthermore, a Ptolemaic mummified male from Egypt (150–30 BCE) with widespread dental disease had an interproximal carious cavity between a lower second premolar and first molar packed with textile material, possibly linen, suggesting an attempt at treatment (Pantazis et al. 2020).

Further evidence of dental treatment comes from Etruscan populations living in Italy over 2,500 years ago where gold bridges, dentures, and individual false teeth are noted (e.g., Becker 1994; Barnett 2017, 36; and see Fig. 3.15 as a denture example). Indeed, Seguin et al. (2015) described a wealthy female buried in Iron Age France with an antemortem or postmortem dental implant (an iron pin in the place of a tooth); they suggested that Celtic mercenaries—hired professional soldiers—returning from Italy may have brought the technique with them. Whittaker (1993, 53–59) also described fillings and dentures in nine individuals from the postmedieval (eighteenth–nineteenth century CE) crypt population of Christ Church, Spitalfields, London. The dentures were composed of porcelain, ivory, or bone and fitted using metal base plates and other stabilizing features, such as gold pins. Such interventions were likely available only to the wealthy. From antiquity to the late eighteenth century and beyond, dentistry was mostly confined to tooth pulling (Barnett 2017; Jones 2014). Evidence exists in both written records and artistic representation for tooth extractions in the past, but identifying deliberate removal using skeletal remains needs careful differentiation: the socket of a tooth lost antemortem of whatever cause may have healed. In their detailed analysis of an aristocratic female (Anne d'Alègre) living during the sixteenth–seventeenth centuries in France, Colleter et al. (2023) showed how her dental diseases (caries, periodontal disease, calculus, tooth wear, and bruxism) produced fascinating information about her personal life. One

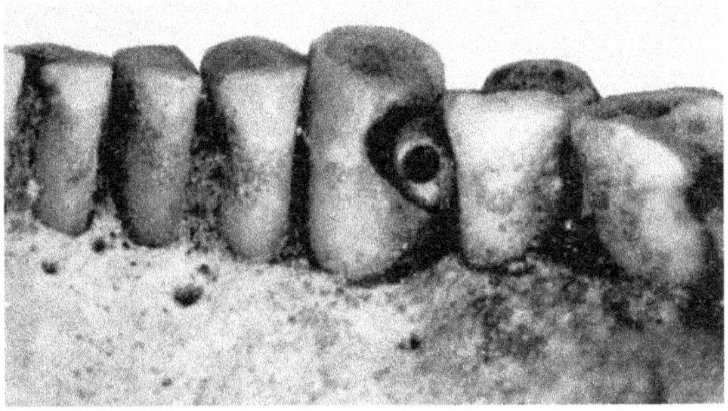

Figure 3.14. Rosary bead used as a filling in a carious canine tooth in a mature adult, from fifteenth century CE, Denmark.

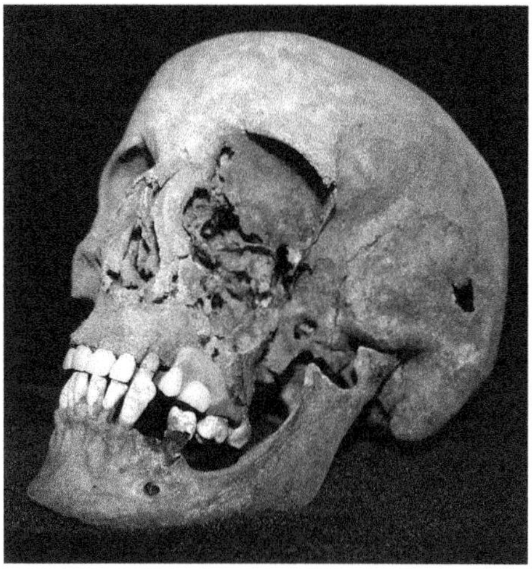

Figure 3.15. Left maxillary denture in a mature adult female from St. John's Church, Redhill, Surrey, England, 1750–1850 CE. Photograph by Mary Lewis.

tooth had been replaced with an ivory prosthesis held in place with wires, perhaps indicating its importance for her visual appearance.

Historical records and artwork document evidence for oral hygiene in the past—for example, in the writings of Dame Trota of twelfth-century Salerno, Italy, and of Pierre Fauchard (1679–1761 CE) of France; the latter emphasized prevention, conservation, and hygiene and coined the word *dentiste* to distinguish his profession from tooth pulling (Bifulco et al. 2016; Jones 2014, 84–87). However, there is very little archaeological evidence for oral hygiene practices. For example, grooves on adjacent teeth have been interpreted, controversially, as evidence that toothpicks were used as early as the European Middle Paleolithic (250,000/300,000 and 35,000 years BP—see Bahn 1989; Christen and Christen 2003; Estalrrich et al. 2017; Ricci et al. 2016). The use of chewing sticks has been described in some societies (Cook et al. 2015), and enslaved African people who arrived in Brazil during the eighteenth or nineteenth century probably used chewing sticks prior to their enslavement, as seen in abrasive marks on the roots of their teeth.

Methods of Recording Dental Disease

As we have seen, dental disease and modification of the dentition, through whatever means, provide the paleopathologist with a wealth of information about people's lives. However, use and comparison of these data are only possible when all researchers engage with the same methods of analysis. Dental data are often presented in a variety of forms, summarized here:

1. Teeth/tooth sockets affected as a percentage of the total teeth/sockets available for examination
2. Individuals affected as a percentage of the total individuals examined; this assumes all teeth and sockets are preserved
3. Number of dental pathological lesions per individual (again, assuming all teeth and sockets are preserved)

As with all pathological conditions, it is essential to present these data with reference to the age and biological sex of the individuals being studied. If a person lives longer, dental disease will naturally be more likely to occur and increase; therefore, a population composed mainly of older people would be expected to have higher rates of dental disease than a younger group. However, we cannot assess the age at which the person developed these different dental diseases (a debatable exception being enamel hypoplasia); we can identify only those dental diseases present when they died. Recorded differences between populations, when put into context (e.g., access to diet or status of the person in the population), allow inferences to be made more easily.

Epilogue

Teeth are usually remarkably well preserved in the archaeological record, both in human and nonhuman remains, making their study a major component of paleopathology. Since the third edition of this book, major advances in the study of dental calculus have appeared and seem set to continue as more complex questions about the past are asked and answered using an ever wider range of evidence types and analytical methods. Increased knowledge of the oral microbiome, both past and present, will further enhance our understanding of the links between what we have in our mouths and to what that might predispose us in the rest of our bodies (comorbidities), not only different dental diseases but also nondental diseases such as cardiovascular problems. Paleopathologists have developed a range of recording methods for all the dental diseases we may observe, but there is a need for consistency. All researchers must come to some agreement about how dental disease can be effectively recorded, first, to provide a primary and true record of the past, and second, to enable realistic comparisons between time periods and between (and within) regions of the world.

4

Trauma

Life without injury can hardly be imagined.

—C. Wells, Bones, Bodies, and Disease

The World Health Organization reports that accidental and violent injuries kill over four million people a year, with young males more often the victims of suicide, homicide, and road-traffic accidents (Global Burden of Disease 2021). In modern times, preventing injuries is often promoted, reflecting the high economic costs associated with trauma and its potential longer-term physical impairment (e.g., Peterson et al. 2021: costs in the USA in 2019 were $4.2 trillion). In the past, a plethora of paleopathological evidence has revealed that people were not immune to being injured, often in circumstances not unlike our own. The difference in outcomes would, nevertheless, have been much more challenging to manage without the often-complex interventions the medical profession has at its disposal today, from antibiotics to surgery. Trauma is much more than the injury it causes; it is now recognized that it can have a profound effect on a person's psychological state long after the injury has healed, and no two people will react to injuries in the same way. Indeed, people may be traumatized without any physical injury.

In paleopathology, trauma is defined as any injury or wound to the body. This could be of the soft tissue alone, the skeleton, or both. Any injury to bones will always be associated with injury to the adjacent soft tissue, but the majority of injuries to soft tissue in the form of a deliberate external physical assault or an accident will not necessarily impact bone. The bones of our skeleton provide a supporting framework, protect vulnerable organs and viscera in the body cavities (e.g., the ribs protect the lungs), store minerals, make blood cells, and allow movement of the body through muscle, ligament, and tendon relationships. Damage to the skeleton can therefore affect these functions. It is self-evident in a consideration of injuries in skeletons that the anatomy and physiology of the related body organs, including potential nerve and blood vessel dysfunction, are examined and proposed even when these soft tissues are usually no longer preserved.

Trauma can be subdivided into four categories (Redfern and Roberts 2019, 211; Grauer 2019):

1. A partial or complete break in a bone (fracture)
2. Abnormal displacement or dislocation of a bone or joint
3. Disruption in nerve and/or blood supply (e.g., trauma-related circulatory disorders such as osteochondritis dissecans)
4. Artificially induced shape or contour (e.g., deliberate cranial modification)

The first category also includes the amputation of limbs and trepanations (surgical removal of a piece of the skull). Trauma (especially fractures) is one of the most common pathological conditions seen in human skeletal remains, along with dental and joint diseases, and is routinely reported in the paleopathological literature (e.g., Redfern 2017a; Lovell and Grauer 2019; Byrnes and Gaddis 2023).

The complexity and variety of injuries seen in any given group will increase with the complexity of their lifestyle (Huang et al. 2021). Further, some people experience repeated trauma throughout their lives, and as they age the number of fractures experienced increases (also termed recidivism), a concept that is often incorporated into paleopathological research (e.g., Redfern et al. 2017; Mant 2019; Antunes-Ferreira et al. 2021; Biehler-Gomez et al. 2023). For example, Redfern et al. (2017) studied evidence for single and multiple injuries in skeletons from England, Siberia, and Sudan (third–nineteenth centuries CE). They found that males and people aged 26–35 years at death were the most likely to have experienced trauma and to have multiple fractures.

What is of interest to the paleopathologist is not merely the presence of isolated traumatic lesions, but rather, the change that has occurred in the patterning of human trauma across time and place and its interpretation in relation to archaeological context; the long view or deep-time perspective. By observing the precise morphological characteristics of traumatic lesions, we can begin to assess the cause and clinical severity of these injuries. Indeed, they may shed light on the everyday activities of the afflicted individual. For example, the Paleolithic hunter, the medieval farmer, and the modern factory machine operator may all exhibit traumatic evidence of working in their trade. Young and old alike are subject to injuries characteristic of their age group, and the influence of biological sex on fracture patterns is clear, as we will see. Paleopathologists are, and should be, increasingly considering intersectionality in their interpretations, such as how social inequalities of class, gender, sexuality, religion, ability, and ethnicity shape one another (Collins and Bilge 2020). Using this approach, in their study of trauma in a tenth-to-thirteenth-century population from Poland, Betsinger (2023) emphasized that this particular approach provides a more nuanced appreciation of the impact of interpersonal violence. How successfully these injuries heal also provides us with information about that individual's dietary status, the availability of care and treatment, and the occurrence of complications.

We should at this point highlight the potential for a person being impacted by structural violence within their community—that is, social structures that harm people (Farmer et al. 2006). For example, generally speaking, the poor are more likely to experience trauma (Huang et al. 2021) and will have less ready access to treatment. Further, homicides are more common in countries or regions with greater social inequality (e.g., the US) (Wilkinson and Pickett 2009, 135, 136). Paleopathologists have started to address the impact of structural violence on health. In a study of nineteenth-century African American and Euro-American females of low socioeconomic status, de la Cova (2012) found African American females experienced higher frequencies of trauma to their head, nose, and fingers, while Euro-Americans had more hip and forearm (radius) fractures. It was concluded that, because the former were incarcerated in psychiatric hospitals, their injuries were probably related to interpersonal and structural violence (also see Blevins et al. 2023; and Lewis 2018, 122–123, regarding children). Addressing questions about the impact of structural violence on past peoples contributes knowledge to the United Nations Sustainable Development Goals 16 (Peace, Justice and Strong Institutions), and 10 (Reduced Inequalities).

Trauma may not, of course, be purely accidental, and warfare on an ever-increasing scale and complexity seems to have been a recurring theme throughout history (e.g., see Martin and Frayer 1997; Harrod et al. 2012; Schulting and Fibiger 2012; Knüsel and Smith 2014; Martin and Harrod 2015; Fibiger et al. 2023). Even in recent times, conflicts in Afghanistan, Africa, Iraq, Israel, Palestine, and Ukraine remind us that human populations have not learned to live in harmony. Indeed, and as Hazer and Gredebäck (2023) have intimated, the effect of warfare and displacement can be associated with poor mental health and developmental delays in children.

The Neolithic arrowhead, the medieval battle-axe, and the later musket ball have all left their evidence in the paleopathological record (e.g., see Novak 2001 for cranial wounds of soldiers from the fifteenth-century Battle of Towton in England). Surgical practice also results in intentionally inflicted wounds, albeit without the aggression of violent attacks, and the orthopedic and neurosurgeons of antiquity also left their mark on the archaeological record (Verano 2016; X. Zhang et al. 2021).

Injuries to Soft Tissues

Before considering bone injuries themselves, it is important to understand that the paleopathological evidence of trauma is but a very small part of the total spectrum of injury affecting populations. By and large it is the gross injury that is in evidence, and the multitude of commonplace cuts, abrasions, and bruises so familiar to us all are lost in the archaeological record. Evidence of soft tissue injury is sparse and merely inferential in skeletal remains, although more obvious in preserved bodies. For example, trauma in the form of strangulation or a cut throat has been identified in association with the bog bodies of northwestern Europe, the former evidenced by a ligature around the person's neck (Giles 2020). We must therefore acknowledge that skeletons represent once-living people like us, people who not only had bones but also soft tissues.

One example of a soft tissue injury is myositis ossificans traumatica. This is caused by injury and then ossification of the blood associated with this muscle (hematoma), and researchers have identified examples of affected muscles in specific locations on a particular bone (Fig. 4.1). To recognize such an injury it is thus necessary for new bone formation to have occurred within the hematoma, as seen on the pelvis of a seventeenth-century Royalist soldier from England in whom a severe muscle tear of the rectus femoris muscle must have occurred (Manchester 1978).

Clearly, any injury that penetrates bone must also involve the surrounding soft tissues. One may also infer damage to soft tissues by examining the location of the injury closely. Some fractures at specific sites in the body may lead to damage to blood vessels or nerves. For example, fractures to the shaft of the humerus (upper arm) can cause radial nerve palsy, the most common nerve lesion associated with long bone fractures (Shao et al. 2005). Obviously this would have implications for the individual's motor and sensory functions.

Likewise, a rib fracture can result in a perforated lung injury with bleeding into the pleural cavity surrounding the lungs, along with pain on breathing. A spinal fracture, if involving the spinal canal directly, may result in restricted or reduced blood flow to the spinal cord due to injury to the arteries supplying it and to the segmental spinal nerves. Such an outcome would incur peripheral neurological damage leading to a disturbance in function of one or more nerves that supply various organs (i.e., the bowel, bladder, and reproductive organs, which may be variously associated with persistent diarrhea or constipation, urinary incontinence, and sexual impotence). In considering soft tissue injuries and sequelae of specific orthopedic fractures in paleopathological studies, it is essential to understand the total pathophysiology of the injuries encountered to be able to make a diagnosis and interpret how these injuries affected the life of the individual.

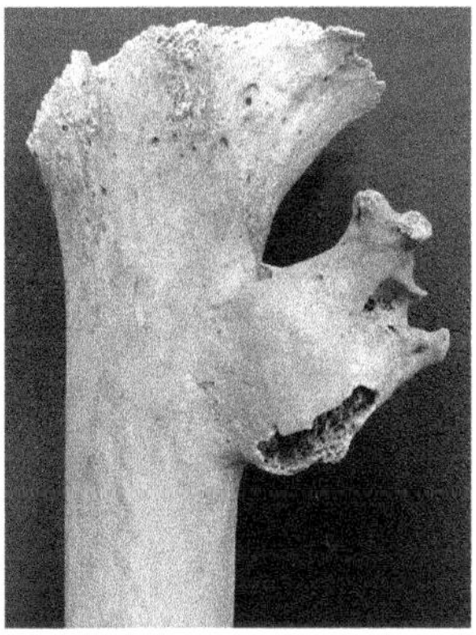

Figure 4.1. Soft tissue injury causing ossification on a femur (myositis ossificans traumatica) from postmedieval Spain. With kind permission of the Fenwick Human Osteology Laboratory, Department of Archaeology, Durham University.

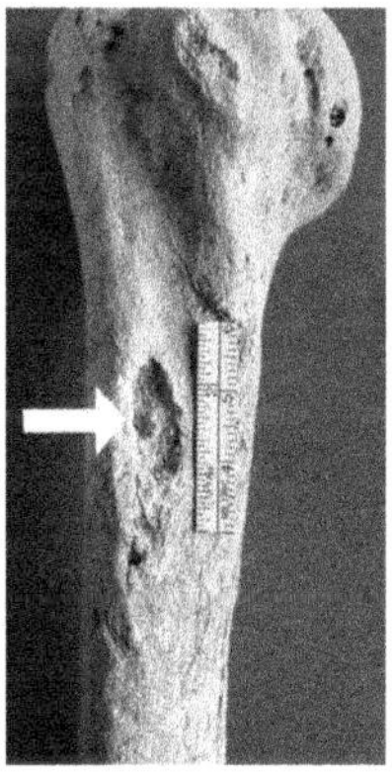

Figure 4.2. Humerus from commingled remains with a cortical defect from Ermida de Nossa Senhora da Conceição, 1500–175 BCE, Seixal, Portugal. Photograph courtesy of Francisca Alves Cardoso.

Destructive (or lytic) lesions may also occur as a result of stress or strain of an associated soft tissue structure. It is likely that these lytic lesions are the result of injury and interruption of the arterial blood supply to the specific anatomical region, eventually causing death of the cortical bone and soft tissue attachment at the site (Fig. 4.2). For example, in the posteromedial aspect of the distal femur, Resnick et al. (2024, 1223) identified cortical defects, irregularities, and excavations. The most common of these lesions in clinical contexts, cortical irregularity, was found to be more frequent in children and adolescents and associated with stress of the adductor muscle (see also Stern et al. 2020: association with skiing). Less common in living populations, but seen archaeologically, are the cortical lesions associated with stress—although care should be taken to distinguish these lesions from nonossifying fibromas (see Chapter 8).

Culturally Related Modification of Bones

The cultural practice of artificial cranial modification (Fig. 4.3), or shaping, was first described in written texts in the fifth century BCE by the Greco-Roman writer Hippocrates (*Airs Waters Places*, 14; Hippocrates 2022), and the earliest recorded evidence in a skeleton was found in Shanidar Cave, Iraq, and dated to 45000 BCE (Gerszten and Gerszten 1995). There are several methods and materials used to change the shape of the cranium of a newborn, such as bandages, boards, stones, and pads (see Püschel et al. 2020, and references within). The application of boards is believed to be the most effective method, usually involving applying them to the frontal and occipital bones. These devices were usually kept in place for three years and then removed, with growth of the skull then continuing in the direction established by the shaping apparatus (Weiss 1958, in Aufderheide and Rodríguez-Martín 1998, 35–6). One reason for cranial modification was to signify identity and a belonging to a particular social group.

This practice has been noted in skeletal remains in Europe (e.g., Fernandes et al. 2019), the Middle East (e.g., Fletcher et al. 2008), Asia (e.g., Ni et al. 2020), the Americas (e.g., Torres-Rouff 2020), and Africa (e.g., Ricci et al. 2008), and probably developed independently across time and space. Notably, it is believed to be effective only if undertaken in the very young, when the bones of the skull are "plastic" and easily shaped (e.g., see Özbek 2001: Türkiye; Khudaverdyan 2011: Armenia). Of interest here is that a flat area on the cranium (plagiocephaly) also occurs unintentionally in babies, and has recently increased in frequency after pediatricians recommended they sleep on their backs to prevent sudden infant death syndrome (Jung and Yun 2020). Many resulting different cranial shapes have been documented in the archaeological record, and some concurrent conditions have been recorded, for example, alteration of the normal closure pattern of the cranial sutures (C.D. White 1996: Lamanai, Belize; Dean 2004), the number of ossicles occurring between modified and unmodified skulls (Wilczak and Ousley 2009), and overlapping of the temporal bones leading to a prominent border and necrosis of bone (Gerszten and Gerszten 1995). Nothing of a serious nature has been suggested to co-occur. Some research has intimated, however, that modification might affect the lobes of

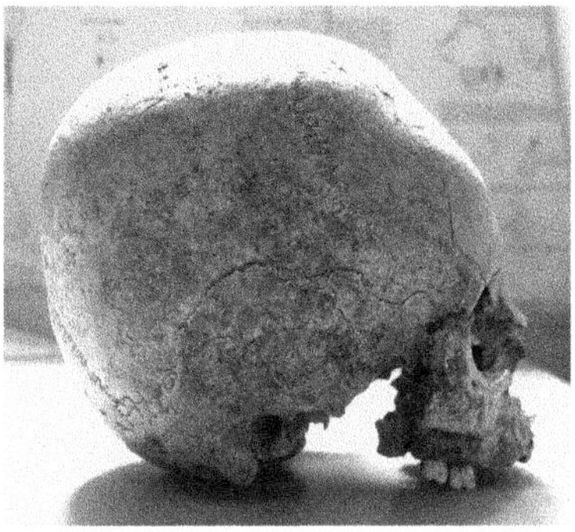

Figure 4.3. Intentional cranial modification in an adolescent male from Osijek, Croatia, fourth–fifth century CE. Note flattening to the frontal bone suggesting a circular band was used to give the cranium an accentuated erect profile. Photograph courtesy of Mario Novak.

the cerebral cortex and could lead to problems in vision, hearing, concentration, learning, memory, and behavior (O'Brien et al. 2013).

While cranial modification has been frequently reported in past populations, especially in South America, evidence is rare for other forms of intentional skeletal alteration, such as female foot binding. This cultural practice began in China in the Song Dynasty (960–1270 CE) and lasted until the Cultural Revolution in the 1940s. Evidence for foot binding is viewed as reflecting "a society's past values placed on women in marriage, sexual attraction, social status, physical beauty, and filial duty" (Lee 2019, 9). In a known (nonarchaeological) example of foot binding described by Mann et al. (1990), the heads and shafts of the metatarsals were atrophied and distorted, and the phalanges had constricted shafts, while the metatarsophalangeal joints were partially dislocated. The practice was usually performed by mothers on their daughters every two weeks, using silk bandages up to ten feet long until the full growth of the foot had been achieved (Mann et al. 1990). Linhuan and Fajun (2021) identified a female who may have experienced foot binding in a cemetery in Taohuayuan, Tianjin, China, in the fourteenth–nineteenth centuries CE. In an extensive review paper on foot binding, Lee (2019) documented evidence from Xuecun in Henan province in China. Eleven females had alterations to foot bones consistent with the practice. Berger et al. (2019) also described evidence in four elite female skeletons from the Ming Dynasty (1368–1644 CE) in Shaanxi province, China.

The two final examples of bone alteration involve the thoracic cavity. In a fifteenth century CE female skeleton buried within Ripon Cathedral, England, Groves et al. (2003) described a sternal deformity (pectus carinatum). It was hypothesized that this female was high status because of the location of her burial. As people with pectus carinatum today can be stigmatized, which may impact their identity, body image, and mental health (e.g., see Steinmann et al. 2011), it was suggested that this anomaly was treated by compression of the upper chest, which led to flattening of the spinous processes of some of the thoracic vertebrae (Figs. 4.4 and 4.5). Wearing a corset can also affect the thoracic cavity. While corsets have been fashion items, they were also used for treating spinal tuberculosis (TB) (Moore and Buckberry 2016). In nineteenth-century Europe, tuberculosis was rife, and at the same time the number of women wearing corsets increased. Aside from this, at that time it was felt that having TB made them more attractive (thin, pale, and "sickly") (Day 2017). Corsetry can cause restricted lung function and affects how much oxygen can reach other body tissues. Organs may be compressed, including the uterus, which can cause problems for childbearing and even lead to abortion of the fetus (Roberts 2020c). Bone changes from corset wearing include "anterior displacement of the ribs and antero-lateral deviation of the spinous processes of the vertebrae" (Moore and

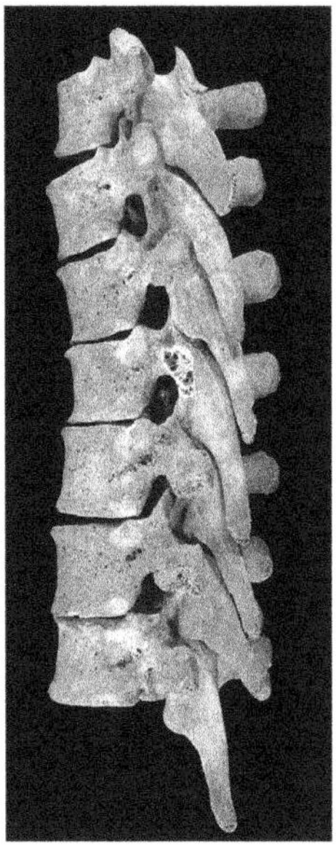

Figure 4.4. Part of the spine from a female from Ripon Cathedral, Yorkshire, England (twelfth–sixteenth centuries CE). Note the flattening of the spinous processes, which may be the result of compression treatment for a sternal deformity. Photograph by and courtesy of Jeff Veitch.

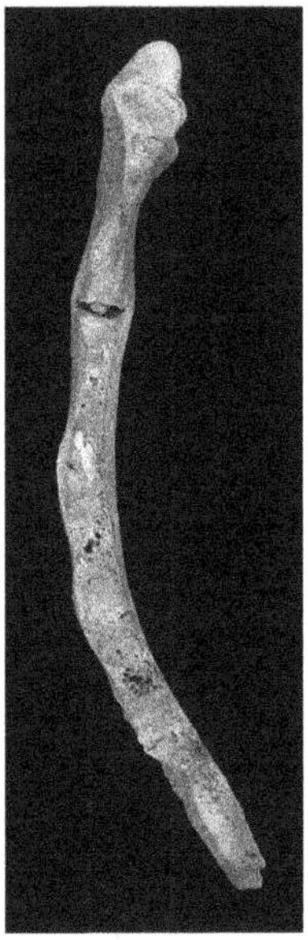

Figure 4.5. Bowing of sternum (pectus carinatum) in the female from Ripon Cathedral. Photograph by and courtesy of Jeff Veitch.

Buckberry 2016, 75). Today "waist training" using a corset has come into vogue, with consequential effects on breathing. Noticeably, most of these body modification practices were carried out by, or on, women, and Stone (2012) discussed the skeletal evidence for such "binding" of women (including foot binding) as representing chronic and indirect cultural violence.

Types and Causes of Fractures

The most common type of trauma to the skeleton are bone fractures. A fracture can be defined as the result of any traumatic event that leads to a complete or partial break of a bone. In theory, then, injuries to the cranium caused by a bladed weapon, piercing injuries, and surgical procedures, such as trepanation, are all classed as fractures under this definition. The fractures that occur a short time before death or may be coincident with it (perimortem), and which show no evidence of healing, can be very difficult to distinguish from postmortem breaks of bone (see later in this chapter). A further subdivision of fractures, and one that throws light on the mechanism of the injury, is the type (and, by inference, direction of force) of the break in the bone (Fig. 4.6). The types of stress or force that a bone may be subject to are tension, compression, twisting, bending, and shearing (Redfern and Roberts 2019). Fractures result from both direct (at the point of impact) and indirect (not at the point of impact) injuries (Lovell and Grauer 2019).

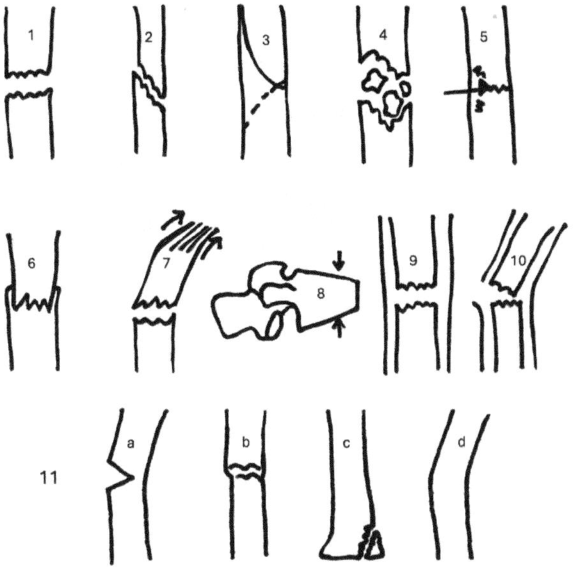

Figure 4.6. Types of fracture. 1. Transverse (direct force); 2. Oblique (direct force); 3. Spiral (indirect torsional force); 4. Comminuted (more than two fragments); 5. Penetrating; 6. Impaction (fractured ends forced into each other); 7. Traction/avulsion (tendon or ligament stressed; bone fragment pulled away); 8. Crush (force applied to one [depression] or both sides of a bone [compression]); 9. Closed/simple (fractured bone closed to the external environment); 10. Open/complex (fractured bone broken through skin and exposed to external environment); 11. Pediatric fractures: a: greenstick; b: torus or buckle; c: metaphyseal (physeal); d: plastic deformation. Created by Charlotte Roberts and edited by Mary Lewis.

The simplest fracture in mechanical terms is transverse, resulting from a force applied at right angles to the bone. Oblique or spiral fractures are due to an indirect and/or rotational force. A further feature of fractures may be multiple splintering of the broken bones. These comminuted fractures are common in road-traffic accidents today, usually need surgical intervention, take longer to heal, and may have an outcome that is not functionally satisfactory. Impaction fractures result in the two fractured ends being forced together, producing a rather stable fracture that may heal readily, even though some length may be lost on the affected limb. A traction/avulsion fracture is the result of a sudden strain of a tendon or ligament. In this case the soft tissue pulls a small piece of the bone away. A common avulsion fracture is that of the distal fibular malleolus, resulting from an acute inversion injury of the ankle joint. A complication of such a fracture, apart from the pain and ankle joint instability, is the disruption of arterial blood supply to the dislocated malleolus, and subsequent failure to reunite with the fibula shaft. The crush fracture may be due to depression or compression of a bone, a typical example being of a vertebra (Fig. 4.7). Often associated with osteoporosis in later life, it causes underlying weakness of the bone structure, and the individual vertebral body collapses into a wedge shape. Crush fractures are also commonly found on the joint surfaces. A further type of direct trauma is that of penetration, where the cortex is completely or partially penetrated and fractured, possibly into many

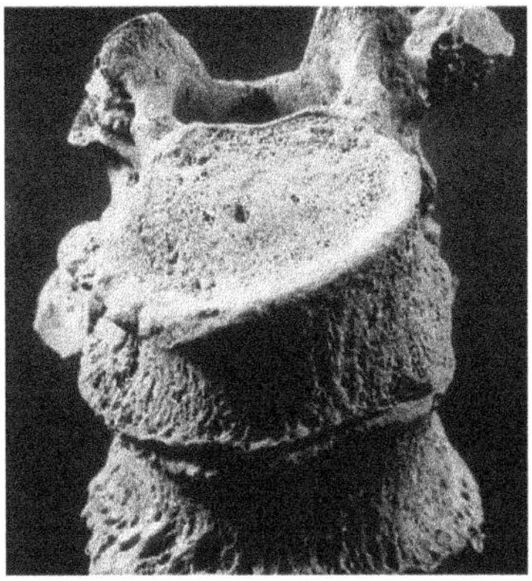

Figure 4.7. Compression fractures of the vertebrae in an individual from twelfth–sixteenth centuries CE, France. Photograph by and courtesy of Jean Brown.

pieces; this would then be called a comminuted fracture. These injuries are the result of the impact of a "large force to a small area" (Lovell 1997, 141), for example, injuries from the metal blade of a weapon or a flint projectile point.

In children, the pliable, or plastic, nature of immature bone means long bone fractures are usually incomplete and tend to heal rapidly without deformity (Lewis 2018, 91). The most common fractures occurring in children are greenstick, plastic deformation, torus or buckle, and metaphyseal (or physeal) affecting the cartilaginous growth plate (Lewis 2018, 92; also see Verlinden and Lewis 2015). Angular or rotational forces produce greenstick (incomplete) fractures; these partial fractures develop bowing on the compressed side, with the fracture on the tensile side. Plastic deformation is caused by excessive vertical compression; torus or buckle fractures involve "buckling" of the cortex due to compression along the diaphyseal/metaphyseal junction; and physeal (or metaphyseal) fractures can affect the cartilage or both cartilage and bone within a joint. Particular age-related fracture patterns can be present in children (e.g., birth trauma, or when children become more mobile; Lewis 2018, 110). The adolescent growth spurt also makes the growth plate more vulnerable to damage and slippage of the epiphysis (Resnick et al. 2024, 53–54). Children and adolescents who are obese, and the physically active, are more vulnerable to increased shearing stresses on the epiphysis. There have been few reports of slipped epiphyses in the paleopathological literature (see Lewis 2018, 112, for a summary in nonadults), although Knüsel et al. (1992) described the condition in the femur of an adult skeleton of a priest buried in the cemetery of a late medieval hospital in North Yorkshire, England.

All fractures belong to one of two categories, closed or open. Closed fractures are those in which there is no connection between the outer skin surface and the fractured bone itself. Open (or compound) fractures are those in which there is an open connection between the fracture site and the skin surface. This communication allows transmission of pathogenic organisms to the bone and development of acute painful osteomyelitis. Fractures can therefore potentially be infected, a problem even in modern medical practice. In the past, without the benefit of antibiotics, such an infection in a severely injured person may have been transferred to the bloodstream (sepsis) and caused death. Well-healed infected fractures have been noted in the archaeological record, and those individuals fortunate enough to survive may have been left with a chronic osteomyelitis (see Chapter 6). In studying of skeletal remains, the absence of the soft tissues means that placing a fracture into one or another category is largely inferential unless clear evidence of associated infection is present. Care should be exercised in diagnosis because infection may have been present in the bone before the fracture occurred.

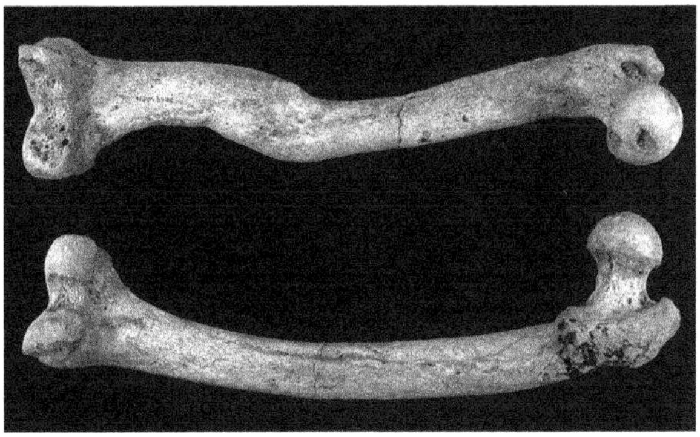

Figure 4.8. Healed fracture to the left femur (top) in a male with underlying Paget's disease, shown with the nonfractured opposite femur (bottom) (eighth–tenth centuries CE, Jarrow, Tyne and Wear, England). Photograph by and courtesy of Jeff Veitch.

There are three major causes of fractures: acute injury (e.g., a skiing accident, in a modern context); underlying disease (pathological fracture), which weakens the bone and makes it more susceptible to fracture (e.g., tumor of a bone, osteoporosis); and repeated stress (e.g., in athletes; see Resnick 2024, 34, for a list of activities that lead to stress fractures at specific locations in the body). In people with stress fractures, there is often no history of direct injury, and pain will increase if the activity continues. Many stress fractures are "hairline" in nature and are difficult to diagnose, even using radiography. Further, once they heal there may be no evidence left to see, and in an archaeological context identifying this type of fracture may be difficult, if not impossible.

Pathological fractures may be induced by general or localized disease in the body. A good example of a pathologically weakened bone with an associated fracture was found in the femur of an individual from the cemetery associated with Jarrow monastery, northeast England (Wells and Woodhouse 1975: early medieval, seventh century CE; Fig. 4.8). The skeleton also displayed Paget's disease (see Chapter 7), although one must consider the possibility that Paget's disease developed after the fracture had occurred, which may have been unrelated to the disease. Examples of a stress fracture related to repetitive activity are those that affect the fourth metatarsal bones. These can develop during long-distance walking or marching ("march fractures"). Small transverse fractures of localized cortical areas of the tibial shaft are today also associated with repetitive brisk walking, running, and cycling. These are clinically insignificant and do not lead to prolonged tibial pain, although localized cortical tenderness and swelling may be a feature. These lesions, known colloquially as "shin splints," are unlikely to be diagnosed without radiography.

Fracture Healing

Following a fracture, healing normally takes place through three phases of differing duration. In general terms, the time taken for a fracture to heal depends on the bone fractured and the type and position of the fracture. It is also affected by the fracture's severity, the relative apposition of the fractured fragments, stability of the fragments during healing, age and nutritional status of the individual, presence or absence of infection or other pathological processes, blood supply to the area affected, and access to treatment. Fractures in the young tend to heal faster and more efficiently than in adults. This is because their bones are constantly growing with osteoblasts continually laying down bone. If they sustain a fracture, osteoblasts are immediately directed to the break. Once healed, they may not be visible even macroscopically or radiographically (Kleinman and Walters 2015). Upper limb fractures also heal faster than those of the lower limb, and long bone fractures heal more rapidly than cranial fractures.

The three phases of healing, and the relative percent of the healing process that they contribute, are (1) inflammatory (ca. 10%); (2) reparative (ca. 40%); and (3) remodeling (as much as 70% of the healing process) (Resnick 2024, 27–28). Initially, blood seeps out from the fractured ends of the bone and forms a hematoma around and between the fractured bone ends. Severed blood vessels contract and become sealed with blood clots; this occurs within approximately 12 hours after the fracture. Bone adjacent to the fracture dies (necrosis). The reparative phase consists of invasion of the hematoma by fibrovascular tissue, which lays down collagen fibers that are mineralized into a primary callus (Latin: *callum* = hard). The callus stabilizes the fracture by uniting the bone ends. The final phase (remodeling) involves realignment and remodeling of the bone along the lines of stress. Excess callus is absorbed, and bone trabeculae develop. Lamellar bone eventually replaces the fiber (or woven) bone that had formed the primary callus. Remodeling occurs over many years, with eventual restoration of the normal architecture of the bone to its original appearance, even on a radiograph. The three dynamic phases overlap in time, and the healing process is completed at different times for different bones of the body. Radiography aids considerably in the interpretation of fractures in both the living and the dead (Roberts 1989), particularly in assessing the mechanism behind the injury (i.e., type of fracture) and the state of healing of the fractured bone (Fig. 4.9).

In archaeological contexts, taking accurate measurements of angulation, apposition (how much of the fractured fragments are in apposition, or side by side),

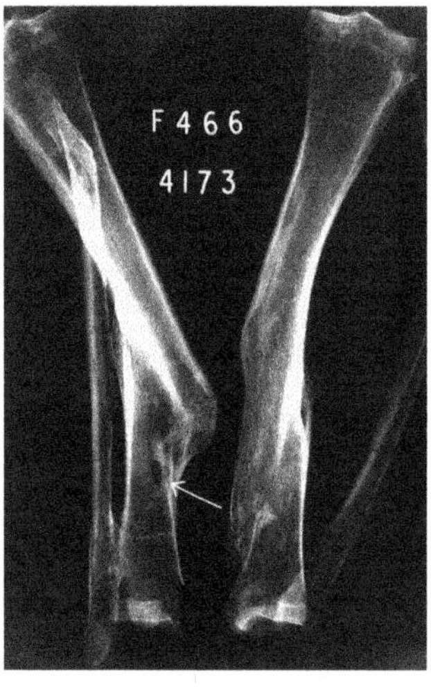

Figure 4.9. Radiograph of fractures to the tibiae and fibulae in an adult male showing healing, but with associated angulation and osteomyelitis (hole arrowed), indicating this was originally an open fracture. The tibial fractures, both of which are oblique, are associated with contrecoup fractures at the proximal ends of the fibulae (fourth century CE, Baldock, Hertfordshire, England). Photograph by and courtesy of Jean Brown.

and overlap of the fracture fragments is possible using radiographs (see Grauer and Roberts 1996 for an example). DeBoer et al. (2015) provided a detailed list of the features to identify in the healing process in adults using a combination of radiography and histology, along with time since fracture. They recommend using (destructive) histological analysis to assess time interval since fracture. Lewis (2018) advised using a reduction of these healing times if studying skeletal remains of children. However, there is little information on how much the healing time of different bones is reduced for children compared to adults; Lewis (2018, 98) recommended using DeBoer's (2015) table as a "rough guide."

Fracture Complications

Several fracture complications can occur at the time of the injury or years later, some of which can be assessed through analysis of skeletal remains. Compound fractures can lead potentially to (nonspecific) infection of the fracture site (e.g., osteomyelitis), which can delay healing. If a fracture is not adequately reduced manually or by traction (i.e., the bone ends are not pulled apart and "set" in the correct anatomical position), shortening of the affected limb and malalignment of the fractured ends can occur. This could lead to joint degeneration and osteoarthritis (see Chapter 5) due to altered stresses through the affected limb. Osteoarthritis may also occur if a fracture line extends into a joint (Waldron 2021, 214). It is also worth noting, however, that joint degeneration, like infection, may have already been present in the bone before the fracture occurred. It is also possible to confuse a cloaca (draining sinus) resulting from osteomyelitis associated with an open fracture, with a hole left after the postmortem decay of soft tissue that was originally incorporated into the fracture at the time of the injury, or during the healing process. Damage to the blood vessels and nerves can also occur in relation to fractures in certain parts of the body (Hamblen and Simpson 2007). For example, a fracture to the neck of the femur can interrupt, to varying degrees, the blood supply and cause avascular necrosis of the femoral head and delay to the normal healing process, or even non-union. A fracture to the mid to mid-distal part of the humeral shaft can damage the radial nerve and cause weakness (palsy) of the forearm and hands, as well as sensory dysfunction; this can happen in around 12% of these humeral fractures (Schwab et al. 2018). Two fracture complications are specific to children: premature fusion of the epiphyses with subsequent growth arrest (shortening), and in cases of metaphyseal trauma where the epiphyses are spared, accelerated growth of the bone (overgrowth) due to an increased blood supply to the area of fracture during healing (Lewis 2018, 96–97).

In archaeological contexts, many of these fracture complications cannot be observed directly and are only surmised from the position of the fracture. For example, in some fractures fat globules can be released from the medullary cavity, causing fatty deposits (fat emboli), which pass into the bloodstream and may cause obstruction of arteries and arterioles in the brain, lungs, and viscera, with death of tissues. Non-union of fractures in antiquity has been observed, but care must

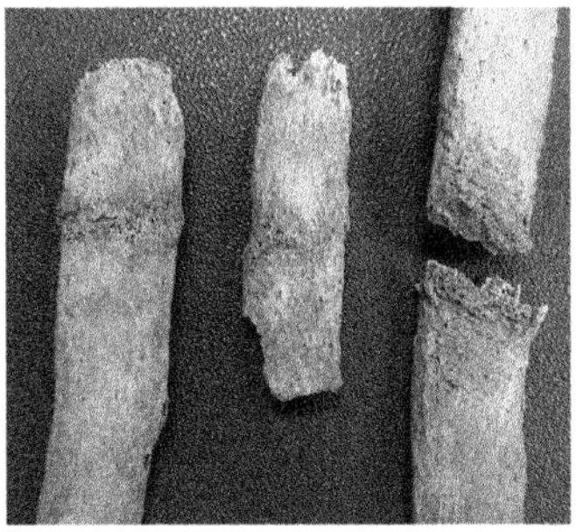

Figure 4.10. Healed, healing, and non-union (right) of rib fractures. Note the formation of new bone at the fractured ends indicating the person died during the healing process before the rib on the right had the chance to heal (twelfth–sixteenth centuries CE, Fishergate House, York, England). Photograph by Charlotte Roberts.

be taken in differentiating between true non-union (i.e., not healed in the time expected for a specific bone) and *delayed* union at the time of death, the latter suggesting that there had been insufficient time for the fracture to heal before the person died. Today, non-union is commonly seen in fractures to the femoral neck and in the shafts of the forearm bones; the most common causes include malnutrition, infection, poor blood supply, and inadequate reduction of the fracture and/or immobilization while the fracture healed. The bone that suffers most frequently from non-union is the ulna shaft, probably because of imperfect immobilization (Hamblen and Simpson 2007), but other bones such as the ribs can be affected (Fig. 4.10). Recognition of non-union is possible, particularly if the fracture fragments display new bone formation of an attempted callus at the ununited ends or some opacity of their fractured ends on a radiograph, indicating the body's attempt to heal the fracture. A false joint, or pseudoarthrosis, may occur in some cases too.

Limitations of Trauma Study

There are several limitations to note in the interpretation of fracture data in paleopathology. Modern population studies can look at the real age distribution of fractures, but in archaeological groups this is not possible. Even though an individual with a healed fracture would have died at a certain age, this does not mean that the fracture was sustained at that age. The fracture could have occurred many years before the death of the individual, although if the fracture displays early stages of healing, then the age at death will be close to the age when the fracture occurred. Of course, people who live into later life have more time to experience multiple instances of trauma (recidivism), and so might be expected to display more fractures. By contrast, nonadults have had less time to become injured and, when they do, their fractures are more subtle or partial (greenstick) and tend to heal without deformity. Hence the pattern of trauma seen across a group may be more a reflection of the age profile of that group than the true rates of trauma experienced. To try and combat some of these limitations in younger individuals, Glencross and Stuart-Macadam (2000) and Glencross (2011) first identified childhood fractures in adults where the trauma led to fusion of the growth plate, and Verlinden and Lewis (2015) provided a list of new features to help identify the more subtle signs of trauma in the young. Perimortem fractures (at or around the time of death) are also a challenge to interpret. If there was no time for healing to take place before the individual died, these fractures may look like postmortem breaks and thus not be identified as antemortem injury.

In published studies of fractures in living populations, each fracture usually represents one individual, and rates of fractures per 1,000, 10,000, or 100,000 individuals can be produced. In an archaeological context, fracture rates are usually presented as (1) the percentage of the total bones affected that were examined; (2) the frequency of individual skeletal elements affected (e.g., percent of total femora observed—TPR); and (3) the percentage of individual skeletons with fractures (CPR). These measures, however, assume that all bones of the skeleton were present to be recorded. It is also difficult to know whether, if an individual has a fractured radius, for example, there was an associated fracture to the ulna if this bone has not survived burial to be examined. Therefore, problems arise with comparing fracture prevalence between ancient and modern populations; clearly, for modern groups all the bones of the skeleton are usually present to observe, whereas in an archaeological population they are not.

Fractures: Early Humans and Living Populations

Studies of trauma in much earlier humans have been limited, possibly because of the relative lack of skeletal remains recovered for these distant time periods. There have been some focused studies of Neanderthal populations. In 1995, Berger and Trinkaus suggested that trauma patterns they observed had the greatest similarity to rodeo performers, with a high risk of head and neck injury. Berger and Trinkaus suggested interpersonal violence, attacks by wild animals, and the fact that these hunter-foragers were always on the move as the key underlying behavioral risk factors contributing to the observations made. In collating the evidence for cranial trauma in western Eurasia (80–20,000 BCE) from Upper Paleolithic early modern humans (37 sites) and Neanderthal remains (30 sites), Beier et al. (2018) found similar levels of trauma in both groups, dismissing the hypothesis that Neanderthals alone were highly traumatized.

Fracture rates in both ancient and modern human populations reflect both intentional violence and accidental injury (see Judd 2004, on a comparison of past and present injury). Technological advances have changed rapidly through time as we have transitioned from being hunter-foragers to being farmers, and then become urbanized and industrialized. Clinical studies illustrate the complex nature of variables underlying the patterns of trauma seen today in different populations. We have been, and are, subject to many different risk factors for injury, varying across time and space, but high-impact road-traffic accidents and injuries sustained through work particularly face populations today.

In their classic early study of fracture patterning across the life course in over 8,500 admissions to an Oxford hospital in England (1953 and 1957), Buhr and Cooke (1959) divided their data into four fracture pattern groups: (1) the "wage-earners": mainly males; with fractures to the hands and feet; (2) "post-wage-earners": older people of both sexes who had a high frequency of proximal humerus and femur fractures; (3) the "pre-wage-earners": mainly young males with tibial shaft fractures; and (4) a "composite group" made up of people in their youth as well as older males and females. This study confirmed that people of both sexes in the 1950s were differentially affected by fractures through their life span. In a later study by Fife and Barancik (1985), of 8,177 people from northeast Ohio, United States, 11% (n = 877) had fractures, and 59% of these were in males. Researchers identified fracture rates of 26 per 1,000 for males and 16 per 1,000 for females. Two peaks of age-related trauma were found, at 10–14 years and in people over 60 years, although male fractures exceeded female fractures until the age of 50 years. Some 46% of the injuries were caused by falls, but in the over-65-year-olds this rose to 87% of the fractures. Other causes were road-traffic accidents (9% and mostly in the younger age groups), work-related accidents (8%), assaults (5%), and bicycle accidents (3%). However, 18% of fractures were sustained in the context of sport (by falls or being struck by objects).

While age, biological sex, and "occupation" in its broadest sense clearly have an effect on fracture patterns, the impact of climate and the weather may also generate risk for fractures. One could argue that people in countries with particularly harsh climates have probably adapted to these situations by introducing measures to prevent accidents, whereas people who do not usually experience those hazards may be caught out by rare weather conditions. For example, in Cardiff, Wales, in 1978 and 1979 the streets were sometimes covered with ice and hard-packed snow, predisposing people to falls (Al-Azzani et al. 2016). During that time, fractures were three times greater when compared to a control group, and forearm fractures were 16.5 times more common.

Today, fractures represent a serious economic burden in most countries across the world, resulting in work absences and decreased productivity, as well as high health care costs, disability, and an impaired quality of life (Global Burden of Disease 2021). A global, regional, and national review of the incidence and prevalence of fractures sustained between 1991 and 2019 showed a 33.4% increase in fracture rates (n = 178 million) over time. Fractures occurred with increasing frequency in three anatomical sites: the patella, tibia or fibula; the radius or ulna, or both; and the clavicle, scapula, or humerus (Global Burden of Disease 2021). Males overall had the higher fracture rates, but equally high rates were seen in the older females (likely related to postmenopausal bone loss; see Chapter 7). Males were more likely to sustain sports-related injuries, be subject to interpersonal violence, and have road accidents. The highest prevalence rates by country were in New Zealand, Slovenia, and Australia. The three regions with the lowest age-standardized incidence rates were central, western, and southern sub-Saharan Africa, and the lowest rates overall were seen in North Korea, Liberia, and Zimbabwe (Global Burden of Disease 2021). Many epidemiological factors contributed to these patterns, but taking a broad view of fractures brings together a lot of data that can be used to inform future health and social care policies.

In a more focused retrospective study of patients seen by the Orthopaedic Trauma Unit of the Royal Infirmary of Edinburgh, Scotland, in 2000, there were almost 6,000 fractures in patients aged 12 years and above (Court-Brown and Caesar 2006). The average age of those affected was 49.1 years, with half being male and half being female patients. Incidence rates were 11.67 per 1,000 per year in males and 10.65 per 1,000 per year for females. Females had similar fracture rates for all age groups until menopause, while males had more fractures at a young age, which gradually declined until 60 years of age, at which point they rose again. Fractures of the distal radius, proximal femur, hand phalanges, and ankle bones contributed 60% of the total fractures observed. Similarly, in exploring fractures in 550,000 people between 2015–2018, Bergh et al. (2020) used data from the Swedish Fracture Register, which collects data at the point of seeking care for a fracture. Mean age at fracture occurrence was 57.9 years (range 16 to 105 years), and females represented two-thirds of the fractures.

Genetic differences may also influence who experiences trauma. Bao et al. (2023) carried out the first study of the quantitative evidence for the association between genetic ancestry and the risk of fractures. They demonstrated that White Americans in the United States had a higher fracture risk than African, Hispanic, Asian, and Indigenous Americans. African Americans in particular had a low risk of fracture. Differences in life expectancy at birth and greater bone mineral density in people of African ancestry were suggested as explanations, but it is important to note the limitations of the analytical side of this study. (1) There was substantial to considerable heterogeneity in all of the analyses; (2) the meta-analyses pooled several measures of effect sizes together; (3) most studies did not account for many established confounders known to influence fracture risks; (4) the study focused on ancestral groups in the US only, which may not be applicable to other countries and have different degrees of fracture risk (Bao et al. 2023, 13). There are also clinical data from populations who live in different environments. For example, Jónsson et al. (1993) studied lifestyle and fracture prevalence in Swedish populations from urban and rural environments and found a lower fracture rate in the urban environment. This was explained by the increased risk rural populations would have been exposed to during their everyday activities. Jónsson et al. (1992), however, showed an opposite trend and attributed the lower rate of fractures in their rural population to continued physical activity and its preventive effects against low bone mineral density and fracture. In a further study of urban and rural differences (Olmsted County, Minnesota, United States, 1980–1989), Madhok et al. (1993) found that hip fractures were 36% more common in the urban group from the city of Rochester. They suggested that urban populations were less healthy generally and had more medical problems, which could have led to loss of bone mass, osteoporosis, and the risk of falls.

Although we can use some of these clinical data as a comparison for our archaeological populations to try to understand why they sustained fractures, specific data that relate to the causes of fractures in the past are harder to determine because modern technological advances causing fractures are not relevant. The closer interaction between animals and humans in past societies would also have had its dangers. Nevertheless, studies of injuries sustained by people as a result of encounters with animals do appear in the clinical literature. Jones (1990) studied three years of admissions to the hospital by the Amish community of mid-eastern Ohio. The Amish are a group of people whose religious beliefs disallow the use of many modern conveniences, including cars and electricity, and thus they may be, to a certain extent, considered closer to our archaeological communities in terms of health than a "typical" rural population. Of the injuries observed, 26.7% were cattle or horse related. Another study in the United States of agriculture-related injuries, this one in Wisconsin over 12 years, found that a majority of trauma was caused by animals (30%)—falls from horses and encounters with uncontrollable horses and cattle. Some 22% of the 739 individuals affected were left with significant neurological, pulmonary, or orthopedic disability (Cogbill et al. 1991).

Fractures to Different Bones: Past and Present

Starting with the long bones, the humerus may be fractured at its neck, greater tuberosity, shaft, supracondylar area, the condyles, or the epicondyles. Fractures to the humerus are not frequently seen archaeologically compared to some other bones, but in populations today the shaft (usually mid-third and caused by an indirect twisting/direct injury) and neck (seen in older women with osteoporosis and caused by a fall on the limb) are most commonly affected (Hamblen and Simpson 2007). In children aged between birth and seven years, fractures to the distal humerus made up the majority of fractures (65%) in 6,493 children from modern-day Hong Kong (Cheng et al. 1999). Today, fractures to the radius and ulna (wrist) are the most common upper limb fracture (Pradhan et al. 2022). Fractures to these bones are also common archaeologically. Various parts of these bones may be broken (e.g., the head, shaft, and distal end of the radius; and the olecranon, coronoid process, and shaft of the ulna). Fractures to the shaft of the ulna may represent interpersonal violence caused by raising the arm to shield a blow to the face or head, or a so-called parry fracture (see later in this chapter), or they could equally be caused by a fall on the arm (Judd 2008). Colles (distal shaft) fractures to the radius, again often with underlying osteoporosis, are usually the result of a fall on the outstretched hand (Hamblen and Simpson 2007). They have posterior displacement and are the most common fracture in adolescents and adults in the Western world (Longo et al. 2023). They are also frequently seen in skeletal remains (Mays 2006).

Fractures of the femur may occur at the femoral neck, between the greater and lesser trochanters, the shaft, the condyles (rare), or the supracondylar area of the shaft (Crawford-Adams 1983, 204). Fractured femora at the neck or trochanteric region are common in older females with underlying osteoporosis, often as a result of a fall. Fractures in this region today can be repaired with internal fixation, using screws, plates, and rods, or with hip replacement, none of these options being available for our predecessors. Fractures to the shaft of the femur follow severe trauma and can occur at any age—for example, in a road-traffic accident (see a clinical study of pelvic and femoral fractures by Lundin et al. 2021, and hip fractures in urban eighteenth- and nineteenth-century urban England by Ives et al. 2017). Shaft fracture fragments can be very displaced, and muscle can become interposed between the fragments as the fracture heals (Hamblen and Simpson 2007). Fractures to the patella are caused by a force hitting the knee, a fall, or a sudden violent contraction of the quadriceps muscle while trying to maintain balance during a fall. They are rare in archaeological populations, and in people today, making up only 1% of all skeletal injuries (Henrichsen et al. 2018). Fractures of the tibia and fibula can occur together; fractures to the fibula alone normally affect the distal end/ankle (Hamblen and Simpson 2007). After the age of two years, when children begin to walk, "toddler's fractures" may occur in the distal tibia as a result of a fall twisting the ankle while the knee is fixed (Heinrich 2001), but these injuries are subtle, heal well, and are easy to miss in the archaeological record. High-velocity motorcycle accidents are by far the commonest single cause of major fractures to the shafts of the tibia and fibula today (Hamblen and Simpson 2007), not something that would have been a problem in the past. Fractures to these bones tend to be focused on the ankle, and so the very distal parts of these bones are the most fractured parts; ligament injuries occur alongside the fractures. Fractures of both bones may be at the same level if there is a direct blow to the bone, but if it is a spiral force (indirect twisting injury) then the opposite ends of the two bones are usually affected. These diametrically opposite fractures of the tibia and fibula are termed contrecoup fractures.

Of course, fractures to parts of the skeleton other than the long bones are observed in living and ancient populations, but reports of fractures to the hands and feet are infrequent in the latter; this may be partly explained by the relatively poor survival or incomplete excavation of these bones in archaeological contexts. The scaphoid bone, however, can be fractured by falling on an outstretched hand (usually in young adults). The rest of the carpals are rarely fractured (Hamblen and Simpson 2007), although Wakely and Young (1995) described a fractured hamate bone of the wrist in a late medieval male from Abingdon, Berkshire, England. These fractures are usually caused by a crushing injury from a fall onto the hand, or today from "gripping and swinging a golf club"—(Wakely and Young 1995, 53). The base of the first metacarpal can be fractured in boxing, as can the other metacarpals, and may involve the proximal joint surface or not (Hamblen and Simpson 2007). Metacarpophalangeal fractures may also indicate defensive wounds from interpersonal violence. Fractures to the tarsal bones include compression injuries to the talus and calcaneus caused by a fall from a height and landing on the feet (Hamblen and Simpson 2007). Axial loading to the calcaneus due to a fall frequently causes a crush fracture and destruction of the medullary trabecular bone structure, and does not heal well. The metatarsals can be fractured through their shafts, usually by a weight dropping on the foot, a twisting injury, or by repeated stress (the march fracture). Fractures to the shafts of the phalanges of the foot are also usually caused by heavy objects landing on the toes (Hamblen and Simpson 2007), and several examples have been identified in past populations (Lorentz and Casa 2020; Dittmar et al. 2021a).

Fractures involving the pelvis are rare in paleopathology, probably because today they occur most frequently following high-impact road-traffic accidents. Nevertheless, Guimarey Duarte et al. (2023) have described two females excavated in Aswan, Egypt, with pelvic trauma (1980–1760 BCE). Damage to the abdominal structures, particularly the gastrointestinal and genitourinary viscera, was a serious complication potentially experienced by these females. Sternal fractures (especially associated with anterior rib fractures) and scapula fractures are also rare in paleopathological studies, but, when they are seen, they may indicate a blow to the back or chest of the individual as a result of interpersonal violence (Morgan et al. 2022; Fig. 4.11a–b). Sternal fractures in clinical contexts tend to be associated with deceleration injuries and blunt chest trauma, often occurring in road-traffic accidents (Khoriati et al. 2013). Scapula fractures comprise around 1% of all fractures (Cole et al. 2013). Unfortunately, in archaeological contexts the scapula is often damaged during burial or excavation, especially in the scapula blade area (where the majority of fractures occur). Therefore, the frequency of this fracture is probably underestimated (but see Blondiaux et al. 2012). Fractures to the acromion of the scapula have been recorded in archaeological contexts, but distinguishing between a true fracture and non-union, and developmental nonfusion of the acromial epiphysis (os acromiale), perhaps because of a specific physical activity, is challenging (see Chapter 5).

The clavicle is usually broken by falling onto the shoulder (Hamblen and Simpson 2007) or as the result of a birthing injury (Ahn et al. 2015). This fracture is seen regularly in paleopathology. Along with rib fractures (again, commonly observed), even in modern contexts clavicle fractures are often left to heal without therapeutic intervention, that is, conservatively, although today surgical intervention is used when the fracture is displaced (Frima et al. 2020). The two main causes of rib fractures are falls and a direct blow to the rib cage, although constant coughing or sneezing can break ribs. Damage to underlying soft tissues, such as the lung, may be a complication. Fractured adult ribs are commonly observed in paleopathology (see Brickley 2006 and Matos 2009a, for two of the few population studies). While rib fractures are rarely reported in nonadults, Lewis (2018, 108) notes that they are frequent in children today who have been subject to caregiver violence; the posterior aspects of the ribs are usually affected as a result of squeezing the chest. On the other hand, anterior rib fractures are usually related to accidental injury in children.

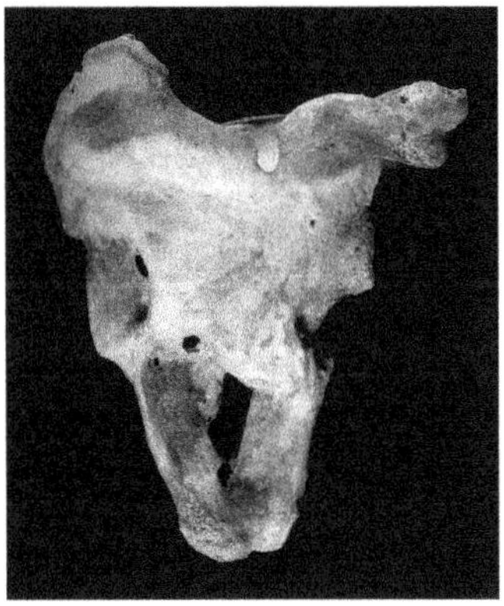

Figure 4.11a. Healed fracture of the scapula blade in a mature male from postmedieval St. Bride's Lower Churchyard, London. Anterior view. © Museum of London.

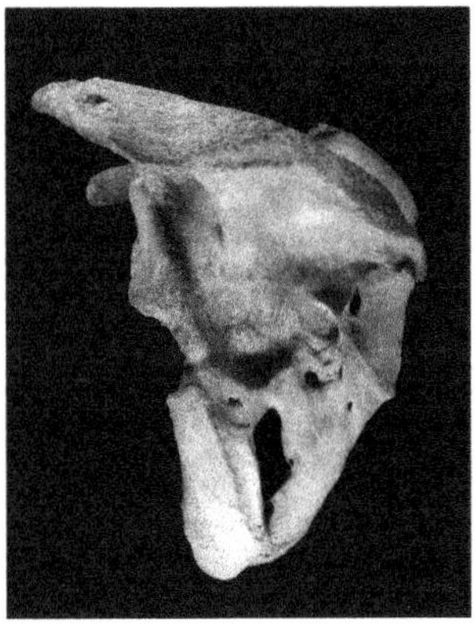

Figure 4.11b. Healed fracture of the scapula blade in a mature male from postmedieval St. Bride's Lower Churchyard, London. Posterior view. © Museum of London.

Trauma in the vertebral bodies of the spine can result from a vertical-force-induced hyperflexion injury, such as jumping from a height onto the feet, causing compression fractures, and ultimately scoliosis and/or kyphosis (Hamblen and Simpson 2007). Often, underlying osteoporosis may lead to weakness and subsequent fracture through these mechanisms. Merbs (1983) reported that 36 of 80 adult vertebral columns of Sadlermiut Inuit individuals (Hudson Bay, northeastern Canada) had vertebral compression fractures (third thoracic to fifth lumbar vertebrae). The frequency was higher in females. The reasoning suggested for this finding was that females traditionally rode on sleds and toboggans over rough terrain, which led to compressive forces that were transmitted through the spine. Females also carried their children on their backs. Postmenopausal females may also have had underlying osteoporosis that predisposed them to trauma and subsequent fractures. Legge (2010) also found similar damage in the spines of Alaskan Inuit from Golovin Bay and Nunivak Island, Alaska, and particularly in females. Using kayaks and umiaks (open skin boats) on rough seas was suggested as a potential cause for the patterns seen.

Compression fractures can also occur in the cervical spine and, although less frequent, they are more serious (Hamblen and Simpson 2007). Often associated with subluxation, or partial dislocation of vertebrae, they convey an increased risk of damage to the spinal cord in the neck. Fracture-dislocation to the second and/or third cervical vertebrae (C2 and C3) has been consistently referred to as the "hangman's fracture" (Resnick et al. 2024, 1265). As Resnick et al. (2024, 2853) noted, despite its popular name, the injury today "typically results from a motor vehicle accident or a fall." No examples have been reported archaeologically, but examination of three series of criminals executed by hanging between 1882 and 1945 (34 bodies) revealed that fracture-dislocation of C2 and C3 (or traumatic spondylolisthesis of the axis) was the "exception rather than the rule" (James and Nasmyth-Jones 1992, 91). Fractures of the spinous processes at the levels of the seventh cervical and first thoracic vertebrae are termed clay-shoveler's fractures (Knüsel et al. 1996) because the combined actions of the trapezius and rhomboid muscles during shoveling initiate this fracture. Such a finding may help identify occupations using this action in the archaeological record, although there have been few reports to date in paleopathology (e.g., see Jordana et al. 2006). Fig. 4.12 shows an unhealed example.

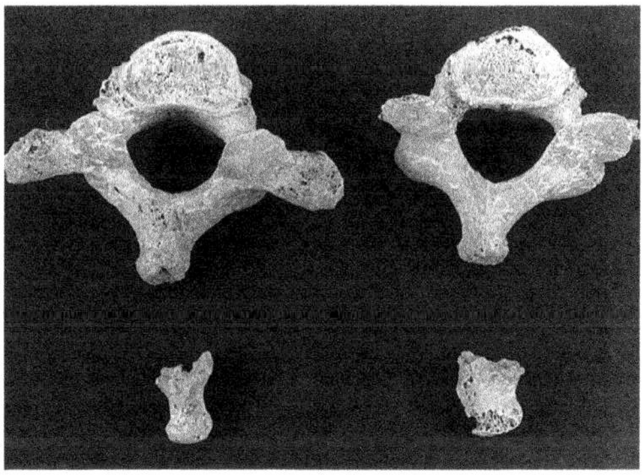

Figure 4.12. Unhealed "clay-shoveler's" fractures to the spinous processes of the seventh cervical and first thoracic vertebrae of an adult male from fourth century CE, Baldock, Hertfordshire, England. Photograph by and courtesy of Jean Brown.

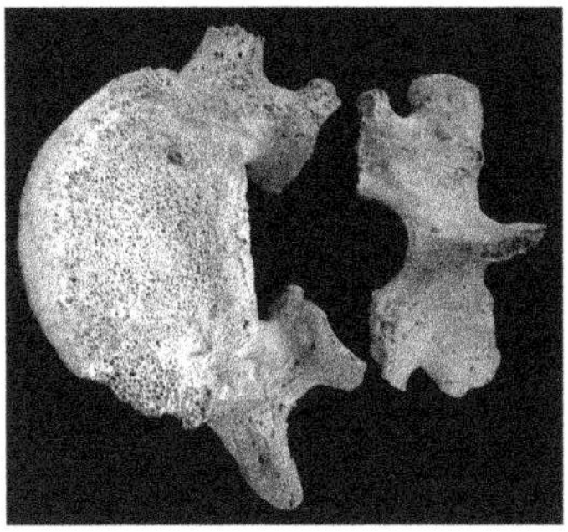

Figure 4.13. Unhealed spondylolysis of a fifth lumbar vertebra in a young, possibly male individual from Mis Island, fourth Nile Cataract, Nubia (500–1500 CE). Photograph courtesy of Sam Tipper.

A special type of vertebral fracture, which is seen in many periods of antiquity, may have its roots in a congenital weakness of a small area of bone on the vertebrae. This condition, known as spondylolysis, is recognized in skeletal remains as the separation of a single vertebra into two parts (see also Chapter 2). It is essentially a stress or fatigue fracture, and the weakness of the bone is at the position between the upper and lower joint surfaces on the neural arch, or that part of the vertebra lying behind its solid central body and surrounding the spinal cord (Leone et al. 2011). Today, it is most frequently seen in the lumbar spine of adolescents, and especially in athletes. It is thought to be caused by developmental or acquired stresses at the site of weakness—for example, bending and lifting with an upright posture. It is only seen in humans and is related to bipedalism and an erect posture (Plomp et al. 2020a). In their study of the fifth lumbar vertebra, Plomp et al. (2020a) found that the shape of healthy vertebrae was different from those affected by spondylolysis, and the researchers concluded that spondylolysis is an adaptive evolutionary trait that developed as humans became bipeds. It develops after a child starts to walk, and it is more common in males, although with increased participation of females in sport its incidence in females is rising (Li et al. 2022). Spondylolysis results from repetitive, vigorous movements of the lower back—for example, in football, weightlifting, dancing, kayaking, wrestling, and gymnastics. Ultimately, the bone at the site fractures partially or entirely, with the neural arch separating from the vertebral body. The only link remaining is ligament and fibrous tissue. Generally speaking, many of these fractures do not heal, probably, as Merbs (1989, 170) suggested, because of continual stress at the site, although today conservative treatment has led to healing (Choi et al. 2022). Most evidence occurs at the fifth lumbar vertebra, less commonly at the fourth, and occasionally elsewhere (Fig. 4.13).

Merbs (2002, 156) noted that asymmetrical spondylolysis is "part of the earliest picture of spondylolysis." If this happens, the right side is most affected, which, Merbs suggests, may be related to handedness. The end result, asymmetrical spondylolysis, may develop into a bilateral lesion, the asymmetrical lesion may heal, or it may develop into spondylolisthesis (discussed below). The modern incidence of the condition has been reported to be around 3–6% of populations, with variation in subgroups such as males, females, and African Americans (Standaert and Herring 2000). The incidence in Inuit groups may be up to 50%, a frequency that has been attributed to their usually physically arduous existence. Numerous bioarchaeological studies of spondylolysis are synthesized in D'Angelo del Campo et al. (2017). For example, in their study of southern Patagonian hunter-forager skeletons, they found a mean frequency of 20%, and a range of 11–25% across sites. Comparative site frequencies from four North American, three European, one African, two Asian, and five Oceanian sites ranged from 0 to 71%; these compare to a range of 3–5% for living populations. In a study of 515 skeletons from the Meroitic period of Nubia (350 BCE–1500 CE), Tipper et al. (2023) found 6.6% of individuals with spines preserved for analysis were affected (crude prevalence), and a frequency of 1.2% of preserved lumbar vertebrae (true prevalence). As D'Angelo del Campo et al. (2017) explained, reliably comparing frequency rates for spondylolysis is challenging because not all authors use the same methods to record and present their data.

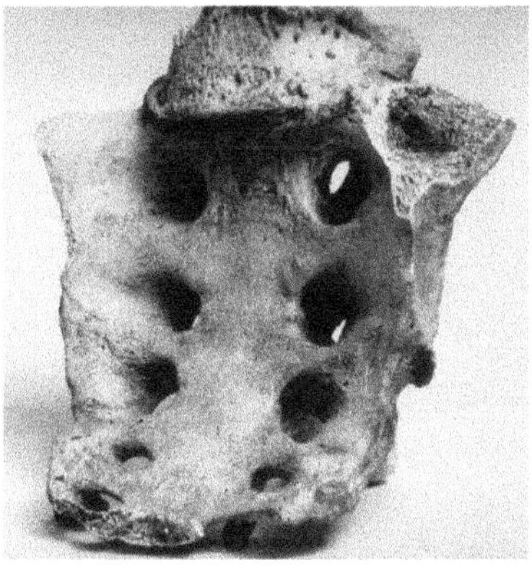

Figure 4.14. Spondylolisthesis with fusion of the fifth lumbar vertebra to the sacrum in an adult female from Eccles, Kent, England (sixth–eighth centuries CE). Photograph by and courtesy of Jean Brown.

Apart from slight, constant, lower back discomfort, spondylolysis causes no symptoms unless it is associated with a dislocation of the now unstable vertebral body. This condition, termed spondylolisthesis, is a serious abnormality and a complication of trauma. Although uncommon, it was no doubt present in the past and can cause compression of the corda equina and neuropathic consequences, such as problems with bowel and bladder function. The corda equina is a group of nerve roots that leaves the lower part of the spinal cord in between the vertebrae to serve other parts of the body. The recognition of the abnormality in skeletons from archaeological sites is difficult and rests upon the observation of bone formation along the rims of the displaced vertebral bodies (Gagnet et al. 2018), or eburnation (polishing) that suggests movement between the joints. Fusion by bone of the displaced vertebra upon its neighbor may also occur. A rare example of spondylolisthesis (Fig. 4.14) shows the condition in an early medieval individual from Kent, England, in which bony fusion between the anteriorly displaced fifth lumbar vertebra and the sacrum has occurred (Manchester 1982). This natural process occurring in antiquity has achieved fusion, albeit in a poor position, a process that modern orthopedic surgical practice sometimes endeavors to do.

Recording Long Bone Fractures

As we turn to a consideration of archaeological data on trauma, we should first talk about recording of fractures. If fracture frequencies are to be compared between skeletal populations on a local, regional, national, or global scale, it is essential that methods of recording used by researchers are the same (as with any other pathological lesion). First, a detailed description of the fracture should be made, including the bone affected, side if appropriate, position of fracture on the bone, type of fracture, any evidence of underlying pathology, features of healing including any problems visible (e.g., linear angulation, spiral deformity, poor apposition and overlap of fragments), and complications evident (see table 9.4 in Redfern and Roberts 2019, 234). It is also particularly important to describe whether the apparent injury is antemortem (healed), perimortem, or actually a postmortem bone change (i.e., taphonomic). Complementary to macroscopic recording, radiographic and histological analyses can be used to detail the inside of the bone at both macroscopic and microscopic levels (if available). They are also helpful for revealing features related to healing: linear angulation, spiral deformity, poor apposition, and overlap of fragments. Radiography includes X-ray and other imaging techniques, such as computerized tomography (CT) and micro-CT. Histological analysis, which requires a sample from the bone, is destructive, but has been used to explore the healing process in fractured bones (e.g., De Boer et al. 2015) and other features (see Lovell and Grauer 2019, 336). Radiographic methods, which are nondestructive, are commonly used for visualizing various features in healed bones. Different radiographic views or angles may also provide more information, as a number of different fractures of a single bone may be visible by using more than one view. It is therefore advisable to take a minimum of two radiographic views of a bone fracture—anteroposterior (AP) and mediolateral (ML).

Comparing the macroscopic and radiographic features of an affected bone is essential. For example, linear angulation can be measured on a radiograph using a protractor and ruler (along the longitudinal axis of the bone, as done in Roberts 1988); in this case the degree of angulation of the distal fragment is measured in relation to the proximal fragment. The direction of angulation of the distal fragment (lateral, medial, anterior, or posterior) should also be assessed. In recording deformity of fractured fragments in spiral fractures, comparison between affected and unaffected paired bones is required. In this case recording whether the distal fragment is rotated internally (medially) or externally (laterally) is achieved by comparing the two bones. Nevertheless, 3D digital images of bone fractures may equally enable details of deformity to be assessed (e.g., Digitized Diseases 2024). We should remember that a basic radiograph is in two dimensions despite a bone being 3D, and we therefore lose the full "image" of the bone by using only two dimensions. Apposition, again, can be measured on a radiograph, and the measurement taken should be of the amount of bone apposed between each fragment as a percentage of the 100% of total possible. In effect, horizontal displacement of bone fragments can occur in a mediolateral or anteroposterior direction, thus emphasizing that a minimum of two radiographic views are required. Overlap of fracture fragments (which means that there would be no apposition at all) can also be measured on a radiograph. By measuring the maximum length of the bone and its pair if available, it is also possible to see how much length has been lost on healing of the fracture (see details of recording in Grauer and Roberts 1996).

The preceding are basic features that would be recommended for recording fractures. More detailed methods of analysis of long bone fractures have been described and tested by Judd (2000, 2002) and have particular relevance for recording fractures in bones that are fragmented postmortem. When testing five different methods of recording long bone fractures, Judd found that some methods allowed for differential preservation and raised the fracture frequency, compared to methods that did not. All methods used true prevalence rates. Judd (2002, 1263) also noted that fracture frequency would decline as more poorly preserved (i.e., fragmented) long bones without trauma were included in the sample. If only complete, well-preserved bones were included in the assessment, then 21% of the fractures would have been missed (n = 6 of 28). This study, and the selection of a specific method of analysis for long bone fractures, has implications for final analysis and interpretation of population samples, as well as their comparison with others, including modern clinical studies. With respect to age at death and clinical data on fractures, Milner et al. (2015) have produced a method for correcting for age at death so that modern and ancient frequencies of trauma can be more reliably compared. They also recommended that using a method that takes into account differential preservation—for example, when analyzing cremated remains—will produce more information about trauma patterns in a wider variety of burial contexts and population samples.

Cranial Injuries

Three types of head injury are identified archaeologically: sharp, blunt, and projectile. Sharp injuries are usually the result of an edged weapon (Fig. 4.15), while the blunt injury, caused by a blunt instrument or a fall, usually results in a depressed fracture (Fig. 4.16). Blunt force injuries can be recognized by concentric radiating fractures on the external cranial surface (Figs. 4.17), a light blow producing a linear fracture, and a heavier force causing a comminuted injury with radiating fractures in the immediate area of the trauma, or on the opposite side of the cranium (Boylston 2000). The projectile injury is characterized by the velocity with which the weapon contacts the body (Novak 2001, 91). In this type there are very obvious entry and exit wounds and extensive fracturing.

The type of cranial fracture produced will depend on the direction, velocity, force, and time taken to produce it, the area of cranium involved, and the size and shape of the weapon used to produce it—if a weapon is involved (Gurdjian et al. 1950; Polson et al. 1985; Leestma and Kirkpatrick 1988). In addition, the individual characteristics of the cranium, hair, and scalp can ultimately affect the resulting fracture pattern (Gordon et al. 1988). Bone is nearly twice as strong and stiffer in compression than it is in tension (Hart et al. 2017), and if force is applied slowly, then

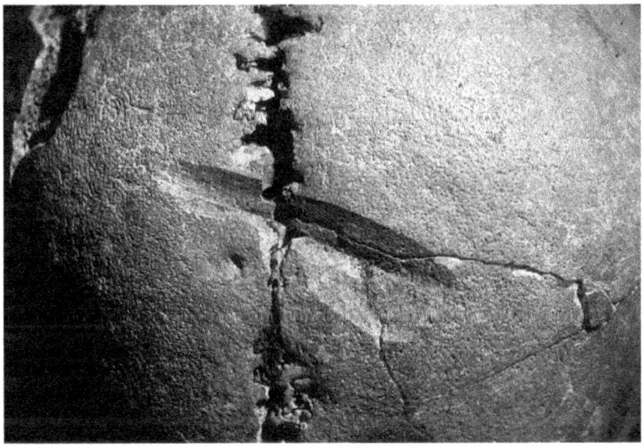

Figure 4.15. Unhealed perimortem blade injury to the cranium in an adult male from late Iron Age/early Roman, Beckford, Hereford and Worcester, England. Photograph by and courtesy of Jean Brown.

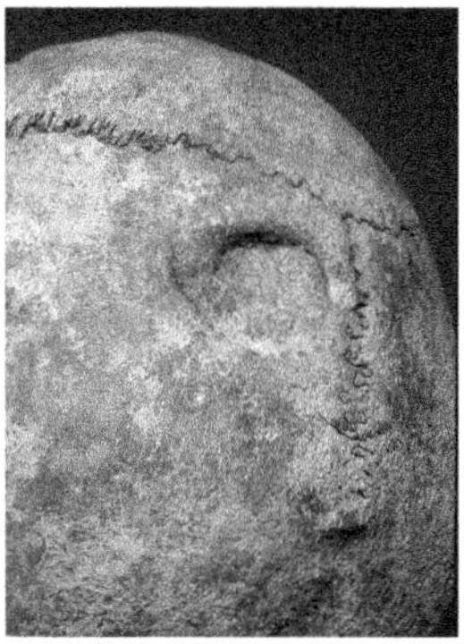

Figure 4.16. Healed depressed fracture to the parietal bone of an adult male from St. Oswald's Priory, Gloucester, Gloucestershire, England (twelfth–sixteenth century CE). Photograph by and courtesy of Jean Brown.

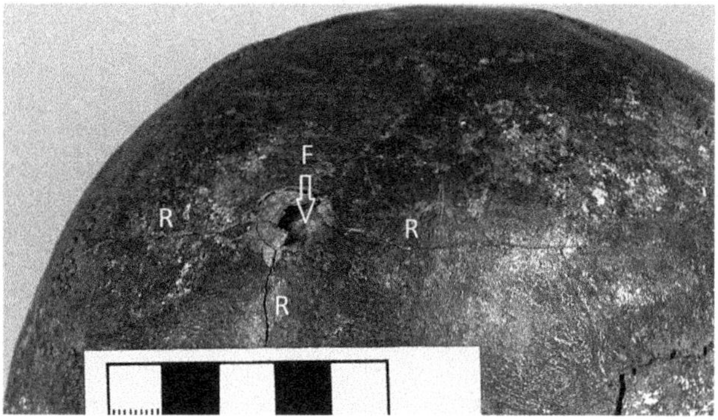

Figure 4.17. Unhealed blunt force injury to the cranium of a young adult male from Arbeia Roman Fort, South Shields, Tyne and Wear, England (second century CE). Radiating fractures can be seen around the lesion (R), and a depressed fragment (flap) of bone protrudes into the endocranial aspect (F). Photograph courtesy of Jeff Veitch, with kind permission from Anwen Caffell.

the bone can withstand a greater load. The configuration of the cortical and cancellous bone and structural buttressing result in lines of lesser and greater resistance; fractures will develop along the former. Whether the person was moving or stationary, on horseback or on foot, or wearing protective armor (Boylston 2000) are other factors to consider in the interpretation of head injuries, but these can be overlooked in archaeological contexts where specific behavioral evidence is lacking. Each cranial fracture may be caused by direct or indirect trauma (e.g., a blow to the back of the head versus falling from a height). Lovell (1997, 149) notes that the most common fractures to the cranium are from directly focused low-velocity injuries, which are usually linear or depressed (blunt trauma) or penetrating (e.g., from a projectile). In blunt trauma the cranial vault curve flattens and the force is distributed over a large area; the outer table of the cranium is compressed and the inner table is under tension (Berryman and Haun 1996). The area around the impact bends outward and the center is depressed inward. In some cases, associated fracture lines develop, usually in the weakest areas of the cranium. The position of the fracture lines may indicate the impact point: star-shaped fracture lines occur at the point of impact, while radiating lines run away from it (Lovell 1997, 154).

The penetrating injury has a much higher velocity, and the entry wound is small, circular, and discrete, with beveling of the inner table of the cranium. The exit wound, however, is larger and irregular, and may include comminution and loss of some bone fragments, with outer table beveling. Differentiating between postmortem loss of a cranial ossicle (normal variant) and a penetrating injury such as from a gunshot wound in an archaeological context may be tricky (Machado et al. 2016). Forensic experiments conducted on cadavers have produced data on cranial fracture patterns with forces applied from different directions (Gurdjian et al. 1950; but also see Kroman et al. 2011); subjected to evolving ethical guidelines, this research is important for paleopathological studies. The study of cranial trauma in relation to interpersonal violence is discussed in more detail later in the chapter.

Trauma to the head may result in a brain injury (Maas et al. 2022), which will vary according to the fracture type. Depressed fractures often lead to brain damage both directly underneath the fracture and at a distance from it, while a linear, blade injury has potential for causing brain damage directly below the fracture site. Of course, brain tissue in the majority of archaeological contexts is not preserved, and therefore the extent of brain damage can only be inferred on the basis of the type, pattern, and position of the fracture on the cranium. Brain damage may include necrosis of some of the brain's tissue; this is due to increased pressure from blood collecting inside the cranium that leads to a lack of oxygen supplied to the tissue (subdural or extradural hematoma). Infection is also a potential hazard following cranial trauma, and it would likely have been a major problem in antiquity, affecting the brain and possibly the entire body of the afflicted person (e.g., via septicemia). Individuals in the past who developed brain infection may have died well before bony change had time to develop at the fracture site. Some paleopathological studies have attempted to assess the impact of a traumatic brain injury using the Bioarchaeology of Care process (Tilley and Cameron 2014), including Li et al. (2021) and Tornberg and Jacobssen (2018). In a study of an individual from the Neolithic battle-axe culture in Sweden (2475–2334 BCE), Tornberg and Jacobssen (2018) inferred that two antemortem injuries to the cranium caused sensory and motor constraints, and particular difficulties with spatial orientation and doing complex activities. Li et al. (2021)—in their research on an adult male from Sampula, an Iron Age (55 BCE–335 CE) cemetery on the edge of the Tarim Basin in the Xinjiang Uygur Autonomous Region of China—found a well-healed antemortem injury to the right side of the frontal bone caused by blunt force trauma. This population subsisted on oasis pastoralism and hunting and foraging. It was suggested that the man would have experienced physical and psychological impairment, including compromised cognitive function, and yet he survived possibly owing to community care. Notwithstanding these interpretations, we can never be certain whether, and exactly what, complications resulted from head injuries.

A cranial injury may be healed (Fig. 4.18), healing, or unhealed, the latter suggesting that the wound may have contributed to the cause of death. Cranial fractures usually heal with fibrous union, but bony union can also be found. Bone formation during the healing process is present but is less important than in fractures of the postcranium (Sevitt 1981, 231). A detailed study of 135 crania from American Civil War casualties (i.e., with an associated documented history and curated at the National Museum of Health and Medicine, Washington, DC), considered the evidence of healing of traumatic lesions (Barbian and Sledzik 2008). The information linked to each cranium documented when the injury had occurred and how long it was before the person died after the injury. The authors found that the earliest bone response to cranial fracture was after five days, but in most cases no osseous response was evident during the first week following the trauma. By the fourth week all injuries had some osteoblastic response and by the sixth

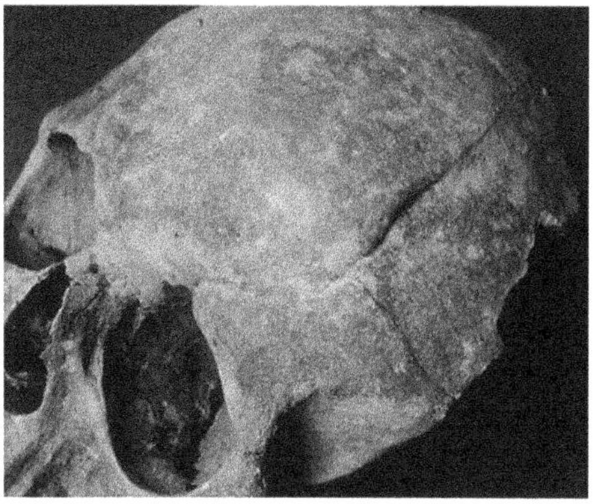

Figure 4.18. Healed injury to the frontal and left parietal bones in an individual from later medieval York, England. Photograph by and courtesy of Jean Brown.

week all had osteoclastic response. The expression of these responses was similar on both the endocranial and the ectocranial surfaces, but generally speaking, the more extensive expression was on the latter. Other features noted were lines of demarcation establishing a boundary between dead and living bone—probably where the periosteum had been torn away from the bone during the injury—and sequestration, or the development of dead bone. Kaufmann et al. (1997, citing a 1956 chapter by Ham and Harris) also highlighted that evidence of a healing cranial fracture would be seen by just over one week following the injury, although within 48 hours proliferation of the osteogenic layer of the periosteum will be visible microscopically.

Head injuries require detailed description to reveal more specifically the type of force that was directed at the skull and whether the trauma is healed. Descriptions of the bones of the cranium affected, including any deformation, and the characteristics of the fracture lines, should be provided. Cranial injuries can produce radiating fractures away from the site of impact; this occurs when the impact distorts the bone beyond its maximum elastic properties. In addition, a study of the intersection of the fracture lines allows a reconstruction of the sequence of injuries. For example, research has used scanning electron microscopy to analyze cranial wounds. This enabled a reconstruction of the order and direction of injury in individuals from an early medieval cemetery from Kent, England (Wenham 1987).

Specific studies of cranial trauma have revealed interesting information and fascinating stories about populations both temporally and geographically, and in some cases large datasets covering a long period of time have been produced in specific regions of the globe to illustrate temporal trends in the impact of violence (e.g., Europe: Baten and Steckel 2019; Middle East, on human populations: Baten et al. 2023). In North America, Walker (1989) identified 144 individuals with one or more cranial fractures (19.3% of 774 crania) from prehistoric sites on the north Channel Islands and adjacent mainland of Southern California. Both accidental and interpersonal violence injuries were identified. The fractures were common on the left side of the head and on the frontal and parietal bones, males being more affected than females (ratio of 12:5). Injury was rarely seen on the occipital bone, suggesting that interpersonal violent injuries were sustained by frontal combat and not when the victim was fleeing. More injuries were seen in the island groups than on the mainland (perhaps because of competition for scarce resources), and frequencies increased through time (possibly the result of increased population density and tension).

Antemortem, Perimortem, or Postmortem?

Often one of the most common questions asked of bone injuries is how long ago did the person sustain the trauma before they died? Unfortunately, it is usually impossible to say. Studies such as Barbian and Sledzik (2008) can provide some information on the time between the injury and death, bearing in mind the many factors that can affect healing rates, and of course these will vary for each individual affected. Healing, identified as rounding of the wound edges, indicates survival of the person following the injury, but little can be said of what complications were present. Distinguishing recent antemortem or perimortem unhealed injuries from postmortem breaks may also be difficult, requiring detailed observation and more objective criteria (Figs 4.19 and 4.20) (Cappella et al. 2014). Lovell (1997) provided a useful summary of how to distinguish between antemortem injuries and perimortem breaks (Table 4.1).

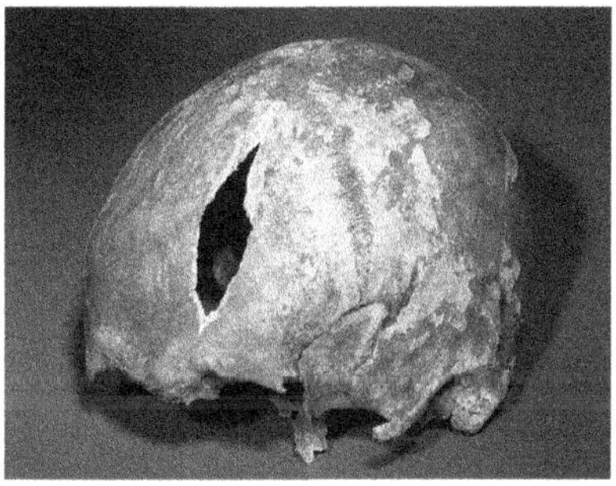

Figure 4.19. Postmortem "wound" to the cranium, probably due to damage during excavation. Note the jagged white edges of the "lesion." Photograph courtesy of Jo Buckberry, Calvin Wells Photographic Collection, University of Bradford.

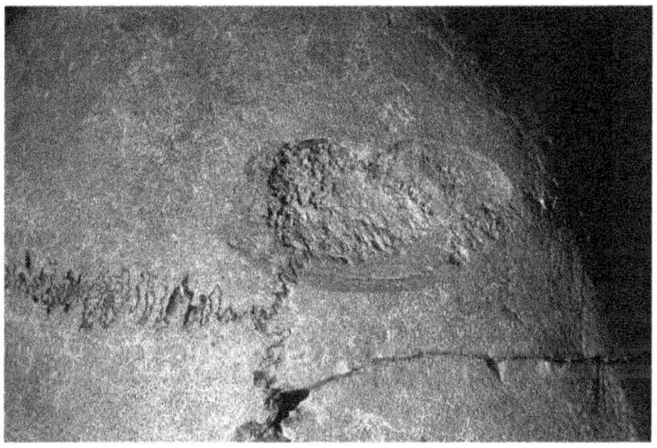

Figure 4.20. Perimortem (unhealed) wound to the cranium of an adult male from late Iron Age/ early Roman, Beckford, Hereford and Worcester, England (first century BCE–first century CE). Photograph by and courtesy of Jean Brown.

Table 4.1. Differences between antemortem or perimortem trauma and postmortem trauma (from Lovell 1997, 145)

Antemortem/perimortem	Postmortem
Any evidence of healing or inflammation	Smaller fragments
Uniform presence of water, soil stains, or vegetation on broken or adjacent surfaces	Nonuniform coloration of fractured ends and adjacent bone surface
Presence of greenstick, spiral, depressed, or compressed fractures	Squared fracture edges
Oblique angles on fractured ends	Absence of fracture patterning (dry, brittle bone shatters on impact)
A pattern of concentric circular, radiating, or stellate lines	

Other authors have provided information to help make the distinction between perimortem and postmortem fractures. Hutchinson (1996) reported that fractures occurring in fresh bone are usually uniform in their cortical and noncortical coloration, and the edges of the wounds have acute or obtuse angles, while dry bone fractures are usually perpendicular to the long axis of the bone and have irregular surfaces because, as the collagen has disappeared from the bone, it becomes more brittle and is likely to shatter on impact (Kaufman et al. 1997). Ubelaker and Adams (1995) and Quatrehomme and Iscan (1997) emphasized that the cortex of the ends of bones fractured postmortem have a lighter color than the rest of unaffected bone.

Trauma is not just confined to fracture of the long bones and cranium. Next we consider other forms of traumatic injury identified in the archaeological record, and what inferences we can make about people's lives from them.

Dislocation

In a dislocation there is loss of contact between two osseous surfaces that normally form a joint. This can also be associated with a fractured bone—for example, the Monteggia fracture, a fracture of the ulna with radial head dislocation (Konrad et al. 2007). A dislocation may be total or partial (subluxation) and, in archaeological contexts, is recognizable usually if the bones remained unreduced during life (i.e., out of alignment) for a relatively long period of time. This may be why so few dislocations are identified in paleopathology. Should a joint remain dislocated for long enough, a new joint surface (pseudoarthrosis) may develop away from the original joint or adjacent to it (Fig. 4.21). Joint degeneration, as well as damage to bones, ligaments, tendons, and joint capsules at the time of the dislocation, may also be recognized. Dislocations are most commonly caused by trauma, but people can also be born with them—for example, the congenitally dislocated hip (see Chapter 2). A dislocation may also arise as a complication of another condition; for example, in rheumatoid arthritis, loss of bone leads to partial dislocation of the metacarpophalangeal joints (knuckles) (Resnick 2024, 216). Dislocations generally tend to affect the hip and shoulder joints, but potentially any other joint could be affected. Sometimes a dislocation can reduce naturally, especially if it is an unstable joint, such as the shoulder, where its anatomical structure makes it particularly susceptible to dislocation.

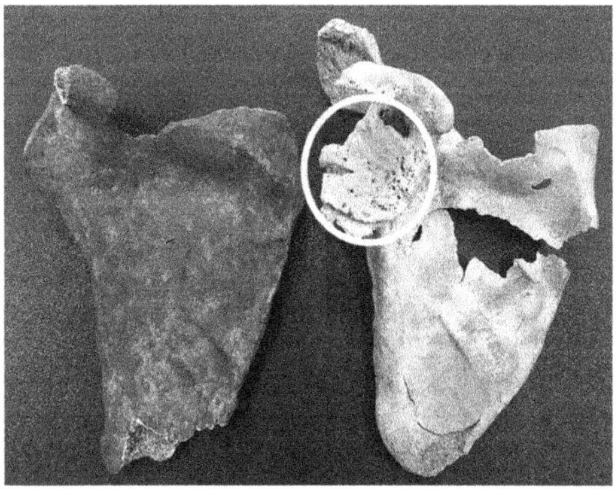

Figure 4.21. Dislocation of the shoulder showing a new joint surface near the glenoid cavity (right) with a normal scapula for comparison (left). Postmedieval Spain. With kind permission of the Fenwick Human Osteology Laboratory, Department of Archaeology, Durham University.

Osteochondritis Dissecans

There is another condition in skeletal remains that is related to trauma, that of osteochondritis dissecans (Chau et al. 2021). It is classified with other so-called osteochondroses, such as juvenile kyphosis (Scheuermann disease) of the spine, Osgood-Schlatter disease of the knee, and Perthes disease of the hip (Resnick 2024, 1008, see table 41.5). All these conditions involve fragmentation and collapse of a small but variable area of the articular surface of a joint (cartilage and bone). They all affect young individuals, especially males in their first decade of life. The lesion of osteochondritis dissecans presents as a localized and circumscribed area of necrosis of the articular surface, due, probably, to localized lack of blood supply to the affected area and subsequent ischemia (death) of the bone; repetitive loading of the joint is suggested to be responsible (Fig. 4.22). This is an insignificant lesion clinically, with transient joint pain but no symptoms in the long term.

Normal variation of bone morphology has also been suggested to predispose people to developing this condition (Wechter et al. 2014). The knee and ankle are most affected, usually with an underlying traumatic etiology in people who are physically active in sports; there may also be an inherited component (Chau et al. 2021). The necrotic fragment of bone separates and may remain loose in the joint (loose bodies), may become absorbed, or may heal back into the defect. Few papers on osteochondritis dissecans appear in the published paleopathological literature (Wells 1974a; Loveland et al. 1984; Anderson 2000), and most observations are confined to the "gray literature" and skeletal reports. However, two important population studies have been published. Lewis (2016) conducted a large-scale study of 2,549 adolescent skeletons 7 to 17 years of age and found 38 had the lesion (0.15%). Urban rather than rural individuals had more lesions, and occupation-related risks were suggested as a cause. A study of 140 skeletons, with approximately equal numbers of males and females from a nineteenth-century farming community in the Netherlands found a 12.9% prevalence of osteochondritis dissecans in foot bones (Vikatou et al. 2017). They suggested the

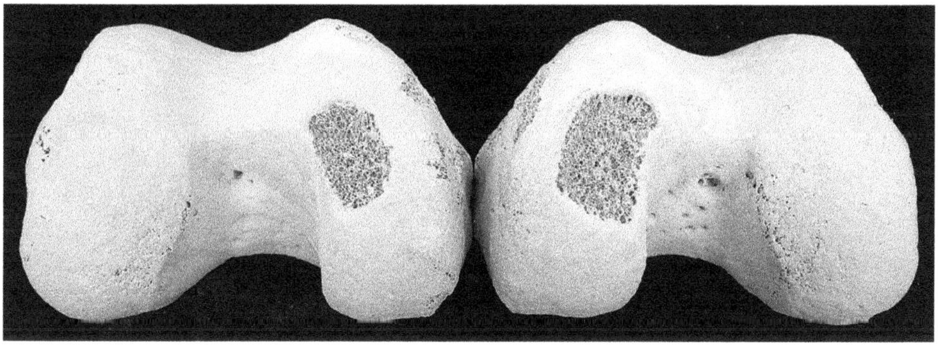

Figure 4.22. Osteochondritis dissecans in the distal femoral joint surfaces of a 15- to 17-year-old individual (fourth century CE Roman Poundbury, Dorset, England). Photograph by Mary Lewis and taken with the kind permission of the Natural History Museum, London.

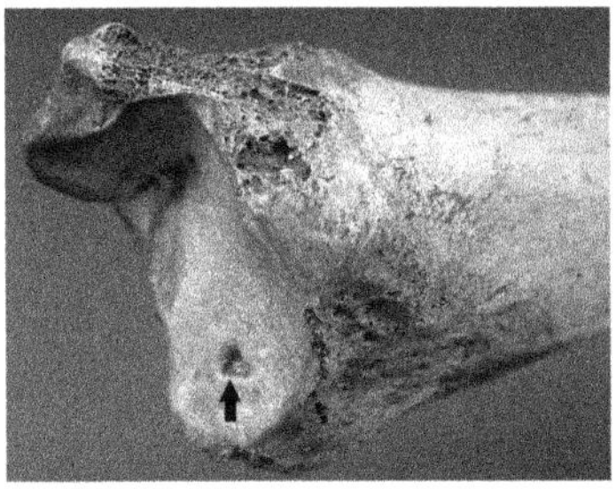

Figure 4.23. Joint lesions that may be confused with osteochondritis dissecans on the distal articular surface (talar facet) of the right tibia. Photograph by and courtesy of Jean Brown.

data reflected repetitive stress, acute trauma, and especially the wearing of wooden shoes (clogs).

It is important to appreciate that paleopathologists also note defects in the joint surfaces, which may be mistakenly attributed to osteochondritis dissecans (Fig. 4.23), and there is a danger of overinflating prevalence rates if these are counted as such. True osteochondritis consists of a well-defined, porous, often circular defect, usually lower than the joint surface, and most often on a convex joint (e.g., the distal femoral condyles and the capitulum of the humerus).

What Can Evidence for Trauma Tell Us About the Past?

Notable studies of trauma in past populations are seen in work on skeletons globally (see Larsen 2015, chap. 4, for a comprehensive summary), and since the third edition of this book many more studies have been published. Many thematic approaches related to trauma have been and are being explored through paleopathological studies—for example, climate and environmental change (Harrod and Martin 2014; Schug 2021); social status (e.g., Redfern 2017a, table 5.1); political instability (e.g., Tung 2012); subsistence (e.g., Cohen and Armelagos 1984); terrain (e.g., Judd 2006); and migrant populations (e.g., Meyer and Steyn 2016). With increasing global warming, climate and weather pattern change, increased food insecurity, and subsequent migration, it is predicted that violence will increase. Further, alongside increasingly advanced techniques of analysis, more nuanced understandings of the underlying reasons for trauma in the paleopathological record are now being achieved. For example, using stable isotope analysis, Meyer et al. (2018) identified non–locally born and raised victims of violent trauma found in a Neolithic mass grave in Halberstadt, Germany.

It is impossible to discuss the totality of these studies in an all-encompassing way, but this section provides a few highlights of the work to reveal the ways in which evidence for trauma is used to understand the impact of injury on populations living on different continents in the past. Studies on interpersonal violence then follow.

Europe

Many studies of trauma have been carried out on European skeletons. Focusing on the skeletons of people buried in three medieval cemeteries in Cambridge, England (St. John the Evangelist, All Saints by the Castle, and the Augustinian Friary), Dittmar et al. (2021b) studied long bone and cranial fractures. Eighty-two, or 31%, of the individuals with preserved long bones (n = 267) had fractures: St. John had the lowest fracture rate (27%; 42/155) and All Saints the highest (44%; 37/84). Of the 179 crania preserved, 10 (6%) had antemortem trauma, but there was no evidence for perimortem trauma. The highest frequency was again at All Saints (9%; 4/47), and males experienced more fractures than females. The poverty linked to the people buried at All Saints most likely predisposed them to a higher risk of fracture, although the other two cohorts of burials were not free from risk. Nevertheless, there was no convincing evidence for interpersonal violence, with the fractures considered the result of accidents (e.g., falls, work related).

Grauer and Roberts (1996) concentrated on five late medieval English cemetery sites and one from Scotland. At St. Helen-on-the-Walls, York, fractures were evident in 2.9% of individuals (n = 30/1,014 skeletons examined) with 0.8% of bones affected (n = 41/4,938). The majority were healed fractures of the radius and/or ulna. Fracture complications included linear deformity on healing, but there was no significant shortening of affected bones. Documentary sources for medieval York indicate that this cemetery population was poor and exposed to risk factors for injury during their everyday lives. Comparison of fracture rates among eight other medieval sites (one Scottish and seven English) show similar rates for six of them, between 0.3% and 1.1% (Table 4.2). The two sites with higher prevalence rates dated to the eleventh–twelfth century—the lay cemetery of St. Nicholas Shambles, London—and the twelfth–seventeenth century—the leprosarium cemetery at Chichester. The higher rates in London may be explained by the hazards of living in a large city (but see St. Mary Spital, also in London, at 1.1%; Connell et al. 2012). The rate for those buried in Chichester may reflect its use as a hospital (for leprosy initially and then for any illness), with the likelihood of people being admitted for care following a fracture. In addition, people with leprosy can develop osteoporosis, and leprosy can affect the senses, including sight; compromised sight could have precipitated falls and fractures. Therefore, both these risk factors may have been responsible for some of the fractures identified in individuals buried in this cemetery (Judd and Roberts 1998).

Table 4.2. Long bone fracture prevalence in eight late medieval English urban populations

Site	Number of fractures	Total bones	%	Sources
Whithorn, Wigtownshire, Dumfries and Galloway, Scotland*	27	9,563	0.3	Cardy (1997)
Blackfriars, Gloucester, Gloucestershire*	11	1,861	0.6	Wiggins et al. (1993)
St. Helen-on-the-Walls, York, Yorkshire*	41	4,938	0.8	Grauer and Roberts (1996)
St. Andrew, Fishergate, York, Yorkshire*	26	3,235	0.8	Stroud and Kemp (1993)
Chichester, Sussex*	41	1,554	2.6	Judd and Roberts (1998)
St. Nicholas Shambles, London*	18	296	6.1	W. White (1988)
St. Mary Spital, London	550	48,749	1.1	Connell et al. (2012)
Wharram Percy, Yorkshire	16	3,338	0.5	Mays et al. (2007)

* denotes the Grauer and Roberts (1996) study sites

Examination of the pattern of fractures in the skeletons from these sites (Fig. 4.24) revealed that the arm, especially the radius and ulna, was the most frequently affected limb, a pattern seen today, except at Chichester, Fishergate, and Whithorn, where the fibula rate was higher. Rates for the strongest bone in the body, the femur, were particularly low in all groups. Femoral fractures today are associated with high-impact trauma and increased longevity linked to osteoporosis; consequently, their relative absence in antiquity is probably explained by the absence of these risk factors. Fractures to the tibia were also rare. In one retrospective Danish study of tibial shaft fractures between 2009 and 2010, the incidence was 16.9 per 100,000 per year, with males being more affected than females, and both sexes sustaining them during physical activity, such as sports (Larsen et al. 2015). While this was a study of people doing sports, it is somewhat surprising that there was a low frequency of such fractures in ancient populations who would also have been very active, at least more active than many people today.

Connell et al. (2012) documented fracture prevalence in a large skeletal population from London (n = 5,387, St. Mary Spital, a hospital and Augustinian priory). Because of the availability of narrow date ranges for the four time periods, it was possible to look at time trends in injury. Overall 22.5% of individuals (n = 1,214) were affected by trauma (21.4% of adult females, 32.4% adult males, and 3.4% children). Frequency increased with age and through the time periods, the latter suggesting:

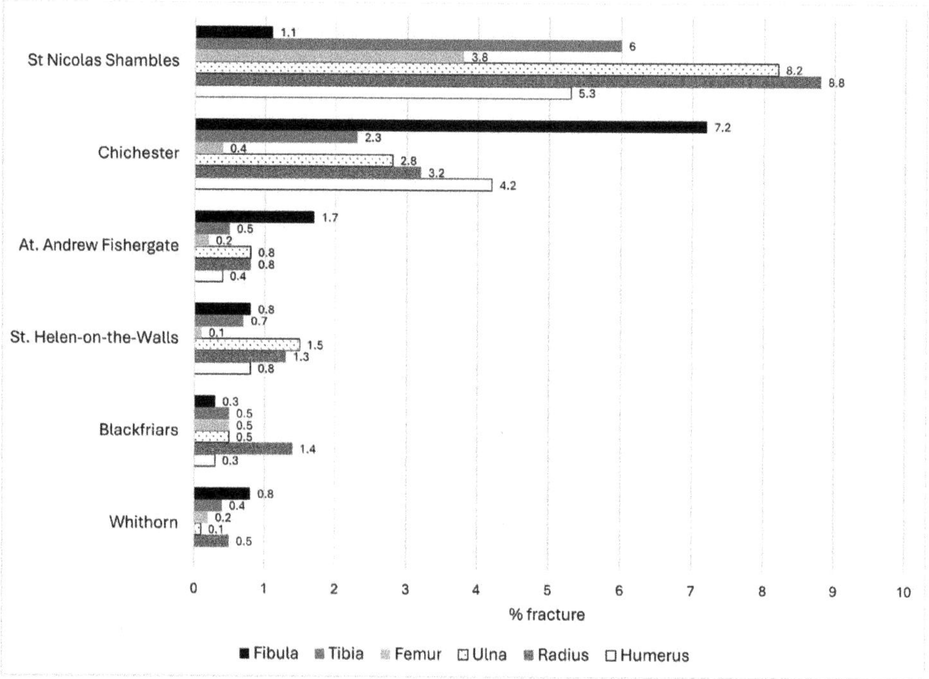

Figure 4.24. Long bone fracture prevalence in six late medieval English populations. Figure created by Mary Lewis.

"London became a more dangerous place to live throughout the course of the medieval period" (Connell et al. 2012, 89). Long bone fracture frequency was 1.1% (*n* = 550/48,749), and forearm bones were most affected, especially the ulna. Recidivism was seen more in males than females. Fractures increased into early adulthood, and later analysis revealed the youngest child affected was 2 years of age (Lewis 2016).

A study of skeletons from a Central European admixture of populations (fifth–eleventh century CE), buried at Säben-Sabiona, Bozen-Bolzano, Italy, revealed that the majority of the injuries sustained were likely work related and linked to political instability and social changes following Roman rule (Tumler et al. 2021). In this research, on high-social-status burials, 16.4% of 226 individuals sustained fractures (*n* = 37/226), with more males than females affected. A few individuals with perimortem injuries to their crania indicate that people were also exposed to interpersonal violence. A study of limb bone fractures in a population buried in Pannonia in the northern provinces of the Roman Empire also invoked the impact of Roman rule (Gilmour et al. 2015). The authors emphasized that the lives of Roman provincial populations are not well known, even though they were important for providing resources and services. In the Graphisoft cemetery, 11% of individuals had fractures (*n* = 23/210). This cemetery was linked to the first-to-fourth-century civilian settlement of Aquincum, Budapest, Hungary. The patterning of fractures suggests that they were the result of falls, and that males experienced more high-impact hazardous activities than females, indicating that they followed traditional gender roles.

Urban-rural fracture frequencies have also been a focus for study (e.g., see Judd and Roberts 1999, England), and a good summary of medieval urban and rural studies in the UK is provided by Redfern (2017a, table 4.1). A comparison of trauma affecting people buried in a rural (Tjaerby, *n* = 225 individuals) and an urban cemetery (Randers, *n* = 170 individuals) in Denmark (1050–1536 CE), showed no significant difference in fractures between the urban and rural groups (Collier and Primeau 2019). However, when using the common odds ratio to calculate relative risk or susceptibility to injury (e.g., in relation to age or biological sex), Randers carried a 1.13% higher risk of trauma. This is contrary to the findings of Judd and Roberts (1999). Finally, a study of almost 4,000 skeletons of children and adolescents (6–25 years) from urban and rural medieval England (900–1700 CE) revealed 137 examples of trauma. While the crude prevalence rates were similar for urban and rural areas (6.4% and 4.6%, respectively), the pattern of injury was broader in the urban adolescents, with males showing more signs of interpersonal violence (fractures to the nasal and cheek bones and ribs) and urban females sustaining injuries to their legs and spines, perhaps reflecting the rigors of domestic service. By contrast, while rural males started to develop injuries by 10 years of age, fractures occurred in rural females only after 17 years of age; however, the number of rural adolescents studied was small (Lewis 2016).

North and South America

Like Europe, there are a plethora of studies on trauma in skeletal remains in North America. For example, in the southeastern United States, Lambert and Welker (2017) considered evidence for long bone fractures in skeletons of low-intensity farmers located in three floodplain sites (11 sites in total); the date range was around 1000–1525 CE for most sites. They also considered published comparative data from six hunter-forager, and four low-intensity and six high-intensity farming sites. They concluded that low-intensity farming was the most risk-averse subsistence strategy for the occurrence of trauma, compared to foraging or high-intensity agriculture, indicating that the methods and intensity of agricultural production were most important for fracture risk at this time and in this place.

Other studies have documented trauma patterning in South America (see Murphy and Juengst's 2020 review of trauma studies in Andean South America, 1800 BCE–1600 CE). What follows are a few specific studies. In research focused on a northern Chilean population of 144 individuals, a hunter-forager culture that concentrated on coastal resources, complemented by wild plants and camelids (Standen and Arriaza 2000: 4,000-year-old Chinchorro), only 1 of the 55 nonadults showed any evidence of trauma (a quartz lithic point tip in a vertebra). However, 30% of the adults (*n* = 27/89) had some evidence of trauma, mainly to the cranium (17 people, or 63% of the trauma), with three times more evidence in males. This finding was suggested to be more likely the result of interpersonal aggression than accidental or work-related trauma. Unfortunately, the number of bones available for this study were not provided, and therefore, true prevalence rates of bones fractured could not be compared with other studies. Another study of a prehistoric population from the region of San Pedro de Atacama, also in Chile (250–1240 CE), provided data on a population that relied on camelids and small garden cultivation in oases for subsistence. Here, 244 individuals (161 adults) were examined (Neves et al. 1999); 1.9% of the 2,471 long bones observed (humerus, radius, ulna, femur, tibia, and fibula) were fractured, and yet again, the most frequently fractured bones were the radius and ulna.

Finally, through extant and newly collected data, Lessa et al. (2011) considered fractures caused by accidents in two groups from precolonial coastal Brazil (prior to 1500 CE): Sambaqui (shell mound builders). There were 119 adults from nine published and unpublished sites and 96 fisher-hunter-forager adults from two sites. The former group, who subsisted on intensive collection of seafood, revealed a fracture prevalence of 19% of individuals, while for the latter it was 27% (people who relied on a more diverse subsistence, including seafood, but also land fauna). Male and female frequencies were similar. It was concluded that the main cause for the fractures observed were falls while navigating along the rocky coastal areas, and falls onto outstretched arms—radius and ulna fractures—were most common for both groups.

Africa

Fewer studies of trauma in Africa and Asia have been published compared to Europe and North America. Judd (2000) found 2.7% fractured bones (*n* = 47/1771) at Kerma in Nubia (1750–1500 BCE). These data can be compared with a study by Alvrus (1999), who found a prevalence of 1.6% fractured bones (*n* = 48/3013) at Semna South, Nubia (300 BCE–300 CE), and with Kilgore et al.'s (1997) research at Kulubnarti, Nubia (550–1450 CE), where a higher 4.3% (n = 66/1526) of bones were fractured. Judd (2000) compared the frequency of fractures at urban Kerma with rural Dongola, 70 km away. At both sites, the radius and ulna were among the most frequent bones affected. At Dongola, however, fractured tibiae were also common, while at Kerma the overall rates of trauma were lower. It was suggested that the fractures in the rural population were the result of accidents related to cultivation and herding activities. This pattern was also found in the study by Judd and Roberts (1999). In a further study of rural (2500–1700 BCE) and urban (2050–1500 BCE) adults from Nubian sites, Judd (2006) noted evidence for interpersonal violence (cranium, ulna, and multiple injuries). However, the rural population had more nonviolent injuries (likely related to the work they did or hazards with navigating their environment), while the urban group had more severe injuries. This, it was suggested, could have been related to interpersonal violence possibly due to increasing tensions during the seventeenth dynasty.

In a rather different study, this time in South Africa, alongside historical accounts Meyer and Steyn (2016) analyzed thirty-four skeletons of people who had migrated from China to South Africa in the early twentieth century. They became indentured mine workers—contracted to work without a salary for a specific number of years. From 1904 to 1910 CE they worked deep in the Witwatersrand gold mines and experienced occupation-related injuries. Most fractures were perimortem, with very few antemortem (healed) fractures. It was proposed that the latter were likely sustained in China before they moved to South Africa.

Asia

Some research on trauma in Asia has documented injuries in very early humans. One such study by Beier et al. (2021), based on published literature, describes cranial trauma in Upper Paleolithic individuals dated from 40,000 to 10,000 BP. The study comprised over 200 crania (1,285 cranial bones) deriving from 101 sites. Males were affected more than females, and older people were more affected than younger. The data were interpreted to be a result of warfare and generally riskier situations, and for males and females, different activities and behaviors.

In a study on more recent, but still prehistoric, skeletal remains, nonvertebral fractures were the focus in 299 individuals from four prehistoric Thai sites (Domett and Tayles 2006). Dated to between 2000 and 400 BCE, two were on the coast and two were inland. Over time, fracture frequencies increased, from the Neolithic period (0.3%) to the Bronze Age (3%), and craniofacial and ulna fractures became evident in the Bronze Age. The small hand and foot bones, clavicle, and forearm bones were most affected. It was suggested, based on archaeological evidence, that subsistence patterns changed, which affected fracture frequency.

Injuries Associated with Interpersonal Violence

In the twenty-first century, we are all familiar with aggression in societies, and "in some ways patterns of violence are remarkably consistent across time and space"

(Wilkinson and Pickett 2009, 131). While there can be, and has been, a general "tendency to stereotype women as non-aggressive" (Redfern 2017a, 25), recent research is changing those ideas. As Redfern stated, this "non-aggressive" presumption goes alongside debates and discussions about biological sex, gender roles, and social behavior in many different cultures. Nevertheless, the majority of violence is perpetrated by young men, and inequality is linked to acts of violence, such as homicide. In the United States, states with greater inequalities of socioeconomic status have more homicides, and more unequal countries encompass more children experiencing bullying, fighting, and conflict (Wilkinson and Pickett 2009, 135, 139). Even within a single community, one section may live in peace with only sporadic and infrequent episodes of aggression, while in a neighboring area, an undercurrent of continuous violence may be the norm. Often the most dramatic injuries are to the head, and in crime scene investigations, where the cause and manner of a victim's death are being evaluated, it is usually the head and neck that reveal most of the trauma. The head is the most common target for violence, and injury to the brain is often a consequence of a cranial fracture leading to increased intracranial pressure from bleeding (Knight 1991, 156). It should be remembered that cranial fractures can occur if a person falls on the ground, for whatever reason; hence the injury may not always be violence related.

Since cranial injury often represents an intentional blow, the enumeration of such injuries may indicate the peace or otherwise within and between communities. In forensic contexts, the interpretation of cranial fractures has often followed the "hat brim line rule" in differentiating trauma caused by a fall or a direct blow (Kremer et al. 2008). The hat brim is defined as a 3 cm band above the top of the eyebrows. Kremer et al. (2008) revealed intentional blows occurred above the hat brim line, and more commonly on the left side. Right-sided cranial injuries were also revealed to be more likely to be the result of a fall, unless the assailant was left-handed. In reviewing this and two other relevant studies (Kremer and Sauvageau 2009; Guyomarc'h et al. 2010), Fracasso et al. (2011, 1662) noted that these authors had concluded that the hat brim rule "had limited validity" and should not be utilized. In challenging the rule Fracasso et al. (2011) emphasized that a blunt force head injury cannot occur above the hat brim line if the person was in a kneeling or sitting position before the fall or if the fall was from a height, down the stairs, onto an irregular floor, or involved intermediate obstacles such as furniture or walls.

Occasionally, blows are delivered from behind and, accepting that the majority of the world's population is right-handed (Jing 2020), an occipital bone injury at the back of the head on the right side would be expected. The skeletal remains from the Battle of Wisby, Sweden (1361 CE), showed frequent occipital wounds, suggesting that blows were delivered to a fleeing enemy (Courville 1965) or that people were struck while lying face down on the ground. While males generally display more injuries than females in the past and present day, this pattern is most striking when it comes to head injuries (Knüsel and Smith 2015).

Injuries to the neck caused by strangulation and severe trauma or suffocation may cause fractures of the hyoid bone and/or calcified thyroid cartilage (Ubelaker 1992). For example, Jiménez-Brobeil et al. (2011) reported a healed fractured hyoid bone in an individual from prehistoric Spain, probably due to neck trauma. As these elements of the skeleton are rarely preserved or excavated, this type of injury has been rarely documented in paleopathology. Generally speaking, wounds of the facial skeleton are less commonly observed, suggesting that in the past, blows to the head were purposefully delivered to the cranium to produce maximum damage. It may be, however, that in archaeological contexts the fragile facial bones, being commonly damaged during burial, do not survive well or often enough to identify injury to this part of the body. Nasal bone injuries are sometimes seen, and these, no doubt, are due to fistfights, an age-old and continuing method of solving minor disputes (Fibiger et al. 2013). Walker (1997) found a 7% frequency rate of nasal fractures in populations from the United States, Europe, and Asia (106 of 1506 individuals). Walker also found nasal fractures to be more common than other cranial injuries. Furthermore, in a study of three documented early modern Portuguese skeletal populations, Magalhães et al. (2023) identified nasal fractures in 10% of males compared to 6% of females. This higher frequency in males was interpreted as being the result of sociocultural factors that provided men with more opportunities to be involved in violent behavior.

Dental trauma includes damage to the teeth, jaws, and associated soft tissues (e.g., complete or incomplete fractures to the root, crown, or dentine); subluxation (a loose tooth that remains in place in the jaw); avulsion (displacement of the tooth from its socket); and antemortem loss (Bastone et al. 2000). Nevertheless, dental trauma is often difficult to identify and, importantly, while dental trauma may reflect interpersonal violence (Loe et al. 2014), it could be caused by other behavior-related factors (e.g., sport, accidental falls). In addition, fractures to teeth may be postmortem, although observation under a microscope can help to identify healing (rounding of the edges). Because the permanent teeth stay longer in the jaws than the deciduous teeth, the former are usually more affected by trauma. In an archaeological context, differential diagnosis of trauma to teeth must include possible cultural modification and ritual-related tooth removal. Lukacs (2007) studied antemortem tooth loss and dental fractures and found an overall 9% rate of antemortem tooth loss in a pre-sixteenth-century Guanche population of Tenerife, Canary Island (Spain). Maxillary more than mandibular teeth were lost, and similar rates were found for males and females. Five maxillae and six mandibles contained, primarily, incisor and premolar teeth that appeared to have been fractured, based on location of the fracture consistently at the alveolar margin, reparative dentinogenesis, relative root integrity, and some proliferative alveolar bone growth over the broken root. Two specific causes were suggested: falls while navigating very steep valleys on volcanic terrain, and conflict (e.g., wrestling and stick fighting).

In addition to craniofacial trauma, fractures to the ribs, scapula, forearm and hand bones (defense injuries) are all considered potential indicators of interpersonal violence. It is therefore important to look at the patterning of injuries in any skeleton (see Jurmain 1999 and Judd 2002). There have been many reports of directly induced "parry" fractures of the mid or distal third of the ulna. Smith (1996) noted a high frequency of parry fractures in females buried at the site of Eva in Tennessee (2500–500 BCE). In order to understand this pattern, they conducted a review of forearm fractures in individuals from eight prehistoric Tennessee sites (hunter-foragers and farmers). The limited evidence for cranial fractures associated with arm injuries led Smith to caution against overinterpreting these fractures as the result of female-directed domestic violence; instead, Smith explained the apparent high prevalence in females as an artifact of the ratio of females to males. Nevertheless, if the blow was successfully defended then perhaps we would not expect the cranium to be fractured. In reflecting on the conundrum of reliably identifying parry fractures, Judd (2008) refined the parry fracture diagnostic criteria to the following: (1) an absence of radial involvement; (2) a transverse fracture line; (3) a location below the midshaft (<0.5 adjusted distance to the lesion's center); and (4) either minor unalignment (<10°) in any plane or horizontal apposition from the diaphysis of <50%. In addition, Jurmain (1999, 217) had advised that when a parry fracture was suspected, evidence for dislocation of the radial head should be ruled out, as this usually accompanies an ulnar shaft fracture resulting from a fall (also called a Monteggia fracture).

Temporal Evidence for Warfare and Political Upheaval

Generally speaking, males are and were more involved in warfare. Not that females do not, and did not, fight, but males still vastly outnumber females today in the world's armies, although this is changing (Rank and Heroux 2018). For example, Price et al. (2019) discussed the tenth-century Birka burial found on the island of Björkö in Lake Mälaren, Uppland, modern-day Sweden. This high-status warrior burial has until very recently always been presumed to be that of a biological male since its excavation in 1878. Using aDNA analysis in 2017, it was confirmed that "he" was actually female (Hedenstierna-Jonson et al. 2017). Concluding their study, Price et al. (2019, 189) emphasize that the weapons in the grave, and an absence of jewelry or weaving equipment, were originally taken to indicate a male burial, and that "it is important to remember that when [the individual] was recorded, male biological sex was not only conflated with a man's gendered identity, but also that warriorhood was presumed to be an exclusively masculine pursuit; the same interpretation would undoubtedly have been made had no human bone survived at all." While it is not possible to present a detailed survey of recent work in this fascinating area of study, the reader is directed to a number of publications that provide that detail (Martin et al. 2010; Matić and Jensen 2017; Scherer 2021). Another example of female involvement in warfare comes from Morton Village and Norris Farms 36 cemetery, central Illinois, United States. Bengtson and O'Gorman (2017) identified females as active defenders of their late prehistoric community and not passive victims of violence.

In reconstructing methods used by people to inflict interpersonal violence, the skeletons of males who died at the Battle of Wisby revealed many cutting wounds to the cranium and postcranium as the result of obliquely directed downward blows (Courville 1965). Less frequent is the vertically directed blow, and even more rare is the horizontal blow. This merely reflects the manner in which a heavy sword or axe is wielded. As would be expected with fatal wounds sustained in combat, many cranial injuries consist of a single cut. In those crania possessing several cuts, the direction of the blows is often variable. Microscopy has been suggested to provide greater detail as a complementary analytical tool in the study of injuries, particularly in these contexts (Boucherie et al. 2017).

Projectile injuries are rare in the archaeological record, although examples of such injuries have been noted from as early as prehistoric contexts (Jurmain 1999, 211–214; Lockau et al. 2016 on buckshot injuries). However, in these contexts blunt force cranial injuries may actually be sling shot trauma (i.e., blunt force projectile injuries; Linda Fibiger, pers. comm., 10/6/2024). The weapon used to produce the projectile injury may also be interpreted from the injury observed, but only rarely is the weapon found in situ in the wound. Nevertheless, a flint arrowhead was found in the humerus of an individual buried in the Tollense Valley, Germany, in 1200 BCE and, using micro-CT, researchers discovered evidence of healing around the wound (Flohr et al. 2015). Another survivor, this time from Neolithic Turuka in Siberia (8000–6800 cal. BP), was reported by Lieverse et al. (2017) where a lithic projectile point penetrated the spine of a young adult male (Fig. 4.25). A similar injury from a quartz lithic point tip in a lumbar vertebra was reported by Standen and Arriaza (2000). There was no evidence of healing and the wound was probably the cause of death. Finally, Tur et al. (2016: Koitas, central Kazakhstan) reported that a seventh–sixth century BCE aristocratic nomadic male also survived a spinal injury caused by a bronze arrowhead.

With weapons preserved in situ in bones, it may be possible to surmise the direction of flight of the projectile, and even associated soft tissue damage and complications. Armed with this knowledge, and with an understanding of anatomy, the soft tissue and skeletal damage can be assessed and the clinical effects of the injury reconstructed. Consider the Neolithic arrowhead in the anterior aspect of a lumbar vertebra described by Wells (1964a). The weapon, entering the body of the victim from the front, would, on reaching the abdomen, perforate the gut and transfix the aorta, the largest artery of the body, lying immediately in front of the vertebra at this level. The resultant hemorrhage would have been catastrophic, and death would have ensued within minutes. In contrast is the early medieval example of a metal arrowhead that came to rest on the posterior aspect of the third lumbar vertebra (Manchester and Elmhirst 1980). Its horizontal position suggests

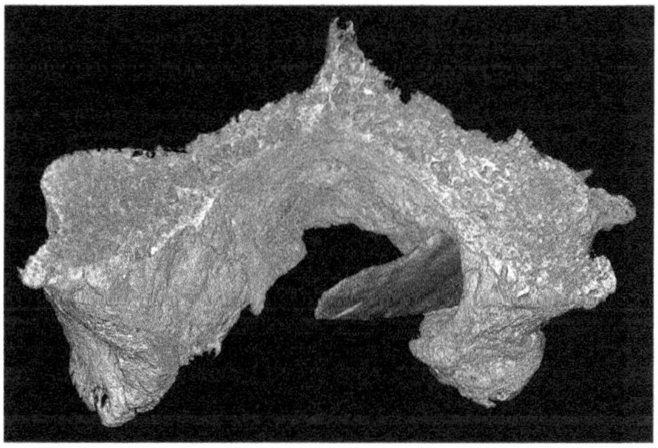

Figure 4.25. Quartz lithic projectile point in the neural arch of a lumbar vertebra in an adult male from Turuka, Baikal, Siberia (8000 BCE). Photograph courtesy of David Cooper.

that the weapon was shot at the upright victim, probably from a fairly close range to his right. The perimortem injury probably did no more damage than create pain, some bleeding, and in this instance at least, a minor opening in the spinal canal. As it turned out, this injury was insignificant because the victim also became subject to a tremendous blow to the right side of the back of the head. Bennike (1985) also reported in situ weapons in the pelvis, palate, cervical vertebrae, and sternum of skeletons of various dates from the Neolithic (4200–1800 BCE) to the Viking period (800–1050 CE) in Denmark. All the injuries were unhealed and the presence of the weapons suggests they contributed to the death of the individuals concerned. The availability of different materials to produce projectile weapons changed through time from, for example, flint to metal, and these changes would have affected the type and severity of resulting injuries. Therefore, as we move later on in time we see more injuries resulting from metal weapons, and even gunshot wounds.

With reference to gunshot wounds, although common in forensic contexts today, archaeological examples are rare. Nevertheless, four lead-shot balls were found associated with a cranium with evidence of an unhealed fracture from a postmedieval cemetery in Glasgow Cathedral, Scotland (King 1994), and Willey and Scott (1996) reported gunshot wounds to the cranium and postcranium in 60% of individuals (n = 6/10) from the Battle of Little Bighorn (1876 CE). Here, radiographic analysis provided evidence of metal fragments at the site of some wounds, and the direction of the shot was ascertained by the characteristics of the injuries. The medieval knight encased in metal armor from head to toe may be the classic, or rather popular, soldier of antiquity; for example, see Gurdjian's 1973 discussion of head protection through time. The rank and file, the ancestors of our armies today, were rather less fortunate. Body and head protection for these people may have been no more than leather garments, although there are more sophisticated examples. Even these would have afforded some defense against an aggressive blow. The protection, or otherwise, of the victim must be borne in mind when examining skeletal remains of victims of suspected interpersonal violence. While the fifteenth-century King Richard III of England had his arms and hands protected, he seems not to have been wearing a helmet when he was attacked. Perhaps he originally wore a helmet when he went into battle, but his aggressor may have taken it from him to inflict the fatal injuries (Appleby et al. 2015), and he probably died from one or more of the nine perimortem head injuries found on his skull.

Not only do cranial wounds throw light on the actions of the aggressor; they may also give an indication of the type of weapon used, where it does not survive. Indeed, experimental research has helped to identify the marks left on bone by specific weapons (e.g., Downing and Fibiger 2017; Forsom and Smith 2017). Dyer and Fibiger (2017) further described experimental research that has helped us understand the mechanisms behind blunt force trauma and violence in Neolithic Europe. A sharp blade will produce a clean cut, usually with smooth, straight, polished edges, and a blunter instrument may cause splintering of the edges of the wound. The war-hammer or mace tends to produce blunt force depressed fractures and puncture wounds (Moodie 1927; Wells 1964a). One of the most malicious hand weapons of all times was the medieval "morning star" or "holy water sprinkler." This weapon consisted of a wooden shaft with a metal spiked ball attached to it using a chain.

Forensic research can help paleopathologists in assessing marks of injuries. For example, Andahl (1978) considered the effect of different saw types on a range of materials, including bone. Later work (Humphrey and Hutchinson 2001; Tucker et al. 2001) examined the characteristic macroscopic and microscopic effects of machetes, axes, and cleavers on fresh pig bone and found that they produced different appearances on bone, thus indicating that the outcomes of this piece of research could be applied to studying human bones. Paleopathologists have also made attempts to determine the weapon type that produced the wound.

At the Battle of Towton (1461 CE) there were many victims, but only around forty individuals were found and excavated (Fiorato et al. 2001). Novak (2001) considered the evidence for cranial and postcranial trauma. Of the thirty-nine discrete burials, thirteen had postcranial trauma (average of 2.2 wounds per individual). Most of the trauma occurred on the forearm bones (both blunt and sharp force), and defense injuries were suggested as the mechanism behind these injuries. Nine of twenty-eight crania displayed healed injuries (32%), with twenty-seven also having perimortem trauma (average of 4.2 wounds per cranium). Some 65% of injuries were sharp, 25% blunt, and 10% puncture wounds. Most of the sharp and blunt injuries were probably the result of blows from the front in face-to-face combat. The twelve puncture wounds (eight people) were mostly square-shaped (three sharp, two projectile, and seven blunt), and arrowheads, poleaxe top spikes, war hammers, and crossbow bolts were suggested as weapons that could have produced them.

Perimortem trauma was also identified in twenty-one of the skeletons of thirty soldiers (70%) buried on the Napoleonic battlefield of Aspern (1809 CE), Austria (Binder and Quade 2018; Quade and Binder 2018). Here, lead musket balls were found within some of the graves, with seven of them potentially originally embedded in the bodies of the soldiers. The authors concluded that much of the perimortem trauma was caused by projectiles, although nine people were affected by blunt force trauma. These soldiers appeared to be infantry who were subject to injury from muskets and canons, but also possibly from being trampled by cavalry horses, remains of which were found at the site. In the Czech Republic at the site of Teplá, a monastery that functioned in the thirteenth–fifteenth century CE, a study of trauma in thirty individuals revealed almost half had injuries, and of those almost two-thirds displayed convincing evidence of violence. In considering associated historical accounts of the site, Pankowská et al. (2019: 919) concluded that these medieval monastic "clients" may have been trained to defend the monastery because its location was on a "military strategic land-road from Prague to Bavaria,"—that is, they were monastery warriors. An alternative explanation is that the cemetery received burials of laypeople killed in monastery attacks. Another example of violence directed at civilians comes from the Michelet necropolis of the fourth–eighth centuries CE in Lisieux, France (Timmins et al. 2017). Of 109 nonadults excavated, four aged between 2 and 7 years had evidence of perimortem cranial trauma. On the basis of the evidence, and knowledge of the political tensions experienced by the population through barbarian raids as the Roman Empire declined, it was surmised that these children were likely victims of related violence.

Directed violence in Oslo, Norway, has also been highlighted through the excavation of human remains from the high-status cemetery of St. Mary's (royal) Church, dated to 1040–1540 CE. Analysis revealed cranial trauma in some individuals, including some perimortem lesions; middle-aged and older men were most affected, but females and children were not spared (Brødholt and Holck 2012). Analysis of historical records for the site suggests that some people buried there were casualties of the civil wars in Oslo in the twelfth–thirteenth centuries. Finally, fourteen nonadults buried in 5 of 10 Gran Canaria caves in Spain were victims of violence. The largest proportion (9 of 42 burials) derived from a cave at Guayadeque dated from the sixth–seventh to the twelfth–thirteenth centuries CE (Velasco-Vázquez et al. 2018). While there was evidence for violence in adults too, the most affected age group studied comprised 5–6-year-olds. This may have been the outcome of the group trying to protect/secure resources, the authors emphasizing that this was an insular community subject to social instability.

In Asia a number of studies have included cranial trauma; three are illustrated here. In Iran, Afshar et al. (2018) documented cranial trauma in individuals buried at Tepe Hissar (fifth to second millennium BCE). Of the 129 individuals studied, 60 had cranial trauma (46.5%). Evidence for burning, mass burials, and destruction of buildings when this population was living support the hypothesis that cultural and economic changes led to tension and interpersonal violence. In southern Siberia, a nomadic second–fourth century CE site located at Tuva revealed 22 individuals (of at least 87) with 130 perimortem traumatic lesions to cranial or postcranial bones (or both). Chopping and slicing marks, along with penetrating and blunt trauma lesions, were seen. Males were more affected, with the evidence suggesting hand-to-hand combat, raiding, execution, violent rituals, throat slitting, and scalping (Milella et al. 2021). Contextual evidence indicated political instability at that time in this region. In a further study, this time in China (Turpan Basin, Xinjiang Uygur Autonomous Region), 129 intact crania from three Bronze to Iron Age Subeixi populations dating from 1000 to 100 BCE were studied (W. Zhang et al. 2021)—60 adult males, 54 adult females, and 15 nonadults. Of the 21 individuals with violence-related injuries to their crania (16.3% of 129), 81.6% of the injuries were perimortem. This suggests that these people may have been subject to nomadic invaders from the steppe attempting to secure resources, such as food supplies. Also in Asia, two studies in the Levant (eastern Mediterranean region of West Asia) have shed further light on fracture patterns indicative of interpersonal violence. The first was based on over 700 skulls from 47 sites in the southern Levant spanning 6,000 years (4300 BCE–1917 CE). There were 387 males, 223 females, and 145 nonadults, and overall 25% of individuals were affected. A similar frequency was seen across time, but based on the lesions observed, weaponry changed—from blunt to sharp to projectile. Twice as many males were affected as females, and most injuries had healed. Cohen et al. (2014)

concluded that as frequencies did not change over time, that might suggest that the violence was not related to changes in subsistence (farming to urban living) or to warfare, but rather to local interpersonal encounters. The second study was a literature review of evidence for antemortem trauma in Mesopotamia (present-day Iraq) based on published and unpublished sources (Sołtysiak 2017). Twenty-five sites with evidence were identified dating from 10,000 BCE to 1500 CE. Of the 1,278 individuals from these sites, 28 had 31 lesions between them (2.2%); few sharp force lesions were seen, and frequency was higher in earlier periods. Again, the author interpreted the data as reflecting intragroup violence and accidents, rather than intergroup warfare, and suggested that the consequences of state formation and the creation of professional armies were also likely risk factors for the trauma identified in some areas of the region (see Fibiger et al. 2013).

Like Europe and North America, South America has seen many studies of interpersonal violence in a variety of skeletal populations. Four are illustrated here. Juengst et al. (2017) explored the impact of sociopolitical change on the severity and extent of trauma when the Wari and Tiwanaku states in Bolivia lost power in 600–1000 CE. It was a time when people were constructing defensive buildings on the north shore of Lake Titicaca, but not on the south shore. All nine individuals excavated from the Copacabana Peninsula in the south shore area (1000–1250 CE) had interpersonal violent injuries that had healed. In the same time period, an increase in skeletal trauma was noted in the central and southern Andes. The authors of this study suggested that the injuries sustained at Copacabana were nonlethal, possibly because community care enabled people to survive. Clearly, the violence experienced by people living in this part of the Andes was not universal. Scaffidi and Tung (2020) focused on a pre-Hispanic (200–750 CE) site called Uraca in Arequipa, Peru, for their study of interpersonal violent cranial trauma. Of the 145 adult crania studied, 67% had injuries and two-thirds of those had more than one injury. More males than females were affected, and elite males in particular were victims. Both males and females had trauma to the anterior part of the cranium, while females had a higher frequency of trauma to the posterior area. Scaffidi and Tung (2020) concluded that these injuries were the result of raids against other groups and possibly aggression within their community in Uraca.

Two further studies, from Chile, complement this section. The first focuses on the oasis site of San Pedro de Atacama and 682 crania (Torres-Rouff and Costa Junqueira 2006). The research tested the hypothesis that environmental stability and affluence there would be associated with low rates of cranial injury, while environmental extremes and state collapse would result in high cranial trauma rates. Frequency rates increased from 5.1% in the earliest period to 10.9% in the Middle Horizon (600–950 CE), and then again to 35.6% in the Late Intermediate period (950–1400 CE). The occurrence of major droughts, poverty, and evidence of fortified buildings are used to argue why cranial trauma rose. Frequencies then declined a little in the Late Intermediate period. This was followed by a major decline in the Terminal phase of this period when environmental conditions improved (7%), and again in the Late Horizon period (1400–1532 CE) that encompassed the Inka occupation (3.4%). The second study is of skeletal remains of 10,000–4000 cal. BP Chinchorro hunter-fisher-foragers living on the Arica coast of the Atacama desert, Chile (Standen et al. 2020). Twelve sites revealed a total of 262 mummified remains and skeletons for the study of evidence of injuries due to interpersonal violence (136 adults and 126 nonadults). Two hypotheses were tested: that violent behaviors increased through time due to increased population density and social complexity; and that violence was more common between local Chinchorro groups than groups from other inland locations. Results showed a constant presence of violence over time, which was considered a normal part of these communities' behaviors, and males were more affected than females. The study therefore rejected the idea that increasing social complexity and density over time led to increased interpersonal violence.

Finally, studies from the African continent are considered, one from South Africa and the other from Sudan. Pfeiffer (2016) provided evidence for trauma, including accidental and interpersonal violent injuries, in 446 later Stone Age Cape skeletons (third millennium BCE). Healed and unhealed injuries were identified, and nonadults were not affected. However, perimortem injuries were only found for a specific period of time (ca. 2500 BCE) and in the southwest region, mostly in females and children: cranial trauma, embedded projectile points, and injuries caused by arrow points. This was at a time when there was a decline in height in the northwest and south, but not in the southwest. Changes in subsistence and land use were identified as precipitating violence, presumably to counteract pressure on resources. Pfeiffer suggested that when some populations were under stress, their reaction was to turn to violence, but that handling of that stress varied, with some groups experiencing a stature decline. Also related to social stress, Buzon and Richman's (2007) research explored evidence for interpersonal violence in Sudan as a result of aggressive Egyptian colonial campaigns in Upper Nubia, including the building of defensive structures, such as fortresses, in the Middle Kingdom (2050–1650 BCE). Buzon and Richman studied skeletons from Tombos (New Kingdom; 1550–1050 BCE). Their data were compared to those of Judd (2000, 2004) from nearby Kerma dating to a later time period (1750–1550 BCE). There was more evidence for cranial and parry fractures at Tombos than at Kerma. They concluded that in Kerma there appeared to have been more diplomacy and cooperation with the Egyptian administration, thus explaining less evidence for trauma; this may be because the population had come to terms with being colonized.

While we have seen the methods used for distinguishing antemortem and perimortem from postmortem marks in skeletal remains is very important, this is especially the case in the following sections where specific interpretations are being made in paleopathology (decapitation, scalping, defleshing, cannibalism, and domestic violence). We should also be cautious when presenting research that addresses these scenarios in the past. Discussing interpersonal violence in communities through these scenarios can be damaging to descendant communities.

Decapitation

Beyond sharp force injuries to bones, another type of sharp force injury that has been identified in the archaeological record focuses on a particular part of the body—decapitation. Evidence may be identified from cut marks on the cervical (neck) vertebrae and occasionally the mandible, or from the method of burial of the body, although the former is a safer interpretative context (direct rather than indirect evidence). Decapitation may be suggested when the skull of the skeleton is placed elsewhere in the grave—for example, near the feet. Although evidence for decapitation is usually considered to be a deliberate act carried out by someone else, and the result of corporal or capital punishment, self-decapitation has been noted in a modern forensic context (Hejna et al. 2012). Several other reasons for decapitation have also been suggested. These include interpersonal aggression aimed at the neck, subsequently leading to decapitation, a mismanaged hanging, trophy taking, as a form of bloodletting, or for reliquary collection (Boylston et al. 2000).

In the UK, a number of sites have revealed evidence for decapitation. At third–fourth-century Kempston, Bedfordshire, England, 13% (n = 12/92) of the Romano-British individuals had been decapitated (Boylston et al. 2000). Both females and males were equally affected, and one child. In all cases the skulls were placed near the legs or feet in the grave; eight had been buried in the main cemetery and four were placed in a ditched enclosure and classed as "other." Five of the twelve individuals were buried in coffins and five had evidence of cut marks on their cervical vertebrae. It was hypothesized that the decapitations were performed on incapacitated individuals, or on already dead individuals, and that some may have been casualties of armed conflict (Boylston et al. 2000, 250). The late first–fourth century CE Roman cemetery of Driffield Terrace in York revealed that over half of the eighty young to middle-aged males had been decapitated (Müldner et al. 2011; Fig. 4.26). Various interpretations of these findings have been suggested for this burial ground, including that these men represented "high-status Roman citizens" executed during the power struggle that followed the death of the Emperor Septimius Severus at York in 211 CE (Müldner et al. 2011, 280). Stable isotope analysis of eighteen of these men also revealed that whether they were locally born and raised or nonlocal had no bearing on whether they were decapitated, or whether they were interred together in a multiple grave. Other sites in the UK that have reported evidence for decapitation include the tenth–eleventh century CE Viking mass grave in Weymouth, Dorset, England (Loe et al. 2014), and Musselburgh, in East Lothian, Scotland (Moore et al. 2020). At the latter site, four Roman period (25–253 CE) skeletons were identified with evidence of decapitation. Stable isotope analysis indicated that they had all migrated to the area, but they did not have a common origin. Decapitation has also been reported elsewhere in Europe—for example, from first century BCE Celtic Sarliève-Grande Halle, France (Ardagna et al. 2005), second–first century BCE Israel (Dittmar et al. 2022); and of Swedish soldiers in seventeenth century CE Krakow (Kępa et al. 2013). Finally, Gao et al. (2023) reported a mass decapitation event in a Neolithic Chinese settlement site (4100–4000 BCE), intimating a culture of head-hunting at that time.

We also include skeletal evidence in this section of being hanged, drawn, and quartered, a fourteenth-to-nineteenth-century punishment (execution) for various crimes in England, Ireland, and Wales. Lewis (2008) reported the first evidence in skeletal remains for this practice in a male buried in the cemetery of the Cistercian monastery of

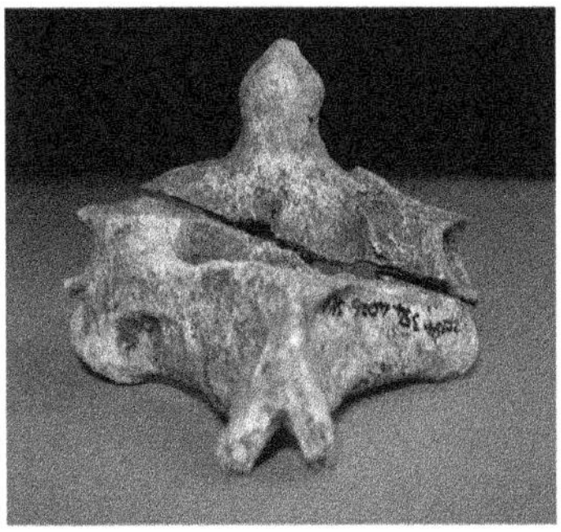

Figure 4.26. Evidence for decapitation on the axis vertebra of a young adult male from third century CE, Driffield Terrace, York, England. With kind permission from York Archaeology.

Hulton Abbey, Staffordshire, England (1219–1538 CE). Using historical records, the person was identified as Hugh Despenser the younger, a supposed lover of King Edward II (Fig 4.27). Evidence for torture has also been reported in the bioarchaeological record by Osterholtz (2012), who examined 14,882 commingled bone fragments representing thirty-three individuals at a settlement site at Sacred Ridge, in the Southwest United States (710–825 CE). Social control through torture was inferred from injuries to the plantar surfaces of foot bones, which it was thought resulted from direct blows to the feet. Termed "falanga" today, this practice can be life-threatening, and people may require surgery to recover (Dickson-Lowe et al. 2021).

Scalping

The culturally induced practice of scalping, resulting in cuts to the head and ultimately marks on the cranial bones, is defined as "the forcible removal of all or part of the scalp" (Owsley 1994, 335). A sharp implement was used on living (but

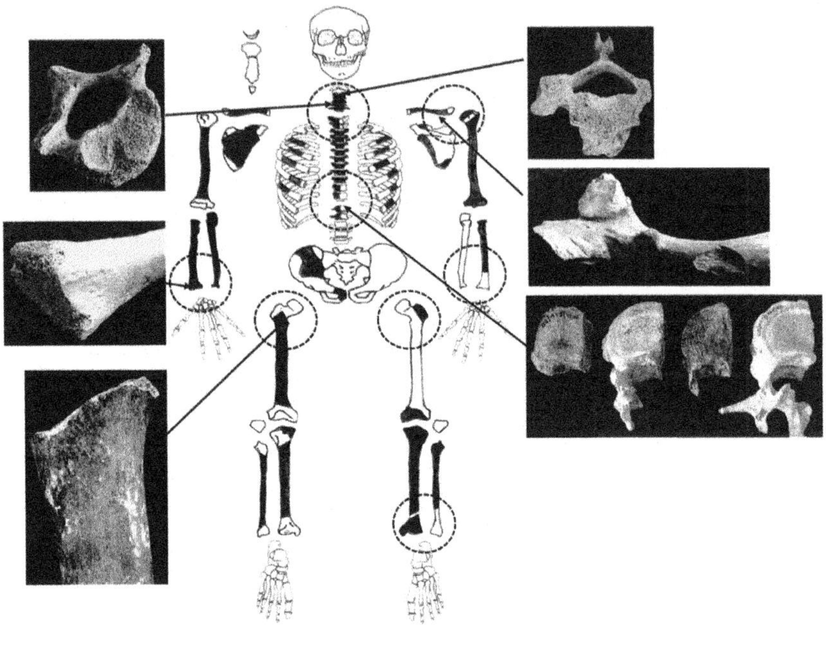

Figure 4.27. Distribution pattern of perimortem cut marks and the bones affected in a mature adult male from Hulton Abbey, Staffordshire, England (1219–1538 CE). He was hanged, drawn and quartered. The shaded black areas are the bones that are preserved. Figure produced by Mary Lewis.

mostly dead or dying) people, leaving short, straight, or slightly curved cut marks on the frontal and parietal bones. In some cases, fragments of the implement used for scalping have been found in the resulting wound (Olsen and Shipman 1994). During scalping, the periosteum and covering skin are removed, usually across the forehead, thus depriving the cranium of its periosteal blood supply. This resulted in death of the outer table of the cranium. If the person survived the process, which has been noted (see later in this section), inflammatory granulation tissue develops in the diploic space and the dead bone becomes separated from the living tissue next to it (Smith 2003, 308). Smith observed these changes in three individuals from Late Mississippian sites in the southeastern United States. New bone formation eventually occurs if the person survives, and the healed surface appears depressed, smooth, and variable in thickness. Another feature that has been identified is a groove around the circumference of the cranium, which indicates the area of skin and scalp incision (Hamperl 1967, 632). As Bueschgen and Case (1996) pointed out, the changes seen on the cranium vary according to whether the whole or part of the scalp is removed, and whether it is removed in bits or in one piece.

Reasons suggested for scalping in the past include violent interpersonal aggression, the wish to collect human trophies (to prove an enemy had been killed), intragroup sacrifice, medical treatment of a head wound, primitive autopsy, the removal of the scalp as a keepsake before burial (Redfern and Roberts 2019, 264–266), and even an accidental encounter with a wild animal, identified because of the irregular margins of the area involved (Ortner and Ribas 1997). The practice was first described by the Greek writer Herodotus in the fifth century BCE, and it has been seen worldwide in both prehistoric and historic periods. Bueschgen and Case (1996) indicate that the earliest evidence for scalping in North America dates from 5000–1500 BCE, and the majority comes from the Northern Plains of the Midwest, where tribal warfare was evident; males, females and children were all affected. There are also reports in South America—for example, in the pre-Hispanic Peruvian site of Kuelap, Chachapoya, where two individuals had probably been subject to scalping; one survived for a short time but the other revealed a more advanced state of healing, suggesting long-term survival (Toyne 2011). The Old World has also produced evidence, summarized in Murphy et al. (2002), with the earliest evidence coming from Neolithic Denmark (4500 BCE), and Jordana et al. (2009) report an individual buried in Mongolia, Asia, who had been scalped (fifth–third century BCE Pazyrk, Altai Mountains).

Defleshing and Cannibalism

Defleshing of soft tissue from the skeleton may also leave marks on the bone, and distinguishing between scalping and defleshing may be undertaken by examining the distribution of cut marks. Cut marks located on the cranium can usually be attributed solely to scalping (Williamson et al. 2003), while cut marks located more widely over the body could be due to defleshing, the latter indicated by cut marks around the joint surfaces, indicating disarticulation. A complicating factor for identification may be postmortem damage to areas of the skeleton revealing cut marks before and after defleshing, which could indicate that the body had been exposed prior to mutilation (Olsen and Shipman 1994).

Cannibalism as a cultural practice also should be differentiated from defleshing as part of secondary burial. Most evidence for cannibalism comes from the American Southwest and especially late prehistoric Anasazi groups (see the special issue of *Int. J. Osteoarchaeology* 10 (1) in 2000). The sites concerned date from 900–1650 CE, and a small proportion of the burials are multiple interments with many disarticulated and broken skeletal elements representing males, females, and nonadults (Larsen 2015, 146–148). Turner (1993) provided useful criteria for identifying cannibalism in the archaeological record, based on an assemblage of eight Anasazi individuals from Chaco Canyon, New Mexico. Perimortem cranial and postcranial bone breaks, cut marks, anvil-hammerstone abrasions, burning, bone fragment end polishing, and missing vertebrae were suggested as evidence. T. D. White (1992) also provides detailed data on the Mancos Canyon skeletal remains where human-induced toolmarks (indicating defleshing, percussion, chopping, and disarticulation) and thermal modification were identified on bones. Long bones were also extensively longitudinally fractured with patterns similar to those seen in animal bones where defleshing, disarticulation, and marrow extraction had been undertaken. Other data from elsewhere in the world include those reported from Fiji (50 BCE–1900 CE; DeGusta 1999, 2000), a Pleistocene hominin from Kenya (Pobiner et al. 2023); Europe (e.g., Villa et al. 1986; Boulestin and Gomez de Soto 1995; Fernando-Jalvo et al. 1999; Santana et al. 2019), and from the 1845 Franklin expedition to the Canadian Arctic (Mays and Beattie 2015).

Domestic Violence: Infanticide, Child Abuse, and Elder Abuse

The presence of traumatic lesions on the skeleton may represent other cultural practices, such as infanticide, physical abuse, and elder (caregiver) abuse. Domestic violence has been increasingly of interest to paleopathologists. Redfern (2017b) provided a review of the identification and interpretation of domestic violence, based on the criteria outlined in the clinical and social sciences. While paleopathology uses a clinical base for recording disease and injury in skeletal remains, Redfern cautioned that these data may not always be the most appropriate for interpretative purposes. Nevertheless, archaeological evidence has been published on child and elder caregiver violence, recognizing that “what is regarded as child abuse varies cross-culturally, and similar ambiguities are likely to arise at the older margins of the life course” (Gowland 2016, 521).

Infanticide is defined as the practice of killing unwanted infants in the first year of their lives (Craig 2004) and is essentially a specific type of child abuse. Infanticide in the past may have been practiced in a community because the child could not be provided for, or to contribute to birth spacing, or it may have targeted diseased children. It was also normally undertaken on females in cultures where males were considered more valuable. As Elmahi (2000) noted, contemporary hunter-forager and pastoral groups still practice infanticide, although accurate data on the number of victims are virtually nonexistent. Scrimshaw (1984) identified two main methods of disposing of infants: deliberate (through direct violence causing death) and passive infanticide (i.e., abandonment and/or exposure to a dangerous situation without emotional or biological support).

The evidence for the practice of infanticide at archaeological sites remains controversial (Lewis 2007, 90–91). Some have used the age-at-death distributions for perinatal individuals alongside their burial context (Smith and Kahila 1992; Mays 1993), where an unnatural peak in babies dying at 38–40 weeks (rather than baby deaths spread more widely across weeks) suggests death at childbirth and hence infanticide. The sex distribution of these perinates may also provide clues. Smith and Kahila (1992) analyzed the remains of one hundred 1–2-day-old infants from Ashkelon, Israel, found beneath the fourth century CE Roman bathhouse in a sewer. Ancient DNA analysis of nineteen of these babies revealed that 74% (fourteen) were male (Faerman et al. 1997). This led to an interpretation that the well was used by a brothel, and that female children were kept to be raised, while the male babies were "disposed of." Conversely, a natural death may have been responsible for the thirty-one perinates discovered in villas in Roman Sussex, England; at Beddington and Bignor, nine of thirteen babies (69%) analyzed for mitochondrial aDNA were male (Mays and Faerman 2001). At Yewden Roman Villa, Hambleden, 58% (7/12) of the perinates analyzed were female (Hassan et al. 2014). Mays (1993; Mays and Eyers 2011) cited a peak in the deaths of babies at 39–40 weeks' gestation (a full-term birth) as evidence for infanticide being practiced in Roman Britain. Others argue that, unlike at Ashkelon, where babies were placed within a well, the burial of these babies near boundaries or within domestic spaces speaks instead, to a desire to preserve an intimate link with their mothers, whose identities were deeply entwined with their offspring (Millett and Gowland 2015). Such specific burial practices for those who died around the time of birth have also been demonstrated in Spain (Alberto-Barroso et al. 2022: pre-Hispanic Gran Canaria; Rissech et al. 2023: Barcelona).

Of all the different contexts of abuse, the identification of child abuse or caregiver violence in the archaeological record on the basis of the skeleton is a subject that has seen much interest over the past 20 years. Clinical data indicate that today an abused child is usually less than 4 years old (Ragan 2011). The pattern of injuries can include fractures to the long bones (metaphyseal; spiral due to twisting forces), rib fractures (bilateral and close to the spine, caused by grasping/squeezing the child's chest), cranial fractures and widened sutures as a result of subdural hematomas causing pressure inside the cranium, and subperiosteal hematomas (and new bone formation, if survived) as a result of ripping of the periosteum from the bone if a child is grabbed forcibly and/or swung around—this may also result from striking the child. Burns, scars, lacerations, and a failure to thrive and grow normally are also features that may be observed in an abused child, but one of the key features to the recognition of child abuse is the occurrence of traumatic lesions in several locations at different stages of healing, which indicates repeated episodes of violence (Walker et al. 1997; Marine and Forbes-Amrhein 2021; Lewis 2018, table 5.5). If the child dies during the first abusive incident, there would be no evidence of healing. Harris lines of arrested growth, enamel hypoplasia, and shorter than normal long bones for the age of the child may also be indirect indicators of child abuse both present and past (i.e., physical and emotional stress, and a failure to thrive). However, identifying abuse-related perimortem injuries in the bones of the very young can be challenging (Lewis 2018, 139).

Child abuse today is often seen in communities struggling on many fronts, for example, in poverty. As Lewis wrote (2018, 119), some skeletal features recognized for child abuse, such as shorter long bones for the age at death of an individual, are associated with impoverished societies. Several reports of possible child abuse in different times and places have been published, each with very different contexts that helped with final interpretations. The contextual background of each site and individuals studied is needed to understand the potential risk factors, which are key to interpretation. Studies include a 2–4-year-old from Užubaliai, Alytus, Lithuania (Kozakaitė et al. 2018); children buried at the nineteenth-century Kilkenny Workhouse in Ireland during the Great Irish Famine (Geber 2016); a 2–3-year-old from Kellis 2, Dahkleh Oasis, Egypt (Wheeler et al. 2013); and 11 of 242 nonadults from Puruchuco-Huaquerones, Peru (Gaither 2012).

At the other end of the age spectrum, but still an incredibly important part of the demographic, both past and present, skeletons of older individuals are receiving more attention (e.g., see Appleby 2008, 2010, 2018). In particular, elder abuse is a relatively new field of bioarchaeological study. While it is recognized in clinical settings as not a new issue, it is now subject to rigorous scientific study, scrutiny from the criminal justice system, and of medical concern. Gowland (2016) has provided a thorough overview of clinical data on, and risk factors for, elder abuse and has usefully collated the potential generalized and localized injuries that might be encountered in elderly victims of abuse. Gowland noted that clinical data on elder abuse is lacking because research in this area is sparse. Therefore, identification of the practice in clinical settings and in archaeological contexts will remain challenging until more studies are carried out. It is noteworthy that the world's population is aging rapidly, and improvements in medical and surgical care and living conditions for many, but not all, are responsible. The World Health Organization (2024a) reports that about 1 in 6 people who are 60 years and older have experienced some form of abuse in community settings, abuse is higher in institutional settings, such as care homes, and abuse can lead not only to physical but also psychological consequences. Therefore, elder abuse may increase in the future and, one hopes, new research will be to the benefit of older people in both modern and archaeological settings (e.g., see Storey 2020).

Treatment of Trauma

Trauma can be painful, debilitating, and disabling, although inferring these symptoms from skeletal analysis is very challenging indeed. Today, where they can and have the resources to do so, people afflicted with trauma usually try to seek help and have their injuries treated. Trauma has faced all societies in the past, and the treatment of a leg with a simple fracture by reducing and splinting has been adopted by people through time. The evidence for the treatment of trauma is plentiful in historical data, but direct evidence from the skeleton is more rare. The availability of such treatment, however, for all people of whatever status, age, biological sex, or ancestry is generally unknown for the past.

The World Health Organization (WHO 2024g) believes that "all people, everywhere, have the right to achieve the highest attainable level of health." Furthermore, "universal health coverage" is one of the targets for the United Nations Sustainable Development Goals (through Goal 3: Good health and well-being), and in 2019 "countries reaffirmed that health is a precondition for and an outcome and indicator of the social, economic and environmental dimensions of sustainable development" (United Nations 2024b). Inequality of access to medical services affects many across the globe and for a range of reasons, including biological sex, gender, and geographic location. Examples of the disadvantaged include women in Malawi (Azad et al. 2020), rural communities of China (Guo et al. 2020), and remote island dwellers of Jumalig, Luzon, Philippines (Collado 2019). Often, many risk factors for poor health intersect too (e.g., Purnell et al. 2016: United States).

While health care today compared to that of our ancestors is markedly different and more advanced in terms of medicines and surgical procedures, historical sources and archaeological evidence, including that from human remains, show us that people in the distant past did not necessarily sit and suffer. The more obvious treatments of trauma, such as splinting of fractures, trepanation for head injuries, or amputation of traumatized limbs, may be seen in skeletal remains, but complementary medical treatments may be seen only in extant artistic and written sources; for example, maggot therapy (Whitaker et al. 2007; Keene et al. 2019; Zubir et al. 2020) and drug therapy (e.g., see Rawcliffe 1997; Dendle and Touwaide 2008; Van Arsdall 2010). Artifacts from archaeological sites, including surgical instruments and plant remains, may also provide evidence of therapeutic interventions (e.g., see Baker 2013; Bai et al. 2021; Watson and Gilchrist 2021). In addition, observation of wound care in various traditional societies of today may suggest nonsurgical practices of the distant past, even as they are being reappreciated in the present (e.g., Builders and Builders 2016; Salazar-Gómez and Alonso-Castro 2022; Biswas et al. 2023). Treatment of trauma and disease today requires knowledge of the anatomy and physiology of the human body. This knowledge was not always present in past communities. Instead, knowledge of animal anatomy was (and is) applied to managing human problems, including disease and trauma (Franco 2013). Importantly paleopathologists need to be aware of the history of treatment, anatomical dissection, and autopsy, because these interventions changed through time, and they also leave traces on human remains that were not caused by the disease or injury.

Dissection of the human body may go back more than 4,000 years, but human dissection was forbidden at various times and places, including in Greco-Roman antiquity and medieval Christian Europe. Sometimes exceptions were granted to permit autopsies for forensic or clinical reasons when concerns were raised over cause of death (Duffin 2021, 9–38; Bubb 2022; Brenna 2022). Some knowledge of anatomy was essential for surgeons who dressed wounds and set bones. The fourteenth-century French surgeon Guy de Chauliac wrote, "the surgeon who is ignorant of anatomy operates on the human body in the same manner as a blind man works on wood" (*La grande chirurgie*, ed. 1683, 49 [our translation]). In early modern Europe, Italian artists such as Leonardo Da Vinci and Michelangelo, helped put the study of anatomy on a firm foundation; dissections and autopsies became more commonplace, illustrated anatomy texts became more freely available, and anatomical research ensued (Bertoloni Meli 2018; Ghosh and Kumar 2019). While brain function had intrigued the ancients, including Aristotle (third century BCE) and Galen (second century CE), elucidation of its shape, structure, and physiology took some time, until Vesalius, working in the sixteenth century CE, described its anatomy (Martensen 2004; Cobb 2020). The paleopathological record confirms these trends. For example, Flies et al. (2017) found evidence for postmortem dissection or autopsy on fifty-two skeletons from a cemetery associated with a nineteenth-century hospital for the poor in Denmark. Furthermore, Dittmar and Mitchell (2015) analyzed nineteenth-century human remains in the light of dissection manuals to develop criteria for differentiating dissection from autopsy in archaeological skeletons.

Evidence for treatment of disease and injury in the past exists in written and artistic form (e.g., Porter 1997; Duffin 2021, 257–261), and useful comparative data stem from ethnographic and nonhuman studies, such as traditional bone setting in Africa (Ezeanya-Esiobu 2019, 81–96) or self-medication in primates (De La Fuente et al. 2022). Direct evidence for this treatment in the archaeological record relies on identifying amputation, splinting of fractures, and trepanation of the skull (Ellis 2009, 1–6). The following sections explore evidence for these treatments.

Amputation

Amputation of limbs has been carried out since very early times and for various reasons. Apart from the traumatic amputation of a limb during conflict or accident, in the past the deliberate removal of the whole or a part of a limb has been carried out as a surgical procedure for the treatment of disease, such as infection or injury, or for punishment in many parts of the world, including ancient Egypt and Babylon (Mavroforou et al. 2014). One of the earliest examples of amputation, dated to the ninth dynasty in Egypt (ca. 2160–2025 BCE), but one that has been disputed, is the loss of the distal half of the right radius and ulna (Brothwell and Møller-Christensen 1963; Messina et al. 2022). In this case, a bridge of bone between the stump ends and obvious healing and remodeling of their ends indicate that the individual survived the operation. The practice of hand amputation of prisoners of war, practiced in the nineteenth dynasty (ca. 1295–1186 BCE) is pictorially portrayed in the temple of Rameses III, and a recent CT-scan investigation of the mummified remains of Ramses III suggests that one of his toes was amputated (Saleem and Hawass 2017). X. Zhang et al. (2021) also describe a male from China with an amputation that may have been the result of punishment (Fig. 4.28).

Depending on the time and place, skeletal evidence for amputation, however, is rare, probably because unhealed amputated limbs could be mistaken for postmortem

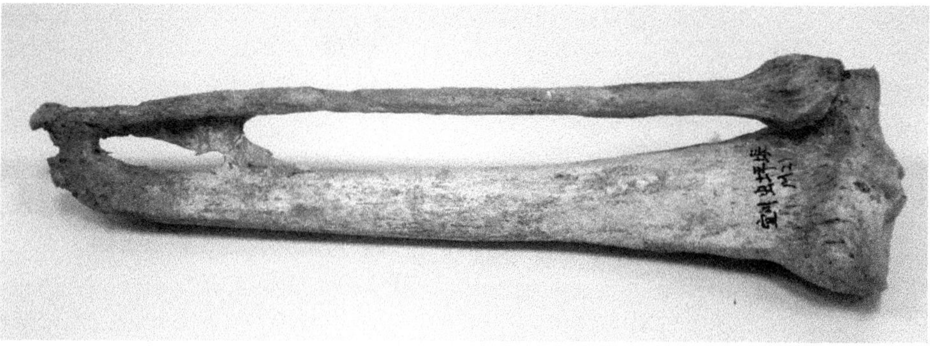

Figure 4.28. Evidence of a foot amputation (healed ends of the tibia and fibula). An older adult male from Chongpingyuan, Shaanxi, Central Plains, China (eighth–fifth centuries BCE). Photograph courtesy of Liang Chen.

breaks of bones. In both cases, whether amputated or damaged postmortem, there would be no evidence of healing; that is, in the former the person died at the time of or very soon after the amputation, probably due to extensive uncontrolled hemorrhage or sepsis. Another differential diagnosis for bones that may appear to have been amputated is a fracture with little or no healing (an ununited fracture); if the distal fragment is missing, an incorrect diagnosis may be made. Microscopic examination of the cut surface of the unhealed bone may reveal marks indicative of the instrument used, thus differentiating between a postmortem break, an unhealed fracture, and an unhealed amputation. Differentiating between perimortem and postmortem sharp force trauma has been discussed earlier in the chapter and is relevant here too. Nevertheless, it may be possible to extend the diagnosis of amputations by assessing the rest of the skeleton and observing abnormal bone change. If a limb has been amputated, a particular scenario could be envisaged. A person may not be able to use the affected limb. Compared to the opposite unaffected side, this could lead to disuse atrophy, or reduction in the size of bones and related soft tissues, associated with reduction in the muscle attachments. For example, Lazenby and Pfeiffer (1993) described overall size, cross-sectional geometry, and mid-shaft histological features in the skeleton of an historically identified nineteenth-century person from Middlesex County, Ontario, Canada. He had undergone a below-knee amputation, which supported the scenario described here. This individual may also have had a prosthesis and crutches to aid locomotion. These artifacts are generally lost to the paleopathologist, being made of organic materials such as wood that do not necessarily survive burial. Nevertheless, these artifacts have been described and illustrated (e.g., Hernigou 2014). Binder et al. (2016) also documented survival of an early medieval foot prosthesis in Austria.

Mays (1996a) made a comprehensive review of the evidence for amputations in the Old World, including detailing the skeleton of an individual from the late medieval English site of Blackfriars Friary, Ipswich, Suffolk, England. Also in the southern part of England, Stuckert and Kricun (2011) reported an individual buried at Lankhills, Hampshire, during the Roman period who underwent bilateral foot amputation, adding a third to two previously reported individuals from the same site with amputations affecting the hands. Elsewhere in Europe, Dorado-Fernández et al. (2021) reported evidence from eighteenth–nineteenth-century CE Spain: an amputated left leg with a comminuted fracture found in a clay vessel partially wrapped in bandages. Finally, Zäuner et al. (2013) described a 6,000-year-old skeleton with evidence for a hand amputation from the site of Tell Yunat, in Bulgaria.

In the Middle East, Bloom et al. (1995) reported on the first amputation evidence from Israel: the skeleton was that of an adult male, dated to 3,600 years old, whose hand amputation showed clear signs of healing. Judd (2023) described evidence of a lower limb amputation from Late Ottoman Jordan. In Africa, evidence for amputations have been described by Brothwell and Møller-Christensen (1963) and Saleem and Hawass (2017); and in the mummified remains of an older adult female from the necropolis of Thebes-West, Egypt (ca. 1550–1300 BCE), evidence for an amputated great toe and its replacement with a wooden prosthesis was documented by Nerlich et al. (2000). This female also displayed evidence of osteopenia of the leg bones (loss of bone mineral density, perhaps leading to atrophy) and atherosclerosis. This latter finding suggests that this female's toes may have been affected by gangrene, thus necessitating amputation. Further evidence from Egypt comes from the site of Dayr al-Barshā reported by Dupras et al. (2010); two individuals with bilateral amputation of the feet and one with an amputation of an ulna, all healed; and one perimortem amputation of the distal end of the humerus. In South Africa, Van der Merwe et al. (2010) documented fractures and amputations in nineteenth-century miners. Evidence from the New World is not as frequent, although three individuals with probable evidence of foot amputation have been documented from Peru and date to 100–750 CE, which correlates well with Moche ceramic depictions of people without feet (Verano et al. 2000). Phillips et al. (2021) described healed amputations of feet in two pre-Hispanic individuals buried at Lambayeque, Peru.

Although the skeletal evidence of amputation is rather scant in the paleopathological record, relatively speaking the records of trepanation are more abundant, albeit geographically biased. When the surgical risks of the two procedures are compared, it is perhaps surprising that, on the evidence available, trepanation appears to have been a more common surgical procedure than amputation. The figures may, however, be biased by the relative ease of recognition of trepanation and the difficulty of finding evidence of amputation, and the picture may change as more evidence for both is found.

Trepanation

Trepanation is a practice known since very early times, being recorded by the Greek medical writer Hippocrates in the fifth century BCE (*On Head Wounds*, 14–21; Hippocrates 1999; Missios 2007); it is also seen today among practitioners of extreme body modification and in a few traditional Indigenous societies (Gump 2010; Mahone 2014). Performed for whatever reason, the operation involves incision of the scalp and the cutting through and removal of an area of the cranium

(Fig. 4.29). The result is the exposure of the membrane (dura mater) covering the brain. Survival of the patient, for individuals must be regarded as patients in this surgical operation, probably depended on the skillful avoidance of perforation of the additional deeper membranes (arachnoid mater and pia mater) and the avoidance, either by luck or good judgment, of the major blood vessels, meningeal arteries, and veins within the cranium. The proportion of survivors of this operation in antiquity was quite high (Moghaddam et al. 2015; Jolly and Kurin 2017). The evidence for survival is the healing and remodeling of the bone around the operation site. Analyzing ninety archaeological examples of trepanation, and on the basis of fourteen modern patients who had undergone trepanation, Partiot et al. (2020) described implications of healing of trepanations for paleopathology.

Several examples exist of individuals having undergone another trepanning operation, having survived a preceding one. A notable individual, represented by the "Cuzco skull" from Peru, shows no fewer than seven trepanned holes, all with signs of healing (Oakley et al. 1959). Perhaps equally surprising is the size of the trepanned areas, particularly where survival has occurred. For example, a crania from an individual from Neolithic Latvia possessed three trepanning defects. The largest single hole measured 68 x 55 mm, and all three merged to produce an opening 120 x 60 mm in size. This individual survived his surgical trauma and died perhaps over a year later, possibly from some other disease unrelated to the trepanation (Derums 1979).

Ancient examples of trepanation number well into the thousands, and their distribution is worldwide (see overview in Arnott et al. 2003). Europe affords many of these examples (e.g., Bennike 1985: Denmark; Roberts and McKinley 2003: Britain; Moghaddam et al. 2015: Switzerland; Riccomi et al. 2017: Italy; Aidonis et al. 2021: Greece). Piggott (1940) suggested that central and northern Europe may be the original home of trepanation. Examples are also found in the Americas (Verano 2016: Peru), Australia (Webb 1988), and Asia (e.g., Sun et al. 2023: China). While the majority of trepanations have been recorded in adults, Lewis (2018, 115–116) has reviewed the more limited evidence in nonadults. A late Paleolithic origin has been claimed, and by the Neolithic period it was an active practice. Although flourishing in the Neolithic period in Europe, perhaps more than at any other time, the operation has been performed during all periods since.

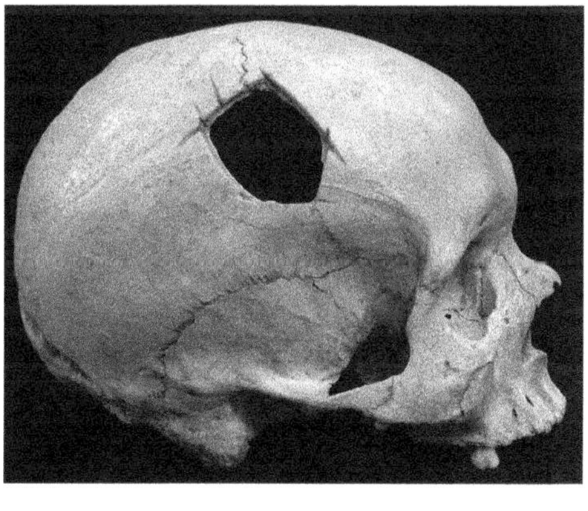

Figure 4.29. Trepanation in the cranium of an adult buried in a cave in Central Highlands, Peru (Late Pre-Hispanic Period). Photograph courtesy of John Verano.

The technical object of the operation was clear, but the actual surgical procedure adopted was variable. Dependent on the era and the technologies available, the operation may have been carried out with a flint scraper or blade, or a metal implement that may or may not have been adapted specifically for the purpose. Initial incision of the scalp is a very bloody procedure, but the hemorrhage can be minimized by turning back the scalp flaps created, a strategy early surgeons may have realized and carried out. Some research has provided evidence for the type of instrument used in the operation. Stevens and Wakely (1993) used scanning electron microscopy to examine a trepanation and, by experimental analogy, suggested that the instrument had been a shell. An experimental study by Yang et al. (2023) on two trepanations from northwest China using electron microscopy and CT imaging suggested that the surgeons were experienced practitioners and that the holes produced could have been done with a variety of tools. By the first century CE, Celsus proposed the operation should be undertaken using a tool he called a modiolus, a hollow cylinder with serrated edges (*De medicina*, book 8, chap. 3, 1; Gross 2009).

After cutting the soft tissues, the outer cranial surface and pericranium was exposed. At this point, the type of trepanation varied. Five methods (types) have been identified from skeletal remains:

1. The scraped type involved removing the bone surface and creating beveled edges on the central hole in the cranium
2. The gouge type entailed removing a larger piece of cranium by delineating a circular area on the cranial surface and gouging it out with an implement
3. The bore and saw type usually involved the use of a drill-type implement to make a series of holes in a circle and a saw to connect the holes
4. The saw type consisted of incising four marks, usually in a square, to enable a piece of bone to be removed from the cranium. A risk, theoretical or real, of the four linear saw actions was the fact that, subject to the size of the quadrangle delineated, the depth of the saw at its greatest point could be deep to the dura mater, potentially entering brain tissue and possibly creating a rapidly fatal injury
5. The final type involved the creation of a small hole with a drill, or trephine, which should strictly be called a trephination

These trepanation types appear in differing frequencies in different parts of the world and in different eras. For example, the scraping method appears more frequently in Europe, including Britain (Roberts and McKinley 2003), and the sawing method in South America. Studies of the site of trepanation indicate that many were performed on the left side of the frontal and parietal bones, and rarely were these operations performed over the skull sutures. Some ancient authors recommended not to trepan over the sutures for fear of lacerating a major vein (Grmek 1991; Aidonis et al. 2021). One can imagine the agony suffered by the patient in antiquity. After cutting the scalp incision, however, the operation is relatively painless, particularly if the patient was comatose or had been given acupuncture, alcohol, or analgesic herbs, such as opium, henbane, willow, or mandrake, all cited as substances used for inducing anesthesia and analgesia in particular population groups (Majno 1975; Eger et al. 2014, 3–10; Hao and Mittelman 2014).

During these processes the bone dust created may have been collected. In more recent periods, human skull dust has been used as a magico-religious remedy (Janssens 1970; Giuffra and Fornaciari 2015). Whatever method was employed by whichever society, the end result was the removal of a piece of cranium and the exposure of the membranes covering the brain. The postoperative care of this bloody and potentially infected operative wound is equally impressive, particularly in view of the survival of many victims. A study by Stewart (1958) found that over 50% of 214 crania with trepanation from Peru had healed. In Britain, the (more common) scraping method was accompanied by good survival rates (Roberts and McKinley 2003). Perhaps the gradual scraping of the cranium allowed more precise and controlled penetration of the inner table and hence less likelihood of brain injury. Osteitis (bone inflammation) and bone scarring surrounding the hole have been attributed to chemical irritants applied postoperatively; however, these features are more likely the result of infection of the wound (Stewart 1958). Doubtless some closure of the skin wound must have been made, either by drawing together the skin flaps or by the application of a dressing, possibly of vegetation. For example, in historic times in Melanesia, the operation site was covered with materials such as wood bark, banana leaf, and coconut shell.

The technique of operation is plain to see. The motive for the operation is not known for certain in most cases (see Roberts and McKinley 2003); it most likely lies in the culture of the societies that practiced it. The popular and somewhat romantic notion that trepanation was carried out solely for magico-ritual reasons may seem hardly credible. Such a reason might have justified the operation on a corpse, and this undoubtedly could have occurred. In these cases, no healing would be expected and postmortem damage rather than purposeful surgery could be implicated; consequently, differentiating perimortem from postmortem wounds is again relevant here. The absence of documentation from the long periods of prehistory permits only speculation. Why would living people submit themselves willingly to such a dangerous operation for ritual reasons? They may have had no choice. And yet, as Oakley et al. (1959) remarked, so many trepanned crania have been found in the chambered tombs of the Seine–Oise–Marne area of France that it is probable that the operation had some ritual significance. Roundels of human cranial bone have also been found in early prehistoric graves, suggesting that such objects were treated as talisman (with magical/spiritual powers), implying that trepanation was also undertaken to produce amulets (Roberts and McKinley 2003).

To the contemporary mind, however, the signs and symptoms of those with mental illness, the uncontrollable seizures of those with epilepsy, and the incapacitating head pain of migraine may have seemed sufficient justification to "let the evil spirit out of the brain." These illnesses are without skeletal manifestation and medical justifications must, therefore, remain speculative. As indicated by Cobb (2020, 15), the concept of the brain as the center of emotion and psychological prominence was a relatively late phenomenon in many societies, superseding the heart as the center. Indeed, some historians emphasize that when confronted with skull fractures, practitioners may have worried more about the broken bone than the underlying brain until early modern times (Rose 1997). Thus, "letting the evil spirit out" may have been a concept unknown in earlier times.

Research has documented the funerary context of trepanned individuals from British burials to explore whether these people were buried in different ways from the normal rite for the period and geographic location (Roberts and McKinley 2003). The hypothesis was that people who had been trepanned might have been regarded as different in some way; for example, they may have had some mental impairment (although there is no direct evidence for this). On the other hand, clear documentary evidence, from at least Hippocratic times, supports the notion that the operation was also carried out for justifiable clinical reasons, even by modern standards; for example, as a release of hematomas (collection of blood) or pus following cranial injuries, as Celsus (first century CE) advised (*De medicina*, book 8, chap. 4, 7). Trepanation may be related to the site of a cranial fracture too (Haneveld and Perizonius 1980; Wells 1982; Parker et al. 1986). A skull with three trepanations, two healed and one unhealed, also displayed frontal sinusitis and intracranial infection, suggesting that infection of the sinuses initiated the trepanation (Zias and Pomeranz 1992). Mogle and Zias (1995) also reported possible evidence of scurvy in an 8-to-9-year-old from middle Bronze Age Israel (ca. 2200 BCE) with an unhealed trepanation. Smrčka et al. (2003) described a late medieval male cranium from the Czech Republic (1298–1550 CE) with a trepanation probably undertaken to treat a meningioma (tumor), which likely led to symptoms of what we would deem increased intracranial pressure. Whatever the ailment being treated in the past, it is clear that ancient people recognized the association of symptoms produced by increased intracranial pressure and head wounds.

To end this section, several other natural lesions of the cranium may also be considered in a differential diagnosis of trepanation; thinning of the parietal bones resulting in a hole (usually in old age), tumors or infections producing holes in the tables of the skull, enlarged parietal foramina, and postmortem damage (Kaufman et al. 1997). With increased use of sophisticated methods of analysis such as the scanning electron microscope and CT imaging, these other diagnoses should be easily confirmed or eliminated.

Fracture Treatment

As we have discussed, satisfactory healing of fractures in adults is a long process taking perhaps many weeks or months, during which time total rest of the injured part is essential. In the past, resting may not have been too difficult to do in the case of an upper limb fracture, when the afflicted individual would have been able to perform some tasks with the opposite limb. It would have been much more difficult in the case of a person from a small community who fractured a lower limb bone. In work-centered groups of the past, particularly in hunter-forager populations, little room would have been created for "passengers." In such cases the injured, if they survived, would have been dependent on the community for welfare. What an enormous reorganization of lifestyle a nomadic group would have had to make to care for a member with a badly fractured femur who may have been totally incapacitated for perhaps three months.

Bone fractures healing in a position of poor alignment are a common finding in skeletal remains from the past. The large bones of the leg, such as the tibia, fibula, and especially the femur, which is surrounded by powerful muscles that contract strongly around the site of a fracture, are the most common fractures for this malalignment. Satisfactory bone healing in a position of good alignment is even less likely in the case of a comminuted fracture. Considering the potentially intense pain of the leg fracture, the long period of total immobility and dependence on others, and the subsequent potential disability because of a grossly shortened leg, and it may be possible to gain an insight into the experiences of the injured victim of antiquity. This is not to say that all healed fractures in the past had such poor outcomes. For example, Gilmour et al. (2019) studied fractures to lower limb bones from two Roman sites in Italy and England. They explored cross-sectional geometric properties of the affected bones, and found that none had outlying properties. They concluded that the people with those healed fractures would not have experienced altered mobility, or impairment, when compared to people who did not have fractures. They therefore stressed that "paleopathologists should be cautious in relying on the anatomical appearance of healed fractures as a predictor of dysfunction . . ." (2019, 127). This is relevant when paleopathologists are attempting to infer impairment and disability (and care) from the skeleton. The care of individuals with trauma has, however, been a focus recently. Dittmar et al. (2023) used plain film radiography and micro-CT scans to analyze three medieval individuals with healed fractures buried in Cambridge, England. They recorded complications of the fractures, the mechanism of injury, and functional consequences, and using the Bioarchaeology of Care model (Tilley and Cameron 2014), they explored what care these people may have needed.

The successful treatment of fractures is suggested in both art and written records contemporary with many historically documented populations worldwide. This is in contradiction to the statement by Wells (1974b, 220), who wrote, "With very few exceptions they [Anglo-Saxons] made virtually no difference to what the natural healing powers of the body would have achieved unaided." Ethnographic studies of traditionally living societies also support the fact, already discussed, that treatment of fractures by reduction and splinting is a simple and logical process to learn and implement. Observations in these societies suggest that some thought is channeled into caring for the injured: reduction by manipulation, or sometimes traction, and splinting of broken bones with natural products such as bark, reeds (e.g., Fess 2002; and see Fig. 4.30), bamboo (Carroll 1972), animal skins (Fortuine 1984), and clay (Szostakowski et al. 2017). Herbal concoctions and bandages, and the use of animal hair and plant fibers, compose some of the methods of treatment of associated wounds. For example, the Yoruba of Nigeria (Oyebola 1980) were conversant at that time with the clinical features of fractures (pain, swelling, deformity, and loss of function) but, having no radiography facility, missed the diagnosis of hairline greenstick fractures and thus identified only the major breaks. Herbal dressings and

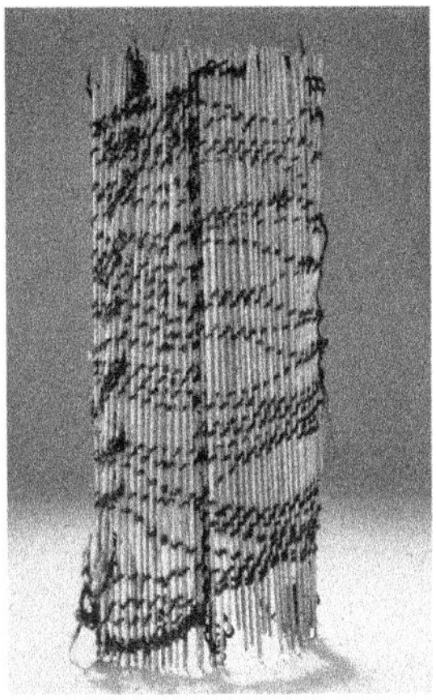

Figure 4.30. Traditional reed splint for an arm lashed together with cord. Science Museum, Science and Society Picture Library; location unknown; Henry Wellcome Collection.

splints were applied and reapplied daily following hot fomentations. The outcomes varied, but observers suggest that delayed healing occurred when patients were mobilized too early and reduction was not maintained consistently. Despite these shortcomings, however, it is clear that relatively effective treatment was practiced by the twentieth-century Yoruba and other traditional societies, and there is no reason to suggest that this was not the case in a distant past.

Authors of the Hippocratic treatises *Fractures*, *Joints*, and *Mochlion* display an intimate knowledge of the bones and joints. They described several methods of treatment of dislocations and fractures, some of which are still used today: reduction and splinting of fractures, maintaining the fracture in reduction with pads and bandages reinforced by clays and starches, including the adjacent joints, and using other bone elements of the limb to splint the broken bone anatomically, for example, radius to ulna and tibia to fibula. Traction was urged for spinal fractures with the use of a device, now called the Hippocratic bench (Nutton 2004, 96). They also recommended a healthy diet to favor healing. Evidence for the use of traction to reduce fractures has been described in Egyptian as well as Greco-Roman antiquity. During later periods in Europe similar fracture treatment methods were advocated by surgeons such as Guy de Chauliac (1300–1370 CE) and Ambroise Paré (1510–1590 CE), both of France, and Hieronymus Brunschwig (c. 1450–c. 1512/1513 CE) of Germany (Brorson 2009; Metzler 2006, 113; Hernigou 2015)

In addition to surgeons, bonesetters were a group of people whose trade developed specifically for this purpose; they seem to have been present in many countries around the world, particularly in the sixteenth and seventeenth centuries CE, and still are today (e.g., see Agarwal and Agarwal 2010). The "natural" bonesetter was the forerunner of the orthopedic surgeon, meeting the needs of those with illness or trauma involving bone, joint, or muscle. The bone-setting skill was handed down through the generations in families. In early medieval England, herbal remedies such as betony, comfrey ("knitbone") and "bonewort" (violet/pansy) mixed with egg white were also recommended for fractured bones (Van Arsdall 2010; Everett 2012, 287). The treatment of wounds associated with fractures, however, varied from what we might now call the relatively reasonable (wine, honey, cautery) to the more drastic, with attempts to make the wound septic, the "laudable pus" of Galen and Guy de Chauliac (Ambrose 2018). In one of the most famous stories of medical history, Ambroise Paré described in 1545 how he accidentally learned that less is more: in treating soldiers wounded by gunshot, light dressings were better than boiling oil of elder (Duffin 2021, 263–264). Stitching wounds was also practiced, the earliest evidence dating to 1100 BCE in a mummified Egyptian (Majno 1975, 93). Linen, catgut, silk, wool, horsehair, and metal clips were used, in addition to cautery of the wound (application of hot irons). Giant biting ants were mentioned for suturing intestinal wounds in the ancient Hindu text of *Sushruta Samhita*, suggesting that their use could be prehistoric; their use has also been reported in the Greek civil war, in traditional societies of South America, and for wilderness explorers (Majno 1975, 304ff; Wujastyk 1998, 111–112; Davis 2019).

Splints made from natural products, such as those identified in traditional societies today, were probably used for fracture treatment but rarely are they preserved in the archaeological record. As most fractures found archaeologically are healed, this probably would preclude the need to bury a body with splints. However, some direct examples have been identified (Fig. 4.31). Elliot-Smith (1908) described splints of bark and wood held in place with linen bandages on broken bones of mummified remains from Egypt. Although there is evidence in Egypt for limbs being broken postmortem during the embalming process and splints being attached, it is known from documentary evidence that splinting as a form of treatment for fractures was practiced at that time. Nevertheless, assessing the state of healing of fractures, including their alignment and presence of complications, can suggest whether fractures in the past were treated with or without splinting (e.g., see Grauer and Roberts 1996; Neri and Lancellotti 2004).

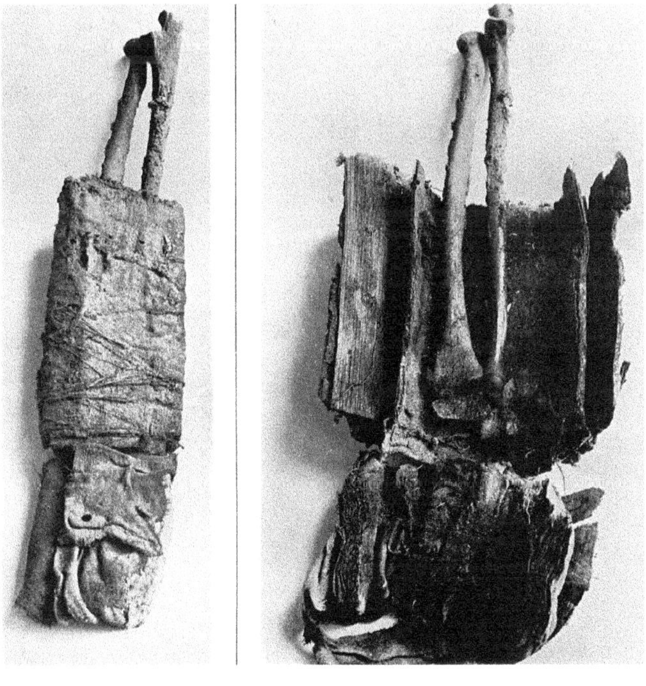

Figure 4.31. Splints made of fibrous wood of date palm, held in place with bandages and cords on the right forearm bones (young female, Christian Byzantine cemetery, Island of Biga, Nubia: 500–1500 CE). Fracture of the distal epiphysis of the radius evident. From Reisner et al. 1907, Plate 39. Left: splint in situ; right: splint opened up.

Any assessment of whether or not a society treated fractures in the past should be undertaken using multidisciplinary forms of evidence (Roberts 1988a, 1989, 1991), and data should be compared with modern clinical data that documents success of healing of fractures treated by simple (conservative) external reduction and splinting (Grauer and Roberts 1996).

Epilogue

The study of skeletal remains from archaeological sites potentially provides a large dataset for considering trauma and its implications for people's lives in the past. Both psychological and physical trauma remain with us today, and while we can detect some traumatic lesions in the past, such as fractures, we are missing most injuries to the soft tissues of the body. As for psychological trauma, we can only surmise that this was a challenge for our ancestors too, especially in periods of stress. For paleopathologists, using clinical data provides a good base for recording and interpretating evidence for trauma, but we have to realize that studying archaeological human remains requires constant awareness of its limitations and that clinical data may not be a "silver bullet" to understanding the trauma landscape in the past. However, the paleopathology of trauma gives us a unique insight into "troubled times" and how our ancestors adapted to them. In addition, paleopathologists have more recently been thinking about how our research on trauma contributes to the United Nations Sustainable Development Goals (3) good health and well-being and (10) reduced inequalities, and particularly (16) peace, justice and strong institutions, and we are learning to take a more thematic approach to our research. Like trauma, the joint diseases were also common in the past and will be covered in the next chapter.

5

Joint Diseases and Skeletal Indicators of Activity

> The diseases occurring in the joints are responsible for a great deal of pain and disability, and are an increasing burden for modern ageing populations. The potential hardships caused by joint diseases make them a very important part of palaeopathological studies.
>
> —J. Rogers, "The Palaeopathology of Joint Disease"

Degenerative diseases are a group of separate and yet related abnormalities. Gradual deterioration with advancing age is a phenomenon of both the animal and plant worlds. In long-lived organisms, such as humans, there is more time for degenerative diseases to appear, advance, and cause increasing disability with older age. The confusion and memory loss of senile dementia (a decline in cognitive function that interferes with daily activities), strokes, coronary thrombosis (arterial degeneration), and the pain and stiffness of joint degeneration are all examples of age-related diseases.

Developments in health care, preventive medicine, and health education particularly in the developed world now allow for people to live well into their 70s and 80s. The global average life expectancy in 2019 was 73.4 years (WHO 2019c). Females have always lived longer than males, and in relatively prosperous countries such as England, the average life expectancy in 2019 was 79.4 years for males and 83.6 years for females (Kings Fund 2024). But along with the benefits of a long life, there are risks. While a male in England might expect to live for 79 years, only 63 of these years will be lived in good health, and the final 19 years of an 83-year-old female's life is often spent in poor health, with people from a lower socioeconomic background suffering the most. For this reason, many countries around the world are turning their focus to healthy aging (e.g., WHO 2023e).

Although paleopathology can contribute to debates on physical degeneration over time and in different environmental circumstances, the prevalence of dementia or the frequency of strokes in the past—conditions of such social and economic importance today—are regrettably unknown prior to the eighteenth century. That cardiovascular disease, including arterial degeneration, was experienced by older people in the past is evidenced by the identification of calcified blood vessels in preserved bodies and with carefully excavated skeletal remains (Binder and Roberts 2014; Roberts 2023b; Antoine et al. 2023; Zink et al. 2023). In fact, aDNA analysis of the 5,300-year-old body of the Tyrolean "Iceman" identified a genetic predisposition for developing coronary heart disease and atherosclerosis. This was supported by the presence of calcifications in the carotid artery, aorta, and right iliac artery identified on a CT scan of his body (Zink et al. 2014).

Along with dental disease and trauma, the joint diseases (or arthropathies) compose most of the evidence for disease in past human groups. Today, it is estimated that around 528 million people worldwide are living with osteoarthritis (OA), and this figure is increasing. Most people with joint disease are over 55 years and are female (WHO 2023c). Looking back in time, joint disease is clearly a very old problem. It has even been diagnosed in the fossilized spine of a Comanchean dinosaur of 100 million years ago (Karsh and McCarthy 1960). Degeneration of joints is also observed in early humans who may not have lived as long as people from more recent times, but who may have put great strain on their bodies throughout their lives (Trinkhaus 1983).

The terminology used for joint disease can be myriad, with *osteoarthrosis, osteoarthritis, degenerative joint disease, arthropathies, spondyloarthropathies,* and *rheumatism* appearing in the clinical and paleopathological literature. Joint diseases are generally separated into two groups, those that are degenerative (they gradually worsen over time) and those that are inflammatory in nature. The first category, degenerative joint disease (DJD), including osteoarthritis, describes milder changes of gradual wear and tear on the joint that we all experience with increasing age, rather than being a disease per se (Loeser et al. 2012). Inflammatory diseases are usually caused by an autoimmune response, where the body fails to recognize its own antigens, triggering an inflammatory response—antigens being a marker that tells your immune system whether something on your body will harm it (or not). Rheumatoid arthritis, ankylosing spondylitis, and psoriatic arthritis are among such conditions recognized in archaeological skeletons (Rogers and Waldron 1995; Burt et al. 2013; Ventades et al. 2018). Rheumatoid arthritis is associated with antibodies in the blood of those affected, antibodies being produced by the immune system to protect the body against antigens (see later in the chapter). Ankylosing spondylitis and psoriatic arthritis are described as "sero-negative spondyloarthropathies" because the antibodies are absent and there is a tendency for spinal involvement of the tendon and ligament insertions (Yamada et al. 2005). For both degenerative and inflammatory arthropathies, bone abnormalities are proliferative (bone formation), erosive (destruction of bone), or both, and they should be considered with regard to their characteristics, causes, and clinical symptoms. Table 5.1 shows a classification for the joint diseases covered in this chapter.

These diseases all affect one or more joints of the body, usually in a clearly defined distribution pattern (Fig. 5.1). The problem with diagnosing specific joint diseases in paleopathology is that many of these numerous diseases leave identical marks on the skeleton. Some also develop subsequent to others—for example, a person may be affected by both osteoarthritis *and* rheumatoid arthritis. This means that a complete skeleton is a prerequisite for any attempts to make a specific diagnosis. Resnick et al. (2024, 144–145) provided a useful view on the diagnosis of joint diseases from a clinical standpoint. Their "target area approach," in which the distribution of joint lesions is mapped in detail, is a good reference point for diagnosing articular diseases in paleopathology. Even with modern technological advances in medicine, diagnosis

Table 5.1. Classification of joint diseases described in this chapter

Type of joint disease	Examples discussed
Degenerative	Osteoarthritis (OA) • Primary (with increasing age) • Secondary (any age in a previously damaged joint)
Inflammatory	Septic arthritis
	Rheumatoid arthritis (RA)
	Psoriatic arthritis (PsA)
	Ankylosing spondylitis (AS)
Metabolic	Diffuse idiopathic skeletal hyperostosis (DISH) Gout

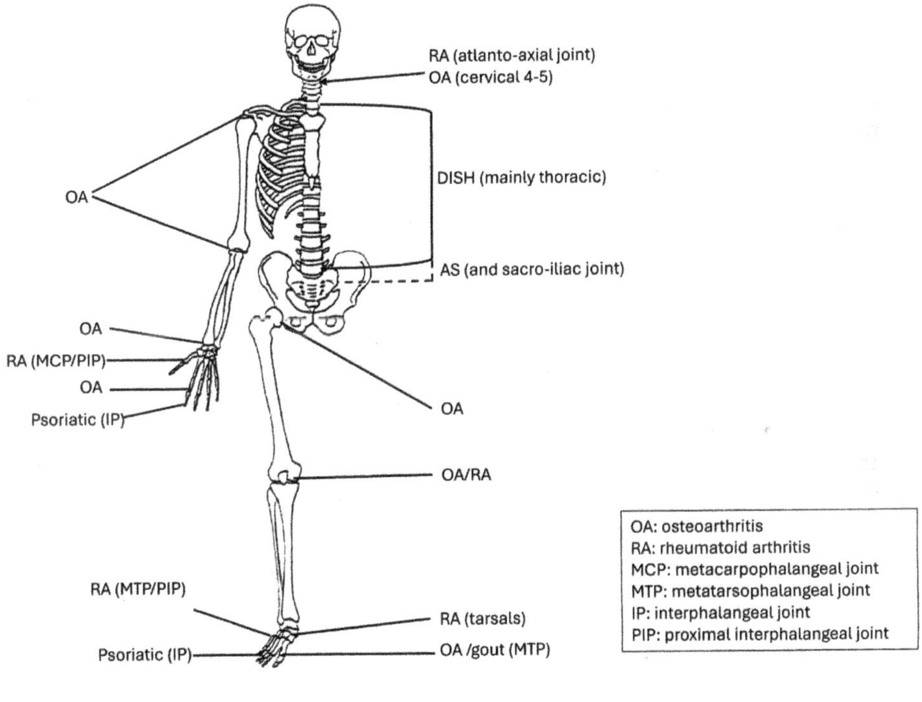

Figure 5.1. Distribution of joints affected by different joint conditions, used to aid a targeted area approach (adapted from Rogers et al. 1987, 184).

of joint diseases is not easy. In fact, despite the great antiquity of arthritic problems, clinical recognition that these similarly debilitating diseases represent different conditions is a product of modern times, as we will see later in the chapter (Buchanan et al. 2003). We should also be aware, when comparing paleopathological data with that of modern clinical medicine, that the number and type of lesions that we can see on dry bones may be greater than what is visible on a clinical radiograph or even a CT scan. For example, Rogers et al. (1990) recorded the features of joint disease in twenty-four knee joints using the macroscopic methods employed in paleopathology, and then radiographically (by a radiologist). The results showed that subtle bone changes were not observed by the radiologist, but the paleopathologist could, on the basis of their findings, diagnose the early stages of osteoarthritis. This study was particularly instructive because it may explain why people today who experience joint pain do not necessarily show radiographic changes of osteoarthritis.

Our understanding of joint disease in the past should not be confined to older people. Inflammatory arthropathies, although less common, also occur in children. The paleopathological literature identifies several examples of juvenile idiopathic arthritis, juvenile-onset rheumatoid arthritis, and juvenile-onset ankylosing spondylitis in individuals as young as 10–12 years old (Lewis 1998; MacKinnon 2016; Riccomi et al. 2021). These include a well-preserved skeleton of a 12–15-year-old from Peru (900–1050 CE) with arthritic changes in the neck, hips, shoulders, and elbows (Buikstra et al. 1990). In arthropathies affecting children, clinical features such as sustained fever, bleeding, and liver or kidney failure are added complications (Ravelli and Martini 2007).

Joint Anatomy and Physiology

To understand how joint diseases manifest, we first need to understand the anatomy of the joints. Joints are classified by movement and by histological features. A synarthrosis (fibrous) is a fixed or rigid joint (e.g., sutures of the skull), an amphiarthrosis (cartilaginous) is a slightly movable joint (e.g., the pubic symphysis), and the diarthroses (synovial) are freely movable joints (e.g., the hip). A fibrous joint may be a tooth in its socket, while cartilaginous joints include the intervertebral articulations, and synovial joints (where the joint cavity is lined by synovial membrane and contains synovial fluid) include the shoulder, hip, knee, and elbow. This latter type tends to be affected more frequently by joint disease (Rogers 2000, 163). The function of the joint depends on the geometry of the bone surfaces that meet each other; its functional integrity in terms of surrounding muscles, tendons, and ligaments; the strength, resilience, and elasticity of the articular cartilage covering the joint surfaces; and the underlying bone. Any changes to these structures may lead to subsequent degeneration. For example, trauma to the ligaments that stabilize the knee may lead to malpositioning of the joint and subsequent degeneration (Loeser et al. 2012).

Cartilage covers the joint surfaces and has several functions: transmission and distribution of loads, maintenance of contact between the bones of the joint with little friction, and absorption of shock. The first stages of joint disease usually involve the cartilage. For example, in osteoarthritis, the normally resting chondrocytes (cartilage cells) are activated as the result of an inflammatory response, leading to cartilage matrix remodeling, hypertrophic maturation (thickening of the cells), and cartilage calcification (Loeser et al. 2012). Repeated biomechanical stress and inflammation causes breaking up of the cartilage structure by fissuring, flaking, and pitting, with the resulting loss of cartilage and exposure of the bone underneath it.

Joint Disease: Pathological Process

Skeletal involvement in joint disease potentially consists of two processes, as we have noted previously: formation and destruction of bone. Osteoarthritis is the only joint disease where bone formation predominates (Waldron 2019, 720) in the form of bony outgrowths called osteophytes (Fig. 5.2). Although the function of osteophytes is still debated, because the buffering nature of the cartilage is lost, rather than being considered a symptom of the disease's progression, they may serve to stabilize and spread the load on the weight-bearing joint (Loeser et al. 2012). Osteophytes may occur on the joint surface, or marginal to it, or bone may form away from the joint, for example, at the margins of the joint capsule. Bone formation under the periosteum in a location away from a joint may occur as a reaction to changes in the joints themselves (Rogers et al. 1987, 180). The extent and character of this new bone formation varies on and around the joint and may indicate a particular joint disease.

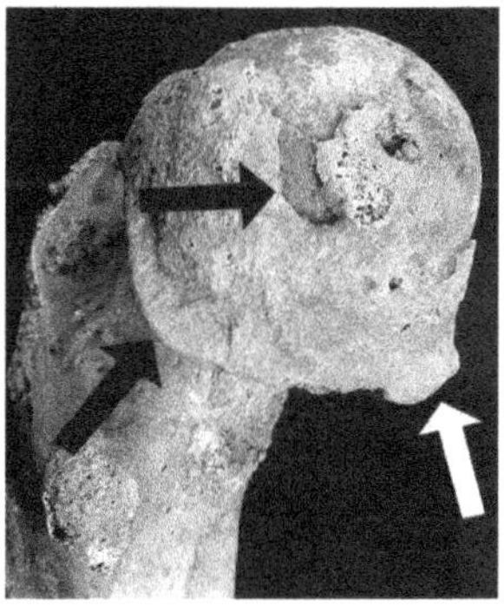

Figure 5.2. Osteophytes on the joint surface (arrowed) and around the margins of a femoral head (later medieval, twelfth–sixteenth century CE, France). Photograph by and courtesy of Jean Brown.

Once cartilage is destroyed, if the individual continues to use the joint, the underlying bone can become very hard (sclerotic) and polished (eburnation—Fig. 5.3). If osteophyte formation is extensive, a joint can become fused (ankylosed). Ossification can occur in cartilage away from the joint itself in some joint diseases. For example, diffuse idiopathic skeletal hyperostosis (DISH) usually involves premature ossification of cartilage in the ribs (costal) and the neck cartilages (thyroid and cricoid surrounding the larynx and trachea). Bone may also be destroyed on the joint surfaces themselves, on their margins, or away from the joint. The patterning and character of these lesions may aid in diagnosis. Destruction of cartilage on the joint surface causes the bone to degenerate and become porous (Fig. 5.4). In a synovial joint, fluid can then infiltrate into the bone directly under the cartilage. The lesions formed are called subchondral cysts and are readily visible on radiographs (Fig. 5.5).

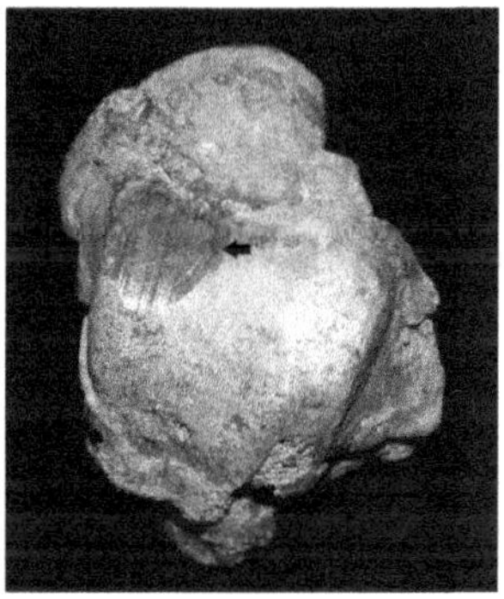

Figure 5.3. Eburnation of the right talus of an adult male (arrow) (late medieval Reading Abbey, England). Photograph by Mary Lewis.

Trying to achieve an accurate diagnosis of joint disease using dry bone lesions in the skeleton is based on evaluation of two fundamental parameters: the morphology of the lesions and their distribution in the body (Buikstra and Ubelaker 1994, 123, and Burt et al. 2013, 72–74, have provided useful recording forms). Comparison between archaeological and modern groups in terms of the prevalence of osteoarthritis is difficult, largely because many of the diagnostic methods are different. For example, the occurrence of relevant symptoms and radiographic changes, such as pain and joint space narrowing, seen in a living patient, are impossible to assess for an affected archaeological joint, whereas a radiograph of a living person may not identify all the degenerative joint changes visible on dry bone (Rogers et al. 1990).

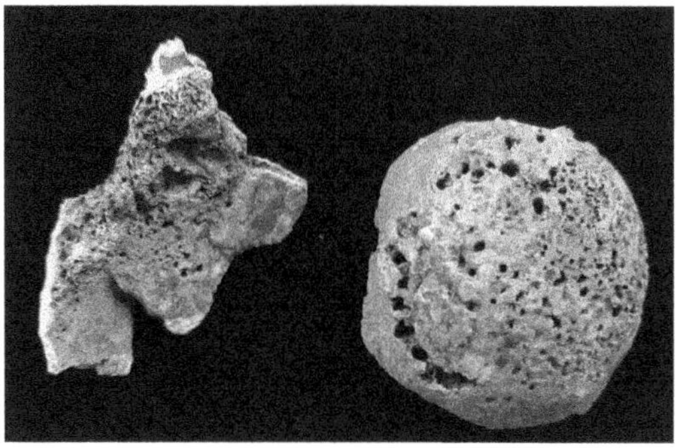

Figure 5.4. Porosity of joint surfaces of the hip joint (femoral head and acetabulum) in an older female from late medieval Hulton Abbey, Staffordshire, England. Photograph by Mary Lewis.

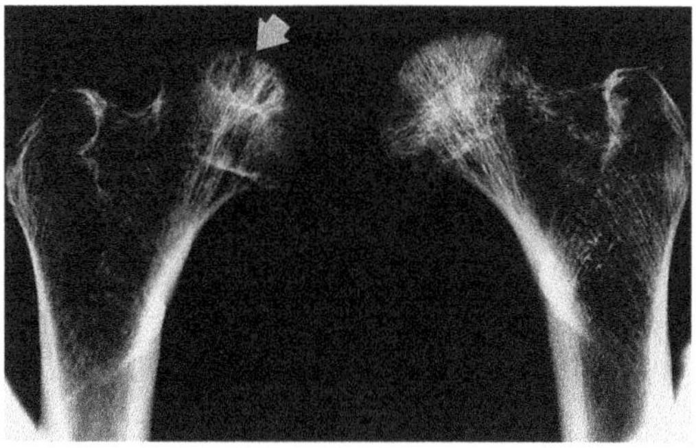

Figure 5.5. Radiograph showing subchondral cysts (arrow) of the left femoral head. Photograph by and courtesy of Jean Brown.

The diagnosis of arthropathies in paleopathology is also hindered by the similarity of lesions, and good preservation of skeletons is needed to allow the distribution of lesions to be accurately observed. Hence, many reports of joint disease merely describe the lesions using broad classifications (i.e., osteoarthritis, joint disease, spondylosis), without reaching a specific joint disease diagnosis. The recording of joint disease in skeletal remains has resulted in many different ways to quantify and classify lesions by different authors. The essential point is that, as with any paleopathological lesion, the basic data must be recorded in a standardized format so that comparisons can be made. Published standards include, for example; also see Buikstra and Ubelaker (1994) and Sager (1969). If standards are not being used, photographs and definitions of severity should be provided so that another researcher can be sure that, for example, their "severe" grade of osteoarthritis is the same as that of another study (Roberts and Cox 2003, 399). Researchers should:

- Report the biological sex and age of the individual
- Present the data according to the numbers of joints affected compared to those observed
- Clarify what is meant by a "joint" (one bone, or all bones that make up that joint)
- Consider the impact of osteoarthritis on the different compartments of the joint
- Indicate whether spinal or extraspinal OA is being recorded

Considering the distribution pattern of changes in different bones of a joint in males and females may help to elucidate patterns for the biological sexes and, potentially, different physical activities (Fig 5.6). Ideally every joint, and all parts of it, should be assessed to ensure realistic reporting of joint disease in groups of skeletons studied. To assist, Ventades et al. (2018) established a stepwise system for recording and diagnosing arthropathies in adults. This involves, for example, establishing

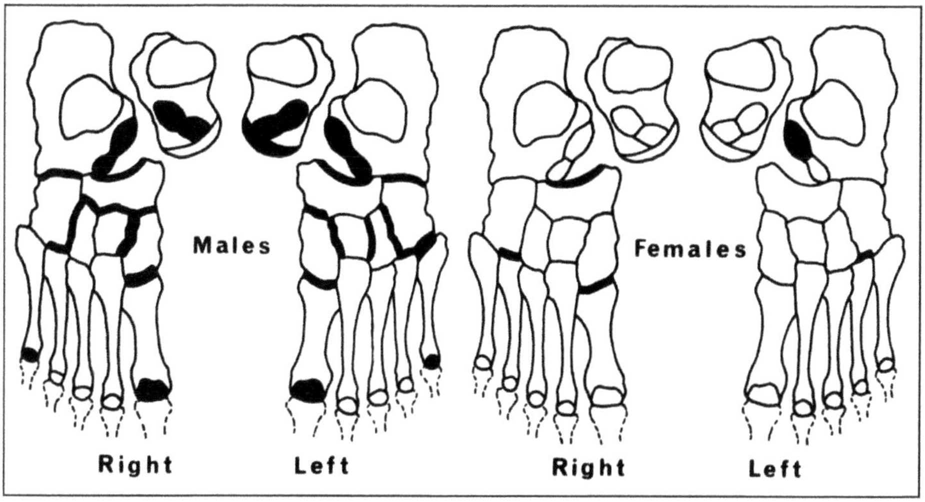

Figure 5.6. Involvement of the bones of the foot in osteoarthritis from males and females in a Canadian Inuit population (originally reproduced with kind permission from Charles Merbs).

which joints or spinal segments are affected, the direction of the osteophytes, symmetry/asymmetry of the lesions, preservation of intervertebral spaces (where the vertebrae are fused), and the presence of entheseal changes. The affected joint is then graded for severity on 1–3-point scale with grade 3 being the most severe (joint fusion and subsequent loss of normal function). The preservation of the skeleton, biological sex, age at death, and context of the archaeological site are also included. In addition, Becker (2019) suggested the use of a specific statistical approach (a generalized estimating equation—GEE) to allow complex OA patterns within and between joints to be more easily interpreted. Scoring osteoarthritic lesions by joint, for example (elbow, knee etc.), can hide patterns of lesions that could be used to help with a specific diagnosis, one individual with multiple lesions may skew the data, and scoring lesions on every articular surface within that joint produces so much data as to render interpretation impossible. When using the GEE approach, each articular surface is given a data point and then scored for lesions. These data can then be analyzed by the surface affected, but also at an individual level, and the data controlled for biological sex and age.

Osteoarthritis (OA)

Osteoarthritis is a complex degenerative disease affecting all aspects of a synovial joint: the synovial fluid, cartilage, bone, joint capsule, and associated ligaments and muscles (Boer et al. 2021). It is the most commonly reported joint disease in archaeological human skeletal remains (Waldron 2019), which implies that it is an easy condition to identify and interpret. Quite the contrary, the disease has a multifactorial etiology that includes obesity (leading to stress on the weight-bearing joints), underlying trauma (the so-called secondary osteoarthritis), specific joint shapes, increasing age, high bone mineral density, ancestry, socioeconomic status, the presence of another joint disease, an occupation with repetitive or habitual movements, and other aspects of lifestyle (Allen and Golightly 2015). In joints of the lower limbs as a result of loss of skin sensation it can lead to increased wear and tear; this can occur in neuropathy from diabetes, venereal syphilis, leprosy, and spinal cord injury. However, "there is no pattern of osteoarthritis that is unique to any one group or to any one occupation" (Waldron 2021, 349). The disease is also related to changes in the body as the result of menopause in women and the presence of osteoporosis (Anderson and Loeser, 2010). Over 100 different genes have been associated with a risk of developing OA (Boer et al. 2021).

Skeletal distribution patterns and rates of OA in people living in urban or rural environments vary, both today and in the past (e.g., see Yadav et al. 2022). In an archaeological study of 7,540 individuals from 103 sites across Europe, Willams et al. (2019) showed an increase in OA in men and women practicing settled agriculture (sixth–tenth centuries CE), with additional peaks as they became more urbanized in the later medieval period (fourteenth–fifteenth century CE). The difference in distribution patterns between men and women remained consistent, suggesting a continuation of gender roles across Europe through time, but also hinting at a greater aging population. Notably, however, the need to consider the age profile of the population being studied and maintaining consistency in recording have been highlighted by Alves Cardoso (2008), who found age, rather than types of activity, had the greatest impact on levels of joint disease recorded.

In clinical contexts, osteoarthritis is characterized by pain and joint narrowing (indicating loss of cartilage), but for paleopathologists these invisible symptoms are replaced by osteophyte formation in combination with joint contour change, pitting of the articular surface, and finally, eburnation. Osteophytes alone are not sufficient to diagnose the condition, as they can form as part of the normal aging process (degenerative joint disease, or DJD), whereas eburnation is considered pathognomonic (Waldron 2019). Waldron and Rogers (1991) recommended that if eburnation is not present on the joint surface, then two other features of osteoarthritis must be present (e.g., osteophytes and porosity). Pain, limitation of movement, swelling of the joint, wasting of muscles, and deformity of joints may also be clinical features associated with osteoarthritis, but some studies have shown no correlation between the severity of joint involvement and these symptoms (Rogers et al. 1990). Any synovial joint of the body can be affected, and some have a characteristic epidemiology. For example, shoulder osteoarthritis is rare, as the shoulder is not a weight-bearing joint; however, osteoarthritis can follow trauma to the shoulder or be related to overuse during a specific habitual activity. It also arises following damage to the rotator cuff soft tissues of this joint (Sankaye and Ostlere 2015).

Osteoarthritis: Skeletal Involvement

In both archaeological and living populations, the hip, knee, and spine are the most common areas affected by osteoarthritis, being the major weight-bearing joints. A global meta-analysis of US populations with regard to osteoarthritis in 2012 estimated that the risk of symptomatic knee arthritis was between 14% and 45% for different age, ancestry, and gender groups, whereas 25% of the population would expect to develop OA of the hip (Allen and Golightly 2015). In an archaeological study, Eng's (2016) consideration of osteoarthritis in 305 individuals from Bronze and Iron Age China and Mongolia (2000–600 BCE), found that 9.8% of individuals displayed eburnation of joints, with the elbow, spine, and knee joints having the highest prevalence at 6.4%, 5.7%, and 3.8% respectively. The overall picture was complex. While signs were evident of an Iron Age transition from walking as hunter-foragers to horse riding with the move to pastoralism, no clear pattern of OA emerged between time and place—perhaps because age was not controlled for. A similar mixed picture in groups practicing different subsistence strategies was found in the people from Ban Non Wat in Thailand (1750 BCE–500 CE), where again, the elbows and knees were the joints most commonly affected (Domett et al. 2017).

In contrast to studies on these archaeological groups, osteoarthritis of the elbow is rare today, except in people with particularly stressful occupations such as mining or pneumatic drilling (Buchanan et al. 2003; Resnick et al. 2024, 176). It is likely that OA in the upper limb is reflecting a past lifestyle that predisposed the elbow to degeneration, a lifestyle that differs significantly from that of today. As for the knee, Western and Bekvalac (2020, 194) found significantly higher rates of knee OA in older individuals living in towns and villages outside London (9.7%, compared to 3.5% in London), before and after the Industrial Revolution, compared to those living within the city. Again, this provides evidence that different physical activities related to work has have an impact on which joints developed OA.

While osteoarthritis of the shoulder is rare (without associated trauma), the hands and feet are affected by osteoarthritis at varying rates in living populations. The joints of the hand (interphalangeal, metacarpophalangeal, and some of the wrist bones) are more commonly affected, especially in middle-aged postmenopausal women (Resnick et al. 2024, 158–159). In the foot, OA of the ankle is rare, but degeneration of the first metatarsophalangeal joint (big toe) is more frequent.

Relatively little work has been carried out on osteoarthritis of the hands and feet in archaeological groups, perhaps because these smaller bones often do not survive burial and excavation. Hand osteoarthritis is a common finding in people today, and may be related to occupation and handedness. In fact, one of the few studies of osteoarthritis of the hands or feet in an archaeological population sample suggests a similar frequency in past populations to modern ones (Waldron 1993). Waldron and Cox (1989) also examined the hand bones of 367 skeletons from the crypt excavations at Christ Church, Spitalfields, London, dated to between 1729 and 1869 CE. The occupations of these individuals were obtained from historical sources. Twenty-nine of the males were weavers, and it was proposed that the effort of weaving on the joints would lead to hand osteoarthritis. However, of the thirteen males with osteoarthritis in their hands, only three were weavers. Instead, there appeared to be a strong correlation with increased age in those affected—demonstrating that increasing age, rather than occupation, was the greater risk factor for OA (see also Alves Cardoso 2008). Molleson (1989) described skeletal abnormalities of Mesolithic/Neolithic skeletons from Syria dated to around 8,000 years ago. She suggested that the abnormalities in the toe and ankle joints were the result of extreme dorsiflexion of the joints of the foot caused by habitual use of a quern stone; robust arm bones and osteoarthritis of the lower spine, knees, and big toes also contributed to this picture.

Osteoarthritis of the temporomandibular joint (TMJ) in the past, mentioned in Chapter 3, reveals rates that reflect those in the clinical literature, around 8–16% of the population (Bansal 2016). Rando and Waldron (2012), however, advised against using eburnation as the overriding diagnostic feature for TMJ osteoarthritis as it is rarely seen, but instead suggest using a combination of features, such as porosity with osteophytes. Using these criteria, Suby and Giberto (2018) recorded TMJ disease in 28% ($n = 7/25$) of hunter-foragers from Late Holocene Patagonia, mostly related to antemortem tooth loss and age. In a later study, TMJ disease was most frequently related to dental wear in prehistoric western Micronesia, potentially associated with the habit of chewing betel nuts (Stone et al. 2020).

Spinal Joint Disease (Spondyloarthropathy)

Today, back pain is considered to be the biggest contributor to disability worldwide, and many resources are spent on understanding its cause (Plomp et al. 2022a). There are normally seven cervical, twelve thoracic, five lumbar, and five sacral vertebrae (that fuse in adulthood to form the sacrum) making up the spine, which is affected by two types of arthritis. Osteoarthritis, affecting the synovial joints (i.e., the vertebral/apophyseal facets) and intervertebral disc herniation (IDH/Schmorl's node) evident on the vertebral bodies themselves (Figs. 5.7 and 5.8).

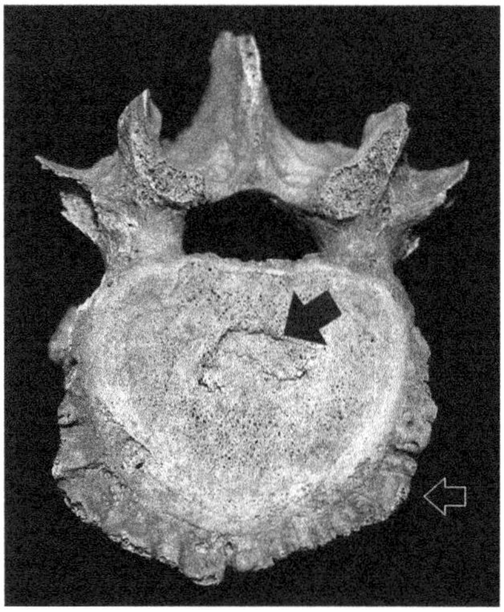

Figure 5.7. IDH causing pitting and osteophytic lipping (white outlined black arrow) on the anterior aspect of a lumbar vertebra (late medieval, St. Oswald's Priory, Gloucester, England). Note also the central Schmorl's node (black arrow). Photograph by Mary Lewis.

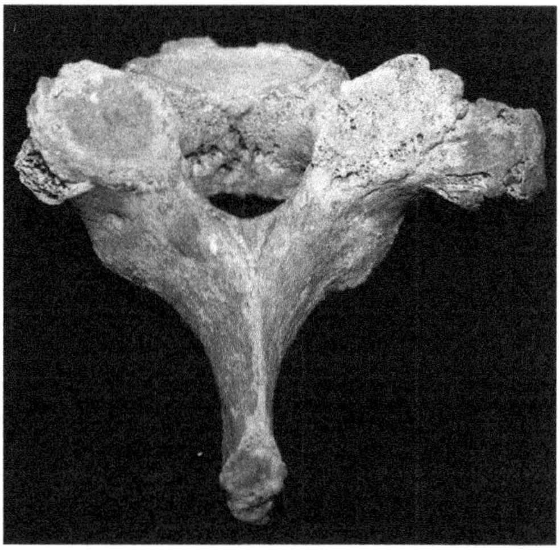

Figure 5.8. Osteoarthritis of the right apophyseal (facet) joint of a cervical vertebra in a mature female. The facet on the left side is normal (late medieval St. Oswald's Priory, Gloucester, England). Photograph by Mary Lewis.

The intervertebral discs consist of a fibrous capsule (annulus) containing a gelatinous substance (nucleus pulposus). With advancing age, a chemical and degenerative change occurs in these tissues. The constant stress to which these discs are subject—for example, in the bending and lifting of everyday activity—causes the internal nucleus pulposus to invade the annulus fibrosus. The rupture of this fibrous capsule stimulates the development of osteophytes at the margins of the vertebral body itself. For reasons of pure mechanics, the anterior area of the annulus and vertebral body are more likely to develop osteophytes compared to the posterior area. With increasing stress and annulus rupture, the size of osteophytes increases (Plomp et al. 2022a). At the extreme, the osteophytes from neighboring vertebrae develop together and unite, fixing the spinal segment affected and preventing movement. This localized and restricted fixation, or ankylosis, is not to be confused with the more generalized diseases of spinal fixation (e.g., DISH, which will be considered later). Along with osteophytes developing around the vertebral body margins, bony outgrowths (syndesmophytes) occur at spinal ligament attachment sites, and the body surface, a cartilaginous joint, also degenerates (known as spondylosis). The surfaces of the vertebral body (or endplates) become porous and pitted, and there may be new bone formed (intervertebral osteochondrosis). This occurs most frequently on the mid-lower cervical spine, upper thoracic, and lower lumbar areas (Rogers 2000, 169; Sager 1969).

Often, rupture of the intervertebral disc will occur vertically (either superiorly or inferiorly), causing depressions on the vertebral endplate known as Schmorl's nodes (Plomp et al. 2022a). These nodes are most commonly seen in the lower thoracic and lumbar spine (Fig. 5.9). In 2008, Faccia and Williams reported on Schmorl's nodes in living patients and their association with pain. They noted that nodes in the center of the vertebral bodies were more frequently associated with back pain, perhaps due to the location of so many nerves in that area, and that 92% of the people in the study found their daily activities were limited by that pain. The cause of Schmorl's nodes is still a matter of debate. Nodes located in the lumbar spine are most frequently associated with IDH, while vertebral morphology, spinal trauma, vigorous activity causing flexion and extension of the spine, an underlying infection, osteoporosis, and neoplastic disease have all been implicated in their formation (Kyere et al. 2012; Plomp et al. 2022a). Using 2D digital shape analysis, Plomp et al. (2012, 2015) found an association between the shape of the lower thoracic and lumbar pedicles in skeletons from six medieval and postmedieval sites from England (a total of 207 males and females aged 18 to 46-plus years), and suggested that in some individuals, the shape of these pedicles failed to provide sufficient support to the lower back. The potential link of Schmorl's nodes with physical exertion, in combination with abnormal vertebral blood vessel development in the growing spine (Mattei and Rehman 2014), may explain why they have also been noted in non-adult skeletons. In a rare study, Lewis (2016) reported Schmorl's nodes in 1.1% (8/732) of English medieval urban children aged 10–13 years, rising to 7.8% (58/736) in both urban and rural adolescents (aged 14–16 years), likely reflecting early strain on their developing spines as they started work.

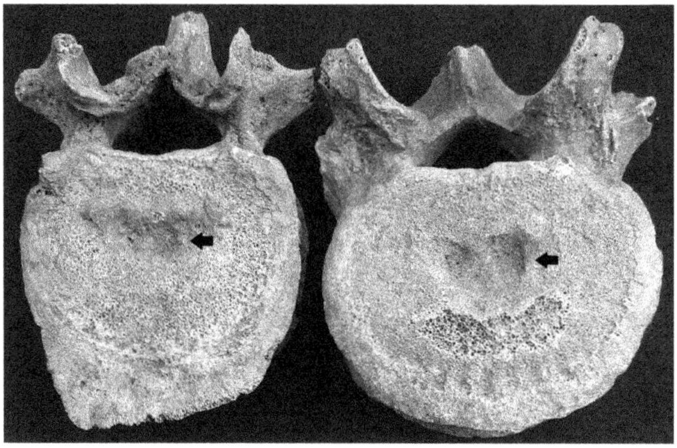

Figure 5.9. Schmorl's nodes (arrowed) on the superior surfaces of the thoracic vertebrae in a 25–35-year-old male from late medieval St. Oswald's Priory, Gloucester, England. Photography by Mary Lewis.

It has long been acknowledged that spinal joint disease, and the pain it may bring, is the price we pay for walking on two legs. For example, while spondylosis has been reported in 48–95% of humans, it only occurs in between 2–5% of other primates who move around using all four limbs (Plomp et al. 2022a). It might be thought that the mechanical stress and strain upon each segment of the spine is constant in the upright posture. However, the spine is not just a straight line and exhibits a backward curve in the chest, or thoracic region, and a forward curve in the lumbar and cervical regions. This causes wedging of the intervertebral discs at the fifth cervical, eighth thoracic, and fourth lumbar vertebrae, and a greater susceptibility to joint disease (Been et al. 2010). The inexorable advance of time results in all people eventually developing the clinical symptoms of spinal joint disease. Intermittent backache, stiffness, and an inability to touch the toes are all too familiar features of this aging process. Just as today, so it was in antiquity. Certainly, the condition is almost universal in adult skeletal remains of the past in all periods, although its frequency varies among groups. Since this is a mechanically induced condition there is, naturally, variation among individuals. For example, Bridges (1994) reported a high frequency of neck osteoarthritis in 125 skeletons from northwest Alabama, United States, and the practice of carrying loads through the use of a tumpline (strap) around the forehead was considered to be the cause, i.e., socioculturally linked.

Activity of a specific kind was also suggested by Stirland (2000) who studied the spines of the 179 men from the Tudor warship, the *Mary Rose*, which sank in 1545 CE off the south coast of England. The original crew comprised 200 mariners, 185 soldiers, and 30 gunners, thus making it possible that activity-related skeletal changes could be linked with occupation. Even though the majority of the male crew were young adults and adolescents, they had a similar frequency of spinal joint disease when compared with a group of older males from a late medieval site in Norwich, England. It was suggested that the activities undertaken on the *Mary Rose*, such as handling heavy guns, accelerated age-related changes in the spine. These people were probably a semipermanent professional crew who had started their work as teenagers (Stirland and Waldron 1997, 335). Another site with specific physical activities, presumed because of its historical context, is that of the battlefield of Towton, North Yorkshire, England. Here, 80% of the thirty-two males excavated (with a mean age of 30 years) had evidence of spinal degeneration, mainly in the form of Schmorl's nodes (40%) and spinal osteophytes (Boylston 2001; Coughlan and Holst 2001), which was suggested to be the result of increased axial loading of the spine.

Exploring the frequency of spinal joint disease as a means to identifying activity, however, has its problems because the spine may also be affected by the activities related to bipedalism that affect us all—walking, running, and so on. This may be the reason why attempts to distinguish between patterns of spinal joint disease, as well as other joints in contrasting groups, show little difference (see Knüsel et al. 1997: medieval York; Domett et al. 2017: prehistoric Thailand; and Myszka et al. 2022: fourteenth–nineteenth-century Radom, Poland). The conclusion must be that joint disease is not the ideal condition by which to observe activity-related stress in the past, unless it is compared with evidence for younger individuals in the same group, hence counteracting the influence of age. If osteoarthritis is seen with a particularly high prevalence or pattern, it may be possible to suggest occupationally induced osteoarthritis. Nevertheless, for occupationally related changes to affect the bones of the skeleton, the person must start the activity young. For these reasons, Domett and colleagues (2017) petitioned for a move away from the study of OA as a marker of activity arguing, instead, for more focus on the debilitating effect of the condition on the quality of life for people in the past.

Markers of Activity and Occupation (Entheseal Changes)

Due to limitations of the study of joint disease alone to help identify physical activity and/or occupational stress in the past, paleopathologists have begun to combine the evidence for OA with multiple skeletal markers of activity in both adult and child skeletal remains. These include entheseal changes (new bone formation at tendon and ligament insertions as a result of an increase in size of associated muscles), trauma patterns, and changes in the size, shape, and robusticity of bones (or long bone cross-sectional geometry) (Villotte et al. 2016; Becker 2020). Of particular relevance for occupationally induced changes in the skeleton is the premise proposed by German anatomist Julius Wolff in 1892, known as Wolff's law of transformation. Although considered controversial by some, this law dictates that bone will adapt to functional pressure or external forces by increasing or decreasing its mass to resist the stress (Ruff et al. 2006). We have already seen how, in OA, the formation of osteophytes will sustain and distribute the load. Hence, if the body is involved in a repeated activity, the bones of the skeleton will respond by becoming larger and denser. Enthesophytes (see later in this chapter) will also develop at muscle attachment sites, and degeneration of the joints may eventually occur (Villotte et al. 2016).

There have also been increasing biomechanical analyses, using long bone cross-sectional geometry, a method that applies the principles of engineering to explore the effects of activity or loading on the bones. Beam analysis is used to measure the geometric properties at cross-sections taken perpendicular to the long axis of the bones, and these measures represent the amount and distribution of the bone at those points (Larsen 2015, 220–221). Features such as the medullary and cortical area and second moments of area (geometric properties that measure bending and torsional strength) are measured. Ruff (2019) provides a useful overview of the field and its use in bioarchaeology. Plain film radiography, CT scanning, and bone sections to allow the measurement of cortical bone width and shape have all played their part in biomechanical analyses, although noninvasive techniques such as the latter are preferred. Archaeological examples of studies using this analytical technique include consideration of the change in shape of limb bones with the transition to agriculture, sex differences in cross-sectional geometry, and the effect of different terrain on the bones. For example, Bridges et al. (2000) measured humeri, radii, ulnae, femora, and tibiae of 372 individuals from west-central Illinois, United States, dating from the Middle Woodland (50 BCE–200 CE) to the Mississippian period (1050–1250 CE); a subsample of eighty bones was also CT scanned. Results showed humeral and femoral strength increased in females when native seed crops were being grown, with females considered key to planting and processing these crops. In the latest period, when maize use intensified, female left arm strength declined, which Bridges suggested could be the result of more efficient crop processing, or because maize is an easier crop to process. Using cross-sectional geometric properties analysis, Cameron and Stock (2018) noted relative differences in humeral strength in females living in the semiarid and desert environments of later Stone Age southern Africa, compared to those living on the coast, perhaps as the result of the greater effort required in gathering resources in those regions.

Studies of asymmetry of limb bone size (length, width, circumference) as a possible indicator of the use of one limb more than the other for a physical activity have also been undertaken using metrical analysis of bones and features on radiographs. Some 90% of humans are right-side dominant when using their upper limb (Ruff 2018), and therefore it seems reasonable to consider whether this was present in past human groups. Steele (2000) provided an overview of the subject of handedness and how it may be recognized in the skeleton, and some archaeological studies have explored the concept of handedness and physical activity (Fig. 5.10). Although in many industrialized groups, some activities required the use of the right arm over the left, enhancing the appearance of handedness (or masking it in left-handers), Fogl et al. (2023) demonstrated that handedness develops during the growth period, with the humerus of the preferential arm increasing in length with age, in the 169 children they studied from medieval Hungary. While biomechanical analyses of skeletal remains from archaeological sites do hold potential for more research, changes in size and shape of bones may be affected by many factors, including diet, biological sex, age, genetic factors, environment (terrain), and activity, as well as the type of loading, duration, amplitude, age at which loading began and stopped, and the bone element involved (Jurmain 1999, 258).

Recent research into the mechanisms behind entheseal changes and musculoskeletal stress markers (MSMs) in bioarchaeology has stimulated debate on their

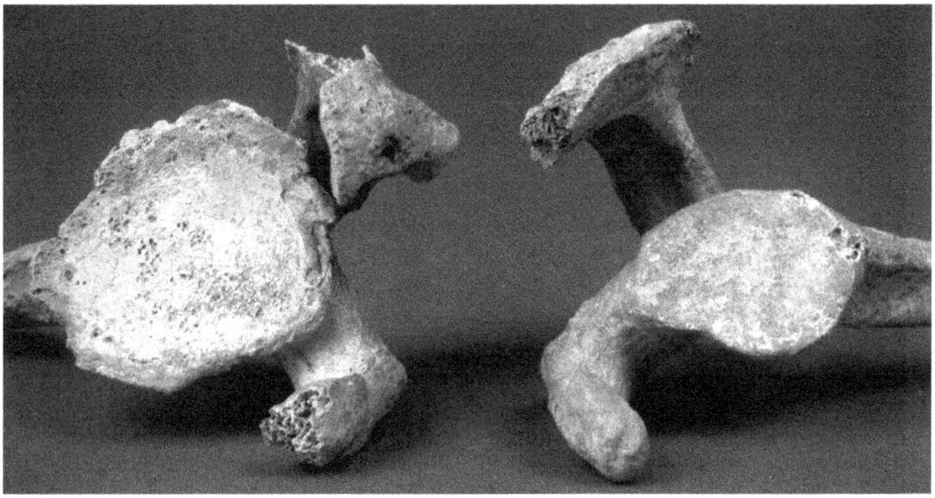

Figure 5.10. Right glenoid cavity of the scapula (with opposite as a comparison) showing enlargement of joint surface with osteophytes and porosity; perhaps this person used their right arm more than their left (early medieval, fifth–seventh century CE, Pewsey, Wiltshire, England). Photograph by and courtesy of Jean Brown.

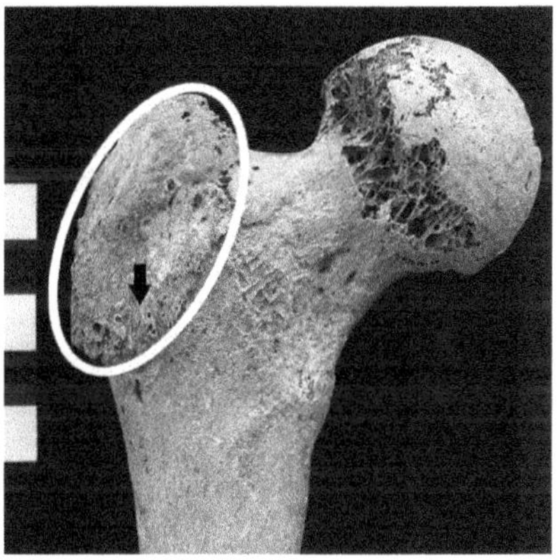

Figure 5.11. Fibrocartilaginous enthesis at the gluteus minimus insertion site of the greater trochanter on the right femur (circled) of an older adult female from late Roman Kültepe in Kayseri, Türkiye. Photograph courtesy of Handan Üstündağ, Kültepe Excavation Archives, with the kind permission of Fikri Kulakoğlu.

reliability as indicators of activity. Highlighted issues are: inconsistency in recording, the time it takes for changes to appear, the influence of age (they become more common with age, eliminating any differences that may have been evident in younger groups), the choice of bones studied, stature, and the unmeasurable influence of hormones and genetics (Miella et al. 2012; Cardoso and Henderson 2013; Albee 2023; Villotte and Santos 2023). When taken in combination with other indicators, however, MSMs are still considered useful in reconstructing habitual movements, although fibrocartilaginous entheses (Fig. 5.11) that occur close to the joints of bones are considered more useful than fibrous ones, which present on the long bone shafts where larger muscles attach (Villotte and Knüsel 2012; Henderson et al. 2012, 2013). Standards to record these changes have been developed—for example, the Coimbra Method, which scores the location and appearance of the attachments, has been widely adopted (Henderson et al. 2016; Albee 2023).

Historical data do exist about occupations in the past and how they may have affected health, but making a direct link to skeletal changes is extremely difficult. We do know that people in the past worked in a variety of occupations—for example, farming, craft industries, food processing, and building; each one of these activities, if pursued for long enough, could have impacted the skeleton and caused changes we can recognize. Furthermore, males, females, and different age groups probably had particular occupations, although we must not assume a direct stereotypical correlation (Panter-Brick 2002). For example, Kinkopf et al. (2023) found no differences in femoral asymmetry according to biological sex or age in medieval Italy. The integration of comparative clinical data, ethnographic analogy, art, and documentary sources, where available, is essential when trying to reconstruct activity. It should also be remembered that a number of different activities can produce the same skeletal changes, and people may have changed their occupations or habitual movements throughout their lifetime. Clearly, cultural context is also important for interpretation of skeletal changes, but selectively choosing factors that fit what is seen in the skeletal data needs to be avoided (for a fuller discussion see Hirst et al. 2023).

Nevertheless, historical literature abounds with examples of occupation-related diseases. Bernardino Ramazzini (1633–1740 CE) was the first author to write a treatise on diseases of workers (Italy, 1700 CE) with an expanded edition in 1713 (Franco 2020). His *De Morbis Artificum Diatriba* (*On Diseases of Tradesmen*) described forty-two occupational diseases in miners, midwives, painters, and sedentary laborers. Ramazzini is lauded as the "father of industrial medicine," and the International Collegium Ramazzini still meets annually in his native Carpi, Italy, to track and prevent occupational disease globally. Notably, while many scholars in clinical medicine have explored the relationship between particular occupations and changes in the body, most studies do not involve the bones of the skeleton. There are certainly some fascinating occupationally related diseases, such as "hatter's shakes," a symptom of poisoning by mercury, which was applied to rabbit skins in the hat manufacturing process, or "potter's rot," referring to the silicosis affecting workers exposed to silica dust in the pottery trade (Cherniack 1992). Furthermore, with the domestication of animals, humans became subject to another set of diseases: the zoonoses. For example, anthrax is contracted through contact with infected domesticated animals and their skins; "wool sorter's disease" became the name applied to anthrax in people working with wool in the nineteenth century (Cullamar and Lutwick 2002). Paleopathologists have also suggested a specific relationship between skeletal lesions and occupation, such as "clay-shovellers fractures" (Chapter 4) and culturally induced dental modifications (Chapter 3).

Kennedy (1986) was one of the first to suggest that auditory exostoses, originally considered a normal skeletal variation (or an "epigenetic trait"), was in fact the result of immersion in cold water (e.g., for pearl diving). A study of ear exostoses in contrasting status groups from first to third century CE Rome, Italy, revealed no evidence for these lesions in females, and found ear exostoses only in the higher-status males (Manzi et al. 1991). It was proposed that these males frequented the thermal baths, including submersion in cold water, which could have induced the exostoses. In fact, it is now considered that many of these epigenetic skeletal traits described previously in the literature may be culturally and not genetically induced (Saunders 1989; Tyrrell 2000).

Os acromiale describes the nonfusion of the acromion of the scapula, which usually fuses at between 15 and 25 years (Hunt and Bullen 2007), but in 1–15% of modern populations it remains ununited. It is particularly common in people of Black African ancestry today (You et al. 2019). There are four ossification centers for the acromion (pre-, meso-, meta-, and basi-acromion). A lack of fusion can occur between any two of these areas, it is thought, as a result of movement at the site, due to flexion of the fragment during arm elevation (Hurst et al. 2019). Os acromiale is usually asymptomatic, but may lead to some discomfort (Fig. 5.12). Few population studies have been published on os acromiale, but Hunt and Bullen (2007) documented the condition in the Robert J. Terry Anatomical Collection (nineteenth–twentieth century CE) at a frequency of 8.3% of individuals out of 1,594 skeletons studied. Because there were differences between the sexes and ancestries (Black male 12.5%; Black female 9%; white male 7%; white female 3%; bilateral expression: Black male 48%; white male 29%), they suggested that an underlying genetic predisposition could be at play, which could be exacerbated by trauma. In the medieval population from Ensay, Scotland, eleven examples of separation (or nonfusion) of the acromial tip were recorded in 220, or 10%, of scapulae (Miles 1994). Stirland (2000) considered the cause of the high frequency in skeletons from the stricken *Mary Rose* Tudor warship (1545 CE). Of 207 scapulae from the *Mary Rose*, 26 had os acromiale (12.5%). When it was possible to pair scapulae, of 52 pairs, 10 individuals had the condition (19%), 6 bilaterally (Stirland 2000). Stirland also observed increased robusticity and size of the left humeri, and argued that non-union of the epiphysis was the result of drawing a long bow using the left arm for archery, which was regularly practiced from an early age. This condition was also found in 3 of 29 individuals (9.2%) buried at the medieval battlefield of Towton, in North Yorkshire, England (Knüsel 2001), where the soldiers may have used the long bow from a young age. Today, this condition is associated with nerve impingement in the shoulder and the development of rotator cuff tears (You et al. 2019), but there is debate as to the exact underlying cause. It may result from both mechanical stress during the development of the shoulder bones and genetic predisposition (Case et al. 2006).

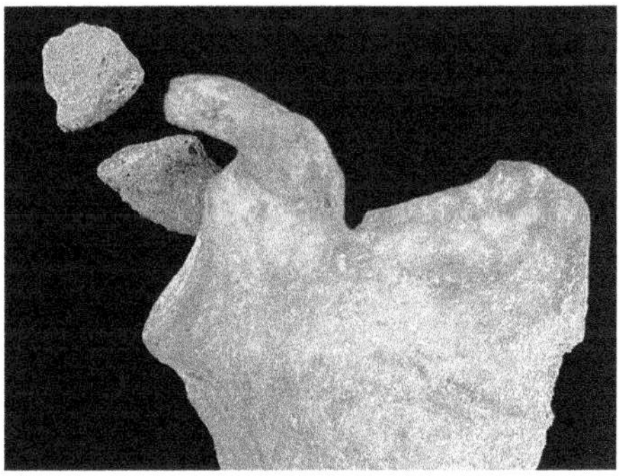

Figure 5.12. Os acromiale of the right scapula bone in a mature adult female from early modern Redhill, Sussex, England. Photograph courtesy of Ceri Falys.

Thinking more broadly about what people did in their working lives, we should consider the effects of pollution in past environments, both inside and outside buildings, that may have impacted the health of people who worked with them or were exposed to them. For example, chronic rhinomaxillary sinusitis has been used in archaeological studies as an indicator of industrial pollution and poor air quality (Roberts 2007;

see Chapter 6), and the inhalation of plant fibers, bacteria, molds, endotoxin, and other organic and inorganic dust (e.g., silica) during plant processing can lead to chronic bronchitis and asthma (Vested et al. 2018). Pabst and Hofer (1998) described deposits in the Neolithic Tyrolean Iceman's lungs (3340 BCE) and probably related to exposure to open fires and threshing residues. The presence of rickets may also indicate the effects of working (or living) in a polluted environment without exposure to sunlight; and tuberculosis may suggest work with diseased animals. Furthermore, developmental conditions (Chapter 2) and neoplastic disease (Chapter 8) may be implicated as responses to environmental pollutants from industries such as mining, metalworking, or textile manufacture. Oakberg et al. (2000) analyzed arsenic levels in individuals from the copper-smelting site of Shiqmim, Israel (fifth–fourth millennium BCE) suggesting people had been working in that industry at that site. A similar study was undertaken identifying high levels of copper in the bones of miners working in the fourth–seventh century Phaeno mines of Khirbet Faynan, Jordan (Perry et al. 2011). Indeed, the effects of prehistoric mining activities may persist today, compromising health in some parts of the world (e.g., in Jordan, see Pyatt and Grattan 2001; Wilson and Pyatt 2007).

At some point in our past, lead pollution may also have compromised health when accumulated in high enough quantities. A classic example comes from the Roman period, when lead pipes brought water to inhabitants of towns, and lead was used to make many items; of course, people would also have mined the lead. Exposure to lead affects a number of chemical processes in the body, resulting in poor intellectual development, anemia, kidney failure, gout, and nerve paralysis, among other conditions (Wani et al. 2015). Environmental lead levels of 0.40 ug/dL, or 40 parts per million (ppm), are associated with toxicity in humans today (WHO 2019b). In 1972, Needleman et al. identified lead concentrations in the teeth of suburban children at 11.1 ppm, compared to 51.1 ppm in children living in the "lead belt" of Philadelphia, which operated in the nineteenth and twentieth centuries. In another example, analysis of lead concentrations in bone from 200 individuals dating from the Neolithic to late medieval periods in Britain and Italy demonstrated a dramatic increase in childhood exposure to anthropogenic lead as a result of industrial pollution in the medieval period, with enamel containing lead concentrations as high as 14.5 ppm compared to prehistoric times at 0.5 ppm (Montgomery et al. 2010). These levels were highest in lead-mining areas, such as medieval Derbyshire, Devon, Durham, and Yorkshire. This study controlled for the effects of postmortem accumulations of lead from the soil, a factor that should always be taken into consideration in chemical analyses. Lewis and Montgomery (2023) identified lead concentration in enamel of up to 17.9 ppm in adolescents from medieval York, with the highest levels in a 10–13-year-old (69.6 ppm), high enough to indicate blood poisoning. This child also had rickets active at the time of death, suggesting a link between the two conditions. A now classic study of the preserved bodies of individuals from Victorian London also found high lead levels that may have contributed to their demise (D'Ortenzio et al. 2018b). Three sailors on the John Franklin expedition to the Canadian Arctic were discovered and excavated in the 1980s. The lead levels in these men were about 133 ppm, and the presumed sources of the lead included solder on tins of food as well as water pipes and medicines used on the ship (Kowal et al. 1989; Farrer 1993). In addition to raised lead concentrations in the teeth and bones, we should also remember that "lead lines" (thick white or radiopaque lines showing lead accumulation in growing bones of children) might be visible at the end of long bones in affected individuals (Gandhi et al. 2003).

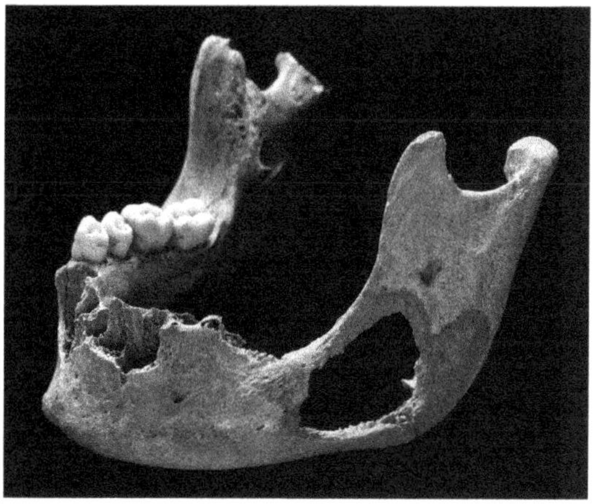

Figure 5.13. Possible "phossy jaw" (hole in the left side) of the mandible of a 12–14-year-old from Coach Lane in Newcastle, England (1711–1857 CE). Photograph by and courtesy of Jeff Veitch.

More direct examples of occupational hazards have been found from industrial contexts. These include osteomyelitis of the jaw in a male adolescent from eighteenth–nineteenth-century Coach Lane in Newcastle, England (Roberts et al. 2016; Fig. 5.13). The area had several matchstick factories at the time. This condition, called phossy jaw, arose in young match makers, usually female, who were exposed to white phosphorus during the production of "strike-anywhere" matches. Phosphorus particles can reach the bony jaw through diseased gums and teeth; and phosphorus poisoning can cause "fragile femur" and "dark lines" at the ends of long bones (Hinshaw and Quin 2015). In the Coach Lane example, however, chemical analysis of their calculus unexpectedly did not reveal high levels of phosphorus (Roberts et al. 2016). Another adolescent—a male aged 16–20 years—from nineteenth-century Gloucester, England, with very similar changes was also identified to have suffered from this painful condition. Gloucester was also a key area of match manufacturing in England at this time (Valoriani et al. 2019).

Reconstructing what people did for a living—occupation or activity—is relevant for interpretations of past human behavior. Work today fills many waking hours, is a major part of adult life, and can create stress; the type of work people do is also determined by many factors such as biological sex, age, ancestry, and socioeconomic status. When scholars of paleopathology are conducting this type of study, we recommend that they use multiple lines of evidence that go well beyond solely relying on joint disease (Jurmain et al. 2012). Jurmain's (1999, 267) warning of more than 20 years ago is still worth heeding, "Story-telling and scenario building may have some (limited) utility [but] without clear empirical controls and [the] application of rigorous means of verification, skeletal biologists can become lost in the . . . intellectual fog."

Now we will turn to a discussion of the more specific joint diseases and the chapter ends with consideration of two metabolic conditions (DISH and gout) associated with them.

Inflammatory Joint Diseases

Septic Arthritis

Septic or inflammatory arthritis is discussed in more detail in Chapter 6 under tuberculosis (TB), but it can also be caused by organisms other than those in the *Mycobacterium tuberculosis* complex (MTBC). Septic arthritis caused by nonspecific infection may have two etiological pathways. Although its precise definition as a distinct entity came after the adoption of germ theory in the 1880s, arthritis associated with venereal disease, in particular gonorrhea, was recognized clinically at least a century earlier (Storey and Scott 1998). The bacteria (usually *Streptococcus* or *Staphylococcus aureus*; Balato et al. 2021) spreads via the bloodstream to the joint cavity, but infection of a joint can also result from the spread of an infection from the skin or bone into the joint (e.g., osteomyelitis). The joint becomes swollen, painful, hot, and red. Today, septic arthritis commonly occurs in young children, with an incidence of 1–5 infants per 100,000 in western countries. The anatomy of their growing bones means that infections can readily travel from the diaphysis (bone shaft) to the epiphysis (growing joint) via the transmetaphyseal vessels that connect them (Erkilinc et al. 2021). It is a serious medical condition, usually affecting a single joint, and needs to be treated with intravenous antibiotics and immobilization to prevent joint destruction, which can occur within days. While it may occur in any joint, the hip and knee are the most commonly affected. In a normal synovial joint, the synovial fluid nourishes the cartilage, particularly with sugars. In septic arthritis, the cartilage is starved of these sugars because of the competing needs of the bacteria. When compared to TB arthritis, chronic, nonspecific septic arthritis is less destructive of the joint surfaces and is characterized by erosion of the bone around the edges of the joint surface. The clinical symptoms include pain, a lack of ability to bear weight on the affected limb, fever, and malaise (Mathews et al. 2010). In the child, the infection may result in limb shortening due to premature fusion of the growing epiphysis (Blickman et al. 2004; Erkilinc et al. 2021), while in adults, dislocation and joint fusion may occur, although fusion is less common in this condition than in TB (Roberts and Buikstra 2019).

Septic arthritis is an infrequent finding in archaeological skeletal remains (Fig. 5.14), and distinguishing between a tuberculous and nontuberculous etiology

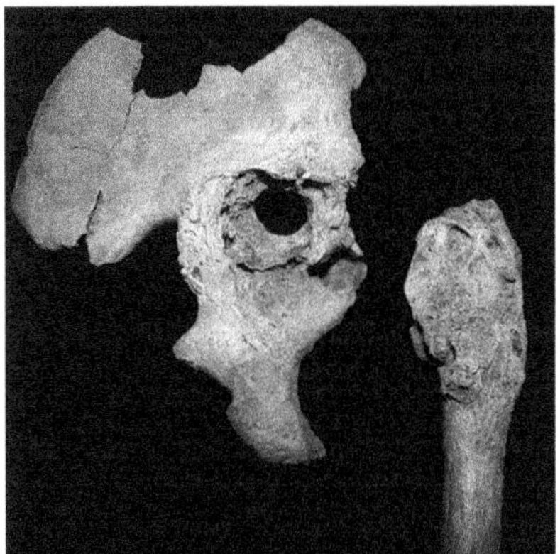

Figure 5.14. Septic arthritis of the hip with loss of the femoral head and lytic destruction of the acetabulum in a 26–35-year-old male from early medieval St. Oswald's Priory, Gloucester, England (900–1120 CE). Photograph by Mary Lewis.

is often problematic without other supporting evidence for TB in the skeleton. Septic arthritis may also be complicated by nonseptic osteoarthritis or other joint diseases so that, in any one individual, a number of joint diseases may be present, making it impossible to differentiate them from one another. For example, polyarthritic changes are also common in the small joints of the hands and feet in lepromatous leprosy (Chapter 6). Zhan et al. (2023) has also described septic arthritis in the left hip of an adult male from the Dapuzi cemetery, Shaanxi, dating to the Western Han Dynasty in China (third century BCE–first century CE). The degree of atrophy suggests that the man had been disabled for many years, probably as a child, resulting in limb shortening and an unusual walking gait.

Rheumatoid Arthritis (RA)

Compared to osteoarthritis and septic arthritis, rheumatoid arthritis is rarely reported in the archaeological record. It is a disease affecting multiple systems of the body, including the lungs and vascular system, but the paleopathologist of course sees only the bony changes (Cotran et al. 1989, 1349; WHO 2024h). It is a chronic immune-mediated disease that causes inflammation of the synovial tissue of the joints. Around 80% of people with the disease have circulating antibodies called the "rheumatoid factor" in their blood. This initiates an autoimmune response where an individual develops antibodies that attack their own body tissues. The IgM antibody (immunoglobulin M) is the initial antibody produced by the adaptive immune system in response to a foreign pathogen. It was discovered accidentally in two different laboratories in the 1940s, but the surprising concept of antibodies attacking the host's own tissues, rather than fighting foreign invaders, took two more decades for full acceptance (Mackay 2010). Another type of antibody (anticitrullinated protein antibody), which is common in RA, was identified in the 1970s. These discoveries allowed for further distinctions to be made among arthritic diseases: those with seropositivity for the antibodies and those without.

The condition has adult and juvenile forms. It is estimated that up to 1% of people in the world have RA and females are affected two or three times more frequently than males, especially in the third and fourth decades of life (Gerosa et al. 2008). Rheumatoid arthritis is now considered to be the result of genetic, epigenetic, and environmental factors (such as exposure to cigarette smoke and air pollution), and even the makeup of an individual's gut bacteria (microbiome) (Yu et al. 2022; see also WHO 2024h). The link to environmental pollution may also account for why it is seen more commonly in industrialized areas, although underreporting in poorer parts of the world may also explain this pattern (Finckh et al. 2022). It is estimated that a genetic component (presence of the disease in another family member) accounts for 60% of disease susceptibility, with 30% of these cases attributable to mutations of genes in the human leukocyte antigen (HLA) class family, and more specifically HLA-DRB*13 alleles (Dedmon 2020; Padyukov 2022). These human leukocyte antigens help code for proteins that differentiate between self and non-self.

Rheumatoid arthritis affects multiple synovial joints symmetrically, especially the small joints of the hands and feet, as well as the wrist, elbow, knee, shoulder, and cervical spine. Less commonly affected are the ankle, hip, and sacroiliac joints. The synovial membrane is affected first. This thickens and forms a layer of granulation tissue called pannus (new connective tissue), which spreads over the cartilage of the joint, eventually destroying it. The bone underlying the cartilage and adjacent to it is also damaged. Ligaments and tendons associated with the joint are involved too, often leading to partial dislocation (subluxation) of some joints, especially the metacarpophalangeal joints. Bone is eroded at the joint edges and, later, on the joint surfaces, and there is usually associated osteoporosis. People with the disease experience weight loss, morning joint stiffness, fatigue, fever, and muscular weakness. Their joints are tender, swollen, and warm, with pain leading to reduced function and severe deformity in later years, such as lateral deviation of the fingers and the boutonniere (button hole—a slit in one of the tendons) and swan neck distortions (Bullock et al. 2019). Fusion of joints is less common than in the seronegative joint diseases.

The first clinical description of RA as a separate entity was made in 1800 by [A. J. Landré-Beauvais] in his thesis Doit-on admettre une nouvelle espèce de goutte . . . ? Should we acknowledge a new species of gout . . . ? Using autopsy evidence, he described a chronic and increasingly debilitating condition that was more common in females and affected multiple joints, particularly of the hands and feet, and he argued that it could be a distinct disease, although earlier descriptions have been claimed—for example, by Sydenham in 1676 (Buchanan and Laurent 1990). Many early medical writers refer to "forms" of arthritis, although nothing in the *Corpus Hippocraticum* (fifth century BCE) reliably matches a description of RA, despite the arguments of a few authors (Byl 1988; Pasero and Marson 2004). Some biographical writings also hint at its presence: for example, it is thought (albeit controversially) that Mary Queen of Scots (1542–1587 CE) had RA (Waldron 2021, 97). It has also been argued that people with the disease are depicted in early modern paintings (Dequeker and Rico 1992; Yeap 2009). Despite these indications, there is much debate on the antiquity of the disease (Entezami et al. 2011).

Primary evidence for rheumatoid arthritis in archaeological skeletal remains is therefore central to our understanding of when the disease emerged in human populations (Leden et al. 2012). For example, was it present in Europe or Afro-Eurasia before European colonial expansion, or did it originate in the Americas (Rothschild and Woods 1990; Kacki 2013; Mant et al. 2024)? Unfortunately, RA is difficult to identify in the archaeological record as its erosive nature means lesions are often obscured by postmortem damage, and the disease may be mistaken for other joint diseases. Its rarity inspired studies of joints from people known to have RA, to ensure diagnostic criteria were correct for identifying affected individuals in the past (Rothschild et al. 1990; Leisen et al. 1991). This heralded an increase in the number of paleopathological reports (in at least eighteen individuals globally, to date). This evidence suggests the presence of RA outside the Americas in the pre-Columbian period (that is, prior to 1492). The earliest example of RA comes from Egypt and is dated to 5500 BCE (May 1897). Bennike (1985) described two people with RA from Denmark dated to 200–400 CE (male) and 1800–800 BCE (female). In England, analysis of skeletons from the medieval site of Barton-on-Humber (Rogers 2000, 174) identified three individuals with RA, a prevalence of 0.2% (Fig. 5.15).

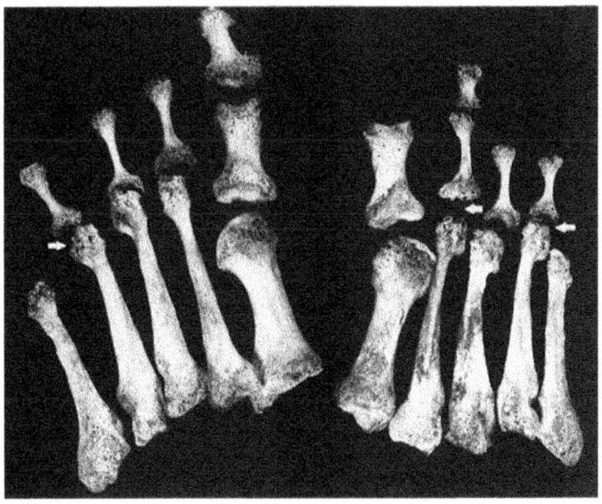

Figure 5.15. Metacarpophalangeal and metatarsophalangeal joints can be affected in RA. Here, erosive lesions of the feet (metatarsophalangeal joints) are visible (eighteenth–nineteenth century CE, England). With kind permission of the late Tony Waldron and Juliet Rogers.

Both Hawkey (1998) and Campillo (1990) have described juvenile-onset RA in adults from prehistoric New Mexico, United States, and third–fifth-century CE Tarragona, Spain, respectively. The male from New Mexico had fused limb bones and severely restricted movement that Hawkey (1998) argued would have developed during childhood and progressed until his death between 30 and 40 years of age (see also Chapter 2). His survival suggests that someone cared for his needs.

The appearance of lytic lesions in the ulna and fusion of the small bones of the hands and feet have been added to the list of criteria that may help us identify RA in skeletal remains (Leden et al. 2012; Craps and Gowland 2015). Despite this refinement, three other joint diseases must be considered in any differential diagnosis of RA: osteoarthritis, gout, and psoriatic arthritis. In osteoarthritis, there are usually no characteristic lytic lesions and the distribution pattern is often more asymmetrical. Gout also has an asymmetric nature, displays "overhanging edge" lesions, and rarely is associated with osteoporosis; it predilects for the great toe joints. Finally, psoriatic arthritis (see next section) is asymmetrical in occurrence and has a distinctive appearance to the phalanges ("pencil in cup"), new bone formation, and involvement of the sacroiliac joints, but rarely osteoporosis. Consideration of these clear differences in character and distribution of lesions should make diagnosis more straightforward. Problems occur either when there are several different joint diseases present on the same joint and/or when the skeleton is not well preserved. For example, osteoarthritis may be superimposed on rheumatoid arthritic joints (Lee et al. 2020).

Psoriatic Arthritis (PsA)

Psoriatic disease is a chronic inflammatory systemic condition that begins in the skin and spreads to the bone marrow and lymphatic system, eventually invading the gut, eyes, joints, and cardiovascular system. Synovial joint synovitis and spinal spondylitis occur (Scrivo et al. 2023), and tendon and ligament attachments to bone may also be involved, with new bone formation (Resnick et al. 2024: 277). It is seronegative. The disease can affect any of the synovial joints, singly or multiply, and usually asymmetrically. While 10–30% of people with skin lesions will develop PsA, there is no direct link between the severity of the skin condition (psoriasis) and the severity of musculoskeletal inflammation (Fitzgerald et al. 2021; Kishimoto et al. 2021). The condition appears to be initiated by trauma to the skin (wounds, tattoos) or stress, which triggers an autoinflammatory and autoimmune response in genetically susceptible individuals (Scrivo et al. 2023). A genetic predisposition to psoriasis has been implicated in around 70% of cases, with variants of the HLA (proteins found on most cells in the human body and linked to the immune system) associated with different clinical subtypes of the disease. Females and males are affected equally, although males are 2–3 times more likely to develop spinal changes (Scrivo et al. 2023), and the age of onset is between 20 and 40 years.

The phalanges of the hands and feet become eroded, with development of a "pencil in cup" appearance in the proximal interphalangeal joints, where the distal end of the proximal phalanx becomes pointed like a pencil and the interproximal phalanx has a cupped proximal surface. Sacroiliac joint lesions are common and often bilateral, and the spine can be affected by ossification of vertebral ligaments. New bone formation on the shafts of the short bones of the hands and feet around the joints is characteristic, and fusion of joints can occur. The erosion of the joint surfaces is normally marginal, as opposed to central (Cantini et al. 2010). Few specific examples of psoriatic arthritis have appeared in the paleopathological literature, and perhaps some evidence may have been misdiagnosed as other erosive joint diseases such as RA or even leprosy (Rogers 2000, 178). Zias and Mitchell (1996), however, reported the condition in two males from the fifth-century CE site of the monastery of Martyrius in Israel.

Ankylosing Spondylitis (AS)

Another of the autoimmune seronegative joint diseases is ankylosing spondylitis, and it was first described in the 1880s. It is a progressive inflammatory disease of unknown etiology affecting the axial skeleton. It is estimated that 70% of people with AS display subclinical intestinal inflammation from a microbial infection, suggesting that the origin of the condition may be in the gut (Hwang et al. 2021). Nevertheless, other factors such as an immune reaction and endocrine disorders have also been implicated in its development. What is clear is that 50–95% of affected people have the HLA-B27 antigen in their blood (Lin and Gong 2017). People with AS risk passing the gene to 50% of their children, and those children have a 30% risk of developing AS. The condition affects males predominantly with a 5:1 male-to-female ratio (Rogers 2000, 176) and has an age of onset of between 15 and 35 years. AS has an incidence of 0.1–0.2% today (Resnick et al. 2024, 256). Erosion and fusion of some joints, especially the sacroiliac joint, occurs; in fact, involvement of the sacroiliac joint (or sacroilitis) is "the hallmark" of ankylosing spondylitis (Resnick et al. 2024, 256). The small joints of the spine fuse, and the vertebral bodies begin to fuse from the lumbar vertebrae upward due to ossification of the annulus fibrosus and bridging between the vertebrae through ossification of the inter- and supraspinous ligaments (Fig. 5.16). Thin vertical outgrowths of bone (syndesmophytes) and ossification of the outer fibrous layer of the intervertebral discs are also evident. As the spine fuses, the bodies remodel and their normal shape is lost; the ultimate appearance is smoothing and squaring of the vertebrae, known as the "bamboo spine" (Takahashi et al. 2023). Lower back pain, limitation of chest

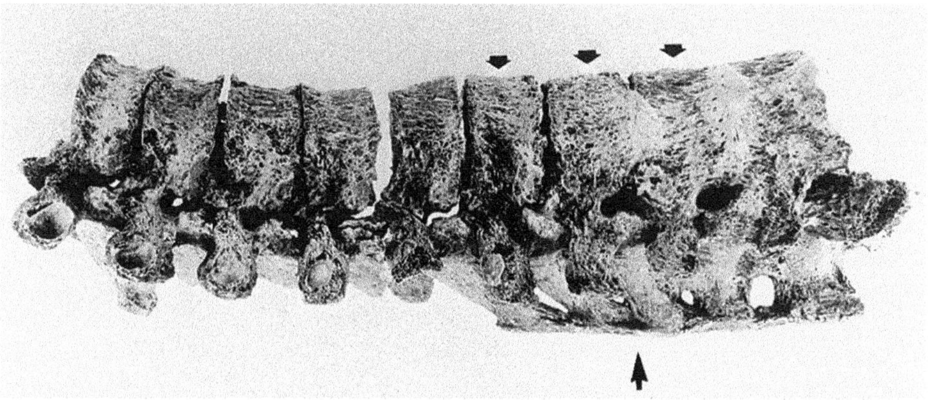

Figure 5.16. Ankylosing spondylitis of the spine showing small syndesmophytes and ossification of the spinal ligaments arrowed (early medieval, sixth–eighth century CE, Eccles, Kent, England). Lumbar spine to the right. Photography by and courtesy of Jean Brown.

expansion, immobility, weight loss, and fever are some of the signs and symptoms. The synovial and cartilaginous joints and entheses are also affected. The hip, shoulder, knee, ankle, wrist, hand, and foot joints are the most commonly affected peripheral joints of the body (Resnick et al. 2024, 258–259).

Individuals with AS in the past have been described from Canada, Croatia, Denmark, Egypt, France, Guatemala, Nubia, Slovakia, Türkiye, the United States, and the UK. Gaľová et al. (2022) suggest a similar prevalence across these regions. While the paleopathological literature commonly reports the condition in males, Khudaverdyan et al. (2021) described spinal ankylosis, potentially AS, in a female from sixth–seventh-century BCE Armenia. It is possible that evidence of AS is underdiagnosed because of the difficulty of differentiating this condition from DISH, but several features can be used to distinguish the two conditions from each other (see later in this chapter). When it comes to differentiating AS from rheumatoid arthritis and psoriatic arthritis, the distribution and nature of the lesions is again likely key (Resnick et al. 2024, 144–57). AS involves significant erosion of the synovial and cartilaginous joints of the axial skeleton, while PsA also involves the synovial joints of the appendicular skeleton, and will have "skip" lesions in the spine (where some consecutive vertebrae are spared). In addition, vertebral spaces are retained in PsA. The sacroiliac joint is rarely affected in RA, and spinal fusion is less common, since it involves only the synovial joints (Cawley and Paine 2015). If a complete, well-preserved skeleton is being studied, it should be possible to differentiate these erosive arthropathies.

Metabolic Joint Disease

Diffuse Idiopathic Skeletal Hyperostosis (DISH)

Diffuse idiopathic skeletal hyperostosis is a progressive noninflammatory bone and soft tissue disease that also affects the spine. It was first described in 1950 by Jacques Forestier, whose name is sometimes used as an eponym (Vaishya et al. 2017). Also previously called ankylosing hyperostosis of the spine, DISH results in characteristic bony abnormalities elsewhere in the body that distinguish it from ankylosing spondylitis. The earliest known evidence was described in a Neanderthal skeleton from Iraq, dated to between 40,000 and 73,000 years BCE (Crubézy and Trinkhaus 1992). Although first described as a spinal disease, it has become synonymous with extraspinal bone changes. The specific cause is unknown, but it appears to be associated with obesity, type 2 diabetes mellitus, a genetic susceptibility, and the metabolic (or insulin resistant) syndrome (Rogers and Waldron 2001). The age of onset is normally 50-plus years, and males are generally more affected than females at a ratio of 7:1, a difference that increases with age (Kuperus et al. 2020; Resnick et al. 2024, 1320). Aufderheide and Rodríguez-Martín (1998, 97) argued that DISH is not a true arthropathy because it does not affect cartilage or the synovium of joints. Furthermore, Resnick et al. (2024, 1319–1320) stated DISH is a disorder of old age of unknown etiology and (in its milder forms) has little clinical significance. Others, such as Rogers et al. (1997) and Mays (2016), have suggested people with the condition are "bone formers"—that is, they have a propensity for excessive bone formation.

Disease or not, DISH results in gradual and complete fusion of the spine (Fig. 5.17), particularly in the thoracic region, with retention of the integrity of vertebral body surfaces and joint spaces, including the apophyseal joints. The anterior longitudinal ligament of the spine and paraspinal tissues ossify, and the osteophytes produced are large and resemble flowing candle wax. These osteophytes are found especially on the right side of the vertebral column at the level of the seventh to the eleventh thoracic vertebra. This is because they are probably prevented from developing on the left side because of the presence of the aorta adjacent to the spine. Fusion of four contiguous vertebrae is necessary for a diagnosis (Waldron 2019). In addition, enthesophytes develop at tendon and ligament insertions; it is not known whether these latter changes occur before or after spinal involvement, but they too are necessary criteria for a diagnosis. Cartilage also ossifies, especially in the neck and ribs. Pain, aching, and stiffness are some of the symptoms of the disease (Resnick et al. 2024, 1320–1322).

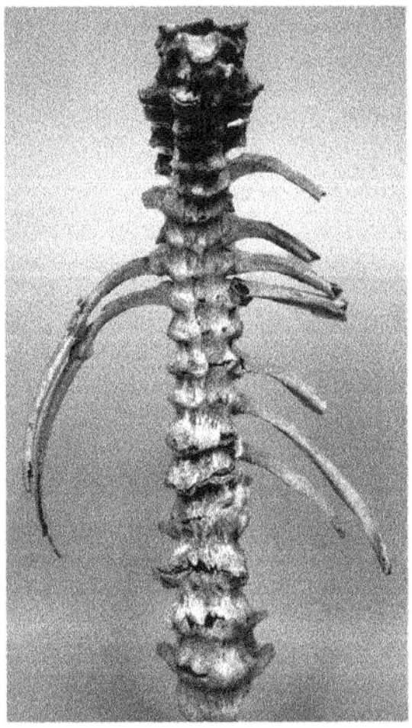

Figure 5.17. Diffuse idiopathic skeletal hyperostosis involvement of the spine; note the ossification of ligaments and tendons causing a flowing candle-wax effect, with fusion of the spine and some ribs. The presence of the aorta has limited ossification on the left side of the thoracic vertebrae (mature male, Roman Droitwich, Hereford and Worcester, England). Photograph by and courtesy of Jean Brown.

Today, DISH is found more often in elderly white populations than in Asians and Africans, but the highest levels are found in Japanese and Korean groups, with rates as high as 24.4% reported in Korea (Ahmed et al. 2022). The prevalence of DISH in older European individuals today is reflected in the archaeological record, but this is not exclusive and more groups from across the world need to be analyzed (see Foster et al. 2018 for possible evidence in a 3,000-year-old Pacific Islander, and the review in Littlejohn 2022). The majority of these individuals are male, with occasional exceptions (Indra et al. 2020). In particular, DISH has often been associated with monastic groups from the medieval and postmedieval periods in Europe (Waldron and Cox 1989; Stroud and Kemp 1993). Its modern frequency is between 3% and 5%, increasing to more than 10% in people over 50 years (Mader et al. 2017). At Merton Priory in Surrey, England, a frequency of 8.6% was reported in the forty-two examined skeletons, dating from the twelfth–sixteenth century CE (Waldron 1985). It was suggested that a rich diet and lack of exercise predisposed people in the priory to obesity and late-onset diabetes. These high-status people may also have lived longer, allowing them to develop chronic signs of the condition. Rogers (2000) argued that at Wells Cathedral in southwest England, high status was more important than age in individuals diagnosed with DISH. Jankauskas (2003) documented the frequency of DISH in 458 skeletons from Iron Age to early modern Lithuania with defined social status, as indicated by grave structure and/or burial location. In agreement with Rogers (2000), Jankauskas demonstrated higher frequencies in individuals of high social status (27.1%) when compared to other urban groups (11.9%) and rural or poor groups (7.1%). The features of DISH were also identified in four mummified Royal individuals from the eighteenth to twentieth dynasties in Egypt (Saleem and Hawass 2014). Stable isotope analysis was used to compare the diets of twenty-five males with and without DISH from the sixteenth–eighteenth century CE Carmelite friary at Aalst, Flanders, France: no association between a protein-rich diet and the disease was found (Quintelier et al. 2014). In fact, Smith et al. (2013) hypothesized that the lower prevalence of individuals with DISH in late prehistoric Tennessee (at 1.0%) compared to European medieval sites argues against a high calorific diet as the main contributor to the disease in their groups, with the genetic component having a greater influence. They suggested that comparing rates of the disease from carefully selected sites with reliable information about different socioeconomic situation and interpopulation genetic differences may help elucidate the causes of this condition in the past.

Differentiating the bony abnormalities in DISH and AS is the first step to identifying the prevalence of both conditions in the past. DISH is commonly found, but by no means exclusively, in older males and consists of characteristic thick, flowing spinal osteophytes and entheseal changes extraspinally, but there is usually no fusion of the apophyseal joints or the sacroiliac joint. AS has thinner, vertically orientated spinal syndesmophytes (bone growth inside spinal ligaments or the annulus fibrosus of disks), fusion of the apophyseal and sacroiliac joints, and no extraspinal bone formation. Complicating the picture, clinical studies have also noted smooth type bridging of vertebrae in DISH and candle-wax type bridging in people with AS (Takahashi et al. 2023). Furthermore, a person may have both DISH and AS, as was proposed by Betsinger and Scott (2023) for a 50-plus-year-old male from seventeenth–eighteenth century CE Poland. They described a combination of both a candle-wax spine, fusion of the apophyseal joints, and inflammation of the sacroiliac joint. In fact, the clinical literature has reported the co-occurrence of these two conditions in around forty individuals to date, stressing that they are two separate conditions and often difficult to distinguish, even when confronted with the entire body of a living patient (Kuperus et al. 2018; Gilio et al. 2019).

Gout

The final metabolic joint disease to be considered is much less common than many of the joint diseases already described. Gout is an inflammatory arthritis with an increasing prevalence today of between 1% and 4% (Singh and Gaffo 2020; Jeong et al. 2023). It is characterized by a high level of blood uric acid (hyperuricemia), caused by an excess of uric acid production or a reduced excretion by the kidneys. Gout affects males more frequently than females in a ratio of between 3:1 and 10:1 (Singh and Gaffo 2020). Its prevalence increases with age and peaks in older age groups (50-plus years) (Resnick et al. 2024, 303). Today, gout is associated with excessive alcohol intake, a diet rich in purines (meat and seafood) and fat, diabetes, and heart disease. There also appears to be a genetic predisposition in up to 20% of cases (Kuo et al. 2015), with Pacific Island populations having a particularly high prevalence (Ling et al. 2023). There may also be a link between high levels of lactose intolerance in this region and the association of restricted cow milk intake and increased hyperuricemia (Johnson et al. 1980; Min and Min 2017) The role of alcohol as a cause may have been greater in the past owing to amounts of lead being added to improve the taste, or to the fact that distillation took place in lead vessels. Lead, after prolonged and repeated ingestion, could cause kidney failure and a consequent rise in blood uric acid concentration: saturnine, or secondary gout. It was not the alcoholic beverage per se but the lead that damaged the kidneys (Steinbock 1976, 309).

During gout, monosodium urate crystals appear in the synovial fluid of joints and cause inflammation and erosion of cartilage and bone (Fig. 5.18). The bone may be eroded on the joint surface, at its margins, or at a distance from the joint, producing overhanging bony lesions shaped like a hook (the "Martel hook" sign is considered pathognomonic of gout; Waldron 2021, 121). The joints affected are mainly those of the feet, hands, wrists, elbows, and knees, with the first metatarsophalangeal joint (big toe) usually involved (90% of people); joints are affected asymmetrically. Urate crystals also accumulate in the tissues associated with the joint (e.g., tendons and ligaments) and away from the joints (e.g., in the fingertips and soles of the feet); these accumulations are called tophi. Without treatment, tophi can occur in 30% of individuals within five years of the onset of gout, while others may never develop this more chronic form (Ko et al. 2013). Gout is an intermittent and extremely painful condition with burning joint pain and swelling and redness of the joints that are tender to the touch. Such attacks can persist for up to three weeks, with massive impact on the quality of life for the affected individual and, in its chronic stages, a higher risk of death (Singh and Strand 2008; Rome et al. 2011).

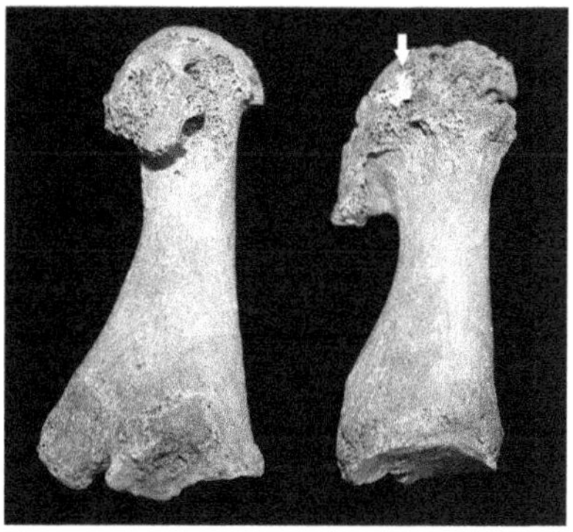

Figure 5.18. Gout in the first metatarsals of a mature male from postmedieval St. Oswald's Priory, Gloucester, England. The white deposit (arrowed) is suggestive of deposits of uric acid. Photograph by Mary Lewis.

The medical historical literature for gout (or "podagra" from the Greek, referring to lesions of the big toe) is prolific and goes back to Hippocrates (*Affections* 31). Because of its exquisite pain and characteristic appearance, gout was likely the first joint disease to be discerned clinically from the undifferentiated morass of arthritic conditions discussed here. The seventeenth-century description of Thomas Sydenham, who had gout, is considered a classic. Colchicine, made from the root of the autumn crocus, is a specific and effective remedy for the pain and inflammation. Known since antiquity and still used today, colchicine's severe gastrointestinal side effects led Sydenham and his followers to avoid it until its revival in the late eighteenth century (Nuki and Simkin 2006; Robinson et al. 2022). Notwithstanding the voluminous historical record, evidence for the disease in archaeological populations is comparatively slim, although it is increasing (e.g., Dittmar et al. 2021c). In a study of 177 adults from different contexts in medieval Cambridge, England, Dittmar and colleagues (2021c) found a prevalence of gout in 3% of the population, with 14% of these individuals buried in the medieval friary. The authors argued that this high frequency was the result of a high alcohol intake and a protein-rich diet in the friary, not shared by those from the hospital or parish sites. Challenging a high-status lifestyle as the only cause of gout in the past, Buckley (2011) carried out a literature review of archaeological and modern clinical evidence for gout and tophi, noting a much higher frequency in Pacific groups (up to 35%). She suggested a greater influence of a genetic predisposition for developing the disease in these less affluent areas. When affluent people were affected, some at least appeared to have sought help. Fornaciari et al. (2019) described gouty arthritis in the hands and feet of a wealthy 50-plus-year-old female from imperial Rome (second century CE). The condition had given rise to ankylosis of the joints and inflammatory cysts in her calcaneus. Evidence for drilling of the bone suggests treatment had been attempted including, perhaps, a postsurgery application of an ointment containing silver. Perhaps the most celebrated early example comes from a fifth dynasty Egyptian mummified individual (2465–2325 BCE) where actual deposits of urate crystals were identified (Elliot-Smith and Dawson 1924). Eighty-six years later scientific analysis had advanced so much that in 2010, Swinson et al. used high-performance liquid chromatography to examine what they also thought was the presence of uric acid in five individuals from various sites in the north of England (1300–1890 CE), two of whom had white powder in their affected joints (both mature males, one from Bromyard Quaker burial ground, Herefordshire (1750–1890 CE), and the other from late medieval Lincoln, Lincolnshire). Both the individuals affected and the white powder tested positive for uric acid, compared to negative results in three individuals without gout (controls). This study increases the potential for the diagnosis of gout and perhaps metabolic syndrome in past populations.

Epilogue

This necessarily brief survey of some of the more commonly occurring and recognizable joint diseases visible in skeletal remains of past humans is but a small part of the total picture of the many hundreds of joint diseases known to medicine today. No doubt more precision in diagnosis of specific aspects of these diseases in the past will be forthcoming, since many of the diagnostic criteria are now better known. Further study of the skeletal manifestations of these diseases in living populations will aid in this goal. In addition, refinement in verifying correlations of osteoarthritis with physical activity are desperately needed to help explore this as an indicator of past human behavior. Significantly, we must control for biological sex and, most importantly, age in our research if we are to truly understand the etiology of the conditions we are recording. The symptoms of joint disease experienced by people today are the same as those experienced by people in the past. Unfortunately for the latter, the medical and surgical relief that we rely on so much, such as specific anti-inflammatories and joint replacements, simply did not exist. Although joint disease is not directly aligned to the UN's Sustainable Global goals [save perhaps for (3) good health and well-being], understanding how well people aged in the past, and the ailments that afflicted them at different rates in different environments, has relevance for modern discourses on the factors that impact healthy aging.

6

Infectious Disease

> In demographic terms, infectious diseases . . . have likely claimed more lives than all wars, non-infectious diseases, and natural disasters taken together . . . as agents of natural selection, infectious diseases have played a major role in the evolution of the human species.
>
> —M. C. Inhorn and P. J. Brown, *The Anthropology of Infectious Disease: International Health Perspectives*

Infectious diseases are caused by several organisms that can be categorized into five groups: viruses (e.g., influenza, smallpox, poliomyelitis); bacteria (e.g., leprosy, brucellosis, tuberculosis); fungi or mycoses (e.g., histoplasmosis, blastomycosis); protozoa (e.g., malaria, leishmaniasis); and helminths (e.g., tapeworms, whipworm). They have accompanied humans and other animals, wild and domesticated, for thousands of years, and paleopathologists have been instrumental in documenting their presence in human remains both at a macroscopic and, more recently, at a biomolecular level. They, like other diseases, are socially constructed but also driven by pathogens (Conrad and Barker 2010).

Since the influential work of W. H. McNeill (1976), infectious diseases have been viewed as major actors in shaping civilizations, and historians continue to embrace or debate his ideas in contemplating their relationship with conquest, geography, and the environment (e.g., Nikiforuk 1996; Diamond 1997; Wolfe et al. 2007; Harper 2021). In the broadest sense, the presence of infectious disease closely reflects the socioeconomic and political environment in which people live, environments that have seen many changes through time. Effective treatments for infections and preventive measures against them have been around for a long time: antiparasitics (quinine, since the seventeenth century); vaccination (since the eighteenth century), antitoxins (since the 1890s), and antibiotic drugs, such as penicillin and sulfone (both in use since the late 1930s). Nevertheless, management of infections remains a considerable challenge in the world today, especially when it concerns "new" infections (ones to which humans have never been exposed); "reemerging" infections (those that have had major declines but are returning); and "emerging" infections (those that have become more common over the past 25 years). In particular, zoonotic infections (those that spread both ways between animals and humans) are prevalent due to our impact on the environment increasing our vulnerability to exposure, caused by factors such as climate change, increased population density, and migration (Baker et al. 2022; Jagadesh et al. 2022). The spread of pathogens between species has most recently been demonstrated by the highly infectious bird flu, which since 1996 has spread to domesticated and wild birds on all continents except Australia (Klaassen and Wille 2023). At the time of writing, bird flu has just been found in the penguins of Antarctica, and fur seals are also dying of it (British Antarctic Survey 2024). Further, the rapid movement of people has exposed "human populations to a host of microbes, insects and other organisms which were previously largely undisturbed" (Connolly et al. 2021, 251). In effect, new ecological niches have developed through time. Movement of people across borders—from urban to rural and rural to urban environments, and even from suburban to urban spaces—provide opportunities for pathogens, humans, and other animals to come into contact, enabling infections to spread.

Overuse and mismanagement of antibiotics in treating infections, in both humans and animals, has led to antibiotic resistance (e.g., Sirota et al. 2024), and new, emerging (e.g., Ebola disease; COVID-19), and reemerging infections (e.g., tuberculosis), as well as new strains of disease, are putting health care services under increasing pressure. Public confidence in vaccination is declining (Larson et al. 2022), and there is global inequity in the distribution of vaccines. For example, barriers remain to the distribution of the COVID-19 vaccine and its uptake (Oehler and Vega 2022; Jackson et al. 2023), while the unvaccinated can face discrimination (Bor et al. 2023). Vaccine hesitancy and low uptake are not new phenomena (e.g., Martini et al. 2022).

Infectious diseases are one of the ten global health challenges according to a range of experts (Lucero-Prisno et al. 2023), and their prevention is relevant to many of the United Nations Sustainable Development Goals, including (1) no poverty, (3) good health and well-being, (6) clean water and sanitation, (10) reduced inequalities, and (13) climate action. Infections are most prevalent in low- and middle-income countries, although high-income countries are certainly not immune. The good news is that advances in health care, improved nutrition, and better living conditions during the past century have enhanced health and well-being and led to a decline in infectious disease and mortality. However, with longer life expectancy comes the risk of noncommunicable diseases, such as diabetes, heart disease, dementia, and cancer. For example, 7 of the top 10 causes of death in 2019 were noncommunicable diseases (ischemic heart disease, stroke, chronic obstructive pulmonary disease, dementia, diabetes, respiratory cancer, and kidney disease), causing 55% of the 55.4 million deaths globally (WHO 2023d). When considered in more detail, however, five of the top ten causes of death in low- and middle-income countries were infectious diseases (lower respiratory tract infections, diarrheal diseases, tuberculosis, malaria, HIV/AIDS). In middle-high- and high-income countries, only one communicable disease featured (lower respiratory tract infections), the rest being noncommunicable diseases.

As we start our journey into infectious diseases in the past, we should remember that many infections we thought had gone away are still with us. The presence and type of infections are impacted by poverty, inequality, and intersectionality (Crenshaw 1991; Marmot 2015), where aspects of identity can intersect to create unique health dynamics and effects. In addition, people can often have several health conditions at once (comorbidities), making them more vulnerable to infection (e.g., see the impact of the COVID-19 pandemic on people with disabilities; Shakespeare et al. 2022). One Health, which considers animals, humans, and the environment (see Chapters 1 and 9), is particularly relevant when studying infections, as will become clear in our exploration of the specific infections identified in the paleopathological record.

While the four major epidemiological transitions occurred at varying times in different parts of the world (Chapter 1), Barrett et al. (1998) identified three periods when infectious diseases increased or decreased. The first encompassed the transition from hunting and foraging to farming (e.g., the Neolithic Revolution), occurring around 10,000 BCE in the Levant, 8000 BCE in North and South America (Doughty 2010), 7500 BCE in northwest Africa, and 4000 BCE in Britain. A transition to farming meant people needed to live in settled communities to maintain their plants and animals. More crowded living conditions and higher population density enabled infectious diseases, including zoonoses, to increase and thrive in humans and their animals. In addition, unsanitary conditions associated with animal and human waste likely led to contamination of soil, water, and, inevitably, what was grown in that soil. The second transition (industrialization), began during the eighteenth century in the Western world (Groumpos 2021). Although the first transition saw an increase in infections, in the second transition infections started to decline. By the early twentieth century, improvements in living conditions along with medical advances, including the advent of vaccines and antibiotics, meant that infections were being eradicated or controlled. We currently live in the third epidemiological transition, globalization, which encourages the rapid worldwide spread of new and reemerging infections. Combined with rising antibiotic resistance and vaccine hesitancy, these infections now pose serious challenges that demand a variety of interventions, not only from medicine, but also from the social and behavioral sciences. Research into the impact of these first and second epidemiological transitions represents a 40-year history of bioarchaeological effort, and by placing our data into context, archaeological and historical information has been used to refine our interpretations (e.g., see Buckberry and Crane-Kramer 2022 for industrial England).

The effect of climate change on infectious diseases has come under greater scrutiny in recent years (Fig. 6.1), and climate hazards are said to worsen the effects of almost 60% of infections that afflict humans today (Mora et al. 2022, this publication includes a link to their dataset). Climate-related hazards can bring pathogens and people closer together, enhancing environmental conditions and opportunities for pathogens to interact with vectors, increasing their ability to cause severe human illness, and weakening the body's defenses. Climate change is clearly affecting ecosystem health, and it can precipitate the migration of infected humans and other animals to new geographic locations, where potential hosts have no immunity to new pathogens (Brooks et al. 2019). At the same time, migrants can be exposed to infections in their new location for which they too have no resistance. Increasing temperatures enable pathogens to spread to locations where they would not previously have survived; this includes mosquito-borne diseases such as malaria and waterborne infections.

Climate can also impact farming. Crop failure can provoke malnutrition, compromised immunity, and increasing predisposition to infectious disease. Further, human manipulation of the environment alongside technological development can create situations that favor the rise of infections. For example, Kyei-Baafour et al. (2020) reported on dam building and its effect on malaria occurrence, transmission, and diversity in a region of Ghana, Africa. Microorganisms can also adapt and change because they are constantly evolving, alongside their environments but also with humans.

The fearful epidemics of plague, smallpox, malaria, and other rapidly transmitted infections were responsible for large numbers of deaths in the past; for example, the fourteenth-century plague that swept medieval Europe is said to have killed 30–50% of the population (Wood et al. 2003). In nonepidemic times, the ever-present and perhaps less spectacular bacteria and viruses would have accounted for a steady and unremitting death rate. Bacteria cause infection today just as they did in antiquity, but with the advent of antibiotics their impact on populations has reduced. Sadly, no antiviral agents, including the new drugs against coronaviruses, are comparable in efficacy to antibiotics. Despite this, one of the greatest medical developments of our time has been the immunization of the young against such viral diseases such as poliomyelitis, measles, mumps, and rubella. Vaccination programs have helped to reduce the incidence of these childhood diseases and thus their impact on the morbidity and mortality of the populations who receive them. Inequality in access to health

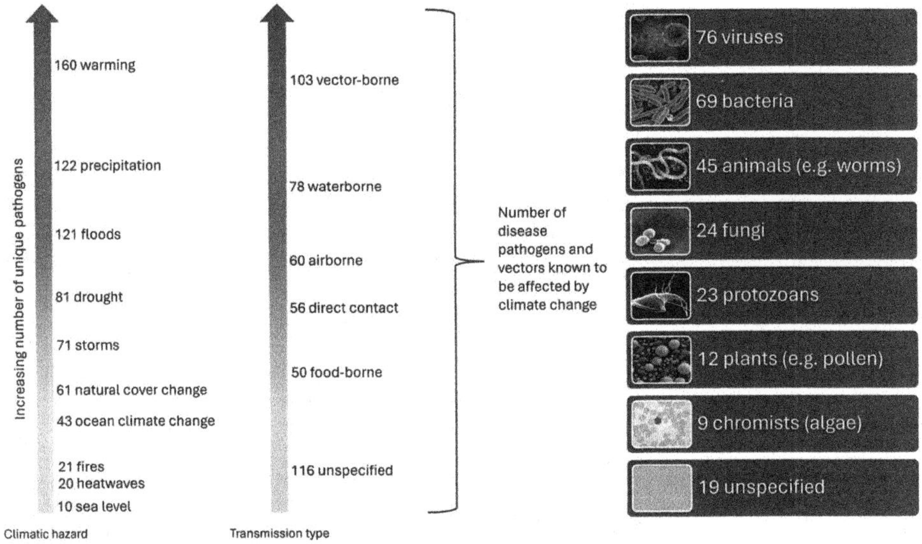

Figure 6.1. Pathogenic diseases aggravated by climatic hazards. The left arrow shows the number of individual pathogens affected by climatic warming from sea level warming (bottom) to global warming (top). The second arrow shows the mechanisms of infection used by such pathogens as the result of the climatic change. For example, the number of infections spread via water increases to seventy-eight as floods become more frequent, and global-scale warming increases the number of infections that use an insect or animal vector to 103 (top). Adapted and modified from Mora et al. 2022.

care means that good health and immunization in middle-high-income countries has considerably reduced the mortality risk of many viral infections, but in low-income countries, viral infections such as measles and influenza, and their sequelae, are still devastating.

Susceptibility to Infectious Diseases

Past or present, whether a person is vulnerable to contracting an infection will be determined by intrinsic and extrinsic factors. Therefore, the overworked and inadequately fed child living in the squalor of an early nineteenth-century industrial town would have been more susceptible to respiratory and gut infections than the child living in a Neolithic village. Intrinsic factors include a person's biological sex, age, immune system strength, the presence of another disease (comorbidity), and genetic predisposition. Extrinsic factors encompass diet (e.g., malnutrition), living conditions, social status, and water and air quality. What follows is a brief introduction to immunity, and the bone's reaction to infection. As mentioned in Chapter 1, the immune system comprises "a collection of cells, chemicals and processes that function to protect the skin, respiratory passages, intestinal tract and other areas from foreign antigens, such as microbes (organisms such as bacteria, fungi, and parasites), viruses, cancer cells, and toxins" (Marshall et al. 2018, 5). There are two forms of immunity: Innate immunity is the first and immediate line of defense, which is non-antigen-specific and has no immunological memory. Acquired immunity is developed through life and includes active and passive immunity where antibodies are produced. Active (adaptive) immunity occurs in response to having a vaccination (artificial) or being exposed to an infection (natural). Active immunity produces the capacity for a strong response to specific antigens and a memory for a future invasion of the same organism. Passive immunity is acquired from somebody else, normally by a child from their mother's milk (natural) or acquired from an immune serum medicine (artificial). Exposure to microbial organisms in early life, including the time the fetus is developing in utero, is essential for developing a strong immune system (Jain 2020).

Even without active treatment, many infections can resolve within a short time. Influenza, measles, colds, and bronchitis are but a few examples. More sinister, and often fatal in the absence of treatment, are infections such as appendicitis, meningitis, and pneumonia. Any infection, be it of soft tissue or bone, is associated with inflammation, although not all inflammation is caused by infection. Agents such as chemical substances and the effects of burning, radiation, or trauma to soft tissues can also cause inflammation. Inflammation is a cellular reaction to the invading organism, be it virus, bacterium, or larger parasite (Ahmed 2011). It first affects the vascular or circulatory system and is manifested in the signs and symptoms of pain, swelling, redness, heat, and, depending on its location, loss of mobility. Inflammatory bone lesions are often, therefore, manifestations of long-standing or chronic infection in a person with a relatively healthy and strong immune system.

Most infectious diseases do not affect the bones, and if they do, they induce bone changes in only a small percentage of untreated people (e.g., 3–5% in TB), with varying frequencies according to biological sex, age, and genetic makeup. This is not to say that the microorganisms causing acute infections mentioned earlier never cause bone inflammation; however, the usually short course of acute soft tissue infections leaves too little time for bone change to develop. By and large, viral infections are more rapidly resolved or are fatal, and do not lead to chronic conditions. Consequently, the infective bone lesions seen in skeletal remains usually resulted from bacterial not viral infections. Furthermore, evidence of infection in a skeleton does not prove that the person died from that infection, unless, perhaps, the lesions observed were unhealed—that is, active at the time of death—suggesting the infection contributed to or caused death. A multitude of causes (related to the disease or not) may have been responsible for death, but most of these are not visible on the bones.

Infectious Disease and the Biomolecular Revolution

Infective lesions of greater or lesser degree are a relatively common finding in skeletons from archaeological sites. However, if we consider the infections that we experience today, it is apparent that the vast majority affect only the soft tissues of the body. That is why studying preserved bodies, such as mummified remains, is important to appreciate the bigger picture of infectious disease in the past, as is harnessing aDNA analytical techniques to detect pathogens in ancient bones and teeth (Sabin et al. 2020; Stone and Ozga 2019). Next-generation sequencing of aDNA (see later in the chapter) has made it possible to identify many infections in the past that were previously hidden to us (e.g., viral infections), including infections that may cause nonspecific lesions. Indeed, infectious diseases have received the most attention from biomolecular analysis, and this is revealing some satisfyingly detailed results. A recent genome study of the early medieval European pathogen landscape, using skeletons from a fifth–eighth-century community that lived in present-day Germany, revealed a large number of infections (Bonczarowska et al. 2022). Not only were several viruses (hepatitis B virus, parvovirus B19, variola virus) and bacteria (*Mycobacterium leprae* [leprosy]) found, but seven individuals had two infections, and one person had three. Tuberculosis has been the target for most ancient biomolecular studies, but leprosy, treponemal disease, plague, malaria, and the influenza pandemic of 1918 also feature prominently. These analyses can provide additional information to macroscopic diagnosis of human remains, identifying infections when no lesions are apparent (e.g., because the person died before bone changes occurred). Furthermore, identifying the particular microbe causing a specific lesion is now technically possible, although directly correlating some bone changes to a positive aDNA result for a microbe is still a challenge. Although these studies represent significant advances for our understanding of the origin, evolution, and paleoepidemiology of infectious disease, they are costly, require specialist equipment and technical expertise, and are destructive in nature. They are also fraught with issues regarding the fragile nature of aDNA and possible contamination with external microbes. These limitations are being explored and addressed, but most paleopathologists utilize macroscopic and radiographic methods of diagnosis as a first (essential) step. For example, certain bone lesions are caused by specific organisms, so that the type of change can be ascribed to a particular infectious disease (termed "pathognomonic"). The specific infections that paleopathologists routinely identify—tuberculosis, treponemal disease, and leprosy—will be considered later in this chapter.

In general, the bone changes of infectious disease are, sequentially, (1) bone resorption mediated by osteoclasts preexisting in normal bone tissue; and (2) bone formation mediated by osteoblasts preexisting in the deep osteogenic (cellular/germinative/cambium) layer of the periosteum in normal bone tissue. Microscopically, this osteogenic layer is clearly differentiated from the outer fibrous layer of the periosteum in non-adult skeletons, but in adults the two layers are fused (Weston 2008; 2009; Tal and Jaramillo 2020). Containing many blood vessels, this inner periosteal layer is essential in repairing bones affected by disease or injury, but its vascularity enables pathogens to spread to other parts of the body. The periosteum is fixed to the cortex by Sharpey's fibers. Because a child's bone is undergoing rapid growth underneath the periosteum (intramembranous growth), these fibers are shorter, less numerous, and more loosely attached to the cortex in children, meaning the periosteum is more likely to be damaged during trauma or inflammation (Lewis 2018, 131–132). Therefore, bone changes of infectious disease may be in the form of bone formation, bone destruction, or a mixture of both. The distribution and characteristics of infection-related lesions, when compared to clinical examples of people with known infections, can help to better identify those experienced in the past. Although most paleopathologists use macroscopic and radiographic approaches for identifying infections, because they are the most cost-effective methods, there has been an increased emphasis on a histological approach, that is, taking thin sections of bone and observing infectious-related features under a microscope (Von Hunnius et al. 2006; for overviews, Schultz 2003; Stout et al. 2019).

In this chapter we consider nonspecific and specific infections (leprosy, TB, treponemal disease, brucellosis) that are more commonly seen in the archaeological record. They are just the tip of the iceberg, however, of the possible infections that may have existed in the past. Nevertheless, space does not allow other types of infections that afflicted humans to be discussed in detail (i.e., parasitic, viral, and fungal infections), and the reader is directed to Grauer and Roberts (2019) for more information. As we will see, infections plagued populations in the past, and we should note that labeling people with infectious diseases such as leprosy, TB, and venereal (acquired) syphilis may be stigmatizing in our world today, especially for descendant populations (Lambert 2012).

Nonspecific Infections

Each layer of bone (cortical, cancellous, and medullary cavity) and the periosteum may all be involved in a bone infection. The terms *periostitis*, *osteitis*, and *osteomyelitis* are usually applied to inflammation of the periosteum, cortex, and medullary cavity, respectively. All of these bone changes are regarded as nonspecific because, if caused by an infection, the invading organism that caused the inflammation is generally not known. These lesions may all occur in the specific infections discussed later, but usually following a specific pattern on the skeleton. Regarding periostitis, although the pathological changes are inflammatory, they are not always associated with infection and may also result from inflammation of the periosteum due to scurvy, trauma, or cancer. Therefore, periostitis should only be used to refer to a condition that is definitely infectious. Waldron et al. (2021, tables 8.9–8.11) listed potential causes of new bone formation in adults and children. For the reasons outlined, subperiosteal new bone formation (SPNB), periosteal reaction, and periostosis are the preferred terms unless the exact mechanism behind the new bone can be substantiated (Klaus 2014a; Roberts 2019b; Waldron 2021, 180–181; Dutour 2023a).

Subperiosteal New Bone Formation

Subperiosteal new bone formation is one of the most common indicators of infection recorded in skeletal populations across time and globally (see Marques et al. 2019, for a review of European data for SPNB on upper and lower limb long bones). Put simply, in response to inflammation, pitting of the bone surface (clastic) is the first bone response, and then dormant osteoblasts on the internal osteogenic layer of the highly vascular periosteum are stimulated to form bone. Nonspecific cellular reactions mean that identifying SPNB is usually straightforward and based on the presence of new bone on the original cortical surface of a bone. The bone formed is initially woven, which is replaced by lamellar bone (including longitudinal striations within it), and plaque-like bone (Figs. 6.2–6.4). Woven (or immature fiber) bone consists of an "initial collagen matrix deposit[ed] in a randomly oriented pattern" (Shapiro and Yu 2019, 137). Some suggest that true woven bone can only be identified using histological analysis (Klaus and Lynnerup 2019, 70), but histological analysis is impractical for most paleopathologists.

There appears to be a predilection for the tibia to be affected. Potential reasons for this include its proximity to the skin surface and exposure to recurrent injury; its cooler surface temperature, which favors infection; its physiologically inactive surface, leading to bacterial colonization; the fact that blood tends to stagnate in the lower legs, allowing bacteria to accumulate; and that the periosteal system supplies 70–80% of the cortical blood supply to the tibia (Waldron 2021, 181–182).

In children who died less than 4 years old in the past, it can be difficult to distinguish new bone formation from normal and rapid appositional growth from bone formed as a response to infection. In this age group, symmetrical and thin deposits of new bone may result from the normal growth processes. Thicker deposits of new bone, however, may be indicative of a childhood infection—of which there are many—and a radiograph of the affected bone may help distinguish normal from pathological new bone. In the latter, a layer of opacity (a double contour) separating the new lesions from the original cortex may be evident (Lewis 2018, 132). In adults, conditions such as varicose veins, venous stasis, and consequent ulceration of the lower leg may also lead to chronic focally induced low-grade inflammation of

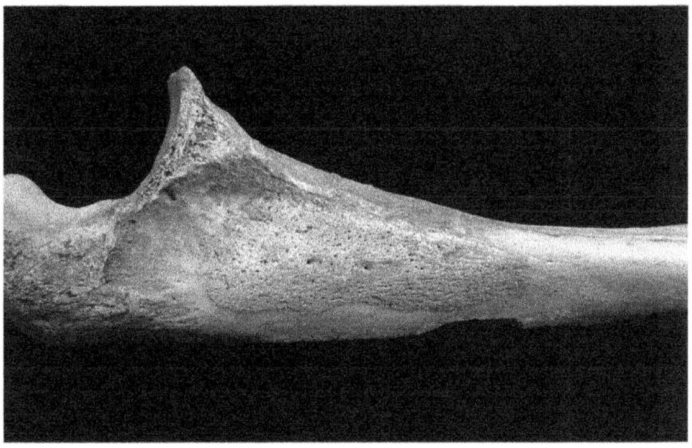

Figure 6.2. Woven bone on a left ulna denoting an active lesion. Photograph courtesy of York Osteoarchaeology.

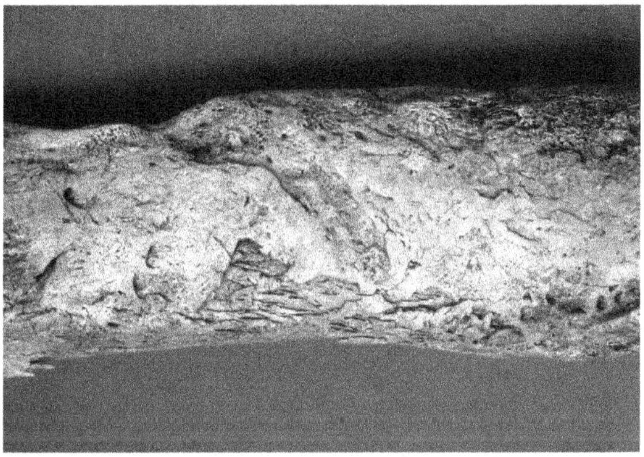

Figure 6.3. Lamellar bone denoting a healed lesion. Photograph by and courtesy of Jean Brown.

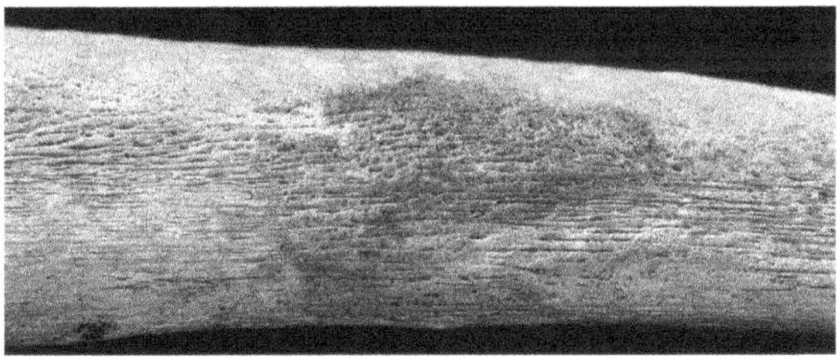

Figure 6.4. Long bone showing striated new bone formation and an area of porous woven bone, indicative of a recurring infection. Photograph by and courtesy of Jean Brown.

the soft tissues and bone, but are unlikely to produce the debilitating symptoms of the more severe osteomyelitis.

Osteitis (Nonsclerosing Osteomyelitis)

Osteitis may be considered based on thickening of the bone cortex as a result of osteoblastic reaction, and subsequent hypertrophy and loss of the bone's (or part of its) normal contours (osteoblastic). This information may be obtained either by observation of the cross-section of the bone, through radiographic techniques, or by comparison of cortical thickness in affected and unaffected paired bones from the same individual. While osteitis may affect the cortex, it can also precede osteomyelitis in the form of the rare nonsuppurative osteomyelitis, known as Garré's sclerosing osteomyelitis (Jain et al. 2021), which presents as a thickened cortex and loss of the medullary canal, but with no signs of an abscess. Resnick et al. (2024, 408–409) acknowledged that using radiography in clinical contexts to differentiate between osteitis and osteomyelitis is extremely difficult. With such severe changes, deciding on whether periostitis, osteitis, and/or osteomyelitis is present is a challenge. However, since bone is a single biological unit, such an arbitrary division of infection into these single terms is, perhaps, artificial (e.g., see Waldron 2021, 148).

Osteomyelitis

If pathogenic organisms invade the medullary cavity, an abscess may form, causing osteomyelitis. Since the pathogenic organisms causing osteomyelitis are not normal inhabitants of bone, they must be transported from elsewhere. They may enter the bone from an external source, as in a compound (open) fracture, or from another site of infection in the body, usually in the soft tissues. In the pre-antibiotic era, relatively insignificant infections of today could lead to sepsis, septicemia, or bacteremia (bacteria in the blood), and the consequent hematogenous spread of the pathogens to more distant organs, including bone. Some of the most common conditions, which often occur together during childhood, are infections of the throat, ear, sinuses, or chest (normally caused by streptococci, staphylococci, pneumococci, or *Haemophylus influenzae)*. Because pathogens require iron to be viable within the human body, the initial site of hematogenous osteomyelitis in a long bone is frequently in the growing metaphysis. In children, this zone of the bone has the most abundant blood vessel supply and is therefore most likely to receive the bacteria and sustain the inflammatory process (Resnick et al. 2024, 388). Indeed, it is likely that infantile hematogenous osteomyelitis was a common and fatal condition in the past—but archaeological evidence is rare (see Lewis 2018, 134).

No doubt individuals with osteomyelitis in the past were seriously ill with fever, pain, and immobility in the affected area. Nevertheless, for observable bone changes to occur, recovery must have taken place. Blood infection is a very serious problem; even today in the antibiotic era it carries a significant mortality risk, and survival in antiquity was probably uncommon. Maybe the evidence of osteomyelitis in the archaeological record testifies to the survival of the fittest. Single or multiple bones can be infected (the latter more so in infants); males are affected more than females for both adults and children. In adults, the axial skeleton is primarily targeted, such as the spine or pelvis, but in children long, flat, and irregular bones are particularly affected today (Resnick et al. 2024, 390). Santos and Suby (2015) examined the remains of children with acute osteomyelitis who were admitted to Coimbra University Hospital, Portugal, during the pre-antibiotic era (1923 and 1929 CE). The most commonly affected bones were the tibia (61.3%), femur (27.3%), radius (4.5%), and humerus/ulna/fibula (2.3%).

Less commonly, osteomyelitis due to direct invasion of bacteria from the skin surface may occur at the time of a penetrating bone injury, such as a human or animal bite, or during surgery (Masters et al. 2022). This is because the normal skin

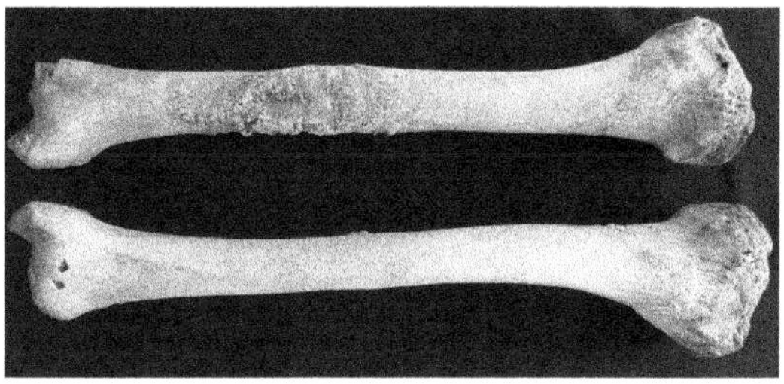

Figure 6.5. Right tibia (top) with focal new bone formation, suggesting an overlying leg ulcer (twelfth–sixteenth centuries CE, Fishergate House, York, England). Photograph by Charlotte Roberts.

surface harbors potentially pathogenic bacteria. In this case, osteomyelitis is located close to the site of the injury. Infection may also spread from a chronic skin lesion such as a deep leg ulcer, eroding through tissues to eventually infect the bone itself (Fig. 6.5).

In both internally and externally derived infection, the longitudinal and transverse spread of the infecting organisms, and hence the inflammatory process in bone, is via microscopic channels known as Haversian (longitudinal) and Volkmann's (transverse) canals, which are found in cortical bone. Thus, the pathogenic microorganisms are spread from their initial focus through the length and breadth of individual bones, producing satellite abscesses that may ultimately come together as one. More rarely, an abscess may remain localized and contained within the bone interior (Brodie's abscess) and will only be detected through radiographic or histological analysis (Resnick et al. 2024, 391–392). Today, osteomyelitis is usually caused by *Staphylococcus aureus* (Masters et al. 2022) but may also be a component of a particular infection like TB, smallpox, or venereal syphilis.

In unresolved and progressive osteomyelitis, gradually and intermittently, the infected bone may extrude pus through to the subperiosteal surface via a draining sinus (or cloaca). The original bone may become surrounded by an enlarged and mechanically less efficient new bone sheath (involucrum), which may be the sole structural support of the specific skeletal part. In such an extreme circumstance, the ensheathed bone—the original cortex—may die (sequestrum) (Resnick et al. 2024, 389–391). The characteristics of osteomyelitis seen on dry bone are a combination of a periosteal reaction and osteitis on the one hand, and resorption and new bone formation in the cancellous tissue of the medullary canal on the other. Three distinct features are required for a diagnosis: a cloaca (draining sinus), a sequestrum (dead or necrosed cortical bone), and an involucrum (a new sheath of bone surrounding the sequestrum). In addition, enlargement of the bone compared to its unaffected opposite may be considered (if preserved). A radiograph may be required to identify a forming cloaca (as a radiolucent area), as well as destruction and formation of bone and areas of increased density. The extent of the involucrum and subsequent hypertrophy of the bone is more severe in an infection sustained during childhood, where the loose periosteum is more readily detached from the cortex (Lewis 2018, 136; Figs. 6.6–6.8).

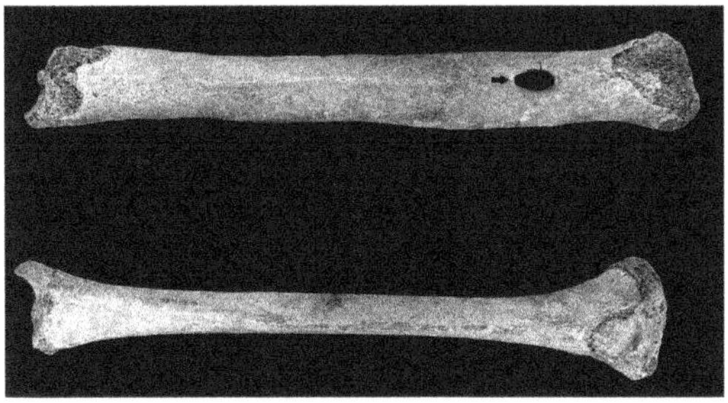

Figure 6.6. Osteomyelitis of the right tibia from an adolescent (top) with opposite (below) for comparison. The affected tibia is enlarged in circumference, longer, and morphologically different. The cloaca is arrowed, linking the inside and outside of the bone and facilitating drainage of pus. The proximal end is to the right (early medieval, sixth–eighth century CE, Eccles, Kent, England). Photograph courtesy of Jo Buckberry and BARC, University of Bradford.

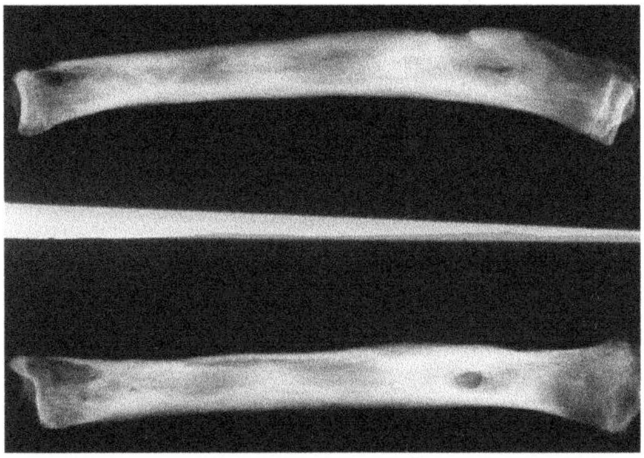

Figure 6.7. Anteroposterior and mediolateral radiographs of the bone in Figure 6.6 showing radiolucent (black) abscess cavities inside the bone. Proximal end to the right. Photograph courtesy of Jo Buckberry, BARC, University of Bradford.

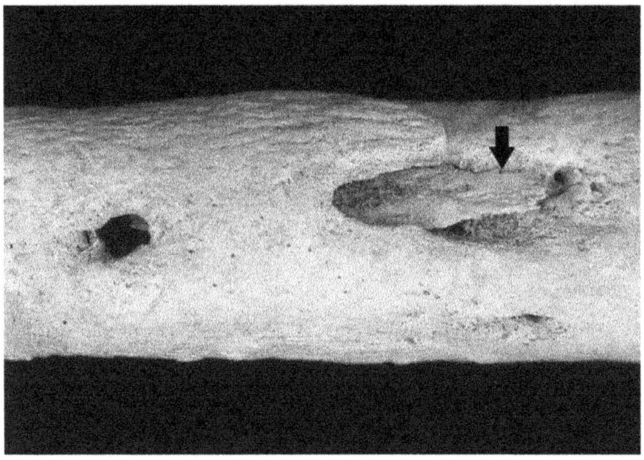

Figure 6.8. Long bone of a non-adult with osteomyelitis, showing the extruding sequestrum on the right (arrow). Originally reproduced with kind permission from Don Ortner.

Before moving onto specific regions of the skeleton subject to nonspecific infection, we will briefly consider the use of copper in the treatment of nonspecific inflammation in four individuals from different sites and periods in Europe. Copper plates were found around the humeri of the following skeletons: from late sixteenth or early seventeenth century in Belgium, but with no evidence of disease underneath the plates (Janssens 1987); from the medieval site of St. Mary Magdalene leprosy hospital, Reading, Berkshire, England (Wells 1964c; Gilchrist and Sloane 2005, 103–104); and from late medieval Sweden (Hallbäck 1976). The latter two individuals had evidence of antemortem disease or trauma. The fractured knee of a male individual from the late medieval cemetery of St. Andrew, Fishergate, York, England (Knüsel et al. 1995: thirteenth–fourteenth century CE), also appeared to have had copper plates applied to it. Copper and its compounds have long been used medicinally and for hygiene. Copper salts were used to aid healing of wounds and sores in the Edwin Smith papyrus (Breasted 1991, 59, 60, 374, 382, 407), by the Hippocratic authors of the fifth century BCE (e.g., *Diseases II*, 25, 20, 33, etc.; *Regimen in Acute Diseases (Appendix)*, 66, 70), and in medieval times (Watson and Gilchrist 2021). Today these virtues are ascribed to its antimicrobial properties (Dauvergne and Mullié 2021; Vincent 2018). Returning to the individual buried in Reading, their copper plates were lined by curly dock leaves—*Rumex crispus L.* (Fig. 6.9). When evaluating the toxicity and antimicrobial, antitrypanosomal, and antiplasmodial efficacy of *R. crispus* extracts, Idris et al. (2019) found *R. crispus* has potency against microorganisms. They also noted that traditional communities use *R. crispus* for the treatment of microbial infections, malaria, and sleeping sickness in the form of decoction or tincture. Furthermore, these archaeological examples reveal primary evidence that proactive treatments were being used to treat infections and other conditions in the past.

Regional Nonspecific Infections

Subperiosteal new bone formation is becoming a common finding in the facial sinuses; the mastoid process and bony components of the ear (upper respiratory tract infections); and on the ribs (a lower respiratory tract infection). Inflammation of the dura mater, the sheath covering the endocranium, has also been implicated in the bone changes referred to as endocranial lesions. All these anatomical locations in the skeleton have received attention, particularly over the past 20 years.

Upper Respiratory Tract Infections

Bone infection induced by blood-borne bacteria was likely very common in antiquity, and the bacteria causing infections probably spread from a primary focus of infection in the throat, ears, nasal sinuses, or lungs. For humans and other animals, the respiratory system is where we let the outside in and provide microorganisms with the ideal (warm and wet) breeding ground. The evidence for these infections in skeletal remains was sparsely reported at the time of the third edition of this book, and we wrote that "documenting of maxillary sinusitis (and rib periostitis) as indicators of respiratory infection needs more attention in paleopathology in the future" (Roberts and Manchester 2005, 176). This situation has

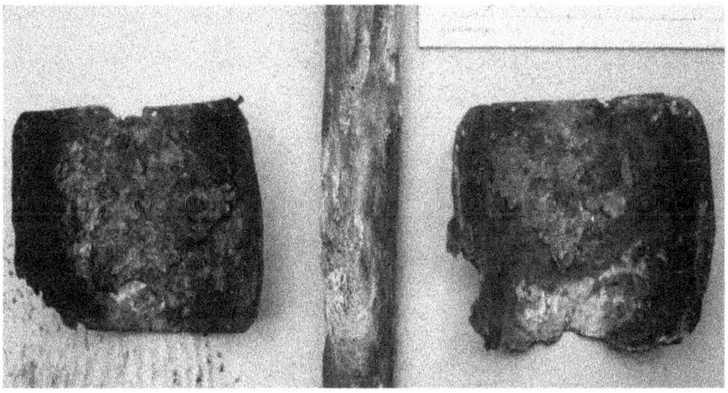

Figure 6.9. Copper alloy plates associated with the humerus of a female with nonspecific infective changes (St. Mary Magdalene leprosy hospital, Reading, England, twelfth–fifteenth century CE). Photograph and permission from Reading Museum.

markedly improved as more researchers have become interested in exploring the impact of poor air quality on health and well-being in the past. After all, we are what we breathe, and we breathe in and out thousands of times a day to stay alive and flourish. If the air we breathe is polluted, the health effects can be profound.

Across the globe, pollutants of many kinds invade the air in our indoor and outdoor spaces, and climate change is exacerbating the situation with impacts on other parts of the ecosystem and other species (e.g., Kessel 2006; Fuller 2018; Barton 2023). Pathogens also abound in our air—for example, those causing leprosy and TB—and can be transmitted from person to person (and even animal to person), something that the world's populations became acutely aware of during the COVID-19 pandemic (e.g., see Dancer et al. 2021a; 2021b).

Indoor pollution can affect the quality of the air outdoors, and vice versa, and even low-level pollution takes its toll (Strak et al. 2021). The World Health Organization estimates that 99% of the global population breathes air that exceeds safe limits, and governments are increasingly recognizing this global challenge and are acting accordingly (e.g., Smith 2023: UK). Within both urban and rural spaces, differences in exposure to pollution according to population affiliation are also present, and their effects on morbidity and mortality have been explored (Ma et al. 2023). Pollution is caused by an array of chemical, physical, or biological particulates. Sources of particulates are either natural (e.g., volcanic eruptions and forest fires) or human induced (e.g., vehicle and industry emissions, agriculture). Farming is a major contributor to air pollution too, such as from livestock waste and dust, field burning, pesticides, and processing crops (Domingo et al. 2021). The very fine particulates that can reach deep into the lungs are the most damaging and can affect respiratory function (i.e., PM2.5–2.5 microns in diameter). Corrosion occurs in the air sacs (alveoli) at the ends of the bronchioles and, because the alveoli are wrapped in capillaries that enable exchange of carbon dioxide and oxygen, that function is affected. While the immune system can become compromised because of air pollution, cardiovascular disease, lung cancer, chronic obstructive pulmonary disease, and lower respiratory disease may also develop (White and Ruparella 2021).

Many people live with constant indoor air pollution from open fires or from stoves that do not work well and are fueled by paraffin, coal, and organic materials (biomass) such as wood and dung (Fig. 6.10). The World Health Organization (2024b) estimated that air pollution in the home led to 3.2 million deaths in 2020, including those of over 200,000 children under the age of 5. Outdoor pollution is estimated to have led to 4.2 million deaths worldwide in 2019, and it is low- and middle-income countries that are affected most. The combined effects of indoor and outdoor pollution are even more deadly, with 6.7 million premature deaths annually.

Susceptibility to air pollution varies for many reasons, some of which will combine to increase vulnerability (e.g., ethnicity, living in poverty, occupation, disability, and wider life experiences). Increasing global attempts to curb pollution and address climate change include incentives for the general public, legal requirements for industry, developing cleaner fuels, and implementing clean air strategies and policies for farming. Nevertheless, the health impacts remain clear. The particulate matter to which our predecessors were exposed may not have been as complex as that of today (e.g., chemicals), but they would not always have been breathing

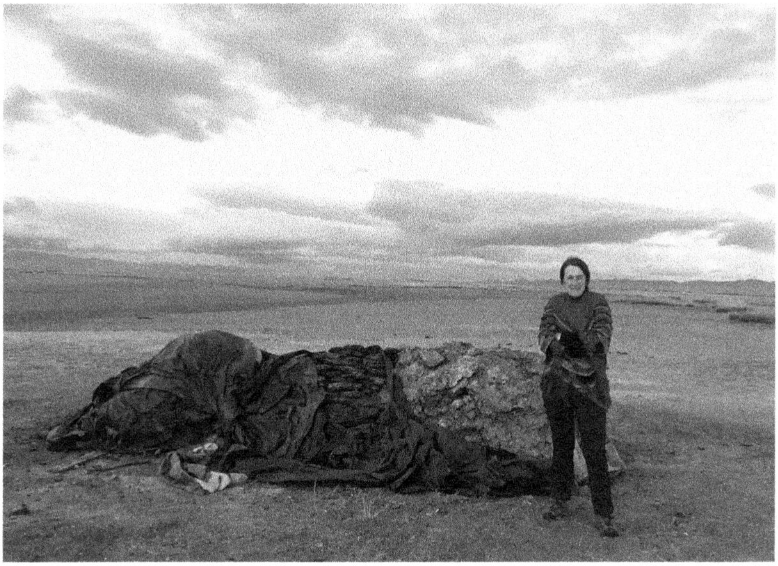

Figure 6.10. Animal dung used in Mongolia for heating and cooking inside gers; it is often the only fuel available. Photograph from Charlotte Roberts.

good-quality air. Prior to living in urban environments and/or farming, hunter-foragers likely breathed air that would have been mostly clean, but urbanization would have increased the inhalation of damaging particulates and subsequent health consequences, perhaps akin to living in a rural community today.

The study of respiratory health in the past has focused on the facial sinuses, particularly the maxillary sinuses, as well as the ribs. It is also worth noting that dental calculus (Chapter 3) can contain soot, microcharcoal, wood dust, and fungal spores that have been inhaled (Radini and Nikita 2023). Five examples illustrate this area of research. Hardy et al. (2016) found microcharcoal in dental calculus in Lower Paleolithic individuals at Qesem Cave, Israel (420,000–200,000 BCE). Hardy et al. (2012) also documented Neanderthals buried in Sidrón Cave, Spain (47,300-50,600 BCE) with the first molecular evidence for inhalation of wood-fire smoke and bitumen. Millard et al. (2020) reported seventeenth-century skeletons buried in Durham, England, with soot particles in their calculus, along with maxillary rhinosinusitis and evidence for pipe smoking. Pabst and Hofer (1998) identified anthracite in the lungs of the Tyrolean "Iceman," probably caused by exposure to wood fires, and evidence in the lungs of twelve mummified bodies suggested pneumoconiosis (Munizaga et al. 1975). These were seventeenth-century coal miners in Chile who had likely inhaled coal dust while they worked. Air pollution inevitably was, is, and will be around us, from our past and into our future.

Maxillary Rhinosinusitis

The paranasal sinuses—frontal, maxillary, ethmoidal, and sphenoid—are air-filled cavities within the bones of the face (Fig. 6.11). The sinuses are lined with mucous

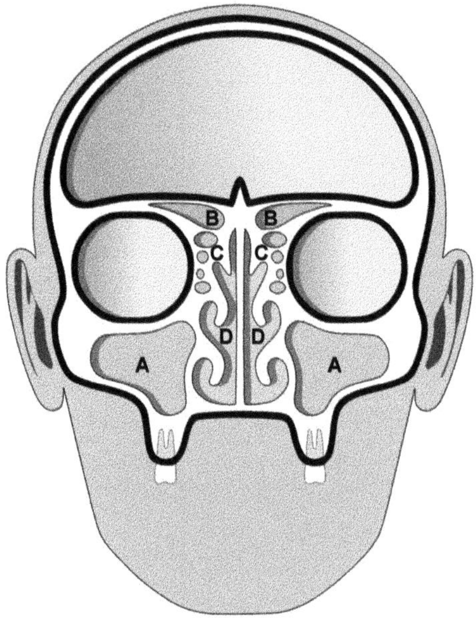

Figure 6.11. Facial sinuses: A, maxillary; B, frontal; C, sphenoid; D, ethmoid. Adapted from Davies-Barrett et al. 2021a, and kindly modified by Anna Davies-Barrett.

membrane that contain cilia, which are hairlike structures on the membrane that brush away or remove mucus from the sinuses. The sinuses are subject to particulates circulating in the air that may provoke inflammation. In the maxillary sinuses, normal drainage takes place via mucus passing through the superiorly placed ostia, but drainage can be inhibited because of inflammatory-related narrowing of the ostia and the mucus becoming viscous (Helliwell 2010). Consequently, lack of normal mucous drainage leads to its accumulation and pain due to pressure.

Sinusitis, or rather rhinosinusitis (Slavin et al. 2005), can be of infectious etiology and is caused primarily by viruses, although *S. aureus* is one of several bacteria implicated (Brook 2011). Other upper respiratory tract infections have been linked to the development of rhinosinusitis, and it can also result from exposure to noninfectious materials to which people may be allergic, such as dust, animal dander, spores, and pollen. In children, in addition to allergies, asthma and developmental conditions such as cleft palate can predispose individuals to rhinosinusitis. Today's preschool children are at high risk for rhinosinusitis owing to close contact that promotes respiratory infections (Lewis 2018, 138); no doubt congregations of children in the past provided a similar context for spread of sinus infection. Researchers have also explored other risk factors for developing this condition. As far as the authors are aware, Calvin Wells was the first paleopathologist to conduct studies on ancient rhinosinusitis (1964c; 1977). In 1964 he reported on evidence of the link between dental disease and rhinosinusitis, in this case a dental abscess. Dental causes of rhinosinusitis were also suggested by Gregg and Gregg (1987) for a fourteenth-century individual buried at Crow Creek, South Dakota, United States, and by Digangi and

Sirianni (2017) in Rochester, New York, for individuals from a nineteenth-century almshouse. As Little et al. (2018) noted, more than 30 million US citizens suffer from rhinosinusitis and a large proportion of their rhinosinusitis is related to dental disease. Magalhães (2018) identified sinonasal variation in nineteenth–twentieth-century Portuguese osteological collections, and Mays (2012) suggested a relationship between nasal septal deviation and rhinosinusitis, an area of study that needs more work. Compared to other health problems, there have been fewer studies of rhinosinusitis in paleopathology. Lee et al. (2024) provided an overview using an online literature search (they found seventy-five studies) and made recommendations for future research.

One reason for this lack of engagement may be the challenges of recording the condition. In clinical practice rhinosinusitis is classified as acute, subacute, chronic, and recurring, based on symptom duration. In paleopathology, only chronic or recurring rhinosinusitis is identified because the duration of acute and subacute rhinosinusitis will not have been long enough for bone changes to occur. The sinuses are also a challenge to record, especially since they can be full of soil on excavation and difficult to clean, while the fragile ethmoid and sphenoid sinuses can be damaged postmortem. Consequently, much evidence of rhinosinusitis from the past has gone undetected, even though inflammation induced by poor air quality was likely relatively common. That said, intact maxillary and frontal sinuses may be accessed by drilling a small hole in the sinus and using an endoscope (Lewis et al. 1995a).

In dry bone, maxillary rhinosinusitis is recognized as destruction of bone, including pitting, and new bone formation on the interior sinus walls and floor (Fig. 6.12). Lesions tend to be situated on the inferior surface (floor) of the sinuses, probably due to mucus accumulating on that surface due to gravity. These bone changes were initially classified by Boocock et al. (1995), whose method is still used, albeit with some modifications (Lee et al. 2024). Recording rhinosinusitis in non-adults under 8 years is problematic because the small size of the developing sinuses makes visualization difficult. In addition, in non-adult skeletons with intact sinuses the developing teeth can inhibit the use of an endoscope (Lewis 2018, 139). Despite the challenges,

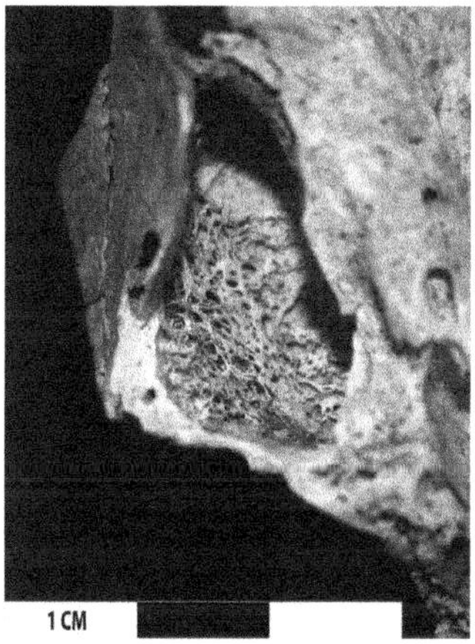

Figure 6.12. Maxillary rhinosinusitis in a male adult from Arnhem, The Netherlands. With kind permission from Gemeente Arnhem and Martijn Defilet (Senior bestuursadviseur Erfgoed en Archeologie).

studies of the rhinosinusitis in nonadults have been reported. For example, Lewis (2002) found almost 10% of sinuses in 0–17-year-olds were affected from sites in medieval and postmedieval England (twelfth–nineteenth centuries CE). Liebe-Harkort's (2012) study of early Iron Age (0–260 CE) non-adult and adult skeletons from the rural site of Smörkullen in Östergötland, Sweden, identified maxillary rhinosinusitis in 50% of the nonadults and 87% of adults. While the sample size was small (*n*=93), the difference in frequency between adults and children may be explained by age at death, with adults having longer to develop a sinus infection or dental disease that may cause it. In a larger sample of nonadults from Poland, Krenz-Niedbała and Łukasik (2016a) reported maxillary rhinosinusitis in 18% of individuals from early urban Cedynia (tenth–fourteenth centuries CE), and in 7.1% of those from rural Słaboszewo (fourteenth–seventeenth centuries CE).

Zubova et al. (2022) focused on climate change and global warming. The study considered chronic maxillary rhinosinusitis in archaeological individuals from five continents and represents the largest meta-analysis of this condition to date (21 sites and almost 2,000 individuals). They noted the importance of climatic changes as a risk factor, especially temperature. For example, lowest frequencies were found in geographic locations with the highest mean annual temperatures. Davies-Barrett et al. (2021a) also explored various risk factors and maxillary rhinosinusitis in a wide-ranging study of almost 500 individuals from thirteen archaeological sites in the Middle Nile Valley, Sudan. These people variously lived as hunter-foragers, pastoralists, farmers, and town/city dwellers (4900 BCE–1500 CE), but urban people had the highest frequencies. In paleopathology it is usually impossible to ascertain what actually caused a person's rhinosinusitis, but patterning can be seen when context is considered, as Davies-Barrett et al. show in their study. However, pathways for irritants to affect the upper respiratory tract are multiple, and it can be difficult to determine how frequent and intense exposure to particulates may have been (Radini and Nikita 2023).

The recognition that air pollution is a contributor to maxillary rhinosinusitis is not a new one. In his second paper on maxillary rhinosinusitis, Wells (1977) took a temporal approach to evidence for sinusitis in English populations. He found an overall frequency of 4% (of 387 sinuses) from the Bronze Age (2000 BCE) to the sixteenth century CE. The highest frequency was 6.8% in the early medieval period (mid-fifth to mid-twelfth century CE). Wells linked this figure to smoky fires and poor ventilation in housing. In the 1990s, Lewis et al.'s 1995a study of contemporaneous medieval rural and urban populations in England found a 55% frequency of maxillary rhinosinusitis in the people buried at the urban site of St. Helen-on-the-Walls, York, and 39% at the rural site approximately 30 km (20 miles) away (Wharram Percy). The cemetery of the urban site served a poor parish in York, where the environment likely harbored atmospheric pollutants, both in the home (burning fuel for warmth and cooking) and externally. A higher frequency in males could have been because they worked in the neighboring parish of Bedern where contemporary historical documents record polluting industries such as tanning, which would have introduced particulate pollution. The occurrence of rhinosinusitis in people buried at Wharram Percy likely related to particulate pollution from the environment (e.g., pollen) and farming (e.g., processing cereal crops). While high urban rates have been seen in medieval England (Roberts et al. 1998a), Roberts (2007) and Lewis (2002) have documented low rates in both adults and children buried in the eighteenth–nineteenth-century urban London crypt of Christ Church, Spitalfields (18% and 3%, respectively). These frequencies may well reflect that these higher-status ("middling sort") individuals were protected from the surrounding urban pollution by their housing, with, for example, chimneys for ventilation. Urban-rural differences in adults were also reported by Casna et al. (2021) in early modern Netherlands (1626–1866 CE): urban Arnhem individuals displayed only slightly higher frequency than individuals who lived in rural Middenbeemster, while Sundman and Kjellström (2013) likewise found little difference between Swedish proto-urban and rural populations from the Viking Age to the early medieval period (750–900 CE). In considering contextual factors for these data, such as documented occupations, it was concluded that living in an urban environment was no more detrimental to respiratory health than living in the countryside.

Some experimental research has addressed the impact of indoor environments on respiratory health in reconstructed ancient houses. Ryhl-Svendsen et al. (2010) documented exposure to daily averages of PM2.5 in seventeenth-to-nineteenth-century houses in Denmark, with a figure that exceeded the WHO guidance. Importantly, the value was comparable to that experienced by females in low-income countries today. In another study, Shillito et al. (2022) worked at the pre-urban UNESCO World Heritage Site of Çatalhöyük, Türkiye, where a replica of a Neolithic mudbrick building was built. Fires using dung and wood fuel were lit inside the building. Again, values for PM2.5 exposure exceeded WHO guidance, and the effects from dung were worse than for wood. These Neolithic houses were likely without windows and entered from the roof, suggesting that there was little ventilation at all and people would have been chronically exposed to air pollution. More studies such as these are needed.

Although relatively rare, extant studies of maxillary rhinosinusitis are concentrated in Europe and North America (Lee et al. 2024). For example, Merrett and Pfeiffer (2000) noted the condition in 50% of 207 individuals buried in a fifteenth-century ossuary at Uxbridge in southern Ontario, Canada, attributing it to pollution in dwellings. Within this group of 207 individuals (114 adults), rhinosinusitis tended to increase with age but had a maximum frequency in nonadults. The study by Davies-Barrett et al. (2021a) from Sudan seems to be the only one published for Africa, and there is only one study from South America (Davies-Barrett et al. 2021b: Peru). In Asia, Mushrif-Tripathy (2014) studied maxillary rhinosinusitis in India, dating from prehistory (1500 BCE) to the medieval period (1700 CE) revealing 9 of 74 individuals affected (12.16%). There are two further studies from Asia (China). Xiong et al. (2021) found rhinosinusitis affected 40% of individuals who had at least one sinus preserved (Heishuihe, Gansu province; Han Dynasty: 202 BCE-220 CE). In the Zaoshugounao Shaanxi province (1400–900 BCE), almost all (n = 24) of the twenty-seven individuals were affected with sinusitis (88.9%). Fu et al. (2023) suggested a number of risk factors: particulate pollution from dry, cold weather patterns, small and poorly ventilated subterranean houses, biomass fuels, and farming.

Prior to the recent wide-ranging reviews by Lee et al. (2024) and Zubova et al. (2022), research that drew together rhinosinusitis data from seven populations who variously lived hunter-forager, farming, and urban lives appeared in 2007. Sites from three continents were considered: North America, Africa, and Europe (Roberts 2007). The lowest frequency was seen in hunter-foragers, followed by rural agriculturists, and then urban dwellers. Surprisingly, the second-highest frequency overall was recorded in hunter-forager Aleutian Islanders (present-day Alaska). The data derived from seven rural sites in the northern Pacific Ocean region. Contextual data indicated that they lived in poorly ventilated semi-subterranean houses lit by seal oil lamps. As these islands are volcanic, perhaps exposure to volcanic dust combined with indoor living conditions predisposed them to the condition.

There are few reports of infections affecting the other sinuses, although frontal sinusitis has been described by several authors: Armentano et al. (1999: Bronze Age Spain); Liebe-Harkort (2012: Iron Age Sweden); Connell et al. (2012: medieval England); and Magalhães et al. (2017: early twentieth-century Portugal). Increasingly, however, researchers are combining different indicators of respiratory disease using a range of methods, recognizing that the upper and lower respiratory tracts are inextricably linked. The middle ear is connected to the sinuses via the Eustachian tube, which is why children who contract an upper respiratory tract infection can develop an ear infection too. Collins's (2019) study of 305 crania from medieval Icelandic skeletons considered maxillary rhinosinusitis, otitis media, and mastoiditis, alongside evidence for tuberculosis, and used macroscopic, microscopic, endoscopic, and CT methods. Krenz-Niedbała and Łukasik's (2020) research on rural and proto-urban nonadults from medieval and early modern Poland also report data on maxillary sinusitis, rib lesions, and otitis media, the latter manifesting as superficial discrete pitting on the surface of auditory ossicles. More commonly studied is the relationship between new bone formation on the ribs and maxillary rhinosinusitis, indicating that both upper and lower respiratory systems can be affected (e.g., Bernofsky 2010: twelve sites in southern England; and Davies-Barrett 2018: twelve sites in the Middle Nile Valley, Sudan).

We anticipate more research on sinusitis now that a strong base has been established. Certainly, from British contexts, maxillary rhinosinusitis appears to increase across time as environments became more complex, especially with urbanization (Roberts and Cox 2003), although to date little evidence has been reported for prehistory in Britain, or globally. People in antiquity, huddled around open hearths in smoky, often ill-ventilated dwellings, would surely have been susceptible to this chronic and irritating condition. Such environments would favor the production and stagnation of pus within the sinuses, creating an opportunity for inflammation and rhinosinusitis along with bone changes that paleopathologists can detect.

Middle-Ear and Mastoid Infection

Otitis media (inflammation of the middle ear) may be caused by viruses or bacteria; these include acute otitis media, otitis media with effusion, or "glue ear," and chronic suppurative otitis media (Schilder et al. 2016). The middle ear connects to the nasopharynx via the Eustachian tube, and with the mastoid air cells via the aditus ad antrum (Vaz et al. 2021). The Eustachian tube maintains equal air pressure across the tympanic membrane, or ear drum, and it ventilates the middle ear. In the

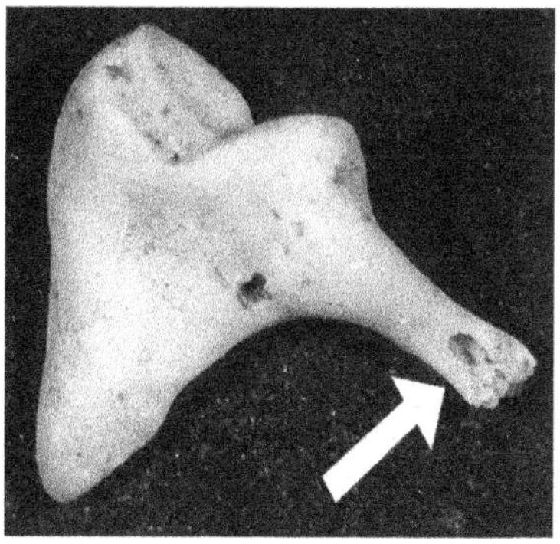

Figure 6.13. Lytic lesions on the lenticular process of the incus in a child from Maastricht, Netherlands (Merovingian period, 480–700 CE). Mean total incus length: 7.04 mm; mean total width: 5.31 mm; mean length of long process (on right of image): 3.27 mm (Kumar et al. 2018). Photograph courtesy of Raphael Panhuysen and Tjasse Bruintjes.

middle ear are the three ossicles: the malleus, incus, and stapes. These bones transmit sound from the ear drum. Otitis media usually results from spread of an upper respiratory tract infection via the Eustachian tube. Today it is particularly common in children under 10 years (Vaz et al. 2021), and 80% of children have usually had otitis media before the age of 6 years (Verhoeff et al. 2006). Inflammation of the middle ear, including the ear bones, ensues and fluid from the soft tissues accumulates. This liquid leaks from blood vessels once inflammation has been established. It can build up in the middle ear, even to the extent that it can perforate the ear drum. Hearing is affected and it is painful. Rare complications include mastoiditis and meningitis. Untreated, otitis media frequently settles following perforation of the eardrum and the discharge of pus, similar to resolution of a painful dental abscess. Although no observable bone changes are seen in acute infection, persistence of the infection turns into a chronic fluid-discharging ear, which induces bone formation and destruction of the walls of the middle-ear cavity and the auditory ossicles (Fig. 6.13; Krenz-Niedbała and Łukasik 2016b).

Otitis media must also have been common in the past. Indeed, the *Corpus Hippocraticum* (fifth century BCE) and sources in the Byzantine period (324–1453 CE) described ear diseases, caused by trauma and what we would call infection, and their treatment (Benmoussa et al. 2018; Lascaratos and Assimakopoulos 1999). Perforation of the eardrum, otitis media, deafness, and hemorrhage from the ear are included in the list of conditions for this period, and herbal, animal, and mineral remedies were recommended and applied via ear drops, poultices, or using special instruments. In skeletal remains of the past, the delicate membranous eardrum does not survive, and evidence of perforation is therefore lost. During the autopsy of the mummified remains of Egyptian Pum II, perforation of the preserved eardrum was noted (Benítez 1988); the pain endured by this man living around 170 BCE may have been relieved by the drainage of the infected middle ear, but he died soon after.

If a middle-ear abscess erodes the surrounding bone and induces inflammation of the mastoid bone and air cells, mastoiditis develops. Unresolved, the infection behind the ear ultimately bursts through the bone surface to either the exterior or the interior of the skull. In this case, the opening in the bone surface should be visible in dry bone, when preservation is good. If the mastoid infection discharged into the interior of the skull, the outcome was probably fatal, but if it drained to the exterior, recovery was possible. Mastoiditis is more common in children today than in adults, and because the mastoid air cells are developing in childhood, this condition can impair normal development. Symptomatically, mastoiditis is associated with unremitting intense pain, fever, sore throat, redness and swelling of tissues behind the soft tissue pinna (external ear), distortion of the ear lobe, and potentially, facial nerve palsy (Cassano et al. 2020).

Paleopathological research on otitis media and mastoiditis have increased just as they have for rhinosinusitis. Wells (1962) documented two individuals with mastoid infection from England, and Schultz (1979) recorded both these conditions in individuals from Merovingian cemeteries in southern Germany (500–700 CE). Schultz (1979) suggested that otitis media was more common in the oldest and poorer members of society, and also that a poor diet and ill health in infancy predisposed individuals to later development of the condition. With regard to otitis media, microscopic examination of ear ossicles has been carried out on skeletons from a medieval leprosy hospital cemetery in England (Bruintjes 1990). Erosive lesions affecting the ear ossicles were recorded in eighty-nine individuals, suggesting chronic middle-ear infection (Fig. 6.13). Of the preserved ossicles, 51% were affected (n = 69/136). For the general population, such a rate of middle-ear infection would be high, and Bruintjes's findings support observations of the frequency of otitis media in people with leprosy today. Dalby et al. (1993) found a lower frequency of 1.5% affected ear bones (of sixty-one studied) in Romano-British individuals (fourth century CE). Future studies may focus on aDNA analysis, which has been found to survive in ear bones, and perhaps analysis may reveal the DNA of pathogens that caused otitis media (Sirak et al. 2020). Studies of ear bones from archaeological contexts need more attention, although survival for examination is impacted by burial and excavation, and extracting the ossicles from the middle ear remains challenging.

Researchers have attempted to record the presence of infection on the bony surfaces of the inner ear of skeletons from the Levant using a variety of methods. Floreanova et al. (2020) used a flexible videoscope and an optical microscope, with microcomputed tomography (μCT) validating the results. Their study resulted in a new diagnostic method for recording bone remodeling on the promontory of the middle-ear cavity. Zhao et al. (2023) reported on two skeletons from China with destruction of bone in the auditory canal and, using macroscopic, microscopic, and micro-CT analysis, the differences between middle-ear and external auditory canal cholesteatoma, which is an abnormal collection of cells in the ear that can favor infection (Mays and Holst 2006). In a particularly interesting study that provided evidence for potential treatment of an ear infection, Olivé-Busom et al. (2021) examined the temporal bones of a medieval Islamic individual from Spain (tenth–sixteenth century CE) with macroscopy, binocular microscopy, radiography, and scanning electron microscopy–energy dispersive X-ray spectroscopy (SEM-EDS). The right bone had changes consistent with otitis media and mastoiditis, including a large sinus. The area of the bone affected had copper staining, which suggests either a copper object in the grave (e.g., an earring) or yet another potential treatment with copper.

Mastoiditis has also received more attention since the 1980s but, while destructive lesions and inflammatory new bone formation may be identified macroscopically, indicating pus had drained from the mastoid process, not all people who experienced mastoiditis would have developed a sinus by the time of their death. Therefore, further evidence of mastoid infection may be found through radiography of the mastoid process, because infection induces changes in the pattern and size of the air-containing spaces within that bone (Gregg and Gregg 1987, 72–74; Dalby 1994). The mastoid air cells are important for the development and outcome of middle-ear disease. During development, epithelial tissue infiltrates the growing mastoid process and produces epithelium-lined air-cell chambers, a process known as pneumatization (Khan et al. 2022). This occurs before the age of 7 years (Scheuer and Black 2004, 84). Therefore, any infection before the age of 7 years will be evident through under-pneumatized mastoid cells, while an infection after 7 years would be present in addition to well-pneumatized cells (Fig. 6.14a and b). Titche et al. (1981) applied radiography to mastoid processes to examine air-cell patterning in relation to mastoiditis using accepted clinical views. They found well-pneumatized air cells in skeletons from Arizona (no infection). Much later, Purchase et al. (2019) developed a handheld X-ray system for recording mastoiditis, which is useful for work in the field and museums. This was tested on around fifty prehistoric skeletons from Cis-Baikal, Russia, revealing two-thirds had mastoiditis, and almost two-thirds of those affected had concurrent maxillary rhinosinusitis. Zhang et al. (2020) documented two individuals with mastoiditis from Shandong province in China dated to 475 BCE–220 CE. They found sinuses on the mastoid bone surface, air-cell fusion, air cells full of sclerotic bone, and asymmetry of the internal mastoid structure. They concluded that these features were consistent with a diagnosis of mastoiditis. With these recent developments and more published studies, mastoiditis may become more mainstream when analyzing human remains.

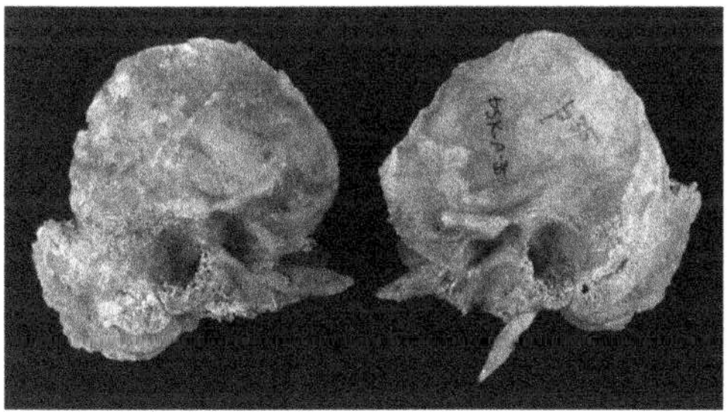

Figure 6.14A. Temporal bones of an 11.5–12.5-year-old from fifteenth–sixteenth century CE Skeljastaðir, Iceland. Both external auditory meatuses have inflammatory changes (new bone formation) and porosity posterior to the meatuses. Photograph courtesy of Cecilia Collins, with kind permission from Ívar Brynjólfsson, National Museum of Iceland.

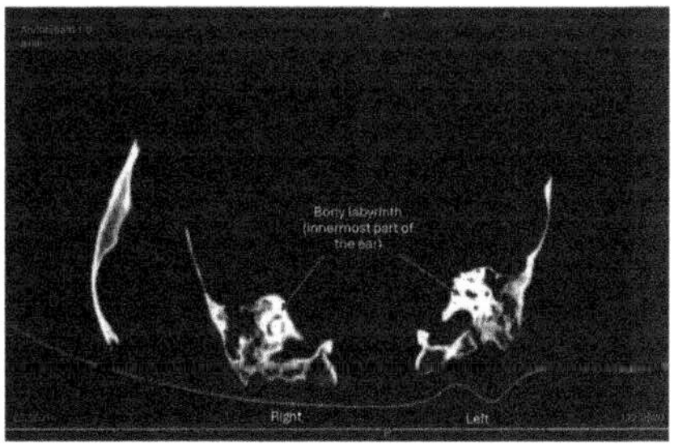

Figure 6.14B. CT image of the mastoid processes of the individual illustrated in Figure 6.14A showing partial sclerotic destruction of the mastoid air cells (white)—there is also some space between the mastoid air cells but some opacity. Courtesy of Cecilia Collins.

Endocranial Lesions

The presence of new bone formation on the endocranial surface of skulls from archaeological contexts has received much attention in recent years (Fig. 6.15). Hershkovitz et al. (2002, 202) published a key study that provoked debate about these endocranial lesions. They described endocranial bone changes as *serpens endocrania symmetrica*, "endocranial area(s) of discolored bone with variant color, texture, and a serpentine branching surface excavation." Examining skeletons from the Hamann-Todd documented collection (Cleveland Museum of Natural History, Ohio, US), they found thirty-two individuals affected, twenty-five of whom had TB listed as a cause of death. The authors suggested intrathoracic disease as a cause of the endocranial pathology, and specifically TB. Nonadult remains with endocranial lesions have been recorded in many locations across the globe and for a range of time periods. The lesions can occur on all the cranial bones and have been noted to follow the lines of venous drainage (Lewis 2018, 142–143).

The appearance of the new bone varies: inflammatory-related pitting; white or gray new bone; new bone organized around vascular structures; and "hair on end" bone formation (see Lewis 2018, 143). Disruption of venous drainage, meningeal inflammation, tumors, or ossified subdural hematomas are among the suggested causes. This is in addition to other suggestions from published research: chronic meningitis, scurvy, vitamin D deficiency, trauma, anemia, and lead poisoning, all potentially causing inflammation or hemorrhage of meningeal vessels. A nonpathological cause may be intimated too when studying infant remains because the skull is still rapidly developing, and new bone is being formed during the normal growth process. As Lewis (2018, 145) stated, the jury is still out about these lesions: "Until we can differentiate between new bone as the result of growth and deposits caused by pathology, we will be limited in our ability to trace infantile disease."

As noted, endocranial lesions have been suggested to represent inflammation of the meninges, or meningitis. Meningitis is a serious infection of the membrane

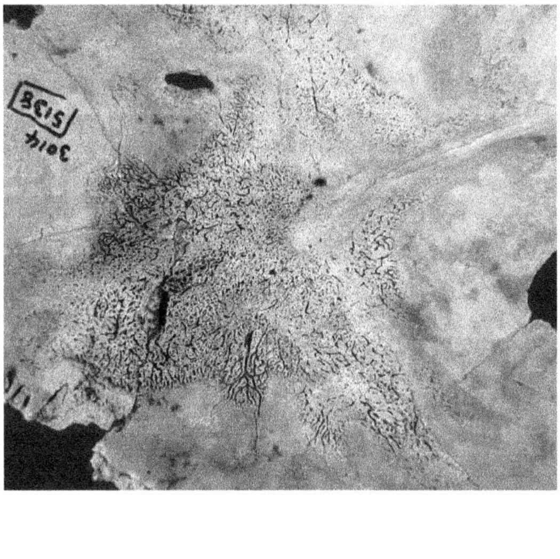

Figure 6.15. New bone formation on the endocranial surface of a nonadult cranium (eighth–tenth century CE, Raunds Furnells, Northamptonshire, England). Photograph by and courtesy of Jean Brown.

covering the brain and spinal cord (Jarman and Vivekananda 2021, 868). It is usually the result of a bacterial or viral infection, such as TB, but it may be caused by noninfectious conditions, such as a tumor. Microorganisms reach the meninges from infection in the ears and nasopharynx, as a result of a head injury, or through the bloodstream. Since the development of antibiotics in the mid-twentieth century, bacterial meningitis can be treated and cured, but this was not an option in the past. In paleopathological contexts, together with Hershkovitz et al. (2002), Schultz (2001) noted that endocranial reactive new bone can be divided histologically into bone formed as a result of hemorrhage (e.g., in a head injury) and as a result of inflammation (e.g., meningitis), but also a mixture of the two.

Even fewer researchers during the early 2000s used histological analyses of pathological lesions; consequently they recorded only new bone presence or absence, and hypothesized potential etiologies. Over time, new research tools have been used to develop our understanding of their etiology. For example, Eerkens et al. (2018) explored the etiology of endocranial lesions in an older female buried in the San Francisco Bay Area between 1250 and 1640 CE. High levels of *Neisseria meningitidis* and low levels of *H. influenzae* were detected in her dental calculus using next-generation DNA sequencing. They concluded that a diagnosis of meningococcal infection, including meningitis, could have been the cause (on next-generation sequencing see Satam et al. 2023). In 2019, Sun et al. recorded that 25.8% of nonadults (*n* = 8/31) from three Neolithic sites in Henan province, China (2448–1700 BCE), had endocranial lesions. They suggested dietary deficiency, lung disease (e.g., TB), and traumatic injury (e.g., "shaken baby syndrome") as potential etiologies, but they concluded that scurvy was the most probable cause due to other bone changes consistent with this condition. Wysocka and Cieślik's (2023) research on individuals buried in Wroclaw, Poland, during the sixteenth–nineteenth centuries used an endoscope to examine the endocranial surface of 144 adults. In around 50% of crania, abnormal endocranial blood vessel impressions and new bone formation were present. Here, meningeal infection and/or hemorrhage were suggested as etiologies. Importantly, they emphasized the use of endoscopic examination for identifying endocranial lesions in well-preserved crania.

Clearly, multiple lines of evidence relying on a range of appropriate methods should be the aim of future work on endocranial lesions. Paleodemographic information and detailed recording of all pathological lesions, along with data on potential contextual factors, are important for exploring what risk factors for these lesions were most important—for example, biological sex, age at death, ancestry, diet, the environments in which people lived (inside or outside; rural or urban), occupations (such as hunting and foraging, pastoralism, farming), and ecological variables such as climate and weather patterns that may promote the presence of particular pathogens.

Soft Tissue Infections

The majority of infectious diseases in the past did not affect the skeleton, as we have already noted, and this makes identification impossible without the aid of more advanced analytical techniques such as aDNA analysis, reference to contemporaneous medical historical documents, or the examination of the soft tissue of preserved bodies. Sadly, as this book is focused on skeletal evidence for disease, we have little space to discuss preserved or mummified remains but refer the reader to other excellent sources (e.g., Aufderheide 2003; Lynnerup 2019; Nystrom et al. 2023; Wilson et al. 2023). That said, some soft tissue infections have been detected in skeletons, such as plague (bacterial; Kacki et al. 2011), smallpox (viral; Crawford et al. 2024), and malaria (parasitic; Smith-Guzmán 2015; Mbouaka et al. 2021).

One of the most devastating of these soft tissue infections in the past was plague, a zoonotic disease found in small mammals (e.g., rodents) and their fleas, which is now treatable with antibiotics. The Democratic Republic of the Congo, Madagascar, and Peru are the three most endemic countries today, but people are at risk anywhere that humans, the bacteria, an animal reservoir, and a vector coexist (WHO 2022c). Plague spreads not only between animals, but also from animals to humans, via the flea vector, which for rodents is *Xenopsylla cheopsis*. There are three main manifestations of this infection: (1) bubonic, which is most common and scientifically linked to the first (sixth–eighth centuries CE) and second (fourteenth century CE) pandemics; (2) pneumonic, which is the most severe and can spread human to human through bacteria-laden droplets; and (3) septicemic, spread via the bloodstream. A very rare fourth form can also affect the pharynx and gastrointestinal tract (WHO 2022a). The pneumonic and septicemic forms are the most virulent and can be rapidly fatal if not diagnosed and treated quickly.

Recent genomic research has indicated that plague was affecting people in Britain 4,000 years ago, much earlier than we had imagined (Swali et al. 2023). Historical sources describe several dreadful epidemics, called plagues, such as the Plague of Athens (Thucydides fifth century BCE) and the Antonine plague (Galen second century CE), although the symptoms suggest causes other than *Yersinia pestis*, such as smallpox, and are as yet unidentified (see a review of the plague and responses to it by Varlik 2017). Traditionally the first pandemic, now reliably considered to have been plague, and for which we have several written sources (e.g., Procopius sixth century CE) is called the Justinian plague, which affected the Mediterranean regions and probably arrived via travelers and traders from the east; it lasted from around 541 to 750 CE (Barbieri et al. 2021; Cilliers 2019, 79–95). Baten et al. (2019, 389) suggested that this outbreak was probably more severe than the plague epidemics of fourteenth-century Europe, although many historians have attempted to challenge its importance (Sarris 2022). While little is known about this early pandemic, improvements in health following its appearance have been noted in skeletons from the time, perhaps due to a smaller population, better labor conditions, higher wages, and generally more equality (Baten et al. 2019).

The second plague pandemic began in the fourteenth century CE, encompassing an initial outbreak of a "pestilence" (ca. 1347–1351 CE) that much later came to be called the Black Death; it lasted with a series of outbreaks until the early eighteenth century (Stone and Ozaga 2019). The previously recorded array of symptoms and extreme mortality prompted cities to keep statistics and enact laws, including the earliest forms of quarantine, and numerous contemporary physicians wrote treatises about its course, nature, and treatment (Jones 2022; Jones and Varlık 2022). This wealth of sources inspires many scholars, and the histories that they generated have themselves become a source of historical interest (e.g., Getz 1991; Varlık 2017; Eisenberg and Mordechai 2020; Martin 2023). Bos and DeWitte (2022) discussed the origin of the name Black Death, and on the basis of relevant research, its appearance in Europe followed decades of declining population health and several smaller outbreaks of the disease as it spread westward. Genetic evidence and textual records of buboes suggests the disease originated in East or Central Asia perhaps as early as the thirteenth century (Hymes and Green 2002; Spyrou et al. 2022). Carried by rats (and their fleas), it may have arrived in Europe in grain imported from Tana on the Sea of Avov, which sits between Ukraine and Russia today (Green 2020; Spyrou et al. 2022). Between a third and two-thirds of the European population were killed, with devastating consequences for those left behind.

An essential first step in studying plague's impacts on its victims is establishing a precise date for any fourteenth-century burial site such as a plague cemetery, using accepted dating methods and exploring extant historical documentation. For example, the historically documented Black Death cemetery called the Royal Mint, situated in East Smithfield, London, has been and continues to be a focus for many researchers since its excavation in the 1980s.

The modern genome sequence of *Y. pestis* was first published by Parkhill et al. in 2001, but prior to this, Drancourt et al. (1998) had detected aDNA in dental pulp in individuals buried in sixteenth- and eighteenth-century graves in France. Since then, paleopathological research has focused on identifying the ancient *Y. pestis* genome in archaeological skeletons (Bos et al. 2011). Rasmussen et al. (2015) provided the oldest direct evidence of *Y. pestis* from Asia and Europe (2,800 to 5,000 BP). By sequencing the genomes, they found that these ancient plague strains are basal to all known *Y. pestis* bacteria.

Harbeck and Seifert (2013) detected *Y. pestis* aDNA in skeletons from Aschheim, Upper Bavaria, Germany (sixth century CE). These data confirmed it was responsible for plague in people buried at this site, the dating being consistent with the Justinian plague. Keller et al. (2019) provide further genetic evidence for the first pandemic across western Europe. Eaton et al. (2023) tracked plague's epidemiology with genomic and phylogenetic analysis of 298 skeletons from thirteen archaeological sites in Denmark (1000–1800 CE), finding *Y. pestis* originating from different European countries in a mean of 8.3% of them (range 3.3–14.3%). Finally, immunological evidence for the Black Death (*Y. pestis* F1 antigen) was reported for three fourteenth-century individuals from a rural eighth–fourteenth century CE cemetery in southern France (Kacki et al. 2011).

Biomolecular analysis has greatly advanced our understanding of the plagues and compensates for the lack of macroscopic evidence. However, there are alternative ways of exploring this infection without the use of aDNA analysis, depending on what questions are being asked. Probably the most relied upon bioarchaeological evidence for interpreting the impact of plague on past populations is demographic: considering differences between the health profiles of known plague and nonplague victims, or whether the bacteria targeted specific age and biological sex groups more than others (e.g., Margerison and Knüsel 1997; Gowland and Chamberlain 2005; DeWitte 2009, 2010, 2015, 2018; Curtis and Roosen 2017; Godde et al. 2020; DeWitte and Hughes-Morey 2021). Naturally, using a combination of evidence from different sources is essential; of course, without the archaeological excavation of skeletons and their study by paleopathologists, there would be no resulting pathogen aDNA evidence.

Specific Infections of the Skeleton

Specific infections are those for which it is possible to identify the exact causative organism (or pathogen). Three such infections have afflicted populations through long periods of our history. They are tuberculosis, leprosy, and the treponemal diseases. These diseases produce similar changes to the skeleton; for example, involvement of the lower leg bones occurs in all three, and facial lesions are seen in both leprosy and venereal syphilis. It is therefore important to consider the nature of the presenting bone lesions and their distribution, as ever in paleopathology. All three diseases increased through time until the advent of chemotherapy in the twentieth century, but patterns of rise and decline in low-, middle-, and high-income countries today vary considerably, relating to inequalities that compromise immunity, including poverty, challenging living conditions, undernutrition, and lack of access to health services. People with these infections were and still can be subject to stigma and marginalization, depending on the region of the world. For example, Zuckerman (2017) examined stigma related to acquired syphilis in post-medieval London, England; and efforts continue to destigmatize leprosy, for which colonies still persist throughout the world (Abdul Rahman et al. 2022).

Tuberculosis (TB)

The Here and Now of TB

Not so long ago, Smith wrote, "tuberculosis is now a conquered disease in the British Isles and the rest of the industrialized world" (1988, 2), but this infectious disease remains with the world today. The World Health Organization (2022b) describes TB as a reemerging infection in high-income countries and as a neglected tropical disease in middle- and low-income countries. It can be prevented and is usually curable. In 1882, the German bacteriologist Robert Koch discovered the bacillus responsible for TB, *Mycobacterium tuberculosis*. Now TB is known to be caused by various bacteria within the *Mycobacterium tuberculosis* complex (MTBC), which contains organisms adapted to both humans (e.g., *M. tuberculosis* and *africanum*) and animals (e.g., *M. bovis, caprae, microti,* and *pinnipedii*) (Brosch et al. 2002). Genomic analyses of *M. tuberculosis* strains in recent years reveal that they can be grouped into eight lineages that primarily affect humans; each lineage indicates direct descent from a common ancestor. The current diversity of animal-adapted strains came from a human strain (Roberts et al. 2022a).

M. tuberculosis is the leading cause of TB in humans. The bacilli spread from human to human when an infected person coughs and another person inhales

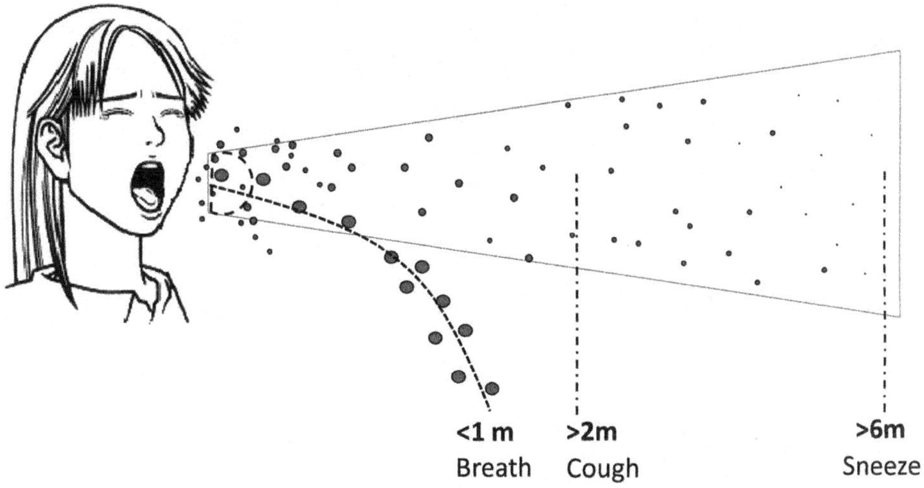

Figure 6.16. The distance exhaled droplets may travel. Adapted by Mary Lewis from Katre et al. 2021.

droplets containing the bacteria (Fig. 6.16). Whatever its source and whatever its evolutionary pathway, the tubercle bacillus has created chronic, endemic, and widespread suffering in human populations throughout time. It was estimated that in 2022, 10.6 million individuals contracted TB, and it killed 1.3 million, a leading killer of all infectious diseases that year and second only to COVID-19 (WHO 2022a). One of the health targets of the United Nations Sustainable Development Goals is to end TB by 2030. Prevention through vaccination, and treatment with a combination of antibiotics, are the mainstays for its management, but variable vaccine efficacy across the globe (BCG: Bacillus Calmette–Guérin) and drug resistance are continuing challenges that hamper the pledge to end TB.

Among many, the main underlying risk factors responsible for its reemergence in humans are HIV/AIDs, poverty, living in urban environments, antibiotic resistance, travel, and migration, often from war-torn areas of the world. The presence of HIV and poverty weakens the immune system and makes people more susceptible to TB, while leisure and business travel, and flight from conflict or ecological disasters, may expose people to the infection in a new location. Aggravating the problem, displaced people and those living in poverty lack access to health care facilities. Smoking tobacco, consuming infected food products such as meat, cheese, and milk, being imprisoned, and working in health care are also risk factors. Furthermore, concurrent HIV, diabetes, particulate pollution, and vitamin D deficiency can trigger an asymptomatic latent or primary infection to progress and become advanced TB (Theron et al. 2021).

Because so many species of animals can contract TB, people who work with animals are also at risk: for example, tanners, veterinary surgeons, butchers, zookeepers, and farmers/pastoralists (Fig. 6.17). Furthermore, as a result of increased travel for leisure purposes, people may be exposed to infected animals and their products. Living in poverty and having contact with infected animals probably contributed most to TB's

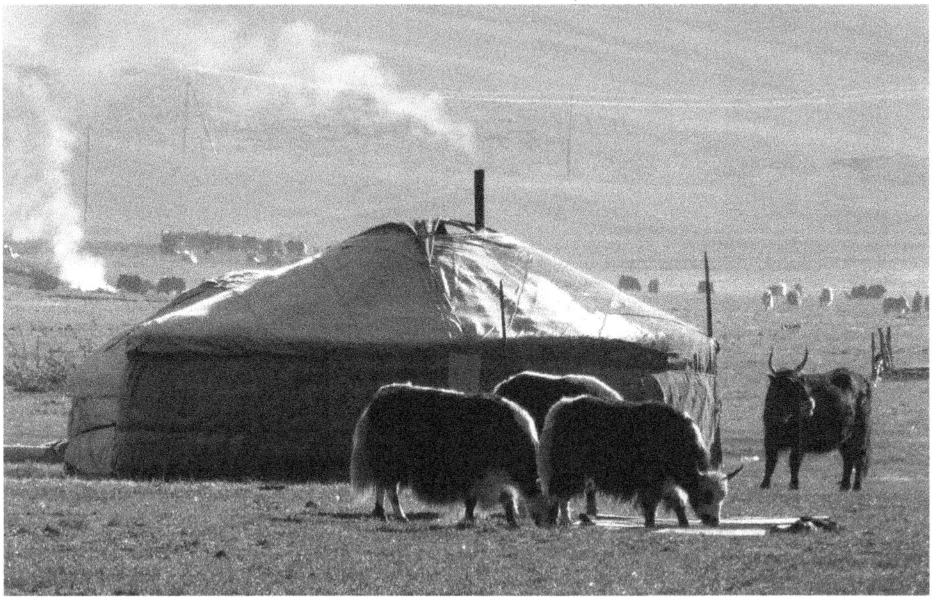

Figure 6.17. Exposure to animals. Yaks can be affected by TB, and in Mongolia they are used for carrying loads, for milk production, and for their meat, hides, and fur. Photography by Charlotte Roberts.

occurrence in past populations. Indeed, it has been found that there are a range of sources that can harbor the mycobacterium in a range of locations, such as soils, water, grazing areas, and in animal excreta (H. Zhang et al. 2022b), and it can survive for months to years outside the body (Martinez et al. 2019). Infected animal dung used for fuel and externally applied to buildings are also risk factors. Symptoms of TB include a prolonged cough (sometimes with blood), shortness of breath, chest pain, weakness, fatigue, weight loss, undulating fever, and night sweats.

Lactose intolerance may also have played a role in animal-to-human transmission. If a person in the ancient past did not have the lactase persistence (LP) gene and experienced symptoms of lactose intolerance (e.g., nausea, vomiting, stomach cramps, diarrhea, and bloating), they may have chosen not to eat dairy products. Therefore, their risk of contracting TB from infected animals would be reduced compared to others (although eating infected meat can also transmit TB). Around 35% of people in the world today have the LP gene (Itan et al. 2010), and its frequency varies from as low as 15% in eastern and southern Europe to above 90% in northern Europe (Gerbault et al. 2011). Combining genetic and archaeological information about LP helps in exploring its origin and evolution (Evershed et al. 2022) and its relevance to TB infection.

The There and Then of TB

Early historical evidence for TB in the lymph glands of the neck dates back to 1550 BCE in the Egyptian Ebers medical papyrus where several "growths in the neck" and their treatments were discussed (Bryan 1974, 142–145; Evans 1998). The classic medical text of *Huangdi Neijing* in China, dated to 2700 BCE, describes a wasting disease suggestive of phthisis (another name for TB), as does the Rig Veda, a Sanskrit hymn of India dated to 1500 BCE (Agarwal et al. 2017). More frequent references to TB appear in classical antiquity from the fifth century BCE—for example, in Hippocratic writings, and later Arabian writers Rhazes and Avicenna (ninth–tenth century CE). With the passage of time, references to TB in writings, drawings, and paintings proliferated. Historical data potentially provide more evidence for TB than is seen in the skeletal record, although it can be difficult to be sure that TB as we know it was being described or illustrated.

A disease of considerable antiquity, the incidence of TB increased over time in places like England. For example, the seventeenth- and eighteenth-century London Bills of Mortality recorded consumption and "tissick" (both believed to be TB) as key causes of death. By modern standards, diagnostic accuracy at this time was probably poor. Even within the "consumption" category, other lung diseases, such as bronchitis, pneumonia, or cancer, could have been included in these records (Robb et al. 2021). The signs and symptoms of breathlessness, coughing up blood, and other respiratory problems would have made diagnosis a challenge without the aid of modern medicine. The "royal touch" and the provision of a "gold angel" or "touch-piece" (a gold coin) was a practice conducted in England and France from the fifteenth through seventeenth centuries, and was mentioned in Shakespeare's *Macbeth*. Possibly originating in the reign of Edward the Confessor (1003–1066 CE), the last Anglo-Saxon king (Krugman and Chorber 2022), this practice of the monarch touching individuals afflicted with various diseases was continued by later royalty in both France and England. It focused on scrofula, or lymphadenitis, a condition of the cervical (neck) lymph nodes often associated with TB. Because of this, TB was also nicknamed the King's Evil (Fig. 6.18). The large number of people touched in the late medieval and postmedieval periods may attest to the extent of the problem, but again whether they all had TB is debatable. Charles II (1660–85 CE) is said to have touched 92,102 people in his reign, and the seventeenth century saw the highest popularity of the practice (Evans 1998). Elizabeth I (1558–1603 CE) ordered that the weight of the gold touch-piece should be reduced, and by the early nineteenth century, the practice had waned. Many people who wanted it no longer received touch-pieces because of cost.

From the mid-nineteenth century to the mid-twentieth century, people with TB were isolated in sanatoria to recuperate (Martini et al. 2018). First appearing in 1854 Germany (Görbersdorf, Silesia—now Sokołowsko, Poland), sanatoria were often situated at high altitude or on the coast, respectively for pulmonary and bone TB. They provided a place to rest, eat nutritious food, breathe fresh air, and gradually regain strength. Sanatoria were also established in other parts of the world—for example, in 1884 at Saranac Lake in modern-day New York state (Gallos 1985)—and sanatoria appeared across Canada's coastal regions, prairies, and mountains (Figs. 6.19 and 6.20). Indigenous people in North America suffered and still suffer more than others from TB, and discriminatory measures are used to control it (Lux 2016; Zwick and Pepperell 2020).

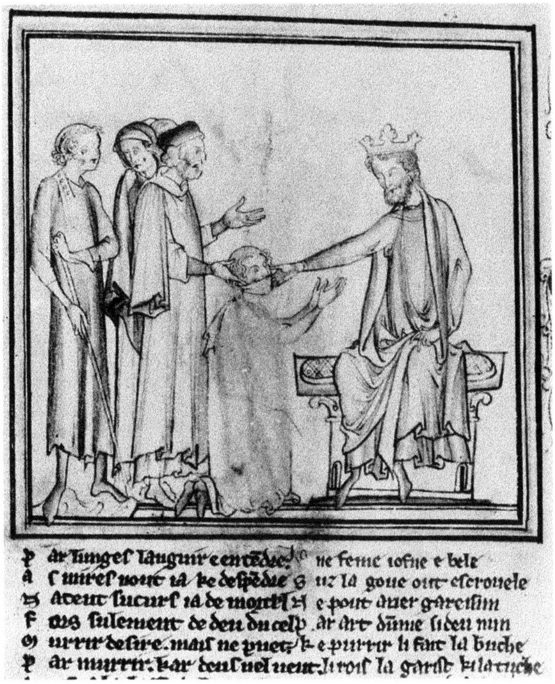

Figure 6.18. Edward the Confessor touching for the King's Evil. Note the person is wearing a mask. Is this early evidence of this practice in prevention of spread of disease? Reproduced with permission from the Wellcome Collection, London.

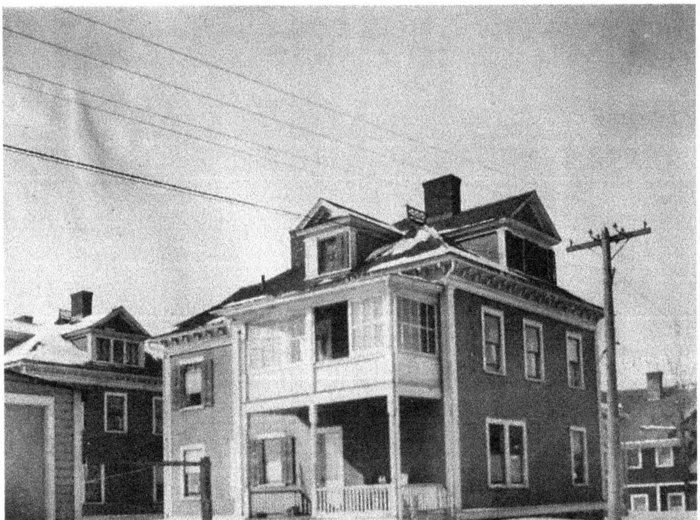

Figure 6.19. Saranac Lake, New York state: the United States' first tuberculosis sanatorium, built in the 1920s. View of Alta Vista Lodge, 48 Franklin Avenue, with "sleeping out" cure porch above the first-floor veranda. Historic Saranac Lake Collection, 2020.2.1.2. Gift of John and Cece Durbin.

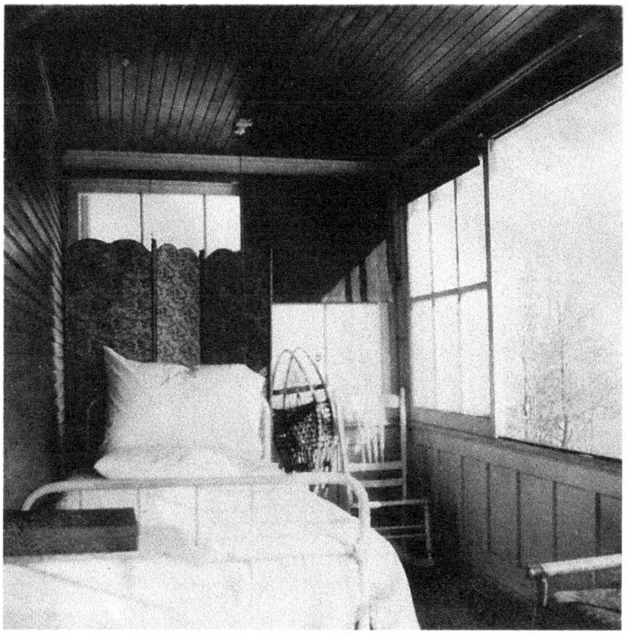

Figure 6.20. Saranac Lake, New York state. The interior of the "sleeping out" porch at Alta Vista Lodge. Historic Saranac Lake Collection, 2020.2.1.8. Gift of John and Cece Durbin.

Hunter-foragers who preceded farmers were likely exposed to TB from wild animals, although there are few reports of TB in skeletons of these populations (e.g., Guichón et al. 2015; Dutour 2023b). During the first epidemiological transition, people in different parts of the world began to settle in larger groups to produce their own food and to domesticate animals and plants (Barker and Goucher 2015). Therefore, population numbers and density increased, alongside mingling with animals. These living conditions enabled TB bacteria to spread between humans and from animals to humans (e.g. see Taylor et al. 2007). The first introduction of any new infection into a human population usually produces severe disease. To what extent this premise applied in TB is not known. If the premise is correct, then the earliest TB infections should have been acute and quickly fatal. The bone changes indicative of long-standing chronic disease would have been unlikely until later generations had developed some immunity, and the infection became less virulent. Therefore, the evidence from that time (e.g., the Neolithic) may not have survived in skeletal remains, although biomolecular analysis can detect infections that are invisible to the naked eye. Wolfe et al. (2007, 280) suggested: "If a disease is acute, efficiently transmitted, and quickly leaves its victim either dead or else recovering and immune to re-infection, the epidemic soon exhausts the local pool of susceptible potential victims, especially if the pool is small."

Infection of the Human Body with TB

TB infects people in three forms: primary/latent, secondary, and miliary. It is usually contracted in children who have never been exposed to TB before. Primary TB is asymptomatic and, whether it progresses or not, the original site in the lung may become inactive and remain as a Ghon focus, detectable radiographically (Stephenson and Byard 2020). Secondary TB occurs when a latent infection in a person is reactivated (perhaps because the immune system has become depressed), or the person is infected again with another dose of tubercle bacilli. It is in the secondary form that skeletal changes occur. Tuberculosis spreads to the bone from its original site of entry via the bloodstream and lymphatic system. The pathological changes of TB occur in several areas and organs of the body, determined, to some extent, by the type of infecting bacillus and its portal of entry. For example, pulmonary TB is the common mode of infection by the human-type bacillus, and the stomach and intestinal tract are the sites common to the bovine type. Bovine infection (i.e., gastrointestinal TB) is more common in children than in adults, a fact possibly relating to the consumption of milk in infancy (Atkins 1992). It should also be noted that bovine TB can be transmitted between humans via droplet infection (Lombard et al. 2021).

Skeletal TB

The skeletal features of TB are primarily osteomyelitis of the spine (Fig. 6.21). The hip and knee joints are the next most commonly affected areas, and particularly in non-adult individuals. This results from spread of the infection through the bloodstream to the joint, or spread from an adjacent TB lesion in a bone (Resnick et al. 2024, 437–439). This osteomyelitic process occurs at the ends of long bones and frequently affects the joint surfaces themselves (Figs. 6.22a and b), producing septic arthritis (see also Chapter 5). Characteristic destruction of the joint surface occurs, progressing ultimately to fibrous fixation (ankylosis) of the joint. A diagnosis of TB made on such evidence is usually tentative and may be confused with the other causes of osteomyelitis and joint disease. Unlike degenerative joint disease, TB involvement is usually of one joint, and the destructive process is more marked than the repair process. In the context of paleopathology, most diagnoses of TB are made on the presence of lesions of the spine consistent with the infection.

In the pre-antibiotic era of the 1940s and 1950s, skeletal damage occurred in 3–5% of all people with TB, and in around 30% of those with extrapulmonary TB (Jaffe 1972). This rate may be much higher, perhaps up to 12%, for children

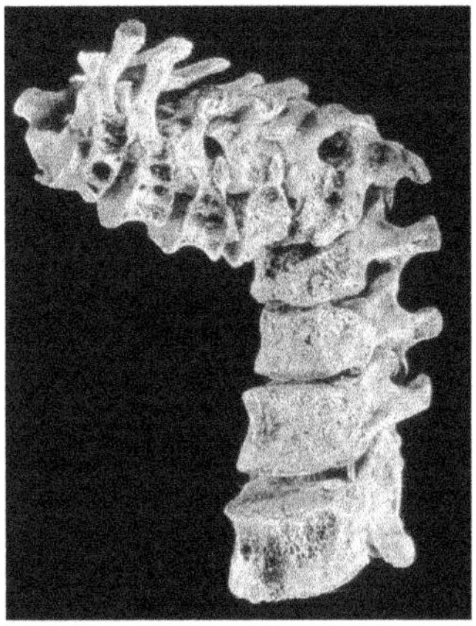

Figure 6.21. Spinal tuberculosis affecting several vertebral bodies of a 16-year-old male who died from enteric tuberculosis (lateral view). C7-T8 affected. Note the kyphotic deformity caused by total destruction of T7. Photograph courtesy of Ana Luisa Santos and the Department of Life Sciences, University of Coimbra. Coimbra Identified Skeletal Collection, Portugal.

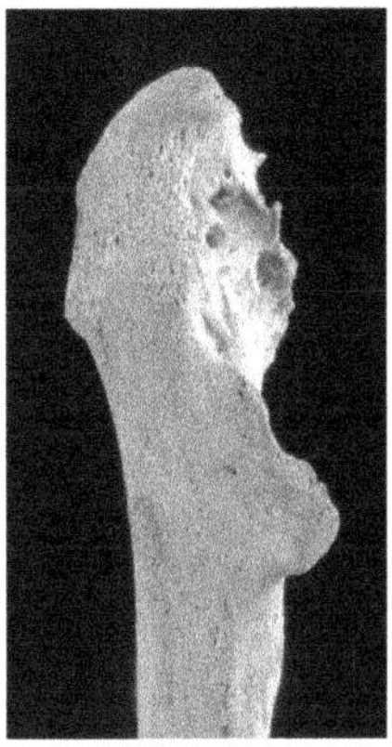

Figure 6.22A. Tuberculosis of the left femur affecting a 27-year-old female who died from pulmonary TB; posterior aspect showing destruction of the neck with healing. The femoral head had become detached but was present and partially eroded. Photograph courtesy of Ana Luisa Santos and the Department of Life Sciences, University of Coimbra. Coimbra Identified Skeletal Collection, Portugal.

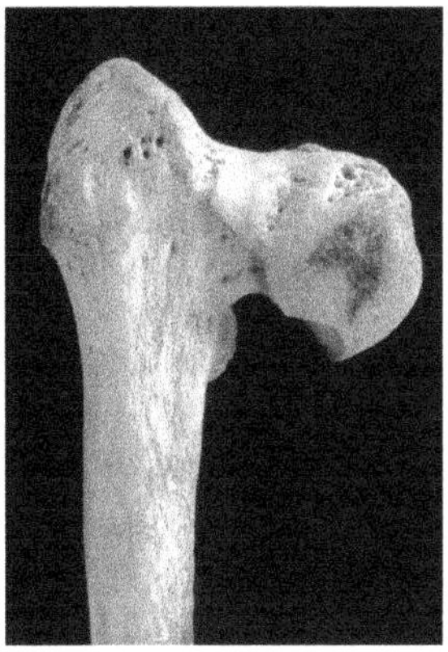

Figure 6.22B. Anterior right femur showing a reduced head–neck angle. The skeleton of this female also displayed rib lesions and spinal TB. Because of the loss of the left femur head, this could have strained the right hip, and caused the consequent head-neck angle. Photograph courtesy of Ana Luisa Santos and the Department of Life Sciences, University of Coimbra. Coimbra Identified Skeletal Collection, Portugal.

(Bernard 2003). Any bone of the body can be affected, but the spine is involved in 25–60% of all skeletal TB (Jaffe 1972). The damage to the spine usually involves between 1 and 4 lower thoracic and upper lumbar vertebrae. Abscess formation within the vertebral body occurs (osteomyelitis), which may perforate into the chest or abdomen, with subsequent collapse and bony fixation of several vertebral bodies of the spine. A characteristic feature of spinal TB (tuberculous spondylitis) is the early destruction of the disks between the individual vertebrae, and the relative sparing of the neural arch (the most posterior part of a vertebra). Paleopathologists should always consider other diseases that cause spinal collapse in their differential diagnosis, such as trauma, osteoporosis, and tumors (see Roberts and Buikstra 2003, 96).

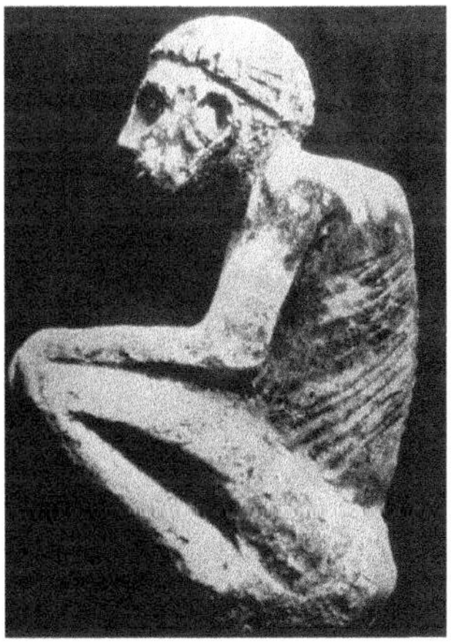

Figure 6.23. Possible TB shown in the spine of this Egyptian statuette found in a clay bowl (height 20 cm); supposed predynastic (4500–3000 BCE); spinal angulation and excessive weight loss may represent advanced tuberculosis. From Morse et al. 1964, 525.

The spinal features of TB are known as Pott's disease after Percivall Pott, a surgeon at St. Bartholomew's Hospital, London, who described the condition in 1779 (Payne 2017, 143–144). The spinal collapse results in angular deformity of the spine and is frequently portrayed by authors and artists (Fig. 6.23), although due to the number of diseases that can also cause spinal collapse, not all of these historic portrayals may have been tuberculous. Spinal TB may be complicated by an abscess penetrating the sheath of the psoas muscle at its attachment to the anterior surface of the infected vertebral body, and by spread of the infection posteriorly into the spinal canal. This latter process can cause compression of the spinal cord and associated nerves, with resultant damage and dysfunction of motor, sensory, and autonomic nerves. Weakness, numbness, paralysis of the lower limbs, and an unsteady gait, with loss of urinary control, may be sequelae of spinal TB (Leowattana et al. 2023). Botha et al. (2024) used data mining and machine learning (decision tree analysis) to help recognize TB in skeletal remains and explore patterns of skeletal involvement, but dramatic bone change does not happen overnight, and we should consider the possibility of identifying TB spinal infection in its early stages before collapse and kyphosis. Baker (1999) described destructive lesions in the vertebral bodies of three individuals, which were suggested to be early evidence of TB. Referred to as "multiple circumferential resorptive pits," they occurred on the anterior aspects of the thoracic and lumbar vertebral bodies; they have also been described as normal vascular foramina (Mariotti et al. 2015). All three individuals had periosteal new bone on some ribs (see below). Subsequent work successfully extracted aDNA of the *M. tuberculosis* complex from skeletons with these lesions (Haas et al. 2000). However, correlation does not mean causation, even if other corroborating evidence is seen in the skeleton. These destructive lesions could be remnant holes of development that eventually remodel as the child ages, but persistence of these resorptive pits into older adulthood could indicate a pathological cause, possibly TB.

Notwithstanding the challenges of interpreting these lesions, more researchers are now recording their presence in both documented and undocumented individuals (e.g., Spekker et al. 2018). In addition, Pedersen et al. (2019) selected eighteen indicators that are considered conventional and unconventional for TB in paleopathology, based on radiographic images and autopsies, modern reference samples, the paleopathological literature, and the authors' experience. They recorded these pits in twentieth-century skeletons from the Robert J. Terry Collection, Washington, DC (with TB as known cause of death) and control skeletons from the William M. Bass Donated Collection, Tennessee. They tested sensitivity and specificity of each lesion and found that resorption pits on the ventral aspect of the lumbar vertebrae occurred more often in the TB group. Masiu et al. (2023), who studied the skeletons of individuals who died of TB or other causes before 1950 in the Raymond Dart Collection, South Africa, reported the same result. We remain of the opinion that these lesions are nonspecific indicators of TB until we can be sure of differentiating pits caused by normal variation. Steyn et al.'s (2013) related research on documented individuals from collections in South Africa who died from TB from the Pretoria Bone (University of Pretoria) and Raymond A Dart (University of the Witwatersrand) Collections included three study groups: (1) people who died before 1950 (assumed no antibiotic intervention); (2) people who died between 1950 and 1985 (assumed treated with antibiotics); and (3) people who died after 1985 (when co-infection with HIV and drug-resistant TB emerged). The overall frequency of skeletal lesions had changed over time, and in the post-antibiotic era skeletal involvement became more frequent, with rib lesions rising and spinal lesions decreasing. Although documented skeletal collections tend to be of people who died prior to antibiotic use, and are thus extremely helpful in understanding infectious diseases, documented causes of death data may not always be accurate.

Nonspecific Indicators of TB

Other skeletal lesions may be considered indicative. Although they are not diagnostic, they are typical of TB (Appleby et al. 2015) and deserve discussion, although to a certain extent they remain controversial even as we write this fourth edition. Many of the studies discussed in this section have suggested aDNA analysis to confirm the association of these nonspecific lesions with tuberculosis. However, as already mentioned, aDNA cannot definitively prove the association of nonspecific evidence to a specific disease. Therefore, details are important when reporting primary skeletal evidence for TB (spine) together with possible (nonspecific) evidence, such as subperiosteal new bone formation on ribs, porosity, endocranial lesions, and hypertrophic pulmonary osteoarthropathy, reviewed here.

Beginning in the 1980s, researchers considered subperiosteal new bone formation on the visceral surfaces of ribs an indicator of pulmonary infection (Kelley and Micozzi 1984; Molto 1990; Pfeiffer 1991; Wakely et al. 1991; Kelley et al. 1994; Roberts et al. 1994; Sledzik and Bellantoni 1994; Roberts 1999; Lambert 2002; Santos and Roberts 2001, 2006; Matos and Santos 2006; Steyn et al. 2013; Mariotti et al. 2015; Davies-Barrett et al. 2019, 2023). This includes the pulmonary infection caused by TB, although these lesions may have a distinct pattern (Fig. 6.24). Santos and Roberts (2006) noted that individuals who died of TB had new bone on the vertebral ends of their ribs, particularly between the fourth and eighth ribs. Notably, in the clinical literature, TB is described as causing destructive lesions of the ribs, with very few exceptions; for example, Eyler et al. (1994) identified enlarged ribs radiologically, presumably because of new bone formation on them. Despite these promising examples, a histomorphological study of rib lesions carried out by Assis and Keenleyside (2019) on individuals with a known cause of death, including TB, from the Luis Lopes Documented Collection, Lisbon, Portugal, found no histological features to distinguish different causes of death. However, they did note that the

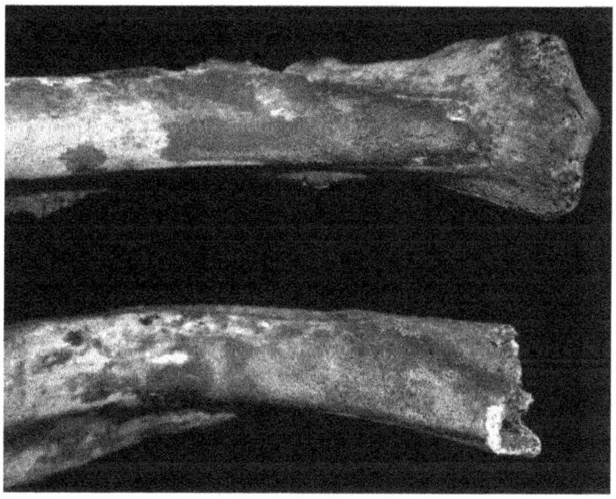

Figure 6.24. New bone formation on the visceral surfaces of two ribs; in a possible male adult from 1626–1866 CE Arnhem, The Netherlands. Photograph with kind permission from Gemeente Arnhem and Martijn Defilet (Senior bestuursadviseur Erfgoed en Archeologie).

microarchitecture of rib lesions was related to the speed of progression and duration of the bone change. Just as for the potential early stage vertebral lesions, making a direct link between visceral rib lesions and TB is challenging, even with aDNA analysis.

However, use of documented collections can offer new insights into pathological lesions on skeletal remains, and new lesions that may be related to TB continue to emerge. For example, using portable X-ray fluorescence, Gomes et al. (2022; 2024) considered the relationship between respiratory disease as a cause of death and porous skeletal lesions (i.e., cribra orbitalia, cribra femoralis, and cribra humeralis) in individuals from nineteenth–twentieth-century Coimbra, Portugal. They found a higher prevalence of cribra orbitalia in individuals known to have died of respiratory infection, especially TB. As pathogens require iron to survive and replicate in the body, and cribra orbitalia is caused by iron deficiency, this correlation may reflect the body's attempt to deny iron to the invading bacteria (Stuart-Macadam 1992).

Endocranial changes, including new bone formation, as a response to tuberculous-induced meningitis, has also been suggested (Schultz 2001), but prolonged survival from this disease in the pre-antibiotic era was improbable. If a person did survive meningitis caused by TB, could they have endured their illness long enough for bone change to occur? If they did survive, were they infected by a less virulent organism? In addition to new bone formation, granular impressions (i.e., not the normally occurring arachnoid granulations) on the endocranial surface of non-adult skulls have been posited to be the result of TB (Schultz 2001). Several studies have focused on these endocranial lesions and TB in archaeological contexts, including in a 9,000-year-old individual from Israel (Hershkovitz et al. 2008) and a Middle Paleolithic *Homo erectus* cranium from Türkiye (Kappelman et al. 2008; see also Roberts et al. 2009); however, to confirm the lesions as tuberculous was not possible. More recently, Abegg et al. (2022) explored the significance of endocranial lesions in skeletons from thirteen Neolithic sites in Switzerland using macroscopic and microscopic analysis; four individuals displayed the bone changes. These individuals all had TB-related lesions on the spine, ribs, and long bones, but aDNA analysis was recommended to confirm the diagnosis.

To address the validity of these lesions as indicators of tuberculous meningitis, Spekker et al. (2020a and b) revealed that granular impressions were significantly more common in individuals from the Terry Collection who died of TB between 1848–1941 CE, than in those who died of non-TB causes. They also considered other endocranial lesions, such as new bone formation and vascular impressions, again finding a correlation between these lesions and people who died of TB. While their research has confirmed previous studies that these lesions might not be pathognomonic of TB, they are helpful when considering a potential diagnosis. Research making use of documented skeletal collections has moved the debate considerably and contributes to developing differential diagnoses of archaeological skeletons.

The bone changes of secondary hypertrophic osteoarthropathy (HPOA) as an indicator of TB have also been studied in paleopathology. New bone formation as a response to pulmonary conditions, including TB, can occur primarily in the long bones (Resnick et al. 2024, 1064–1065). Some work identifying this condition in skeletons with known causes of death has been done (e.g., Assis et al. 2011), and evidence from skeletal remains is increasing (e.g., Anselmo et al. 2016; Binder and Saad 2017).

Paleopathological Evidence for TB

The paleopathological evidence for TB has been extensively reviewed in the literature (Roberts and Buikstra 2003; 2019; Roberts et al. 2022a). Table 6.1 provides a summary of the earliest evidence for TB, accompanied by some more recent studies. Evidence increases over time and becomes more common in historical periods of Europe, such as the late medieval period. Skeletal evidence suggests that TB became a challenge for humans in South America from 700 CE, with examples in human remains found in Chile, but also in Colombia, Peru, and Venezuela, and the earliest derives from the Atacama desert in northern Chile (Allison et al. 1981). Camelids (e.g., llamas) may have been a source of the infection, while the higher frequency in males at some sites suggests that llama herding may have been a male occupation and risk factor. Humans in Peru also contracted TB from sea mammals that they hunted and ate (Bos et al. 2014). One-thousand-year-old mycobacterial genomes revealed that people were affected by a strain of TB most closely related to those adapted to seals and sea lions. The few data from Central America, mostly from its western side, could be a result of trade between South and North America via Central America. More data

Table 6.1 Some of the earliest skeletal evidence for tuberculosis in modern day countries

Place	Date	Source
Israel	9,250–8,160 years ago	Hershkovitz et al. (2008)
Hungary	7,000 years ago	Masson et al. (2013)
Poland	7,000 years ago	Gladykowska-Rzeczyka (1999)
Italy	6,500 years ago	Sparacello et al. (2017)
Germany	6,450–6,775 years ago	Nicklish et al. (2012)
Jordan	5,150–4,200 years ago	Ortner (1979)
Africa, Egypt	6,500 years ago	Morse et al. (1964)
Africa	5,500–500 years ago	Zink et al. (2007)
China, Shanghai	3900–3200 BCE	Okazaki et al. (2019)
China, Shaanxi	202 BCE–220 CE	Li et al. (2019)
Siberia	Fourth century BCE–fourth century CE	Murphy et al. (2009)
Japan	454 BCE–124 CE	Suzuki and Inoue (2007)
Korea	First century BCE	Suzuki et al. (2008)
Thailand	300 BCE–200 CE	Tayles and Buckley (2004)
Chile, South America	700 CE	Allison et al. (1981)
Argentina, South America	905–1030 CE	Luna et al. (2020)
Papua New Guinea and Hawaii	Precontact and eighteenth century CE	Pietreuwsky and Douglas (1994)

after 1000 CE derives from both the eastern and southwest parts of North America. Thereafter, the infection rose in North America as population density increased. Beyond Europe and the Americas, evidence is growing. Archaeological evidence for TB has been identified on all continents except Antarctica, and the infection continues to have a worldwide distribution, but its unfolding story is not yet told.

Stable isotope analysis is now also being used to explore more complex aspects of TB disease transmission and its effect on the body. For example, stable isotope data were used to explore diet and mobility of children with TB in prehistoric Liguria, Italy (Goude et al. 2020). In this study, a local origin was established for Neolithic and Copper Age children, and a nonlocal origin for Bronze and Iron Age children. Vlok and Buckley (2022) examined skeletons from seven prehistoric sites in Japan, Mongolia, and Vietnam with archaeological evidence for varying levels of population interaction; they argue for more consideration of infectious disease per se in relation to networks of mobility and interaction that could have promoted transmission. In a different approach, Sparacello et al. (2016) considered the effects of TB on the skeletons of two individuals (adult and adolescent) from Neolithic northwest Italy. Alterations in growth were studied through stature and body mass evidence, and postcranial strength was assessed using cross-sectional geometry. The adolescent had gracile bones, suggesting that TB took a heavy toll on this individual. Incremental analysis of carbon and nitrogen isotope values in the layers of tooth dentine revealed that nitrogen increased at around 11.5 years of age along with a decline in carbon; these findings suggest that TB triggered a catabolic state in the body and the wasting seen in the bones. In a similar study of documented nineteenth–twentieth-century skeletons in Finland, Mansukoski and Sparacello (2018) found that bones in the TB group had smaller mean total cross-sectional areas when compared to the non-TB group. Finally, Snoddy et al. (2019) applied a life-course multimethod approach to the skeleton of a man who lived with TB in nineteenth-century New Zealand. Beyond macroscopic and radiographical analyses, stable isotope analyses allowed for reconstruction of his diet and mobility history: the results were used to corroborate the documentary evidence that he had started his life in London.

TB and the Biomolecular Revolution

Biomolecular analyses over the past 30 years have also increased our understanding of the origin, evolution, and history of infections, TB being the main infectious disease studied in this way to date. We lack room to document all the outcomes of these studies, but examples of this work follow. The development of aDNA and proteomic analyses are outlined in Chapter 1, and more information can be found in Gagneux 2018, Stone and Ozaga 2019, and Roberts et al. 2022a and 2023a.

This section focuses on the value of aDNA in studying the impact of TB on human populations throughout history. The first work in the 1990s sought to simply identify TB aDNA in skeletons. Studies increased rapidly into the 2000s and continue to multiply. Polymerase chain reaction (PCR)-based techniques were used in the early detection work, but they had and still have limitations. For instance, bone samples may be contaminated by mycobacteria other than TB, such as from the burial environment (Müller et al. 2016; Lawler et al. 2020). Thus, false positives may result. In addition, Nelson et al. (2020) pointed out that PCR does not identify strains within the MTBC and suggested that this could complicate the assembly of MTBC genomes: the resultant data could not be used for exploring the evolution of the pathogen causing TB. However, PCR is still used, and improvements to the method are ongoing. The development of next-generation sequencing was revolutionary because it enabled researchers to look at the molecular complexity of samples, perform whole-genome capture of the DNA present, and "sequence millions of DNA molecules in parallel, which decreases the overall time and cost of obtaining large amounts of genetic data" (Stone and Ozaga 2019, 189). However, as Nelson et al. (2020) stated, aDNA analysis alone is not a simple solution to diagnosis and interpretation of TB; multiple lines of evidence should always be used, alongside contextualizing the data.

The first modern (Cole et al. 1998) and ancient *M. tuberculosis* complex genomes (Chan et al. 2013: mummified lung tissue; Bos et al. 2014: bone) have now been sequenced. A diversity of animal-adapted strains have now been identified—for example, *M. bovis*—which have been seeded by human strains, not the reverse as was once thought (Brosch et al. 2002). Modern and ancient genomic analyses have indicated that TB's origin was in Africa (lineage 8, L8) where there is the most strain diversity. Because we now know where people affected by the different lineages live today and where in the past they were located, it is possible to explore the movement of TB with humans and animals, and hence track transmission. For example, lineage 4 (L4) is seen in Europe, past and present, and was introduced to the Americas with migration, social upheaval, and colonization, and MTBC strains are closely related to European strains. Further, as Vågene et al. (2022) showed, L4 replaced the Indigenous South American TB strain (L6) within 500 years (Bos et al. 2014; see also Roberts et al. 2022a, Fig. 10.1), and Bos et al. (2014) have suggested that the most recent common ancestor of MTBC is less than 6,000 years old. Having access to the information encompassed in modern MTBC genomes enables us to hypothesize how and when TB spread across the globe, learn about the evolution of TB pathogens, and explore the mechanisms at play as humans and other animals coevolved with those pathogens. All this knowledge could potentially be used by practitioners working on this infection as well as those treating people with TB, to better understand the nature and spread of this disease and how TB infection may be prevented in the future.

Leprosy

According to historical literature, few diseases have engendered the same fear of, and cruelty to, its sufferers as has leprosy. Much of the medieval attitude to leprosy in Europe stemmed from the supposed biblical references to the disease, references that today are considered largely incorrect (Grzybowski and Nita 2016). What of the disease itself?

The Here and Now of Leprosy

Leprosy, or Hansen's disease, is a chronic bacterial infection caused by *Mycobacterium leprae* (discovered in 1873), or the less common *Mycobacterium lepromatosis* identified in 2008 (Scollard and Gillis 2016; Deps 2023). Described by the World Health Organization (2019c) as one of the sixteen most neglected tropical diseases in the world, in 2018, 184,238 people were already infected with leprosy, with an additional 208,641 individuals infected in that year. Also in 2018, Brazil, India, and Indonesia reported more than 10,000 newly infected individuals. Thirteen countries reported from 1,000 to 10,000 individuals affected: Bangladesh, Democratic Republic of the Congo, Ethiopia, Madagascar, Mozambique, Myanmar, Nepal, Nigeria, Philippines, Somalia, South Sudan, Sri Lanka, and the United Republic of Tanzania. Ninety-nine countries reported fewer than 1,000 affected people (WHO 2019a), and forty-five countries reported no new cases of leprosy, reflecting progress made on management efforts since 1991. More recently, Brazil, Malaysia, Myanmar, Mexico, the Philippines, and the United States are continuing to report new *M. lepromatosis* infections (Collin et al. 2023a).

The decline of leprosy in recent times is largely due to the use of multidrug (antibiotic) treatment (MDT), a therapy introduced in 1982, and provided free to anyone with leprosy since 1995. As for TB, a One Health approach should be considered to both understand when and where the leprosy bacillus survives (e.g., soil, water, humans, and other animals), and the processes surrounding its transmission (Collin et al. 2023b). Leprosy persists in human populations where risk factors for infection abound, including poverty, under- and malnutrition, lower socioeconomic status, vitamin D deficiency, exposure to infected animals, and contaminated environments (see later in the chapter). For example, a meta-analysis of the relationship between leprosy and nutrition found that people with leprosy had dietary insufficiency that contributed to susceptibility when compared to those without the infection (Velmurugan and Thangaraju 2024).

People with both cured and active leprosy may be physically impaired due to the infection, such as loss of appendages and disfigurement. While treatment with MDT may be relatively straightforward, dealing with the sociocultural consequences of leprosy is much more demanding for individuals affected, their communities, and professionals who care for them. Disfigurements from leprosy are often a consequence of delay in diagnosis, which remains challenging in countries that lack the necessary infrastructure. Furthermore, many parts of the world have limited understanding of leprosy, what causes it, how it is contracted, and if or how it can be treated (Van't Noordende et al. 2021; Fiorin et al. 2023). Related stigma has not gone away despite better education of communities about the nature of this infection. Renewed calls have been made to abandon the words *leprosy* and *leper* in an effort to reduce stigma (Deps and Cruz 2020; Rao and Suneetha 2021). Indeed, these calls, for everyone—from health care professionals to the general public—to stop using the word *leper* have been occurring since the 1948 International Leprosy Congress in Havana, Cuba, repeated in Madrid, Spain, in 1953 (see Roberts 2020d, 4–7). The theme of World Leprosy Day in 2024 was "ending stigma and embracing dignity," with recommendations for educating all people of all ages, patients, professionals, and the healthy public. Changing leprosy's name to Hansen's disease or *M. neurodermatosis* has also been suggested, yet even in Brazil, which uses the name Hansen's disease instead of leprosy, stigma persists (Souza et al. 2024).

While leprosy is largely a disease of humans, it is not exclusively so, and it has been identified in nonhuman primates (Hockings et al. 2021: West Africa), the nine-banded armadillo in the southern United States and South America (Oliveira et al. 2019), the red squirrel in Britain (Schilling et al. 2019), and rodents in Brazil (Lima et al. 2022). Today, because of the presence of infected wild armadillos in the US and South America (particularly Brazil), humans who handle or eat them are at risk of infection (Oliveira et al. 2019). Schuenemann et al. (2018a) revealed that medieval leprosy strains were present in modern red squirrels in England, suggesting they contracted circulating human strains during the medieval period. Keeping red squirrels as pets and for the fur trade, in addition to hunting them, could have enabled transfer of *M. leprae* between human and animal species. The only evidence, to date, for leprosy in archaeological animal bones is a study by Urban et al. (2024), who carried out aDNA analysis on human bones from a medieval leprosy hospital (leprosarium) and medieval squirrel bones, both from Winchester, southern England. They also found the human strain of the disease in the squirrels (Urban et al. 2024).

The There and Then of Leprosy

Leprosy appears to be a late arrival in the history of bacterial disease. The *Sushruta Samhita*, an Indian document from before 300 BCE, described ***kushtham*** with loss of sensation, "falling off" of the fingers, deformity and ulceration of the limbs, and sinking of the nose. The features are almost diagnostic of advanced (low resistant) lepromatous leprosy (see later in this section). Even earlier texts dated to ca. 1500 BCE describe laws restricting the freedom of people with leprosy (Bishagratna 1907–1916, 2, 39–42; Jacob and Franco-Paredes 2008). A similar description was identified in a Chinese bamboo book of the third century BCE (Skinsnes 1980; Skinsnes and Chang 1985). Thus, lepromatous leprosy was established in India and the Far East at an early period, and the clear and accurate contemporary descriptions imply that the authors possessed clinical acumen and familiarity with the disease that may have been prevalent at the time. Possibly of significance for the origin of leprosy, skeletal evidence was found at the Dakhleh Oasis in Egypt in four crania of the Ptolemaic period (250 BCE) (Dzierzykray-Rogalski 1980). Molto (2002) identified a further two early to mid-fourth century CE male burials with leprosy, and stable isotopic data indicated that they lived elsewhere before they died and were buried at Dakhleh Oasis. Although the word *lépra*, denoting a skin condition, appears often in the Hippocratic texts (fifth century BCE), it does not appear to relate to the severe disease we know as leprosy. Some suggest that these findings show leprosy was present in northern Europe and made its entry into the Mediterranean area with the Alexandrian army in 300 BCE, although that theory has been disputed (Grmek 1991, 152–176; Mark 2002), and it still awaits paleopathological and/or biomolecular evidence to refute it.

Medieval images represented leprosy as spots, tumors, and pustules distributed over the entire body (Gron 1973). Early Renaissance artists portrayed limb and facial deformities (Hollander 1913). A sculpture dated to 1250–1350 CE from the site of Burton Lazars leprosarium in Leicestershire, England, also illustrates the facial features of advanced lepromatous leprosy (Marcombe and Manchester 1990). A similar figure is carved on the high altar of a church in Krakow, Poland, and a figurine illustrating both the facial and the peripheral limb features of the disease has been identified in the Abbaye de Cadouin, France (Fig. 6.25; Manchester and Knüsel 1994), inviting the speculation that the sculptor of this poignant figure had an intimate knowledge of a person with advanced lepromatous leprosy. Carvings of less certain diagnosis are known from European and Middle Eastern sources (Grmek and Gourevitch 1998, 247–252), one of which is possibly as old as 800 BCE (Naser Moghadasi 2015).

Infection of the Human Body with Leprosy

The mode of transmission of *M. leprae* and *M. lepromatosis* between people is through exhaled droplets containing bacteria from an individual's mouth and nose during close and frequent contact (WHO 2024d). The bacilli are then spread within the body by blood and lymphatic routes to specific cells (neurons) of peripheral

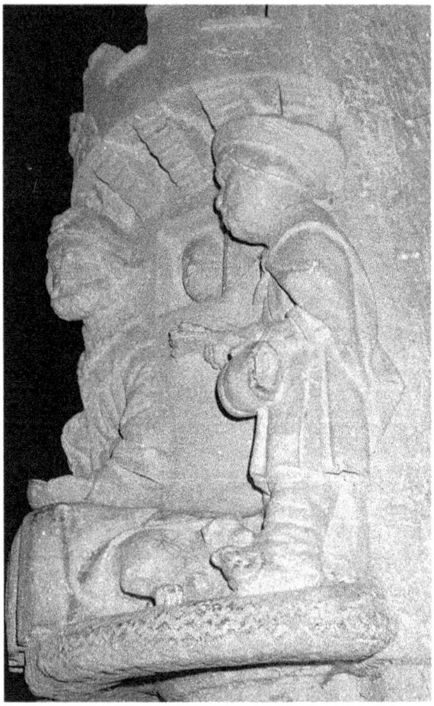

Figure 6.25. A figure depicting leprosy and holding a clapper in the medieval Abbaye de Cadouin, France. Photograph by Keith Manchester.

nerves. Over the years there have been other suggested routes of transmission, including via skin-to-skin contact, from mother to fetus (in utero), insect bites, ingested bacteria, and environmental sources (see Roberts 2020d, 30, for detailed discussion on the viability of these routes). For example, Turankar et al. (2022) found viable *M. leprae* in soil and water and of the same genotypes as those affecting people. Negating prominent medieval thought (Smelyansky 2020, 200–202), the disease is neither inherited nor is it transmitted sexually. Leprosy is often acquired in childhood, and males are affected more than females. Relatively little evidence has been identified in non-adult skeletons compared to those of adults in the archaeological record. Specific information on the clinical and paleopathological evidence for leprosy in children is discussed in Lewis (2018, 164–172). As Lewis noted, children today usually develop tuberculoid leprosy of soft tissue (discussed next), and this may account for a lack of skeletal evidence. However, in areas where the disease is hyperendemic, child incidence is high (Badger 1964).

After transmission there is a variably lengthy incubation period, for example 3–5 years (tuberculoid leprosy) to 9–12 years (lepromatous leprosy), with children having shorter incubation periods and adults much longer (Maymone et al. 2020). The bacterium multiplies slowly, making leprosy difficult to contract and symptoms gradual. Known throughout time as the living death, a medieval pronouncement to the afflicted were the words "*Mundo mortuus sis, sed Deo vivas*" (Be thou dead to the world but alive unto God). The infection affects the peripheral nerves (motor, sensory, and autonomic), a process that is responsible for the majority of its skeletal changes—lack of sensation and motor control leads to extensive unappreciated injury. The skin, respiratory tract, eyes, and bones may also be involved in the disease process. People with leprosy may experience congestion in the nose as well as rhinosinusitis, enlarged nerves, muscle weakness, paralysis, numbness, skin lesions, dry skin, and ulcers on their feet and hands. All five senses can be affected too: hearing, sight, smell, taste and touch. In addition to the skeletal and nonskeletal bodily changes, mental health challenges have been noted in some studies (e.g., Somar et al. 2020). For example, some can develop neurotic symptoms and psychotic reactions probably triggered by the stigma attached to the disease. While detecting the psychological aspects of leprosy through studying archaeological skeletal remains is impossible, clinical data can help us to understand what individuals with leprosy may have experienced. Archaeological context also provides information about what life may have held for those with leprosy in the past, including how they were treated by their communities, with or without, for example, the structural violence embedded in segregation into colonies or leprosy hospitals. The clinical manifestations of leprosy vary in severity, bodily distribution, and infectivity. Because leprosy bacilli have a predilection for cool environments, it is the subcutaneous nerves that are affected. Involvement of the central nervous system is rarely detected. The function of the peripheral nerve modalities of motor, sensory, and autonomic nerves is progressively compromised; it results in motor-nerve-mediated limb and facial paralysis, sensory-nerve-mediated loss of skin and joint sensation, and autonomic-mediated change in perspiration and circulation. The effects of leprosy on the body are individually variable due to differences in the immune status of each infected individual and the strain of the pathogen (Ridley and Jopling 1966; Fig. 6.26). *M. lepromatosis* has a greater proclivity to induce diffuse lepromatous leprosy, which is a more symptomatically severe and extensive disease of skin ulceration and soft tissue damage (Britton and Lockwood 2004).

The variable clinical picture follows a spectrum according to immune status. At one end with low resistance, the disease is highly infective, and the physical signs involve multiple limbs, the face, and body organs (lepromatous leprosy). At the other end of the spectrum with high resistance, the manifestations are fewer, may be unilateral, affecting one or perhaps two limbs, with less severe soft tissue reactions (tuberculoid leprosy). Damage to the bones of the skeleton in leprosy can involve the facial, hand, and foot bones and the tibiae and fibula. Other conditions may lead to the same or similar changes, and therefore the distribution pattern of lesions is key to diagnosis. In paleopathology, lepromatous leprosy is the most frequently identified type, but the low rate of detection of tuberculoid leprosy may be because the less severe bone changes are not recognized. Direct infection of the soft tissues around and inside the nose and mouth by *M. leprae* results in the characteristic changes in the bones of the face, called leonine facies. The facial tissues become nodular, the bridge of the nose collapses and is associated with a persistent nasal discharge, the lower eyelids are paralyzed (lagophthalmos), and, consequently, the eyes become infected and blindness may ensue. Invasion of the larynx produces a hoarse, coarse voice, which is characteristic of advanced leprosy (Velasco et al. 2020).

Skeletal Leprosy

Here, we describe the key leprosy bone changes, but much more detail is provided in Roberts 2020d. Documentation of the bone changes of leprosy in skeletal remains was first undertaken by Vilhelm Møller-Christensen (1961), a medical doctor from Denmark who excavated and analyzed skeletons from Danish medieval leprosy hospital sites, including Naestved (Bennike 2002). Subsequent to Møller-Christensen's seminal work, others refined the diagnostic criteria for leprosy and the specific pathological processes that lead to the bone changes (Andersen 1969; Andersen and Manchester 1987, 1988; Andersen et al. 1992). Like TB, leprosy affects the skeleton in only 3–5% of untreated people (Paterson and Rad 1961), and we do not know yet whether *M. lepromatosis* affects the skeleton in the same way as *M. leprae*.

The macroscopic bone changes of the facial bones of people with leprosy include inflammatory pitting of both surfaces of the palate with possible perforation, loss of alveolar bone around the incisors of the upper jaw and subsequent loss of teeth, absorption of the anterior nasal spine, remodeling of the nasal aperture, and inflammation of the nasal conchae and septum (Fig. 6.27 and 6.28). The bone changes were called facies leprosa by Møller-Christensen (1978) and renamed rhinomaxillary syndrome by Anderson and Manchester (1992), although leonine facies is most commonly used for facial changes in people with leprosy today (i.e., the facial appearance). While the maxillary bone changes are considered pathognomonic for leprosy, other diseases may cause similar changes, including the treponemal diseases

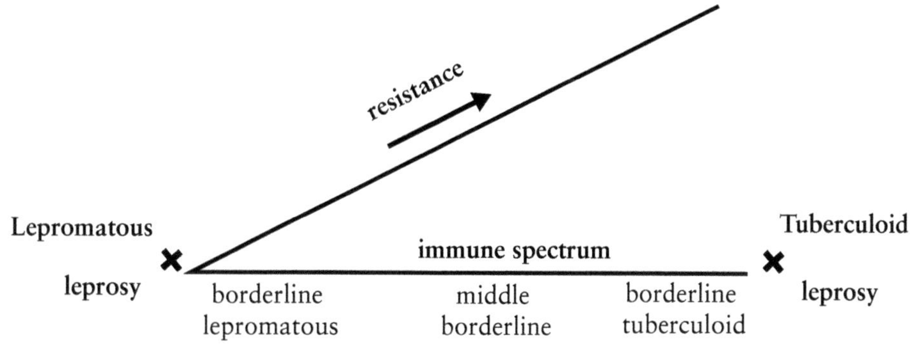

Figure 6.26. Graphic illustrating the Ripley-Jopling immune spectrum of leprosy. Figure drawn by Yvonne Beadnell.

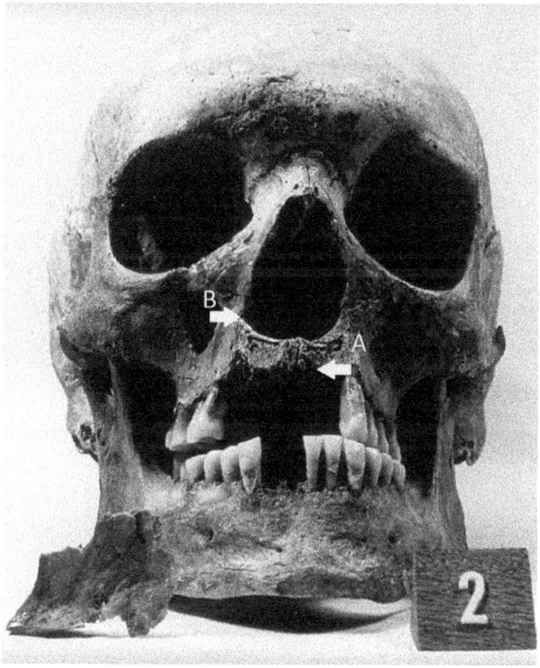

Figure 6.27. Rhinomaxillary syndrome in leprosy. A: alveolar bone resorption of maxilla and loss of teeth; B: remodeling of nasal aperture (twelfth–sixteenth centuries CE, Naestved, Denmark). Photograph by Charlotte Roberts.

and TB. Teeth with short roots (leprogenic odontodysplasia) can also be associated with leprosy and were first described by Danielsen (1970) in skeletons from Naestved in Denmark. The bacteria may stunt the developing roots of the permanent incisor teeth, although this has yet to be clinically proven. They have rarely been identified in archaeological skeletons (e.g., Kjellström 2012; Matos and Santos 2013; Taylor et al. 2024), and never in clinical contexts, as far as the authors are

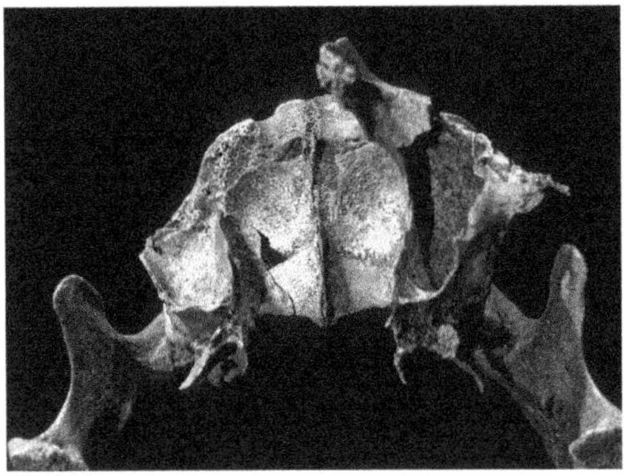

Figure 6.28. Pitting of the nasal surface of the palate (twelfth–sixteenth centuries CE, Chichester, England). Originally reproduced with kind permission from Don Ortner.

aware. It is probably better to consider this dental change as a possible indicator of leprosy; see Lewis (2018, 168–169) for more extensive discussion about potential causes for these dental indicators.

Involvement of the peripheral nerves results in paralysis of muscle groups in the upper and lower limbs, deformity, and functional loss (Figs. 6.29 and 6.30). Loss of sensation particularly affects the hands and feet, leading to damage to the tissues, ulceration, and secondary infection (Fig. 6.31). The bone changes in the hands and feet and the lower leg bones are the direct result of this secondary infection and consist of inflammatory changes to the bones and joints (Møller-Christensen 1961; Andersen et al. 1994), joint fixation and deformity, and bone absorption, particularly in the toes and fingers (Figs. 6.32 and 6.33; Andersen et al. 1992). Interestingly, damage to the hands is less common than to the feet, both past and present, perhaps because soft tissue lesions on the hands are more noticeable than those on the feet and more easily treated to prevent further damage (Manchester 2002). Frequent damage to the plantar surface (sole) of the first and fifth metatarsophalangeal joint areas reflects the areas of maximum pressure in the normal foot architecture. If the arch of the foot collapses (common in leprosy), then the pressure will be redirected to the mid-forefoot, with consequent stress on the ligaments attaching to the dorsal surfaces of the tarsals (Fig. 6.34). Today, in places where leprosy is prevalent, protection of the feet with shoes and the hands with gloves or potholders is part of the educational process for people with the disease (Choudhury 2021).

The subperiosteal new bone formation of the tibia and fibula is a nonspecific inflammatory change in leprosy that can also be caused by many other conditions, such as trauma, treponemal disease, scurvy, and TB. These bones are affected by inflammation spreading upward from the foot through blood and lymphatic vessels; chronic oedema of the lower legs may also be responsible. These lower leg bone lesions are common in skeletons with convincing evidence of leprosy; Lewis (1995b) documented these changes in 38 (76%) individuals with leprosy, compared to 19% of those without leprosy, from the well-studied medieval leprosy hospital in Chichester, Sussex, England (see also Magilton et al. 2008). A small number of radii and ulnae were also affected, which may be the result of inflammation in the hand spreading to the forearm bones. While periosteal new

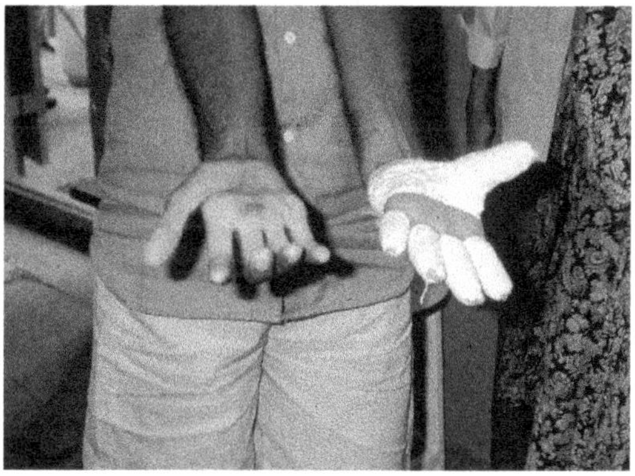

Figure 6.29. Flexion deformity of right hand as a result of motor nerves being involved in leprosy; the left hand is being treated with Plaster of Paris splints to straighten the deformities (Pune, India). Photograph by Charlotte Roberts.

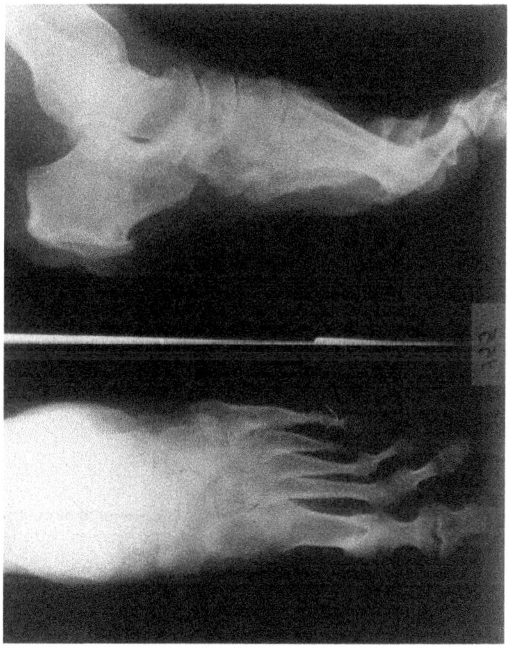

Figure 6.30. Radiograph of feet of a person with leprosy. Top (lateral view) showing flexion deformity of great toe and dorsal tarsal bar. Bottom (dorsal view) showing remodeling of the fifth metatarsal shaft and loss of the head. Courtesy of the late Johs Andersen, and curated in the Calvin Wells Collection, University of Bradford.

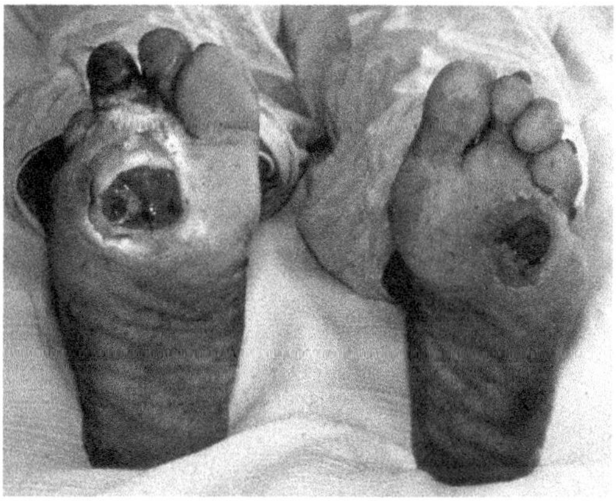

Figure 6.31. Ulceration of the feet in person with leprosy. This is the result of damage to the sensory nerves and loss of sensation. Photography by Charlotte Roberts.

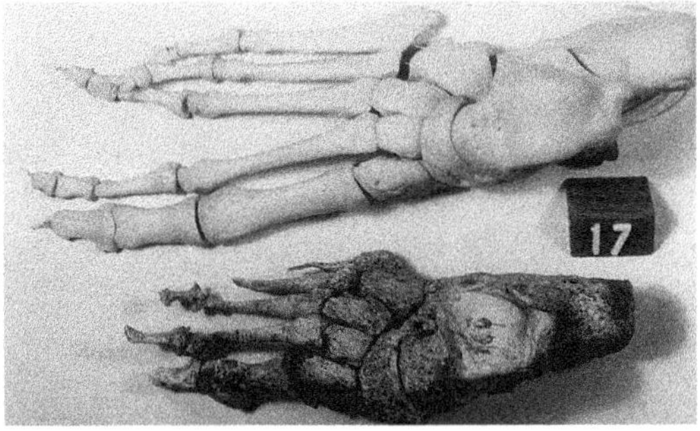

Figure 6.32. Loss of some of the foot phalanges and remodeling of the metatarsals in leprosy, with the normal foot (top) for comparison (late medieval, twelfth–sixteenth centuries CE, Naestved, Denmark). Photograph by Charlotte Roberts.

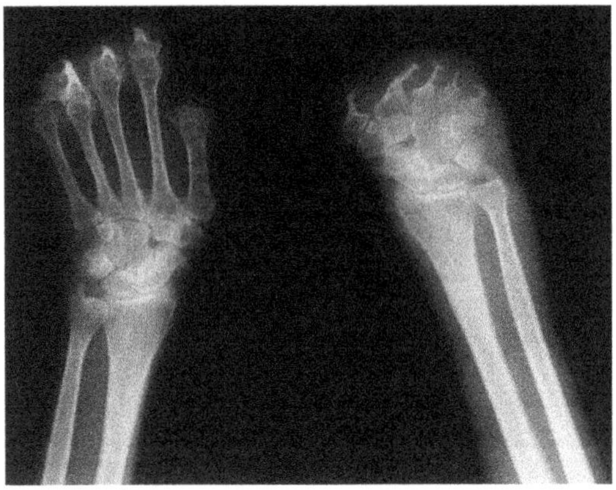

Figure 6.33. Radiograph of forearm, wrist, and hands of a person with leprosy. Left: loss of phalanges. Right: almost complete loss of the metacarpals. Courtesy of Johs Andersen, and curated in the Calvin Wells Collection, University of Bradford.

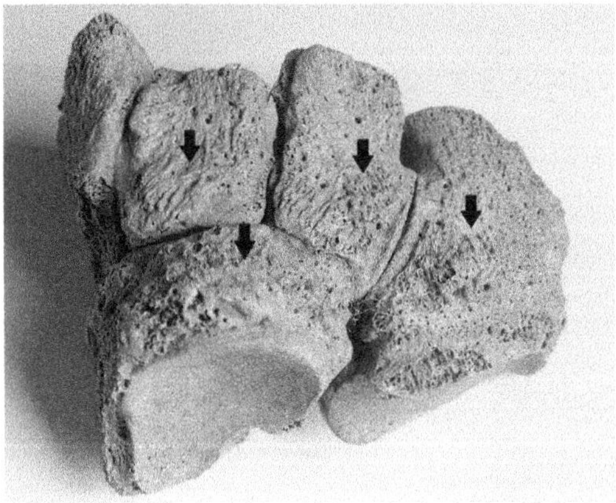

Figure 6.34. Dorsal surfaces of the tarsals of the foot from an individual with leprosy showing new bone formation (tarsal bars) at ligament insertions (black arrows) due to strain following the development of a "drop" foot. Photograph by and courtesy of Jean Brown.

bone is not a specific diagnostic criterion for leprosy in clinical contexts, it appears fairly frequently in archaeological contexts. The lack of recognition may be because the (often) subtle bone changes are not detected on radiographs and therefore not described in living patients (Lewis et al. 1995b, 82).

When should a diagnosis of lepromatous or tuberculoid leprosy be made in paleopathology? Matos (2009b) used medical files from a twentieth-century Portuguese leprosarium and observations of skeletons from a Danish medieval leprosarium cemetery. Matos found that, for a diagnosis of lepromatous leprosy, rhinomaxillary syndrome and bilaterally symmetrical hand and foot bone lesions are characteristic, and for tuberculoid leprosy no rhinomaxillary syndrome would be expected, but bilateral or unilateral hand and foot bone involvement would be needed for a diagnosis.

No wonder that the disfigured, and possibly blind male or female with missing fingers and toes may have provoked fear and cruel reactions. The diagnosis and misdiagnosis of the disease in antiquity has been, and still is, a subject of debate. The extent to which nonleprous diseases of the nervous system, the skin, and eyes were attributed to the "biblical scourge" is surely questionable. Elucidation of the problem comes from the evidence of documents and, more particularly, from the skeletal evidence. For example, some 68% of the skeletons excavated from the medieval leprosarium at Naestved, Denmark, exhibited the bone changes of leprosy (Møller-Christensen 1978).

Paleopathological Evidence for Leprosy

As for TB, the evidence for leprosy in human skeletons has been widely reviewed in the literature, so we will not cover it in detail here (see Roberts 2020d, 191–280; Roberts et al. 2022b). New developments include recording the frequency of leprosy using statistical approaches (e.g., Boldsen 2001; Boldsen and Mollerup 2006) and exploring local versus nonlocal origins for medieval people with leprosy in Denmark (Brozou et al. 2021) and England (Filipek et al. 2022). Researchers have also considered care and treatment of people with leprosy through the study of skeletons; for example, Roberts (2017) used the Index of Care (Tilley and Oxenham 2011), while Fiorin et al. (2024) found evidence of ginger in dental calculus suggesting its medicinal use in a medieval leprosarium.

The following is a summary of the global data that has been recorded, mainly in adult skeletons. Most evidence comes from nonleprosy hospital cemeteries and not from leprosaria, as few of these cemeteries have been excavated (but see Roberts 2020d, 329, where a list is provided). Skeletal evidence has been found on four of the seven continents of the world, with the Antarctic, Oceania, and South America currently having no evidence, while North America has only three reported individuals, to date. Leprosy has been identified in Africa and Asia, with the majority of evidence from Europe, especially northern Europe and the Mediterranean region. Britain, Denmark, and Hungary have the most evidence documented so far.

The earliest evidence comes from Hungary. Köhler et al. (2017) reported on five individuals from 3700 BCE at the Copper Age site of Abony-Turjányos dűlő. Mycolic acids of *M. leprae* and proteins specific to the bacterium were found. Most European evidence comes from the late medieval period (twelfth–sixteenth centuries CE), suggesting an elevated presence at that time. Despite leprosy being an infection of rural areas today, the medieval evidence is from urban contexts where the bacteria thrived in a higher population density of often poorer people. In medieval Europe, measures were taken to control leprosy through various means, including quarantine for travelers and leprosy hospitals to isolate, confine, and care for people with the infection (Blažina Tomić and Blažina 2015; Rawcliffe 2006; Demaitre 2007). Later, in the nineteenth to early twentieth century, segregation on islands was practiced, such as on Robben Island in South Africa, Spinalonga on Crete, and Kalaupapa, Hawaii. In recent years, people who were placed in these locations have begun to tell their stories (e.g., Law 2012; Manes 2013). Leprosy hospitals as a means of segregating and isolating people with leprosy in medieval Europe have been discussed by many. The rules were not strict, which meant that people with leprosy could wander at will and go to markets, enabling the infection to be transmitted to others. Furthermore, not all people with leprosy would have been segregated, possibly because the clinical signs of the infection were not visible and therefore diagnosis was not made or they had high resistant tuberculoid leprosy. They may also have evaded detection, or their community might have accepted them as regular citizens. Overall, a recent global review suggests that when people with leprosy died in the past, they were "buried normally for the time period, culture, and location" (Roberts 2020d, 280). Leprosy hospitals saw their height of popularity, in Britain at least, during the twelfth and thirteenth centuries, with a decline from the fourteenth century onward. Whether this change reflected a decline in the infection is much debated.

Evidence of leprosy in China in 200 BCE–200 CE (Zhenbiao 1994) supports the hypothesis generated by modern *M. leprae* genetic evidence (Monot et al. 2005) that European people took leprosy from its origin in Africa to the east via the northern (Silk Road) and southern routes. Early evidence in Asia too suggests that leprosy could have been taken to the west. In terms of exploring the origin, evolution, and spread of leprosy, our understanding has been increased by Monot et al. (2005, 2009). Using modern and aDNA samples from people who have (or had) leprosy, they proposed an origin in eastern Africa or the Near East 100,000 years ago and spread with movement of people both east and west—for example, via military campaigns, trade, and pilgrimage—with an entry to the Americas over the most recent 500 years via colonization and the slave trade. Comparing the global locations of sixteen different strains of *M. leprae* today with ancient data, it has been possible to observe the phylogeography of leprosy (linking genetic data with geographic location). Knowledge of which strains of leprosy were located, when, and where further increases our understanding of how and when leprosy spread across the world (Donoghue et al. 2015). In fact, the strain of leprosy in the Americas is the same as that in Europe—in ancient Denmark, England, and Sweden. However, apart from two skulls from Vancouver Island, Canada, and from Kodiak Island in Alaska with possible evidence of leprosy and definitive evidence from Mexico City, no evidence has been found for leprosy in North America (Roberts 2020d, 269–274, and references within; see also Ruis et al. 2020 and Schuenemann et al. 2018a for the Mexican evidence). As stated, there is less evidence for leprosy in nonadult remains (see Roberts 2020d, 193–195), although there are nineteenth-century Norwegian illustrations of children with leprosy. However, modern-day Croatia, the Czech Republic, Denmark, Hungary, Italy, Sweden, Türkiye, and the UK have revealed nonadult skeletons with accepted bone changes. Table 6.2 provides a summary of the earliest evidence of leprosy in skeletal remains, with more detailed information provided in Chapter 5 of Roberts (2020d).

Table 6.2 Summary of earliest evidence in modern-day countries for leprosy from a global perspective

Place	Date	Source
Iran	6200–5700 BCE	Tagaya (2014)*
Hungary	3780–3650 BCE	Köhler et al. (2017)
Türkiye	2700–2300 BCE	Angel (1969)
India	2500–2000 BCE	Schug et al. (2009)
Pakistan	2550–2030 BCE	Schug et al. (2013)
Italy	Fifth century BCE	Rubini et al. (2014)
Thailand	300–200 BCE	Tayles and Buckley (2004)
Egypt	250 BCE	Dzierzykray-Rogalski (1980)
China	200BCE–200 CE	Zhenbaio (1994)
Israel	First century CE	Donoghue et al. (2005)
Uzbekistan	First–fourth centuries CE	Blau and Yagodin (2005)
Spain	Second–fourth centuries CE	De Miguel Ibáñez et al. (2011)
France	Fourth century CE	Blondiaux pers. comm. (2013)*
United Kingdom	450–600 CE	Inskip et al. (2015)
Greece	Fifth–sixth centuries CE	Lagia et al. (2006)
Nubia	500 CE	Smith (1908)
Sweden	70–570 CE	Arcini and Artelius (1993)
Czech Republic	Ninth–tenth centuries CE	Strouhal et al. (2002)
Ukraine	Tenth century CE	Inna Potekhina pers. comm. (2008) *
Croatia	Tenth–eleventh centuries CE	Bedić et al. (2019)
Slovenia	Eleventh century CE	Hukeľová et al. (2021)
Iceland	1000 CE	Magnússon et al. (1970)
Guam	Seventh–thirteenth centuries CE	Trembly (2002)
Norway	Eleventh–sixteenth centuries CE	Brødholt (2007)
Poland	Twelfth–fourteenth centuries CE	Kozłowski (2012)
Denmark	Twelfth–sixteenth centuries CE	Møller-Christensen (1969b)
Japan	Thirteenth–fifteenth centuries CE	Hirata et al. (2000)
Germany	Thirteenth–sixteenth centuries CE	Schmitz-Cliever (1971)
Portugal	Fourteenth–sixteenth centuries CE	Antunes-Ferreira (2013)
Cyprus	Fifteenth century CE	Baker and Bolhofner (2014)
Caribbean Antilles	Nineteenth–twentieth centuries CE	Gilmore (2008)
Mexico	Nineteenth century CE	Ruis et al. (2020)
Sub-Saharan Africa	Twentieth century CE	L'Abbé and Steyn (2007)
Kodak Island, Alaska	Not stated	Wilczak and Ortner (2013)
Vancouver Island, Canada	Not stated	Møller-Christensen and Inkster (1965)

* Needs to be verified.
Note: There is new evidence coming from North and South America for leprosy in human remains, and first evidence for ancient *M. lepromatosis*. Lopopolo et al. (2025); Ramirez et al. (2025).

The early history of leprosy in the Near East has, until recently, relied on the apparent biblical references to leprosy. However, a number of researchers have demonstrated that these references are probably false and rest on a mistranslation of the

Hebrew word *tsara'ath*, which describes a range of bacterial and fungal diseases prevalent in the eastern Mediterranean in the first millennium BCE. Consequently, leprosy could have been included in this range of meanings, but *tsara'ath* does not specifically describe leprosy as we know it today (Grybowski and Nita 2016). In any case, the infection was probably known throughout the eastern Mediterranean area at that time. Indeed, the earliest skeletal remains diagnostic of leprosy in Israel is from a first century CE family tomb in a rock-cut grave in the Hinnom Valley, Akeldama (Donoghue et al. 2005). The prejudice against leprosy throughout history may have been due to a tragic error of translation, and attribution of loosely applied names of the past to specific diseases recognized today, but it has resulted in a major pitfall in the investigation of this disease in antiquity.

Leprosy and the Biomolecular Revolution

As for TB, and since the third edition of this book in 2005, biomolecular analysis—mainly focusing on aDNA—has been increasingly utilized for confirming diagnoses of leprosy (although the need for its use is debatable when a clear leprosy diagnosis can be macroscopically made). It has also been employed to detect leprosy infection in individuals who died before the disease affected their bones; and for exploring *M. leprae*'s origin and evolution. The first modern and ancient genomes of leprosy were published in 2001 by Cole et al. and Schuenemann et al. (2013, 2018a), respectively, and the *M. lepromatosis* genome was sequenced by Silva et al. in 2022. This genomic research paved the way for learning more about leprosy's origin and evolution, explored by Monot et al. (2005, 2009). Ancient DNA analysis of skeletons with leprosy commenced in 1994. For a list of studies from 1994 to 2019, most of which have been focused on European skeletons, see Roberts (2020d, table 4.1). Since 1994, studies have increased as laboratory standards have improved, more people are trained to conduct analyses, and more facilities have become available.

Perhaps the greatest advance in these studies, as for TB, has been informative and detailed explorations of the long history of leprosy by looking at the strains of the leprosy bacteria that affected our predecessors. For example, Pfrengle et al. (2021) found a particularly high diversity of *M. leprae* in skeletons from European medieval leprosaria, suggesting that they received individuals infected with diverse strains and from various geographic backgrounds. These people with leprosy may have been travelers on pilgrimage or in search of work or care for their infection. In their study of a fifth–sixth century young adult male from Essex, England, Inskip et al. (2017) found that he had a European strain of *M. leprae* and that he was not born and raised local to the region: stable isotope analysis suggested that he came from outside of Britain. In their similar study of a young adult male who had been buried in the cemetery of the St. Mary Magdalen, Winchester leprosarium, also in England (eleventh–twelfth century CE), Roffey et al. (2017) found a nonlocal origin for this individual; he had also been buried with a scallop shell, a sign that he had been a traveler. In addition, he harbored an *M. leprae* strain that today is associated with south-central and western Asia. All these studies using aDNA analysis show the power of combining archaeology, paleopathology, historical evidence, and biomolecular analyses to make such conclusions.

Doubtless the recognizable clinical manifestations of leprosy were present in antiquity just as they are today, and nothing supports the idea that the disease has changed its features throughout history. From historical sources we might paint the following picture: people with the infection could be poor, marginalized, impaired, disabled, forced to beg for alms and give notice of their presence with wooden clappers. Questions remain. For example, the people who lived in the albeit relatively recent (mid-twentieth-century), Portuguese leprosarium, Rovisco Pais, were not all poor. Was the picture of stigma ubiquitous for all communities and individuals in the past? How was their (or their caregivers') medieval identity shaped by stigma, a field of study that is being explored more closely by both paleopathologists and historians alike (Brenner and Touati 2021)? In answering these questions, caution is needed, because recent historical and archaeological research has changed perceptions of what it meant to have leprosy in the past (Rawcliffe 2006; Demaitre 2007; Roberts 2020d). By combining evidence for leprosy in skeletons and funerary context, Roberts (2020d) found that most people with leprosy were not marginalized in death and were usually buried with the rest of their community. This observation suggests a more accepting community than older sources have led us to believe, a view that is also supported by reevaluating the historical evidence.

The Decline of Leprosy

The decline and elimination of leprosy, particularly in Europe, illustrates the complex and interrelated bacteriological, social, and environmental factors implicated in infectious disease. These factors differ from region to region, and even within individual (modern-day) countries themselves, which may explain the survival of leprosy in one community and its simultaneous disappearance from another. Furthermore, in the medieval period the persistence of leprosy hospitals may not be a reliable guide to the persistence of leprosy within the community in which it was located (Roberts 1986). There is no doubt that by the late medieval period in England at least, people with leprosy were considerably less common. The leprosy hospital, like the TB sanatorium in a later period, maintained its name and dedication but changed its function. By the mid-twentieth century, many TB sanatoria contained few, if any, people with TB, but instead accepted patients with other pulmonary diseases. So it may have been with leprosy hospitals in the late medieval period. Evidence of skeletons from later periods of the medieval leprosy hospital in Chichester, Sussex, England, indicate fewer people with leprosy buried, and people with a wider range of health problems (Magilton et al. 2008). Leprosy was a rare disease in England of the fifteenth century, and by the sixteenth century, it no longer existed. There is also much less paleopathological evidence for leprosy after the fifteenth century; for a list of evidence from prehistory to the postmedieval period in Britain, see Roberts 2020d, appendix 3.

Notwithstanding the vigor with which segregation of people with leprosy was often enforced, it probably contributed little to the decline of the disease, especially as we know that segregation was often lax. In addition, many other reasons for leprosy's decline have been explored but not usually confirmed; for example, not eating fish, not drinking goat's milk, a ban on sexual intercourse, plague preferentially killing people with leprosy, changes in climate, and urbanization. The decline in leprosy has often been linked to a concurrent rise in TB (Manchester 1984; Roberts 2020d, 291–301). To some extent the evidence for an increase in TB in the early modern period is simply assumed, based on an expectation projected back in time from the known high prevalence in the urban centers of the seventeenth century. The reaction of the body at a microscopic level to *M. tuberculosis* and to *M. leprae* is essentially the same (Lurie 1955), and a degree of cross-immunity induced by these two bacteria has been observed. Grmek (1991, 206–209) suggested that there might have been an evolutionary chain of mycobacterial development from the nonpathogenic through and including the human pathogens. In this chain, *M. tuberculosis* is regarded as an earlier entity than *M. leprae*. If bacterial evolution resulted in a decrease in virulence and relatively low pathogenicity of *M. leprae* then, because of biological competition, TB will take precedence over leprosy. Exposure to *M. tuberculosis*, regardless of whether it results in overt TB or rapid self-conquest of infection, may induce a degree of immunity to leprosy, consequently reducing the chances of contracting leprosy (Manchester 1991). As a corollary, because of the cross-immunity of leprosy and TB, leprosy, if contracted, is likely to be of high resistance according to the Ridley and Jopling (1966) immune spectrum and, ipso facto, will present as tuberculoid leprosy. In addition, the Bacillus Calmette-Guérin, or BCG, vaccine, normally used for protection against TB, offers some protection against leprosy, but the success rate varies from study to study (Coppola et al. 2018).

Today and presumably in the past, the primary focus of TB infection in the lungs often becomes arrested early without disease progression. Henceforth, the individual is immune to TB and, by the above reasoning, in part to leprosy. Therefore, an increase in community exposure to TB may result in a decreasing community incidence of leprosy. Exposure to TB needs close human-to-human contact (e.g., in densely populated urban environments). The revival of urban living in Europe, for example, gathered momentum from the tenth century and lasted until the early fourteenth century; at this time there was a decline in new urban foundations. During the later medieval period, the population of England doubled (Dyer 1989), and the fourteenth century saw famine and the Black Death impact population numbers. Thus, to some extent, a decline in population in the fourteenth century may explain the decline in available people to contract leprosy.

The skeletal record may support this hypothesis. The presence of both TB and leprosy in the same skeleton is rare, although skeletons with evidence of both TB and leprosy have been identified, mostly using biomolecular analysis (Roberts 2020d, 298; Table 6.2). The rarity of this combination of diseases is support for the mutually exclusive nature of leprosy and TB and, by inference, for the preceding hypothesis. Research has cast some doubt on the theory of leprosy decreasing while TB increases. Wilbur et al. (2002) analyzed leprosy and TB data from two eras (1938–1980 and 1991–1998) from Texas: they found that leprosy and TB increased and declined together. While admitting that lack of diagnostic accuracy, medical intervention, and underreporting may have affected the results of the study, Wilbur et al. (2022, 255) offered "possible though not conclusive evidence against a model of cross-immunity." Leitman et al. (1997) pointed out that Chaussinand's hypothesis of competitive exclusion of leprosy by TB cannot be tested experimentally, and concluded that "if conditions were such that the basic reproductive rate of leprosy was relatively low, then, as Chaussinand proposed, TB could have played a major role in the disappearance of leprosy from western Europe" (Leitman et al.1997, 1926), but their research indicated that it would have taken centuries for TB to eradicate leprosy. Recent publications continue to address the decline of leprosy. For example, Crespo et al. (2019) revisited the TB and leprosy cross-immunity hypothesis through integrating immunology and paleopathology, and Donoghue et al. (2005) explored coinfections of leprosy and TB in relation to leprosy's decline. Others have considered evidence for the social and biological effects of leprosy on fertility (Blondiaux et al. 2016), and the possibility of increased host resistance with declining pathogen virulence (Henneberg et al. 2021).

Whatever the manifold potential reasons for the decline of leprosy, Europe is now largely spared this most emotive and mutilating of the mycobacterial diseases, but even as new reports of leprosy are declining, it remains a complex challenge. When prejudice, fear, and geographic and economic barriers have been overcome, we hope that leprosy may also disappear from the places it still inhabits and become a disease of purely antiquarian interest.

The Treponemal Diseases

The Here and Now of Treponemal Disease

The treponemal diseases are four clinically different conditions caused by infection with the spirochete bacterium, *Treponema pallidum*. They are thought to have evolved from a common ancestor. However, their history is difficult to unravel and has given rise to numerous hypotheses (de Melo et al. 2010), as we will discuss. Today, the treponemal diseases are found in specific geographical locations and are divided into congenital and acquired conditions (pinta, yaws, endemic syphilis, and venereal syphilis). Pinta is found in Central and South America; endemic syphilis (or bejel) in Africa, the Middle East, and central Asia; and yaws in West Africa and the South Pacific, the latter being the most common of the three (Barlow et al. 2021, 552–553; Stamm 2015). They usually affect people living in poverty. Venereal syphilis, however, has a global distribution, spreads without geographic frontiers, and thrives in crowded urban centers. The World Health Organization estimated that 7.1 million adults between the ages of 15 and 49 years acquired venereal syphilis in 2020 (WHO 2024i). The study of venereal syphilis, in particular, has focused on debate over its origin, evolution, and history. More than an argument of historical or bacteriological nicety, this controversy has global significance, and venereal syphilis is a challenge for the health care professions today.

Yaws, endemic syphilis, and venereal (acquired) syphilis are all associated with inflammatory changes in most tissues, from the body surface to the bones. It was thought that they were purely human diseases, but there have been reports of wild baboons in East Africa being infected by *T. pallidum* (Harper et al. 2012). DNA analysis has revealed that *T. pallidum* strains have affected these animals for a long time and that the strains that infect baboons are genetically diverse and not identical to human strains. Knauf et al. (2013) also suggested that this region may have been a reservoir for human yaws, and Chuma et al. (2018) have revealed that olive baboons, yellow baboons, vervet monkeys, and blue monkeys in Tanzania could be added to the list of nonhuman primates affected. Molecular analysis shows that the most likely infecting organism is the *T. pallidum* subspecies *pertenue*-like strain that is possibly of importance in steps to eradicate human yaws in Africa. This is a good example of the One Health concept in action: yaws flourishes in warm, humid, and tropical forest areas in West Africa, and *T. pallidum* subspecies *pertenue* appears to affect both human and nonhuman primates there. Treponemal disease in humans probably originally derived from an animal infection in Africa or Asia, as suggested by Hackett as far back as 1963 (see later in the chapter). All treponemal diseases are characterized by recognizable clinical stages of development, and the early stage is a relatively mild inflammatory lesion at the site of entry of the bacteria.

The There and Then of Treponemal Disease

The earliest European descriptions distinguishing these four diseases from other skin diseases (and from each other) stem from the early modern period when what we call "classic" descriptions appeared of many different diseases, not only infections. Yaws is thought to have been prevalent in Africa and entered Europe with the slave trade, whereas historical documents attest to the near-epidemic status of venereal (acquired) syphilis around 1500 CE in Europe, suggesting an almost meteoric rise in prevalence (Arrizabalaga et al. 1997). That observation lent support to the theory that the crew of Christopher Columbus brought back from the Americas a virulent strain of *T. pallidum* to an immunologically naïve population, or it may have converted a long-standing and comparatively mild disease, already in Europe, into one of fulminating character. Of course, the exchange went both ways and Columbus left behind Old World pathogens such as smallpox and measles, which wrought dreadful mortality upon Indigenous populations, compounded by deliberate spread (Duffin 2021, 181–182). Some suggest that treponemal diseases were already in Europe prior to the Columbian expeditions (Hackett 1967; Mays et al. 2003), but that they were not distinguished from several other diseases, including leprosy, and they draw support for this confusion in the medieval belief in the venereal mode of transmission of leprosy. Skeletal evidence from late medieval leprosy cemeteries does not support this proposition: Crane-Kramer (2002) reported a lack of evidence for skeletons with venereal syphilis in leprosaria cemeteries studied. In 1940, reacting to the introduction of laws to test for venereal disease prior to marriage, Holcomb examined the evidence for syphilis in medieval Europe. He relied on the writings of observers as early as the thirteenth and fourteenth centuries, among them Gilbert Anglicus and Guy de Chauliac, who described diseases that may now be interpreted as syphilis. These interpretations are dependent on the observations, acumen, and accuracy of recording of these early physicians and sometimes the wishful thinking of observers. No general agreement on them has been found.

The appearance of venereal syphilis prompted more unambiguous descriptions by the Dutch physician Willem Piso and the English physician Thomas Sydenham (*Epistle II*, 1679), and they both considered it a hereditary disease as well as contagious by coitus. Added to the mercury treatment advocated by Girolamo Fracastoro and used into the twentieth century, many therapies were tried, special attention being given to plant remedies from the Americas thought to have been the place of origin. Fear of contagion, moral opprobrium, and horror at the appearance of mutilating lesions prompted the establishment of various special hospitals and coercive measures of control. For example, Hôpital St. Louis in Paris specialized in skin diseases and syphilis; and as recently as World War II female sex workers were confined as a public health measure to keep soldiers healthy (Neary 1998; Parascandola 2009). The advent of penicillin during that time transformed management of these diseases.

The many names once given to venereal syphilis convey blame of enemies or "others," be they ethnically or nationally different, thought to have indulged in illicit sex: Mal de Naples, Arboyne pimple, Scottish sibbens, Swedish saltfluss, French disease (or Morbus gallicus), lues and Spanish pox, to name only a few. The word *syphilis* is derived from the name of a sinning shepherd in Fracastoro's 1530 allegory in which he aimed to present mercury as a treatment (Arrizabalaga et al. 1997; Duffin 2021, 172–173). No finger of rectitude is pointed at pinta, yaws, and endemic syphilis, but moral judgments surrounding acquired (venereal) syphilis remain and have long weighed heavily on the social construction of this disease. As a consequence, much time and thought have been devoted to the question of venereal syphilis and its origin in either the so-called New World (Americas) or the Old (elsewhere)—(e.g., Steinbock 1976, chap. 4; Baker and Armelagos 1988; Dutour et al. 1994; Powell and Cook 2005; Harper et al. 2008, 2011; Baker et al. 2020). Research on this question in paleopathology therefore requires well-studied and interpreted skeletons, with accurate dating (Baker et al. 2020)—information that on occasion has been difficult to establish for several reasons, including poorly preserved skeletons, lack of a clear date, ambiguous bone lesions, and absence of differential diagnostic options.

Infection of the Human Body with Treponemal Disease

The clinical effects of all the treponemal diseases have been known for many years, and basic pathological changes, both gross and microscopic, are identical. Differences between them are purely quantitative and of degree. Pinta may be regarded as somewhat different, despite the identical inflammatory reaction, because it is milder and affects only the skin (Barlow et al. 2021, 552); therefore, it is not manifest in skeletal remains. Pinta is usually acquired during the third decade of life, whereas yaws and endemic syphilis are infections primarily of children; of course, children become adults, and healed lesions will be evident. Pinta usually produces an initial lesion on the hand or foot, with others occurring later, all of which heal with scarring. Its current frequency is unknown, but it is not effectively surveyed for data today.

Venereal (Acquired) Syphilis

Acquired syphilis can be contracted during oral, vaginal, or anal sex (where there is direct contact with infectious lesions), and in pregnancy (mother to fetus), which can lead to stillbirth, newborn death, and babies with congenital syphilis; it can also be transmitted via blood transfusions (WHO 2024i). Ethically unacceptable studies of untreated people in Norway (Gjestland 1955), wet nurses in France (Sherwood 2010), sex workers in Germany (Benedek 2014), and the Tuskegee and Guatemala studies in the United States (Reverby 2009, 2016) generated information concerning its clinical appearance, immunology, bone changes, and involvement of the arterial circulation and the nervous system. Some of these studies were predicated on the search for immune treatment or prevention. They failed, and the information that they provided was already well known.

Venereal syphilis affects the body in four stages. After the infection has entered the body, about 3–6 weeks later a round hard sore (chancre) appears, usually on the external genitalia, and subsequently heals (Marks and Mabey 2020). During this time the infection spreads via the bloodstream around the body. This primary stage usually lasts around 21 days. If the infection is not treated, it progresses to the second stage. Here, a nonirritant generalized skin rash develops, and after 2 or 3 months, lesions occur within the mouth, which may resolve spontaneously (Hook 2017). The infection then becomes inactive with no signs or symptoms (latent stage). About 35% of untreated patients progress to the third (tertiary) stage of the infection, possibly years later (Goldmeier and Guallar 2003). Inflammatory change affects the bones, mainly with destruction but also with regeneration and repair (new bone formation). This stage marks the generalized spread of bacteria around the body. Coexistent with the skeletal damage, skin and soft tissue damage occurs, and inflammatory changes may affect the cardiovascular system, the brain, liver, and spinal cord up to 30 years later. The walls of the major arteries are affected, notably and classically in the thoracic aorta; they become structurally weak and dilate locally as aneurysms, which ultimately rupture with fatal bleeding into other organs of the body (Hook 2017). Inflammatory changes in the brain and spinal cord manifest as a profound psychiatric disorder, and there can be loss of the proprioceptive sense in the lower limbs, causing an abnormal gait (Hook 2017). Proprioceptors mediate position sense, enabling awareness of the location, movement, and action of parts of the body. In the past, this whole clinical picture was termed "general paralysis of the insane," or *tabes dorsalis*, and was an inescapable facet of terminal disease. Now venereal syphilis is treatable with antibiotics and can be prevented by the consistent and correct use of condoms. It is with the evidence of this tertiary stage that the paleopathologist is concerned, and Hackett (1976) documented the skeletal changes well. From this phase alone, the skeletal evidence for the antiquity of venereal syphilis derives.

Congenital Syphilis

There is yet another difference that adds a further dimension to the treponemal diseases. This is the ability of the *Treponema pallidum* subspecies *pallidum* of venereal syphilis to pass from an infected mother across the placenta to an unborn child (Sankaran et al. 2023). This unwelcome infection gives rise to congenital syphilis. It may suggest a difference between the species of *Treponema*, but the absence of congenital infection in endemic syphilis is rather puzzling, except that this is largely a disease of the young who are usually not as yet sexually active. Transmission from infected mother to unborn child was thought to occur only in venereal syphilis, but there is also anecdotal evidence of yaws also being congenital (Engelhart 1959), while Baker (2023) noted that all treponemal diseases can have a congenital component. Thus, finding evidence for congenital syphilis does not mean the underlying cause was venereal syphilis.

Transplacental passage of the bacterium likely occurs in pregnancy during the secondary stage of infection, when there is hematogenous spread of *Treponema*. The bones and teeth of children with congenital syphilis can be affected, and they may have rhinitis, sores at the mouth corners, a skin rash, jaundice, an enlarged liver and spleen, and impaired vision—for example, caused by cataracts, uveitis, or retinitis (Schultz et al. 2021).

Endemic Syphilis and Yaws

In endemic syphilis the bacteria are found in saliva, and the infection enters the body through mouth-to-mouth contact (e.g., kissing), via cuts or abrasions of the skin, or through sharing eating utensils (Barlow et al. 2021, 552). Unlike yaws, there is no generalized rash. The primary lesion is usually small and in the mouth or on the lips, making the diagnosis difficult. In yaws, a person is infected usually before puberty via contact with open skin lesions (Marks and Mabey 2020). Following an incubation period of several weeks or months (Barlow et al. 2021, 552), an inflammatory reaction occurs at the site of infection, usually on the leg, and then the infection spreads. Skin lesions can also occur on the soles of the feet and palms of the hands. Up to 3 months later, a more generalized rash occurs on the extremities, buttocks, neck, and face (Marks and Mabey 2020). After a period of latency, about 10% of people develop the chronic stage of yaws, during which the skeleton becomes affected.

Skeletal Manifestations in Treponemal Disease

Here we describe the key bone changes of yaws, endemic syphilis, venereal syphilis, and congenital syphilis that occur in the later stages of the infection; more detailed descriptions of skeletal changes can be found in Resnick et al. 2024 (447–450) and for children in Lewis 2018 (172–185). Examining different treponemal diagnostic options for paleopathology can be challenging, especially when the skeleton is fragmentary or damaged postmortem such that distribution patterns of lesions cannot be seen.

Generally speaking, the bones are affected with gummatous and nongummatous osteomyelitis, induced in part by an inflammatory reaction specific to *Treponema*. Nongummatous lesions include periostitis, osteitis, and osteomyelitis. However,

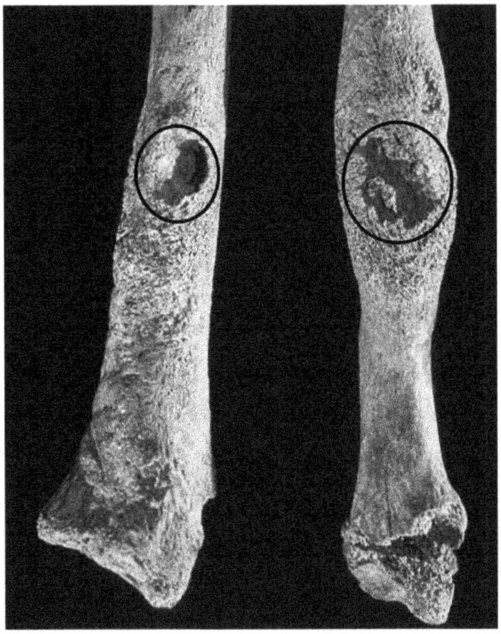

Figure 6.35. Gummatous lesions in the radius and ulna (black circles) (male adult, twelfth–sixteenth centuries CE, Hull Magistrates Court, Hull, England). Originally reproduced with kind permission from Don Ortner.

unlike some examples of nonspecific osteomyelitis discussed earlier, treponemal disease osteomyelitis is accompanied by extensive bone regeneration. In the late stages of yaws and venereal syphilis, inflammation causes gummas (soft tissue growths) that eventually result in bone destruction (Fig. 6.35). Not only can these gummas occur in the bones, but the skin and any of the body's organs may be affected. Initially, these are deep subcutaneous nodules, growing and eventually adhering to the skin, and they can ulcerate and release pus (Shao et al. 2018).

The frequency of bone involvement in treponemal disease was suggested by Steinbock (1976) to be 5–15% of people with untreated yaws, up to 20% of people with untreated venereal syphilis, with endemic syphilis lying between the two figures. However, Marks et al. (2014) pointed out that owing to the wide availability of treatment, these figures cannot be updated as untreated disease is rarely seen. As for congenital syphilis, there are major differences in the frequency of bone involvement in untreated early (birth to around 4 years) and late congenital syphilis (around 5 to 15 years)—in the former, almost all individuals have affected bones, while in the latter, fewer do.

Yaws and Endemic Syphilis

In yaws, the bones of the fingers or long bones (radius, ulna, fibula, and tibia) are the most affected parts of the skeleton (Marks et al. 2014, 2015). *Dactylitis* describes the inflammation of the fingers and their underlying bones. The fingers become swollen and the metacarpals and phalanges are affected by a central, destructive, and expansive lesion, called *spina ventosa* (also seen in TB). The joints may become damaged (erosive joint disease) due to nodular skin lesions causing ulceration and death of bone tissue. The skull is infrequently involved, but when it is, a few irregular crater-like depressions usually appear on the cranial surface, and destruction is generally more severe than in venereal syphilis, particularly in the oral and nasal areas (Manchester 1994). Occasionally the destructive process may be extensive of both bone and soft tissue of the face and results in gangosa, in which the whole nasal area and maxilla may be destroyed (Marks et al. 2014, 2015); this is a severely mutilating stage. More common, however, is osteomyelitis of the tibia, which, due to deposition of subperiosteal new bone along its anterior surface, gives rise to the "saber shin," so called because of its shape. As yaws is contracted in childhood, active lesions are seen at that point, but these may heal if the child reaches adulthood.

As with yaws, cranial involvement in endemic syphilis is uncommon, but may result in extensive destruction of the nasal area and maxilla. In common with yaws, the hand and long bones are the most frequently affected parts of the skeleton, and the saber shape of the tibia is present here too, but bone changes are less severe (Giacani and Lukehart 2014). The difference between yaws and endemic syphilis lies in the timing of the early stages of each disease and geographic location. Both diseases are common and endemic in hot climates, but yaws thrives in the humid tropics whereas endemic syphilis is prevalent in the arid zones lying north and south of the yaws territory.

Venereal Syphilis

Despite the similarities between yaws and endemic syphilis, venereal syphilis displays several differences. The mode of transmission from person to person is the most obvious difference; yaws, endemic syphilis, and pinta are transmitted through bodily contact, or via contamination of fomites, usually in childhood or adolescence, fomites being objects such as clothes or utensils that may carry the infection. Venereal syphilis is acquired, normally in adulthood, through sexual intercourse with a person infected with *Treponema* subspecies *pallidum*. Pathologically the most striking and significant difference is in the severe, incapacitating, and frequently fatal circulatory and central nervous system involvement, features not manifest in pinta, yaws, or endemic syphilis. This most advanced stage of the disease is termed neurovascular syphilis. The affected individual with stumbling faltering gait, given to bouts of irrational behavior, may die dramatically from the rupture of a grossly dilated major artery (aneurysm) and catastrophic hemorrhage. Since the bone changes develop between 2 and 10 years after the infection and as the only truly reliable evidence of venereal syphilis is derived from the study of human remains, it is probable that the prevalence of venereal syphilis in the distant past may be underestimated by as much as 90% (Ortner 2003, 279), and may explain the apparent rarity of the disease in earlier societies.

The bones affected include the cranial vault, the nasal bones, both upper and lower jaw bones, the tubular bones, the spine, and the pelvis. Multiple bone

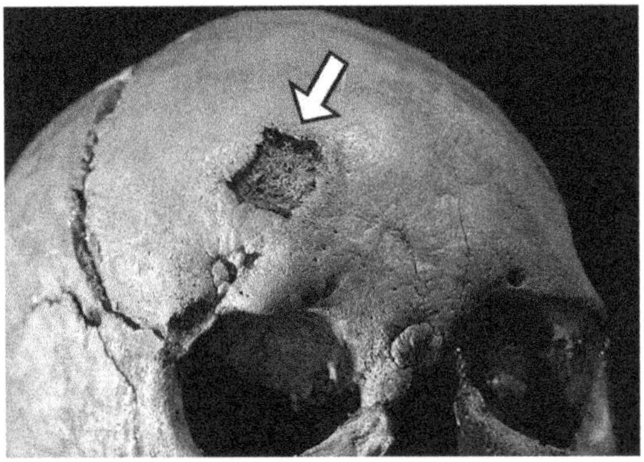

Figure 6.36. Involvement of the cranium in venereal syphilis (caries sicca); note the arrowed destructive lesion on the right side of the frontal bone above the eye socket, with some evidence of healing (twelfth–sixteenth centuries CE, Blackfriars, Gloucester, England). Originally reproduced with kind permission from Don Ortner.

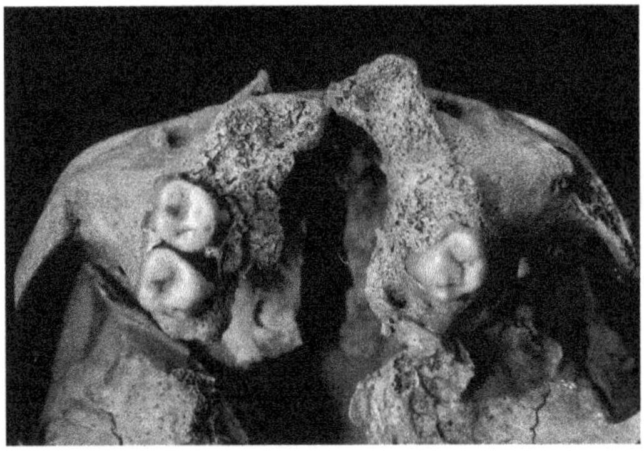

Figure 6.37. Destruction of the bones of the palate, with healing, in the same individual as Fig. 6.36. Originally reproduced with kind permission of Don Ortner.

involvement throughout the skeleton is frequent. Venereal syphilis may also result in destructive changes of joint surfaces, characteristically the knee. The joint itself may be infected or, at a later stage of the disease, may become damaged by the loss of proprioceptive sensation due to nervous system involvement. This so-called Charcot joint further destabilizes the gait. In contrast to yaws and endemic syphilis, however, the cranium is commonly affected in venereal syphilis, and it is upon this change that a paleopathological diagnosis is often reached. The bones of the cranial vault exhibit a characteristic "worm-eaten" appearance, and gummas in the soft tissues infiltrate the bone of the cranium, causing gross destruction, irregular repair, and necrosis (Resnick et al. 2024, 449). This bone damage has been given the name "caries sicca" (Fig. 6.36). Most commonly the parietal and frontal bones are affected. The inflammation commences within the internal substance (diploe) of the cranial bones and gradually spreads both outward and inward. Eventually perforation of the bone may result (Hackett 1981). Although changes also occur in the nasal and palatal bones (Fig. 6.37), they are not as pronounced as in yaws and endemic syphilis.

Congenital Syphilis

The skeletal changes of congenital syphilis are in some respects similar to those of venereal syphilis. In early congenital syphilis (fetus, neonate, and very young infant), osteochondritis, chondroepiphysitis (or inflammation of the joint cartilage affecting the growing ends of the bones), osteomyelitis of the diaphysis of long bones, and subperiosteal new bone formation are described (Resnick et al. 2024, 447). In late congenital syphilis, the early lesions may reduce or disappear, while the residual bone lesions resemble those in venereal (acquired) syphilis. Lewis (2018, 177) illustrated the differences in clinical manifestations. Gummatous and nongummatous osteomyelitis and subperiosteal new bone formation affect the long bones, especially the tibiae, and produce a saber shin, but the flat bones can also be involved, with new bone formation resulting. Destruction of the nasal bones and dactylitis of the hand bones are also apparent. The so-called Hutchinson's triad, which is a combination of dental changes, interstitial keratitis affecting the eye's cornea with possible blindness, and "saddle nose" deformity, is considered diagnostic. A unilateral enlargement of the sternal end of the clavicle, or Higoumenakis' sign first described in 1927, is also seen in a large proportion of children with late-onset congenital syphilis (Frangos et al. 2011). Hillson et al. (1998) noted that Hutchinson's incisors and Moon's molars are likely pathognomonic of late-stage congenital syphilis, but mulberry molars display changes that could be caused by other conditions (e.g., severe enamel hypoplasia). Hutchinson's incisors and Moon's molars will be apparent when the permanent incisors and first molar have erupted around the age of 6 years (Lewis 2018, 179), although radiography can help to visualize them before that time. Recent research has focused on the use of mercury for treating syphilis in the past by analyzing the severity of the dental side effects; Ioannou et al. (2015) described distinct morphological differences between congenital syphilitic teeth and teeth affected by mercury. They also suggested that signs of this treatment for syphilis may be the only indication that a person had congenital syphilis, although it has also been recorded as a treatment for leprosy in the poor. Walser et al. (2019), in studying skeletons from medieval Iceland, described the exposure to mercury for several purposes, including in pigments and for the treatment of diseases, but also the impact of volcanic eruptions on environmental mercury levels.

Mansilla and Pijoan (1995) reported a rare instance of congenital syphilis in a newborn from colonial Mexico, but few other individuals are reported (see next section). The rarity of congenital syphilis in paleopathological contexts may largely be because the disease likely carried a high mortality in the very young. In 2013, Newman et al. estimated that more than 370,000 perinatal deaths and 21,500 additional infant deaths are caused by congenital syphilis today. In archaeological contexts, it is possible that these tiny individuals are not found and may even have been buried outside the local community cemetery. One might also argue that the skeleton of a newborn with congenital syphilis recovered from an archaeological excavation will rarely, if ever, be recognized for what it is. As always, paleopathological diagnosis depends on discovery, preservation of evidence, and identification.

Debate over Treponemal Disease Origins

As discussed, for many years, the search for the origin and evolution of the treponemal diseases centered on venereal syphilis and its relationship to the transatlantic expeditions of Christopher Columbus in 1492 CE (Baker and Armelagos 1988;

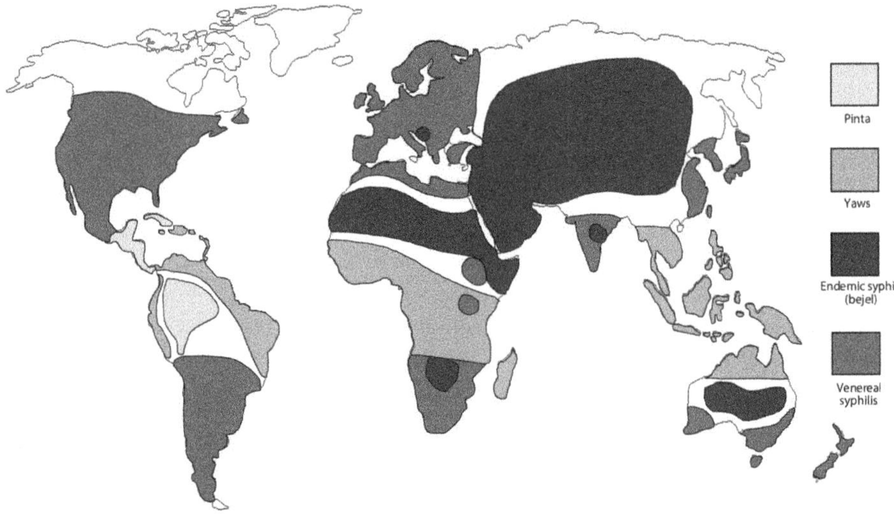

Figure 6.38. The worldwide distribution of the treponemal diseases around 1900 CE, that is, before effective antibiotic therapy (by Mary Lewis and after Hackett 1963, 15).

Crosby 2003). In general, scholars relate the European onset of the disease to the return of the Columbus expedition in 1493 CE. It was said that the crew infected Europe with treponemes originating in North America. Scholars from North America, in turn, have regarded the disease as of Old World, but not necessarily European, origin. Paleopathological evidence suggests that treponemal disease existed in Europe and the Americas before the voyages of Columbus. However, the pre-antibiotic, global distribution of pinta, yaws, endemic syphilis, and venereal syphilis may hold the key to the origin of these elusive ancient diseases (Hudson 1968). Figure 6.38 shows the 1900 CE global distribution of treponemal diseases. Compared to the present day there have been some changes (e.g., see also Melo et al. 2010). Yaws is currently endemic in parts of Africa and Southeast Asia (WHO 2024j); in 1900 CE it was prevalent in sub-Saharan Africa, central Australia, Southeast Asia, and Brazil. Endemic syphilis is now concentrated in the Middle East and southern regions of the Sahara. In 1900 CE it was frequent in North Africa, the Middle East, and into modern-day Kazakhstan and Russia, central Australia, and parts of southern Africa. Venereal syphilis is now ubiquitous globally (WHO 2024i), whereas in 1900 CE it was common in Europe, North America, India, and parts of Russia.

Several theories are debated about the origin, evolution, and spread of treponemal disease (Baker and Armelagos 1988; Powell and Cook 2005; Harper et al. 2008, 2011; Roberts and Redfern 2019; Baker et al. 2020). Essentially, they center around whether the different diseases within "treponemal disease" are caused by different species of the bacterial genus (*Treponema*), or whether they reflect different clinical manifestations of one species (*T. pallidum*). Hackett (1963), supported by Von Hunnius et al. (2007), opined that the different organisms were genetically distinct but were closely related. Hudson (1965) theorized that every social group has a kind of treponematosis that is appropriate to its geographic and climatic home and its stage of sociocultural development. Implicating individual susceptibility, it has also been observed that differing presentations can occur within separate peoples living in the same geographic environment. The relationship between geographic area, climate, environment, host, and treponemal infection is by no means straightforward.

The Columbian hypothesis is now widely discredited (Baker et al. 2020). If it were true, Waldron (2021, 170) argued, then the 50-man crew who returned must have been "extremely busy" in a short time. Given the length of time involved, the crew would have been in a latent state while sailing east and would have been infectious upon arrival in Europe. However, limited but often controversial evidence for treponemal disease in Europe before this date is seen as supporting this Columbian hypothesis (Harper et al. 2011), although this debate still continues (Cole and Waldron 2011, 2012, 2015). A fresh approach to radiocarbon (C14) dating using Bayesian modeling may alter the picture (Baker et al. 2020). Another theory, known as the pre-Columbian hypothesis, argues that one or more forms of treponemal disease, including venereal syphilis, already existed in Europe prior to Columbus's voyage, and his crew took the disease to the New World. According to this view, the disease was unrecognized in Europe prior to 1492 as it was confused with leprosy (Holcomb 1934). The Unitarian hypothesis argues for pinta, yaws, endemic syphilis, and venereal syphilis being the result of a single organism taken by human migration out of Africa and present in both Europe and the Americas pre-Columbus (Harper et al. 2013), with the clinical expression of the disease being determined by the climate, demographic patterns, and sociocultural context of sufferers (Hudson 1946, 1965). Our inability to distinguish between the lesions of yaws, endemic syphilis, and venereal syphilis and the genetic evidence for a near 100% shared ancestry appeared to support this hypothesis, although more research is needed (Baker et al. 2020). The final theory, known as the Evolutionary hypothesis, was championed by Hackett (1963), who suggested that pinta was the earliest global form of treponemal disease, probably derived from an animal infection in Afro-Asia about 15,000 BCE, and that venereal syphilis is its most recent manifestation. Hackett also considered that mutations of pinta after 10,000 BCE may have led to yaws, endemic syphilis, and then venereal syphilis. This theory has now been discredited too, as genetic evidence does not show a basal link between syphilis and yaws (Baker et al. 2020).

Baker et al. (2020, 7) called for "multiple lines of evidence derived from epidemiology, genetics/genomics, archaeometry (including radiometric dating and analyses of stable isotopes and trace elements), and paleopathology to test these theories." For example, linking evidence for treponemal disease in skeletons to stable isotope data and thereby tracking the movement of people in the past may elucidate the impact of migration on the spread of this infection. In a pilot study, Roberts et al. (2013) analyzed the potential and challenges of such a study. Dietary stable isotope studies of skeletons with treponemal disease have also started to appear in the literature, focusing on the bone response to venereal syphilis. Salesse et al. (2019) examined nineteenth-century skeletons with syphilis and offered three possible explanations for the isotopic patterns that they observed: diets prescribed by physicians; nutritional stress caused by cyclical appetite disturbances; or medicinal treatment.

Paleopathological Evidence for Treponemal Disease

There have been many publications on skeletal evidence for treponemal disease, including yaws, endemic syphilis, venereal syphilis, and congenital syphilis. As we are dealing with four different manifestations of treponemal disease, and as there are many syntheses of the data, we decided not to present a summary of the data for each condition as we have for TB and leprosy. The key sources include Steinbock (1976); Baker and Armelagos (1988); Roberts and Buikstra (2019); Baker et al. (2020: global); Dutour et al. (1994: Europe); Powell and Cook (2005: North America); Harper et al. (2008: modern strains of *T. pallidum*); Harper et al. (2011: Old World evidence reappraisal); and Lewis (2018, 182–185: evidence in children). Many of these sources discuss the limitations of the information published and make recommendations for future research too.

Most studies record bone and dental changes macroscopically through observation, description, and the production of differential diagnoses, although histological analysis has been used too (Von Hunnius et al. 2006). Because of confounding factors, such as poor preservation, cremated bone, and so on, that make a specific diagnosis difficult, many scholars are content with making a simple diagnosis of "treponematosis" rather than being more specific. After a controversial and challenging start, biomolecular studies have become a focus (see next section). Developing Hackett's (1976) descriptions of treponemal bone changes, Harper et al. (2011) created a recording system that categorizes treponemal skeletal involvement as pathognomonic, strongly suggestive, or consistent with, but not specific. Baker et al. (2020, 21–22) also provided a list of systematic observations that are recorded as present, absent, or unobservable, to generate a similar guide to the diagnostic status of skeletal changes in treponemal disease: C, consistent with treponemal infection; ST, strongly suggestive; and P, pathognomonic. Zhou et al. (2022) used similar criteria to analyze skeletons from the Central Plain in China (618–1279 CE), concluding that treponemal disease was present in China before 1200 CE.

What then of the skeletal evidence for this infectious disease? Paleopathological evidence of pinta is not found, and recall that only a small percentage of untreated infected individuals will display bone changes of their infection. Taking these facts into account with the often-presumed earlier age at death in antiquity, it is likely that studying the skeletal evidence reveals merely the tip of the iceberg for treponemal (and other infectious) diseases. Most skeletal evidence, to date, comes from North America and Europe, probably reflecting the larger amount of paleopathological research that has been done in those two regions; however, some data have been reported from Africa, Asia, Australia, the Pacific Islands, and South America. The quality of some dates produced many years ago for some archaeological sites has been controversial, not least because of the marine, but also riverine and freshwater, effect on radiocarbon dating. That is, consumption of marine foods can affect the C14 date produced (e.g., see Bayliss et al. 2004; Harper et al. 2011). Dating has been a particular challenge for evidence in late medieval contexts in Europe where diets could include freshwater and marine fish. Harper et al. (2011) also reconsidered previously published evidence of treponemal disease from the point of view of dating, but also their diagnoses: in Africa (4 modern-day countries), Asia (2 countries), and Europe (11 countries). In conclusion, they expressed concern that either the dates and/or the diagnoses of all the skeletons considered had been incorrect: "There is not a single published case from the Old World that can be confidently diagnosed as [both] treponemal and that has a radiocarbon date that places it firmly in the pre-Columbian period" (Harper et al. 2011, 124). This stance has been disputed (e.g., Baker et al. 2020). It is also not proven yet whether all skeletons diagnosed with treponemal disease in the Americas have been correctly dated and diagnosed (Roberts and Redfern 2019).

In paleopathology, continuous reevaluation of previously published studies allows us to reflect on what has been reported and whether diagnoses and dates stand up to scrutiny, especially as newer methods develop to nuance outcomes of previous studies. Nevertheless, we argue that there are indeed skeletons with correct diagnoses and pre-Columbian dates on both sides of the Atlantic, with much more evidence in the Americas, and in recent years, more skeletons have been diagnosed from a greater range of regions of the world (e.g., Marden and Ortner 2011: New Mexico, US; Radu et al. 2016: Romania; Walker et al. 2015: England; Ramos van Raap and Scabuzzo 2018: Argentina; Woo et al. 2019: South Korea; Pietrobelli et al. 2020: Italy; Castro et al. 2020: Chile; Tomczyk et al. 2015a: Poland; and Oliveira et al. 2023: Brazil).

Very rarely reported is the skeletal evidence of the cardiovascular complications in late-stage venereal syphilis (aneurysm, Fig. 6.39). For example, Kelley (1979) described four individuals with venereal syphilis from the early modern Hamann-Todd Collection, Cleveland, Ohio, with characteristic bone changes and signs of aneurysms. A skeleton from prehistoric southwestern Saskatchewan, Canada, with erosion of the posterior surface of the manubrium and the anterior surfaces of the second and third thoracic vertebrae suggested an aortic aneurysm, the rupture of which was probably responsible for the individual's death (Walker 1983). More recently, Castro et al. (2016) reported evidence in an individual from northern Chile of pre-Columbian date.

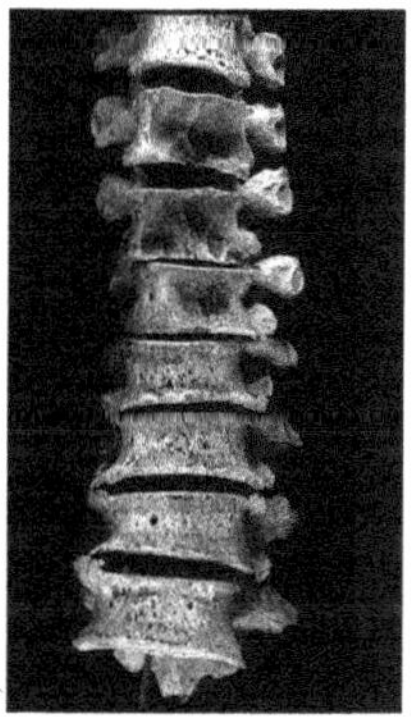

Figure 6.39. Anterior bone destruction of three vertebrae possibly due to an aortic aneurysm in a male who died of tuberculosis. From the Terry Collection, National Museum of Natural History, Washington, DC. Originally reproduced with kind permission from Don Ortner.

Treponemal Infection and the Biomolecular Revolution

The recent use of aDNA analysis for exploring treponemal disease is highlighted here. As an analytical method, aDNA analysis does not always answer the question asked, but it can provide detailed information about a particular infection and may reveal unexpected data. For example, Alves Cardoso et al. (2022) studied a skeleton with evidence for treponemal disease from a hospital cemetery in Lisbon, Portugal, known for treating infectious disease. Between 1511 and 1532 CE, historical data documented that a total of 20,000 patients with syphilis were treated there; however, aDNA analysis showed no evidence for *T. pallidum* in this skeleton. Instead, microorganisms related to respiratory disease, nonspecific infections, dental disease, and leprosy were present.

The first full genome sequence of *T. pallidum* was published by Fraser et al. in 1998, but more than a decade passed until the full genome sequences of *T. pallidum* subspecies *pallidum* and *T. pallidum* subspecies *endemicum* were published (Baker et al. 2020). Prospects for aDNA analysis of the treponemal pathogen looked bleak in the early days of PCR analysis (e.g., Barnes and Thomas 2005; Bouwman and Brown 2005; Von Hunnius et al. 2007). To add to the woes, Von Hunnius et al. (2007) studied archived samples of tissues, including bones, from two New Zealand white rabbits that had been injected with *T. pallidum* subspecies *pallidum* prior to being euthanized. They concluded that treponemal DNA enters the bones during the first stages of the infection, but is absent in the later stages when, in a human, the disease can be recognized in skeletal remains. As a result, researchers have suggested that trying to recover treponemal aDNA from individuals who may have died with congenital syphilis may be more successful, as they may have higher pathogen loads in their bodies and bones (Montiel et al. 2012).

As methods in aDNA analysis developed, including new extraction techniques, library construction, DNA capture, DNA sequencing, the application of next-generation sequencing, and better management of modern contamination, things began to look brighter (Stone and Ozaga 2019). Scholars also explicitly merged paleopathological with phylogenetic evidence (de Melo et al. 2010). As Baker et al. (2020, 7) have said, "advances in genetic and genomic studies are revolutionizing the study of treponemal infections by beginning to remove speculation and subjectivity from analyses of both clinical and paleopathological disease diagnoses." By 2021, over 300 *T. pallidum* full (modern) genomes were available to researchers (Baker 2023), already a large increase from the 150 documented by Beale et al. in 2019; these genomes provide the basis for interpretation of ancient DNA data. In addition, Schuenemann et al. (2018b) published historic *T. pallidum* genomes from skeletons of two infants and one neonate buried in a colonial (seventeenth–nineteenth century CE) convent cemetery in Mexico City. One was affected by yaws and two by congenital syphilis. While the researchers' data were admitted to not be perfect, they sought to apply whole-genome data to consideration of the various hypotheses related to the origin, evolution, and spread of treponemal disease, concluding that the Unitarian theory could be supported. They called for more research to produce greater genetic data from both modern and ancient *T. pallidum* in order to better assess the relationships between strains. Some research has also addressed the common ancestor of *T. pallidum* subspecies and subspecies strains, summarized by Baker (2023). Here again, more data are required from both modern and ancient samples with greater geographical diversity. A recent study of three treponemal genomes from 2,000-year-old human remains from coastal Brazil found that all three had similar (low-variation) genome sequences related to endemic syphilis (Majander et al. 2024). This outcome was interesting because the people whose skeletons were studied did not live in an arid region where endemic syphilis thrives in human populations. A similar situation occurred for a fifteenth-century skeleton from Lithuania, northern Europe, where the outcome of aDNA analysis was a diagnosis of yaws—unexpected in this region of the world with its climate unfavorable to yaws (Giffin et al. 2020). The movement of people in the past enabled infections to move too, and this person may well have moved from a "yaws climate" for a variety of reasons.

Brucellosis

Brucellosis is caused by bacteria of the genus *Brucella* and in animals is a common zoonotic infection today. It causes spontaneous abortions in animals and spreads via reproduction, grooming, and other social activities, so that transmission is promoted by keeping animals in close contact with one another (Uhl and Thomas 2022). Laine et al. (2023) estimated its annual global incidence at 2.1 million people, although some scholars think it is more frequent—between 5 million and 12.5 million (Hull and Schumaker 2018). In a review and meta-analysis, the global prevalence of human brucellosis was suggested to be 15.5% (Khoshnood et al. 2022), with males and females being almost equally affected; however, other studies report males to be more affected (Dean et al. 2012), perhaps reflecting the type of work males do when compared to females. This classic zoonotic infection is relevant to the One Health approach to disease that acknowledges the links among people, animals, and environments (Woods et al. 2017). Infection of the human population occurs through inhaling the bacteria, and via cuts and skin abrasions in people who have direct contact with animals (e.g., farmers, butchers, hunters of wild animals, veterinarians, laboratory personnel), as well as through consumption of infected meat and dairy products (e.g., unpasteurized milk or cheese from infected goats or sheep). Person-to-person transmission is rare; instead, industrial-scale farming of animals and poor hygiene in handling food are key risk factors partly responsible for spread to humans (WHO 2024c).

There are six species of *Brucella*. The first four include *B. suis* (pigs), *B. melitensis* (goats and sheep—the most common and virulent species that affects humans), *B. abortus* (cattle, bison, and buffalo), and *B. canis* (dogs). *B. canis* is a natural reservoir in dogs today, but dogs can also be infected by the other three species (Cosford 2018). Dogs with the infection are commonly euthanized in Western countries because of the public health risk of spread to other dogs or humans. The final two species are *B. neotomae*, found in rodents such as desert rats; and *B. ovis*, found in sheep. Most pathogenic to humans are *B. melitensis*, *B. abortus*, and variants of *B. suis*—that is, caught from pigs, sheep, goats, and cattle (Bendrey et al. 2020)—

and brucellosis affecting domesticated rather than wild animals is considered more virulent (Moreno 2014).

Once infected, any organ of the body can be affected (WHO 2024c). The incubation period ranges from 1 week to 2 months (usually 2–4 weeks). Also known as undulant fever, the symptoms of brucellosis are flulike—recurring bouts of fever, weakness, and weight loss—but symptoms are usually mild and can be treated with antibiotics. Musculoskeletal pain, coughing, gastrointestinal symptoms, blood disorders, and enlarged lymph glands and spleen can also result. As symptoms are mild and nonspecific (they could be caused by any number of conditions), people with brucellosis may go undiagnosed. Following the initial infection, however, the bacteria disseminate in the bloodstream and can cause bone changes. Ulu-Kilic et al. (2014) reported a skeletal frequency of between 10% and 85% today in various studies of living humans, with skeletal involvement being the most frequent complication of this infection (Esmaeilnejad-Ganji and Esmaeilnejad-Ganji 2019).

The bone changes can affect the spine and tend to start usually in the endplates of the anterosuperior parts of the vertebral bodies, which are destroyed in the area of the annulus fibrosus of the intervertebral disk—called the Pedro Pons sign (Mays 2007b). In addition, and radiographically, the pathognomonic sign for brucellosis is a hemi-ring of greater density (indicating repair) around the lower part of the destroyed areas in the spine; this is due to an increase in size of individual trabeculae and their numbers. These bone changes can occur in several other conditions, and differential diagnoses should include Schmorl's nodes, trauma, and, in particular, TB. As a consequence, Mays (2007b, 116) recommended that brucellosis should not be diagnosed on the basis of the Pedro Pons lesion without other supporting evidence in the skeleton. This includes spinal osteomyelitis and spondylodiscitis (simultaneous inflammation of the vertebra and its disk), as well as inflammation of the spinal ligaments. Other joints can also be affected, such as the hip, knee, ankle, wrist, and interphalangeal joints of the hands, but not as often as in the spine. The sacroiliac joint is often involved in *B. melitensis* infections, and in most people, the lower thoracic and lumbar spine are affected. If the infection progresses, then more extensive destructive lesions of the vertebral bodies may be expected. Unlike in TB, reactive new bone forms "parrot beak" osteophytes on the vertebral bodies. Like TB, new bone can form on the vertebrae and visceral rib surfaces, but there is no spinal collapse.

The highest prevalence of brucellosis in humans is in West Asia, the Middle East, Southern Europe, and Latin America. In the eastern Mediterranean, it is endemic, affecting 500,000 people annually. Control and eradication programs over the past 40 years in many parts of the world have resulted in improved training of people who work with animals and better surveillance of animals, slaughterhouses, markets, and transport (Khoshnood et al. 2022). Legislation and animal vaccination have contributed to lower rates of brucellosis in many countries, and eradication in some (e.g., of *B. melitensis*). It is surprising that in archaeological contexts brucellosis is rarely identified in either human or other animal skeletal remains. If we presume that the greater distribution of brucellosis in some parts of the world held true for our predecessors, we might argue that we do not see evidence because regions where brucellosis is endemic have not been subject to much paleopathological research compared to those areas that have (or had) a low incidence. For parts of the globe where paleopathological research is well developed, however, why are we not seeing more evidence? In their helpful review of brucellosis in the clinical and (selected) archaeological records for humans and other animals, including aDNA evidence, Bendrey et al. (2020, 2022) provided ideas for future research to make this infection more visible in the archaeological record. For example, testing of skeletal lesions proposed as indicators of *Brucella* infection could be undertaken in zooarchaeology, because it has been suggested that erosive lesions on the anterosuperior vertebral body could be indicative of *Brucella* in nonhumans, as for humans. Although diagnosis is difficult and reports of archaeological evidence have been few in number, to date, brucellosis in human remains has been reported in Albania, Iran, Italy, Jordan, Siberia, South Africa, and the United States, and there is aDNA evidence for both brucellosis and TB in human remains from Siberia (Bendrey et al. 2020). It has been suggested that brucellosis emerged 86,000–296,000 years ago, and about 6,500 years ago it started spreading in the Fertile Crescent—defined as Egypt (northeasternmost), Iran, Iraq, Israel, Jordan, and Türkiye (Pisarenko et al. 2018). We expect to see more evidence of this disease in future research.

Parasitic Infections

A parasite can be defined as an organism that lives on or in a host organism and gets its food from, or at the expense of, its host. Today parasites affect all climatic regions of the world and are a huge burden on human populations, as well as on health care providers. Many of the sixteen neglected tropical diseases are parasitic infections (WHO 2024f), which affect over 1 billion people globally in low-income countries, the vast majority living in rural areas (Alum et al. 2010). These diseases are very debilitating: they prevent people going to school or work, stunt normal growth, dampen cognitive skills, and weaken the immune system.

The earliest evidence for parasites comes from a cave in France 30,000 years ago (Bouchet et al. 1996), showing that parasites have long been human companions. There are so-called souvenir parasites, which have been acquired recently, and heirloom parasites, which originate in Africa and have been with humans and their ancestors throughout their evolution. A parasite is "symbiotic with other organisms . . . [and] benefits from the interaction while the host is harmed to some degree" (Reinhard and Araujo 2012, 750). However, the host may be benefited by the infection too. There are three main classes of parasites: protozoa (one-celled organisms), helminths (endoparasites: multicellular organisms), and ectoparasites (e.g., ticks, fleas, lice, parasitic flies, and mites that live on the surface of the host or within the skin and do not invade the inner body). While they cause infection, ectoparasites also often act as vectors in spreading infections. Examples of helminths include roundworm, hookworm, pinworm, whipworm, tapeworm, liver fluke, and schistosoma species (see Ledger and Mitchell 2022, 205).

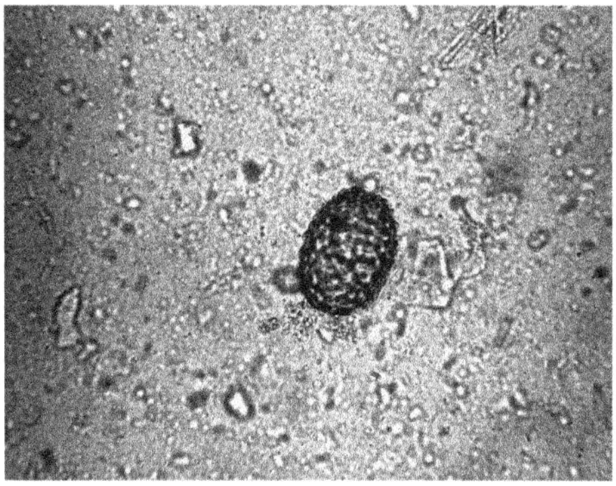

Figure 6.40. *Ascaris lumbricoides* (a roundworm) found in a soil sample from Seokmokri, Puyo, South Korea (Sabi period of the Baekje Kingdom, 538–660 CE). Scale: 75.0 μm (length), 55.0 μm (width). With permission from Min Seo and Dong Hoon Shin.

Endoparasites, which live within the host's body, tend to give rise to chronic disease and are therefore partly responsible for the chronic ill health that characterizes some of the poorer nations of the world today (Fig. 6.40). A similar situation probably existed in the more distant past. Since many parasites not only attack humans but also have animal host stages in their life cycle, a prerequisite for human infection is close animal-to-human contact; sometimes humans are accidental hosts. Many parasites began to infect humans only when, in the evolutionary process, the latter became omnivorous, eating meat as well as vegetables (Abuseir 2021). Several protozoa and helminths live within the flesh of animals either as adults or at some stage in their life cycles (Shanko et al. 2015). By consuming this meat, humans can become infected. This knowledge may explain the origin of the food taboos of certain religious groups. For example, avoidance of pork stipulated by Islamic (halal) and Jewish (kosher) dietary laws may be due to their knowledge in the distant past of infection of pigs by *Taenia solium* (one of the tapeworms) or *Trichinella spiralis* (a roundworm), and their transference to humans by eating infected pork (e.g., see Meyer-Rochow 2009). This knowledge would have resulted from years of conscious experience and careful observation. Parasitic infection of people is likely to have become more widespread with animal domestication, and its increase may therefore have run parallel with TB and brucellosis. Indeed, Hagen et al. (2023) suggested that after contracting parasitic infections through eating meat, early human populations may have found therapy in plants with pharmacological properties.

Evidence for parasites cannot usually be gleaned directly from archaeological skeletons, although they may be inferred indirectly from some evidence—for example, the presence of cribra orbitalia or porotic hyperostosis (Wang et al. 2024; and see Chapter 7). Most evidence in paleoparasitology comes from microscopy of preserved human feces (coprolites) found in the abdominal region of skeletons in sediments in their graves, or from the intestinal contents of mummified remains, rubbish pits, sewers, and latrines preserved in the archaeological record (Ledger and Mitchell 2022). In paleopathological terms, the evidence for these parasitic infections used to be sparse, with few exceptions (e.g., Jones 1985), but since the third edition of this book, many researchers have conducted research on parasites from a wide range of geographic areas, contexts, and time periods. Progress in paleoparasitology has been helped by methodological developments too, such as aDNA analysis (Stone and Ozaga 2019). The gut and oral microbiomes are increasingly a focus, and scholars are reaping many benefits from aDNA analysis, for example identifying once unidentifiable parasites.

Perhaps one of the earliest observations of a parasitic infection was made by Ruffer (1910), who identified eggs of *Schistosoma haematobium* in the kidneys of two mummified Egyptians from the twentieth dynasty (1189–1077 BCE). This condition, or bilharziasis, induces bleeding into the urinary tract and, even today, is a source of considerable morbidity throughout Africa, parts of South America, the Caribbean, the Middle East, and Asia. Another example of an ancient parasitic infection is that of the tapeworm of the genus *Echinococcus,* which lives in the intestines of sheep, dogs, foxes, and rodents. The parasite eggs are passed in the feces of these animals and if, due to food or water contamination, they are ingested by humans, the eggs enter the life-cycle phases of the worm. The larvae of the eggs penetrate the gut wall, spread via the blood, and develop into multiple cystic structures called hydatid cysts, which occupy various organs of the body, principally the liver and, to a lesser extent, the lungs (Torgerson et al. 2020). In a rare example, hydatid cysts calcified in a medieval Danish female with leprosy, and on excavation seventy-two cysts were identified with many cyst fragments in the area of her abdominal cavity (Weiss and Møller-Christensen 1971). *Echinoccocus* infection indicates a close association between humans and their domesticated animals; for example, it is known people have for a long time lived close to dogs (Bergström et al. 2020). Animals may have been used for hunting and herding sheep or may have been kept as pets and companions, as in recent times. The potential for parasitic transfer from dog to human has been ever present, possibly aggravated by squalid and unhygienic conditions in urban environments that increased human population exposure. It is therefore surprising that so little evidence of such cysts has been found, but they are thin-walled and fragile and may not have survived in the environment in which they were deposited.

Malaria is caused by the protozoan *Plasmodium* species and transmitted by the *Anopheles* mosquito species. It is the most burdensome parasitic disease today. In 2022, globally there were an estimated 249 million people affected with malaria and 608,000 malaria deaths across eighty-five countries. The WHO African Region carries a disproportionately large share of the global malaria burden, comprising 94% of malaria cases (233 million) and 95% (580,000) of malaria deaths. Children under 5 years accounted for about 80% of all malaria deaths in the region (WHO 2024e). Malaria may indirectly reveal itself in the skeleton through the bone changes of sickle cell anemia and thalassemia, inherited diseases that are an adaptive response that convey resistance to malaria (see Chapter 7). In all cases the context of the archaeological site needs to be considered. For example, sickle cell anemia occurs in Africa and thalassemia in the Mediterranean area, and while cribra orbitalia can occur in skeletons with both these conditions, iron-deficiency anemia can also be responsible. Consequently, to consider malaria, we might seek environmental evidence for a habitat that would have supported mosquitoes (Gowland and Western 2012). Thanks to developments in analytical methods, researchers have managed to extract and amplify aDNA of the malaria parasite. Consequently, direct evidence of malaria can now be retrieved from the skeleton (Stone and Ozaga 2019; and see Chapter 7). Recent research has identified *P. vivax* and *P. falciparum* across Eurasia dated to several thousand years ago. In particular, data from the Americas suggest colonization and the transatlantic slave trade were likely drivers for introduction to this continent. As for any infectious diseases, it is likely that cross-cultural connectivity helped spread malaria in the distant past (Michel et al. 2024). While aDNA data are being generated, at the same time some research is focused on macroscopic bone changes that may be linked to malaria (Smith-Guzmán 2015).

Of much wider distribution and much less clinical significance are the infestations of humans by ectoparasites. These organisms do not enter the body but live on the skin surface and hair. For survival they suck the blood of the host. Ectoparasites such as the flea, head and body lice, and ticks usually cause no more serious problem than a rash and the social embarrassment of itching. Occasionally, however, these arthropods may be the vectors of serious disease. For example, ticks may transmit Lyme disease, while human body lice transmit typhus (*Rickettsia prowazekii*), which is a serious, sometimes fatal, sequel to life in unsanitary conditions. Typhus was well known as "camp fever" to campaigning troops in recent wars (Polak et al. 2023) and probably was common in earlier times, particularly among the besieged and the besiegers in prolonged medieval warfare. However, only aDNA evidence in lice for typhus can provide direct evidence for typhus. Raoult et al. (2006) studied a grave in Vilnius, Lithuania, from 1812 CE and found segments of five body lice in soil also containing fragments of soldiers' uniforms; they also examined ten Napoleonic soldiers and identified the aDNA of *Bartonella quintana* in seven (trench fever, also transmitted by the body louse) and *Rickettsia prowazekii* in three. Other ectoparasites can be preserved in human remains. Head lice were found on 44% of a small group of mummified remains from North America (El-Najjar and Mulinski 1980), Zias and Mumcuoglu (1991) found head lice in hair combs in Israel, and Capasso (1998) reported head lice at Herculaneum, Italy, in a young female. The eggs of the head lice *Pediculus humanus* var. *capitis* are also common findings in the mummified bodies of Peru (Vreeland and Cockburn 1980). In Table 6.3, we provide some of the more recent research that covers a range of parasitic infection evidence in different times and places—although there is no space to document the many more reports that have been published (Table 6.3).

While parasitic infections have decreased over time with improvements in nutrition, hygiene, and animal management, these infections continue to burden low-income countries in particular. The paleopathological evidence of parasitic infection is becoming more common in the published literature, with approaches that involve new understandings of the environment (e.g., Morrow et al. 2016), theory (e.g., Mitchell 2013; Reinhard et al. 2013; Ledger and Mitchell 2022), and methods (e.g., Reinhard 2017; Barbera et al. 2023). This increase in evidence

Table 6.3. Some recent studies of paleoparasites

Place	Date	Source
Russia	44,000 BP	Slepchenko and Reinhard (2018)
China	9,000–7,000 BCE	Yeh and Mitchell (2016)
Argentina	1050–290 years BCE	Tietske et al. (2023)
Israel	Mid-seventh century CE	Langgutt (2022)
England	Medieval	Wang et al. (2022)
Portugal	Medieval	Knorr et al. (2019)
South Korea	Fifth–seventeenth century CE	Shin et al. (2013)

results from much more research in established laboratories in the Americas, Europe, and South Korea (Reinhard and Araujo 2012). Fortunately, the eggs of parasites from the distant past have particular characteristics that enable a specific diagnosis to be made through microscopic examination, as well as through biomolecular identification. With such knowledge, the clinical symptoms and consequences of these infections can be deduced. For example, abdominal discomfort, diarrhea, and constant blood loss associated with tapeworm infection probably accounted for much morbidity in past populations. Despite being largely controlled, at least in middle-high-income countries, parasitic infections remain common today, and they are also being used in therapeutic applications for the treatment of autoimmune and allergic conditions—for example, inflammatory bowel disease (Ledger and Mitchell 2022)—while a study in Ethiopia found that parasitic infection lowered the risk of developing severe COVID-19 (Wolday et al. 2021). Therefore, parasites clearly are not always (or only) harmful to humans.

Epilogue

Since the third edition of this book much has been written on infectious disease in both the clinical and the paleopathological literature, and the world has experienced the COVID-19 pandemic, an event that brought to the fore how humans are ever more susceptible to infectious disease as our lives become more complex. In this chapter we have focused on the more commonly occurring nonspecific and specific infectious diseases that we see paleopathologically. Specifically, we have emphasized the value of the increased research on poor air quality in the past using indicators seen in changes affecting the bones linked to the respiratory system, and we have acknowledged the advances in identification and interpretation of specific infections. For leprosy, new research shows how people in the past were more accepted by their communities than previously thought. For TB, we highlighted especially the development of research on nonspecific indicators of the disease. For the treponemal diseases, we focused on the need for more accurate dating and diagnosis. For the infections that also affect animals, such as brucellosis, leprosy, and TB, we referred to the One Health approach. For many infections, the biomolecular revolution has enhanced the paleopathological data. In particular, we have shown how infections are still with us and will continue to be so in our world, and we note the relevance of our research to the United Nations Sustainable Development Goals. Well aware of climate change and other risk factors for infectious disease, paleopathologists have produced amazing, nuanced, and informative data from many different time periods, geographic locations, and contexts over the two decades since our last edition. This research about the "there and then" is also relevant to the here and now, and for the future too.

7

Metabolic and Endocrine Disorders

In view of the prevalence of malnutrition in the world today, it is unlikely that it did not occur in the past, despite the vast increase in the world's population.

—D. Brothwell and P. Brothwell, *Food in Antiquity: A Survey of the Diet of Early Peoples*

Unfortunately, classification in clinical medicine is not all-embracing. There exist diseases of paleopathological significance that do not conveniently lend themselves to the categories used in the present volume. These diseases may loosely be considered as the conditions of deficiency or excess, not only of dietary constituents (metabolic) but also of the blood and hormones, the latter being chemicals manufactured by the endocrine glands for the maintenance of the body's health. Understanding the health impacts of food insecurity in the past has relevance today and can provide a deep-time perspective on the 2015 United Nations Sustainable Development Goals (2) zero hunger, (10) reduced inequalities, and (12) responsible consumption and production.

Metabolic Disease

Whatsoever was the father of a disease, an ill diet was the mother.

—George Herbert (1593–1633 CE)

As the quote from the sixteenth-century poet Herbert suggests, the link between nutrition and infection has long been known. Several deficiency diseases, such as pellagra (low niacin, or B_3, intake) and kwashiorkor (low protein intake), were once thought to be infectious because they occurred simultaneously within populations; only in the twentieth century were they shown to be nutritionally related (Goldberger et al. 1914; Williams 1935). There is a growing awareness that poor diets of mothers can have a generational effect on the development of adult chronic diseases in her child (Langley-Evans 2015), meaning our understanding of this situation in the past can help elucidate factors surrounding the developmental origins of health and disease in the past (DOHaD; see Chapter 1). The quality and quantity of food can affect health in two ways. First, if the diet is not adequate and the person is malnourished, then their immune system is weakened, and they are vulnerable to infections. Second, if their diet is lacking in one specific constituent, then the person may develop a dietary-deficiency-related disease. For past societies, population expansion often put a strain on resources, but improvement and refinement of agricultural methods shifted some groups away from starvation, albeit temporarily. This shift sometimes resulted in a greater risk of dietary deficiencies through reliance on a less varied and poorer-quality diet (Cohen and Crane-Kramer 2007). Starvation is still a familiar problem today in the less-developed areas of the world, particularly during conflict or pandemics, with deepening inequality and climate change, and where rain is critical for a successful harvest. In 2015 the United Nations estimated that 9.2% of the world's population are experiencing chronic hunger and 2.4 million fail to access sufficient nourishment. Growing genetically modified (GMO) crops may enable higher yields (Le Page 2002), but some are concerned that these crops may eventually harm biodiversity and exacerbate the problem of feeding the world's population in the future (Jacobsen et al. 2013). However, there is potential in developing GMO crops to combat deficiency diseases—for example, higher iron levels in GMO rice to address anemia (Holmes 1999). No doubt in the past, growing numbers within a community would have stretched the food resource, and famines were a significant threat. It is not just the total lack of food, or the overall starvation problem, that is of relevance. A lack of a quality diet, particularly in respect of essential vitamins, minerals, and chemical trace elements, is just as important. Conditions classed under the "metabolic disease" category in paleopathology can either be traced to specific dietary deficiencies (such as lack of vitamins C and D causing scurvy and rickets/osteomalacia, respectively), or be related to a general exposure to physiological stress brought about by an inadequate diet and/or infection.

Indicators of Nonspecific Physiological Stress

The intricate link between a poor diet and infection is perhaps best measured by a series of lesions known as indicators of nonspecific physiological stress. Many factors are implicated in their development; therefore, a direct causal relationship with an absolute lack of food and/or a poor-quality diet cannot be inferred, as diet is only one of multiple potential causes. The list of such stress indicators includes enamel hypoplasia (Chapter 3), cribra orbitalia, growth faltering, reduced stature, vertebral neural canal restrictions, elevated nitrogen values ($\delta^{15}N$), subperiosteal new bone formation (Chapter 6), Harris lines, and changes in cortical bone structure (e.g., cortical bone thinning, increased trabecularization, and cortical porosity). Mortality rates may also indicate how healthy and adaptive (or not) a population was, always assuming that the ages of adults have been estimated accurately. Infant mortality rates are used today as a measure of how well a population has adapted to its environment. A population is well adapted if they can keep alive the most vulnerable members of their society: the very young and very old (Lewis 2019a). High infant mortality rates may suggest that deadly conditions such as chronic diarrheal disease (where infection and poor nutrition go hand-in-hand) may have precipitated deaths in this age group, as it does today.

The majority of stress indicators represent the individual's adaptive response to stressors impacting the body during the growing years. That response will be determined by a number of factors—for example, the strength of the individual's immune system and genetic predisposition, environmental constraints, and cultural systems (e.g., see Schell 1997). In effect, the environment and the society in which a person lives will generate both the stressors and resources for the population to ward them off (Larsen 2015). Nevertheless, inherent frailty, where the individual has a decreased resistance to stressors, is highly individualistic and usually unrelated to age or the presence of a chronic disease (Fried et al. 2009). Stressors will therefore affect individuals disproportionately, and detecting why, and which people are more stressed (frail) than others can be complex, even in a modern context, something referred to as "hidden heterogeneity" (DeWitte and Stojanowski 2015). Clearly, a skeleton with no indicators of stress may suggest a situation of two extremes (an "osteological paradox"): a person who was immunologically strong enough or privileged enough never to be exposed to stress while they were alive; or someone who lacked the resilience to adapt to the stress, and died during the first insult (Wood et al. 1992). Hence, the idea that skeletal or dental lesions equate to poor health, and that no lesions on a skeleton equates to good health, is far too simplistic (Siek 2013). The age at death of that person may provide some clues, as stressed people will die at a younger age. Paleopathologists are tackling these complexities through a series of indices, such as the skeletal frailty index, which allows the accumulation of stress within an individual or group to be quantified (Marklein and Crews 2022), or weighted according to its severity—the biological index of frailty (Zedda et al. 2021). The list of indices can be long and includes femoral lengths as a proxy for stature, enamel hypoplasia, cribra orbitalia, spinal and joint degeneration, trauma, or osteoporosis. Lewis (2018, 9) suggested an adapted list for measuring frailty in non-adult skeletal remains. These indicators of frailty, however, are proving complex to apply. For example, Zedda et al. (2021) found that individuals in seventeenth-century northern Italy with lower skeletal frailty (i.e., "heathier") were more likely to be found within the plague pits of Imola's Lazzaretto, compared to the likewise "healthier" individuals from the attritional cemetery of Ravenna. But what of psychological stress? Since the mid-twentieth century, it has been clear that psychological stress can also lead to poor health (Seyle 1950), but measuring emotional reaction in past populations is usually beyond our reach. However, we do know that mental stress (along with myriad other causes) can lead to Harris lines of arrested growth in the long bones (Gindhart 1969, and see later in the chapter). In addition, stress may cause reduced cognition and ability to work (Temple and Edes 2022), which could in turn affect the production of essential resources such as food, potentially leading to dietary deficiency disease, a decline in fertility, and ultimately a decreasing population.

The following sections discuss some of the most commonly used indicators of stress in paleopathology, caused by unknown episodes of malnutrition and/or infection: poor growth, stature, Harris lines, and cribra orbitalia. Other indicators, such as dental enamel hypoplasia and subperiosteal new bone formation are discussed in Chapters 3 and 6, respectively.

Childhood Growth and Final Adult Stature

Normal growth of the body (and skeleton) follows two main periods of activity, the first being up to about the age of one year, and the second in adolescence (Crews and Bogin 2010). Intrinsic and extrinsic factors, such as genetic inheritance, nutrition, and the presence of infections, can affect normal growth. Generally speaking, stature has been increasing through time, and much of this reflects better nutrition and less infection due to improved living conditions and medical advances, certainly in middle- to high-income countries. However, normal growth can be intermittently compromised by famines, crop failures, or other crises facing a population. Traditionally, growth in children is estimated by taking mean dental age (considered the most accurate way to estimate the age of a nonadult skeleton), and comparing it to the long bone age (diaphyseal length) to measure whether a child was tall or short for their dental age compared to their peers. Saunders and Hoppa (1993) cautioned that as the children who died (i.e., the nonsurvivors) were the frail section of that population, their study had little to tell us about the growth of the children who survived into adulthood. To test this theory, Spake and Cardoso (2019) used postmortem long bone measurements of 292 modern children under 18 years from Cleveland, Ohio, who died from natural causes (that is, nonsurvivors) to those who died as the result of an accident (as a proxy for survivors). Further, they examined 656 records of girls admitted to the Sant'Anna Sanitorium in Portugal (1904–1953 CE) to test whether their risk of dying was greater the shorter they were in height. In both studies, surviving females in particular were taller and heavier than their nonsurviving peers, but the difference between the heights was not statistically significant. This study was followed by another that tested whether dental development (and hence estimated age) was delayed in nonsurvivors as a result of stress: once again such a mortality bias did not exist, at least not in these groups (Spake et al. 2021).

Research has suggested that reduced appositional growth (cortical thickness), may be a more accurate indicator of stress than long bone length. Mays et al. (2009a) demonstrated that children of lower socioeconomic status from eighteenth-century Birmingham, England, had lower cortical thickness for dental age than those of a higher social status. Using both linear and appositional growth of the femur, Gooderham et al. (2019) demonstrated greater growth faltering in children from the Christian post-Islamic periods in Portugal. They interpreted this outcome as showing a decline in living conditions after the fall of the Islamic Empire. At an individual level, discrepancies in ages derived from dental development, compared to those derived from long bone lengths, can provide insights into the environmental and health conditions experienced by that individual. Roberts et al. (2016) described TB, rickets, scurvy, and phossy jaw in a child from a Quaker burial ground in Tyneside, England (1711–1857 CE). While the dental age suggested that the child died between

12–13 years, the bone length suggested a younger age (under 10 years), demonstrating the toll exacted by the double threat of multiple infections and a toxic industrial environment on the physical growth of this young person, possibly a worker in the local matchstick factory.

Newer methods to assess the impact of stress during growth and development have focused on vertebral neural canal (VNC) size—the area at the back of the spine occupied by the spinal cord in life. A reduced canal size has been linked to stunted neural and immune system development (Fig. 7.1). Adults with smaller VNC sizes have been shown to die significantly earlier than their peers with larger neural dimensions (Clark et al. 1986; Watts 2013). There are two points during growth where faltering due to stress can have an impact on the dimensions of the canal; at 3–6 years when the anteroposterior parts of the neural arch fuse, and around 15–17 years when transverse growth is complete. Newman and Gowland (2015) measured VNC and vertebral body height in a series of children from postmedieval London. They noted a lower age at death in children with smaller transverse diameters. Newman and Gowland also reported reduced vertebral height in the older children who died. Rapid growth of the spine is expected during a normal adolescent growth spurt, making signs of reduced growth here a new and, perhaps, more sensitive measure of environmental stress. However, population differences in the size of the VNC should be acknowledged and may hinder cross population studies (Corron et al. 2023); more research is needed.

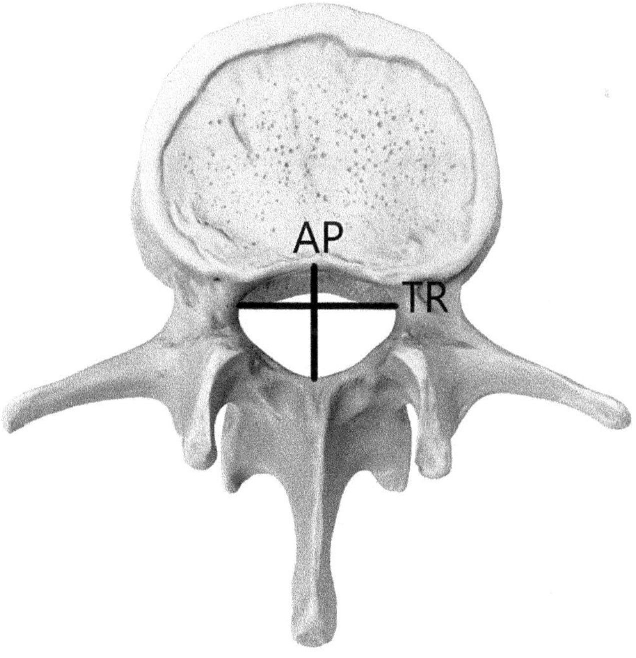

Figure 7.1. Measurements taken to establish vertebral neural canal size along the transverse (TR) and anteroposterior (AP) plane.

The final adult stature of an individual or population will reflect the environment in which they live, in its broadest sense. In addition, a decline in stature compared to what is expected in that particular group may indicate childhood nutritional stress, although a genetic predisposition to be shorter or taller than the norm can be present for some populations. Specific stature equations have been developed for specific time periods and places (Koukli et al. 2023: ancient Greece), but problems may arise using them if they bear little relationship to other groups under study. An alternative approach to evaluating adult height is to simply compare bone length (i.e., mean maximum femoral lengths for males and females) in archaeological groups to gain an understanding of final growth attainment in those populations (Meinzer et al. 2019, 236).

Harris Lines of Arrested Growth

In terms of etiology, less-specific bone changes seen in skeletal remains are Harris lines of arrested growth (Fig. 7.2). They are seen as dense, radiopaque (white) transverse lines on the radiographs of long bones, with the tibia, femur, and radius the most often affected, although lines in the ilia of children have also been observed. These lines have been interpreted as representing periods of slowed or arrested growth as a result of psychological stress, nutritional deficiencies, or infection during childhood (Harris 1931; Dreizen et al. 1959). There have also been suggestions that many may be part of the normal growth process, which naturally slows and accelerates as we grow (Magennis 1990; Lampl et al. 2003; Papageorgopoulou et al. 2011). The mechanism behind line formation starts with the arrest of cartilage proliferation at the growth plate; the thin layer of cartilage cells (chondroblasts) below the plate are replaced by osteoblasts, which begin to form a thin layer of bone, until they too become arrested. When the person has overcome the stress episode, the osteoblasts recover immediately and begin laying down more bone, visible on a radiograph as a transverse line (Park and Richter 1953; Miszkiewica 2015). Eventually, the chondroblasts too recover, and normal transverse growth begins again. Whatever the precise etiology may be, for a line to occur in a bone the individual has to have resumed normal growth (e.g., recovered from the stress episode). Hence they are, in effect, recovery lines.

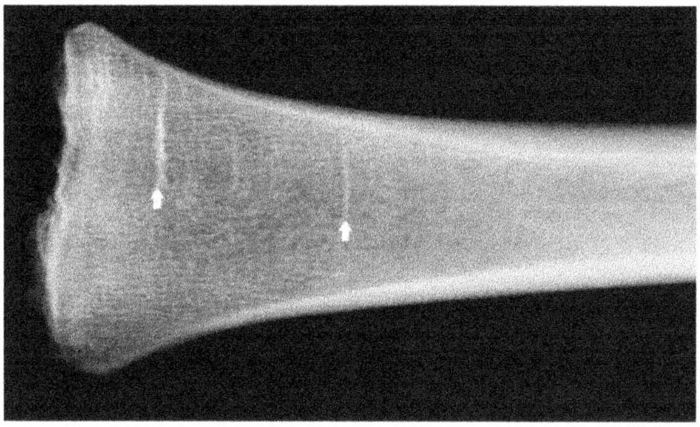

Figure 7.2. Harris lines on a radiograph of a child's bone from St-Helen-on-the-Walls, York, England (1100–1550 CE).

Paleopathologists have used Harris lines to establish the frequency of stress episodes in a population by (1) counting the mean number of lines, (2) estimating the percentage of individuals affected and, (3) estimating the age at which the childhood stress occurred (Lewis 2018, 272). Difficulties in interobserver error, especially in counting the number of lines, inspired Suter et al. (2008) to develop an automated method for recording them using digital radiographs, adding to a variety of methods (Kulus and Dąbrowski 2019). Current opinion suggests an observation of "presence" or "absence" is all that should be attempted (Primeau et al. 2016). While the prevalence of these lines may provide a general indicator of population health, suggesting specific physiological stress events in the past should be done with caution. Lines formed in early childhood will disappear or become line fragments as part of the normal remodeling process, and some modern clinical studies have been unable to associate the lines with any discernible stress episode (Lewis 2000, 2007). Boucherie et al. (2016) suggested that lines that form between the ages of 5 and 9 years are more likely to indicate the impact of a disease, as they do not coincide with a major growth event, while those formed between 10 and 14 years may be part of the normal adolescent growth spurt. However, if considered through the lens of growth, Harris lines can provide insight into a disease process. For example, Ortner (2003, 203) used the space between Harris lines in the infected distal tibia of a 6-year-old from Montgomery County, Maryland (1200–1300 CE), to suggest abnormal and accelerated longitudinal growth as a result of extra blood at the affected site.

Cribra Orbitalia and Porotic Hyperostosis

A diet low in iron, cultural factors such as poor hygiene (leading to parasitic and other infections), subsistence strategies such as farming, dietary choice, social status, preexisting diseases, and biological sex all contribute, together or individually, to anemia in populations (WHO 2023a). Hence, diet is only one of the potential causes of anemia. Porous lesions on the superior surface of the orbits (CO) and on the cranial vault (PH) have been associated with iron-deficiency anemia, or an inherited form of anemia, in archaeological populations for many decades. Iron in the blood may be reduced due to a lack of the nutrient in the diet, as the result of long-standing blood loss, chronic infection (where the bacteria deplete the body's iron stores), or lack of absorption in the gut; hence, these lesions are also regarded as nonspecific indicators of physiological stress. Recently, there has been a renewed interest in the study of cribra orbitalia, and the mechanisms behind it in recent years, especially because of the importance of anemia in the health of modern populations. Current theories will be outlined later in the chapter.

Overall, about 66% of the world's 1.7 billion people who have anemia have been estimated to be iron deficient due to many causes, with the most susceptible being growing children, premenopausal females, and pregnant females (Cappellini et al. 2020; Gardner et al. 2023; Young et al. 2023). Furthermore, it has been reported that maternal anemia has a detrimental effect on birth outcomes (miscarriages, stillbirths, low birth weight). In 2014, the World Health Organization (WHO) pledged to halve the rate of anemia in pregnant women by 2025 (from 38% to 19%), although in 2023(e) the WHO reported a rate of 37%, a decline of only 1%. There are a number of anemias of different causes, but this section deals mainly with the most common form of anemia today, that caused by iron deficiency. For a much more in-depth discussion of this condition, see Brickley et al. 2020.

Anemia can be defined as a reduction in concentration of hemoglobin and/or red blood cells below normal for the age and biological sex of the person, or a reduction in the volume of cells in the blood. Iron is needed for the development of hemoglobin in new red blood cells formed in bone marrow. A person with iron-deficiency anemia has pale and small red blood cells that have a reduced life span of almost half the normal 120 days (Lopez et al. 2016). Iron is usually stored in the liver and the spleen where old or damaged blood cells are broken down. Around 90% of the iron in old red blood cells is needed to form new cells and, as iron deficiency develops, iron stores are depleted while the body attempts to increase absorbtion of iron. As well as being needed for hemoglobin formation in red blood cells, which then transfers oxygen from the lungs to the rest of the body, iron is also necessary for the transmission of nerve impulses and collagen (protein) synthesis, and it contributes to a healthy immune system (Haschka et al. 2021). Fatigue, pallor, headaches, shortness of breath, fainting, palpitations, and an increased heart rate characterize the disease, with more severe forms creating growth and cognitive development problems (Ryan 1997), gastrointestinal disturbances, cardiac failure, and anomalies in the skin and skeleton. Spoon-shaped (koilonychia) brittle nails can also occur. This latter feature has been identified in the arm of a fourth-century CE bronze statue from Gloucestershire, England (Hart 1980).

There are two forms of iron, nonheme, which is mainly derived from cereals and is poorly absorbed by the intestines, and heme iron, which comes from red meats and is more easily absorbed (Brickley et al. 2020, 205). For example, only 1.4% of iron from spinach is taken in by the body, while 20% of iron from red meat can be absorbed (Scrimshaw 2000, 252). Compounds called phytates in staple cereal crops such as maize, as well as nuts and legumes, inhibit iron absorption, whereas vitamin C aids absorption. Cereals are themselves poor sources of iron (Stuart-Macadam 1992), and it is notable that iron is added today to many of the cereals we eat at breakfast. Thus, the transition from a hunter-forager to an agriculturally based economy relying on these crops for an adequate varied diet may have led to iron deficiency in the past (Fig. 7.3). Paleopathological reviews of the impact of agriculture in many areas of the world have shown that, in fact, there are no consistent patterns at this transition, with frequencies of porotic hyperostosis often appearing to increase while cribra orbitalia stayed consistent or declined (Cohen and Crane-Kramer 2007, 343). In British contexts too there seems to be general increase in cribra orbitalia (anemia) through time (Roberts and Cox 2003, chaps. 2–6), although absolute frequency rates were difficult to determine in this study, and a decline was seen in the Iron Age (late 800 BCE–100 CE) and in the postmedieval period (1550–ca. 1850 CE).

Apart from an iron-deficient diet, excessive blood loss through injury, heavy menstruation, cancer, and parasitic infection of the gut probably had a large part to play in the past as they do now. It is known from the survival of parasites in archaeological deposits that humans were subject to parasitic infections as a result of farming methods and poor hygienic practices (Fig. 7.4). Furthermore, advances in aDNA analysis allows for helminths to be differentiated, providing greater insights into human-versus-animal-derived parasites (Flammer and Smith 2020).

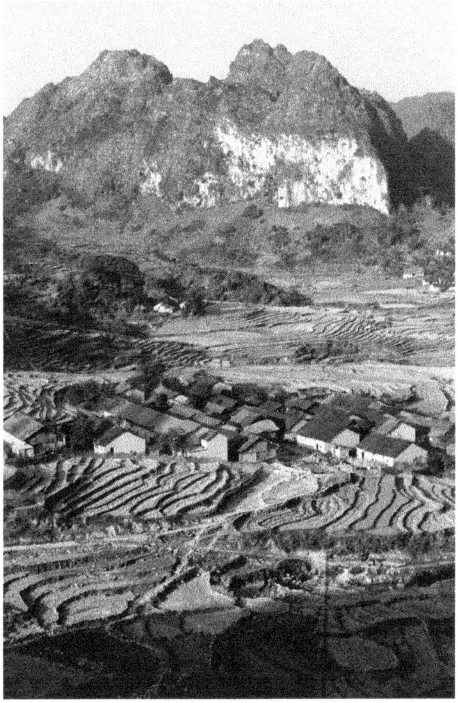

Figure 7.3. China: intensive agriculture, which could generate a less balanced and varied diet. Photograph by Charlotte Roberts.

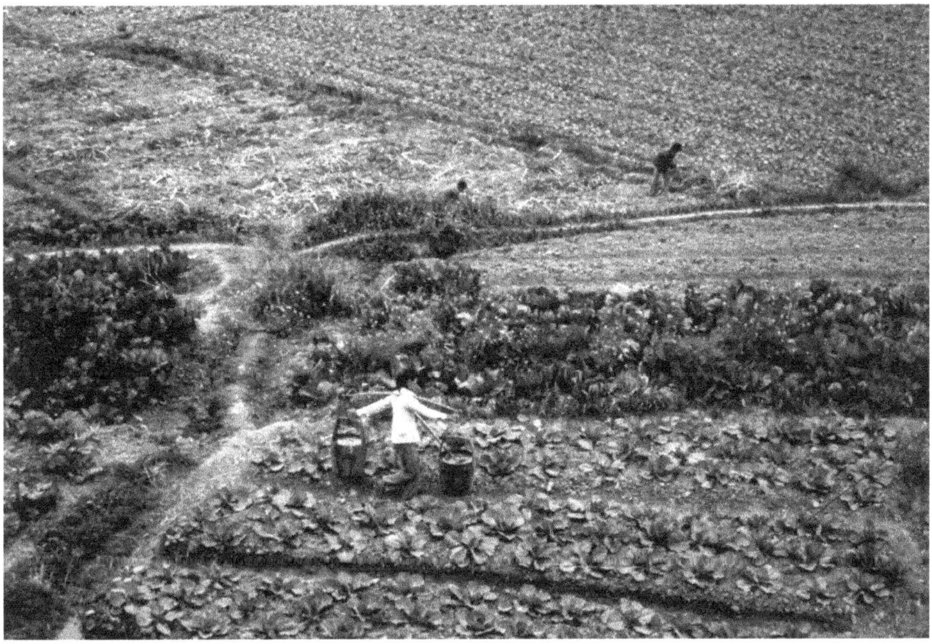

Figure 7.4. China: watering vegetables with "night soil" in an area with little naturally occurring water. Parasitic infections are prevalent from this farming practice. Photograph by Charlotte Roberts.

Last, but certainly not least, is the impact of chronic infection on a population. Most nutritional deficiencies are aggravated by infection, and poor living conditions and sanitation could predispose people to infections. During the process of bacterial infection, the body may withhold iron from the pathogens that need it to survive and reproduce in the body; this makes the body iron deficient and is known as "inflammatory anemia" (Valente de Souza et al. 2021). Work on the medieval skeletons from the Danish leprosy hospital at Naestved indicated that two-thirds of the group with bone changes of leprosy had skeletal indications of anemia. At that time, Møller-Christensen (1953) believed the lesions in the orbits (cribra orbitalia) were indicative of anemia due to leprous infection of the lacrimal tissues within the orbital roof. This theory is no longer supported, but infection is believed to be linked to cribra orbitalia (see p. 214). Cribra orbitalia is the lesion most commonly associated with iron-deficiency anemia in the archaeological record. It is recognized as a porous, pitted area found on the superior surface of the orbits. Lesions in the proximal femur and humerus have also been proposed for iron deficiency anemia (cribra femoralis and cribra humeralis; see Schats 2021), but need further research (Lewis 2018, 194).

Cribra orbitalia is thought to occur due to abnormal proliferation of the red-blood-cell-forming (erythropoietic) tissue within the red bone marrow, provoking a thinned cortex and resulting in "pepper-pot" or "hair-on-end" lesions (Fig. 7.5). As red bone marrow is present only in the orbits of children, up to the age of around 11 years (Brickley 2018), cribra orbitalia is a sign of childhood anemia—although if the anemia persists into adulthood, active lesions may be visible in adult skeletons. In adults, we normally see healed lesions (i.e., filled-in pits or pits with rounded edges).

In some of the earliest work into these lesions, Stuart-Macadam (1989) had proposed that because of the similarity of orbital and vault lesions (porotic hyperostosis) radiographically, both were caused by the same etiological factor. Now, orbital lesions are considered suggestive of severe anemia caused by deficiencies in folic acid and vitamin B_{12} (found in fresh meat and leafy vegetables), while porotic hyperostosis on the cranial vault (Figs. 7.6 and 7.7) is caused by an inherited anemia (Walker et al. 2009; Oxenham and Cavill 2010). Their often distinct etiology was illustrated in 2019 by Papathanasiou et al., who compiled the skeletal data for cribra orbitalia and porotic hyperostosis from different European regions, settlement types, and time periods. Of the 11,330 adults and children

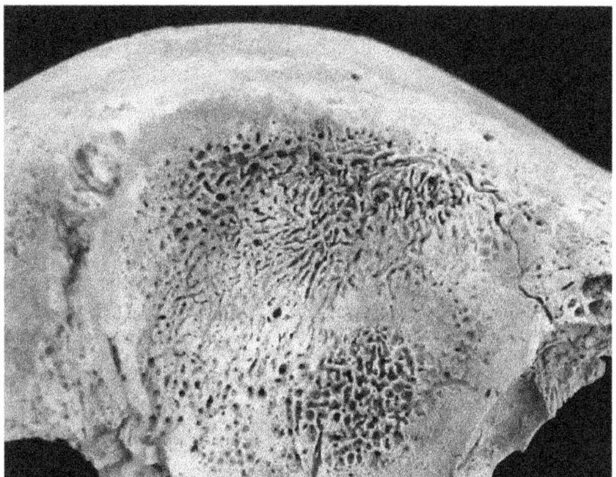

Figure 7.5. Cribra orbitalia on the right orbit of a non-adult from late Roman Kültepe, Kayseri, in Türkiye. Photograph courtesy of Handan Üstündağ, Kültepe Excavation Archives, with the kind permission of Fikri Kulakoğlu.

with both orbits and cranial vaults available for examination, just 3.4% (n = 391) of individuals had both orbital and cranial lesions, while 12.9% (n = 1465) had orbital lesions only; 3.1% displayed only porotic hyperostosis. They also found that farming communities displayed the highest rates of porotic hyperostosis, as well as cribra orbitalia through time (Papathanasiou et al. 2019). Proposing an additional etiology for cribra orbitalia, O'Donnell et al. (2020) noted that children living in New Mexico (2011–2019 CE) with respiratory infections were more likely to display cribra orbitalia and/or porotic hyperostosis than those who did not. They suggested anemia may have predisposed children to a secondary infection, or inflammation as a consequence of the respiratory infection may have caused impaired intestinal absorption of nutrients, and iron-deficiency anemia (also see O'Donnell et al. 2023 on the length of illness and porous lesions).

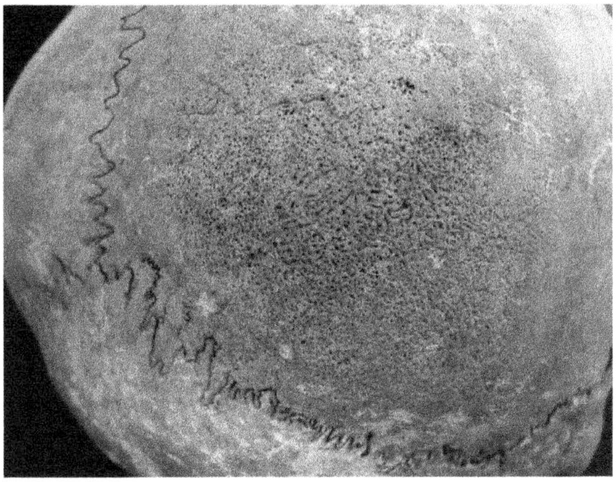

Figure 7.6. Porous cranial lesions on the right parietal bone of a nonadult from late Roman Kültepe, Kayseri, in Türkiye. Photograph courtesy of Handan Üstündağ, Kültepe Excavation Archives, with the kind permission of Fikri Kulakoğlu.

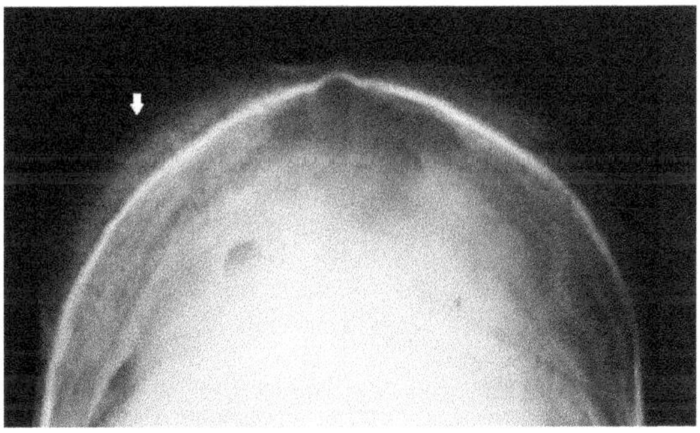

Figure 7.7. Radiograph of porotic hyperostosis showing hair-on-end organization of the trabeculae. Courtesy of the University of Reading Clinical Radiograph Collection.

Brickley (2024) cautioned that porous lesions tend to be age related and have a low frequency in individuals with anemia today, and so may not provide the best evidence for anemia in the past. Instead, she suggested increasing our analytical methods to include measurements of cranial or orbital thickness, and paying careful attention to the appearance of porotic hyperostosis (hair-on-end organization of trabeculae, rather than layering of new bone) (Fig. 7.8). The problem is that porous lesions occur in many pathological conditions—for example, similar porous lesions in the cranial vault may result from vitamin C and D deficiency (scurvy and rickets, respectively, although subtle differences exist), inflammation of the cranium, and some tumors.

Prevalence rates of cribra orbitalia vary considerably in the literature and are often based on small sample sizes, using a variety of recording schemes. A review of the frequency of cribra orbitalia in children from sites around the

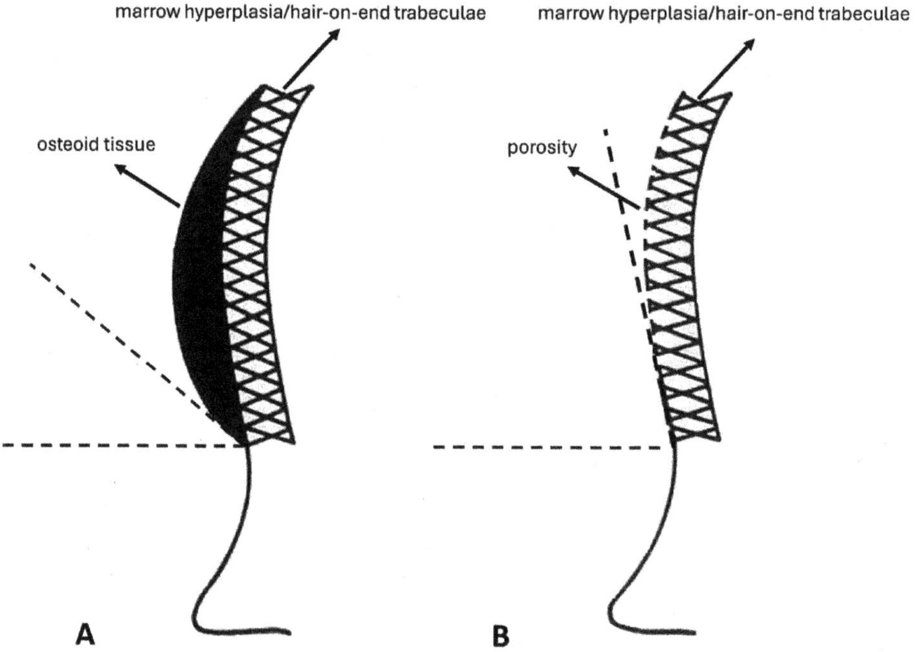

Figure 7.8. Changes to the cranium in an individual with rickets and anemia (A) and anemia (B). Adapted from Lanzkowsky 1968, 23a.

world revealed crude prevalence rates, from 4% in early medieval Gloucestershire, England, to 78% in Iron Age/early Roman Alvastra, Sweden (Lewis 2018, 197). Zarifa et al. (2016) explored carbon, oxygen, and nitrogen stable isotopes values in children with cribra orbitalia in seventeenth-to-eighteenth-century Latvia. Significantly lower nitrogen ($\delta^{15}N$) values in those with cribra orbitalia indicated these children may have been consuming less meat. Marine hunter-foragers in Patagonia (3800–100 BCE) had higher frequencies of porotic hyperostosis than farmers from the same region, which Suby (2014) suggested may indicate a high parasite load from contaminated marine foods. Interestingly, rates of cribra orbitalia were lower than for porotic hyperostosis, with the opposite of the pattern seen in most European groups; this may indicate that a genetic component was influential in Patagonia.

Genetic Anemia

Although iron-deficiency anemia is the most commonly observed anemia today (and probably in the past), two inherited anemias characterized by abnormal hemoglobin should also be discussed: thalassemia and sickle cell anemia. Although strictly congenital conditions, the lesions they give rise to provide a differential diagnosis for iron-deficiency anemia, and so they are considered here.

Both are called hemolytic anemias—that is, they are characterized by increased destruction of red blood cells. They produce bone changes in areas of the skeleton in addition to the cranium but, essentially, the cranial changes are the same for all the anemias (see Hershkovitz et al. 1997 on differential diagnostic features of the anemias).

Thalassemia is genetically determined and caused by a disfunction in hemoglobin synthesis. It is named alpha (α) or beta (β) thalassemia according to which globin chain of the hemoglobin (alpha or beta) has the genetic mutation (Kattamis et al. 2022). It may be polygenetic (caused by the combined action of more than one gene) or monogenic in origin. Failure or depression of synthesis of the chain leads to small, pale cells with low hemoglobin content, which are rapidly destroyed once formed. Thalassemia is the most common monogenic disease, with at least 60,000 severely affected individuals born worldwide each year (Higgs et al. 2012). It is estimated 1.5% of the global population carry a β-thalassemic allele (a mutated gene) and 5% carry an α-thalassemia allele (Kattamis et al. 2020). The classic and most common form of thalassemia is β-thalassemia, which affects groups from the central and eastern Mediterranean (i.e., Italy, Greece, and North Africa). Both beta and alpha thalassemia may be found in other areas of the world, including India, Thailand, Malaysia, and China (Kattamis et al. 2022). There are three types of thalassemia: minor (symptomless), intermedia (moderate form), and major (severe form) (Taher et al. 2018). It is unlikely that children born with T. major would survive beyond infancy in the past. Children with T. intermedia may survive up to the age of 6 years before a blood transfusion—not available in the ancient past—would be needed (Lewis 2018, 200). Over 500 α- or β-thalassemic genetic variants have been described in the online database HbVar (Giardine et al. 2021), and a high variation in the clinical presentation of the disease is caused by this genetic variation. This includes people who are "non-blood-transfusion dependent" who may survive with thalassemia into adulthood, and may have done in the past—although these variants are not without their serious side effects, and today still require transfusions at times of stress (i.e., during pregnancy, surgery, or infection) (Musallam et al. 2021).

Lagia et al. (2006) described the skeletal changes of thalassemia in a 14-year-old girl from a modern documented collection at the University of Athens with hair-on-end-related porotic hyperostosis, absence of the cranial sutures, and an expanded maxilla, widened intraorbital space, protrusion of the upper incisors, delayed dental development, and bony masses on the ribs. The child had undergone blood transfusions and so it is difficult to predict the natural progression of the disease. The first archaeological evidence of thalassemia in England was discovered at Roman-British Poundbury Camp in Dorset (fifth century CE), where expanded masses on the ribs (osteomas) typical of the clinical disease were identified (Lewis 2011). Many more infants at this site had general wasting (osteopenia; see later in the chapter) hinting that they may have died from the more fatal form of the disease (Fig. 7.9a and b). As thalassemia is a condition strongly linked to the Mediterranean, its presence suggests the children were born to wealthy immigrant parents (Lewis 2011).

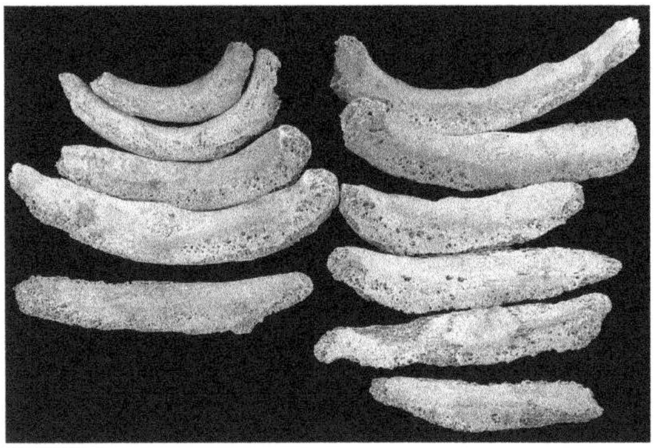

Figure 7.9A. Thalassemia intermedia in an infant from Poundbury Camp Dorset (fifth century CE) with porosity and costal osteomas on the ribs. Photograph taken by Mary Lewis with the kind permission of the Natural History Museum, London.

Rohnbogner (2016) also identified possible ß-thalassemia in a one-year-old infant from Romano-British Colchester, England. Other evidence of thalassemia comes from Thailand in Southeast Asia, presented by Tayles (1996), who described skeletons with indicative changes dating to 2000–1500 BCE. Bone abnormalities in the paranasal sinuses, mastoid processes, and facial bones were seen, in addition to the cranial vault and orbital lesions already described. The long bones and metacarpals and metatarsals were also enlarged, with thinning of their cortices, along with generalized osteopenia of the spine and premature closure of epiphyses. Tomczyk et al. (2015b) used aDNA analysis to identify an Asian ancestry in an adult with cribra orbitalia, porous lesions on the zygomatic bones, and hair-on-end porotic hyperostosis living in Roman period Tell Ashara, Syria (883–859 BCE). It was suggested this individual may have been suffering from ß-thalassemia intermedia, explaining the presence of the condition in a nonendemic area.

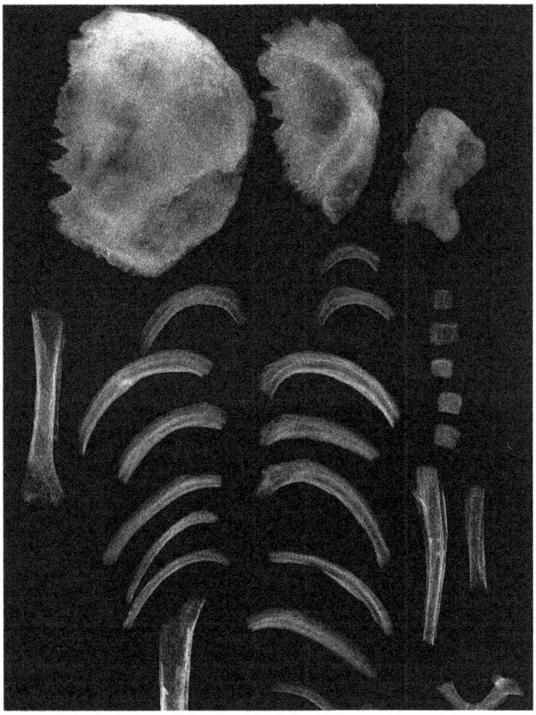

Figure 7.9B. Thalassemia intermedia in an infant from Poundbury Camp Dorset (fifth century CE) with porosity and costal osteomas on the ribs giving a characteristic radiographic "rib-within-a rib" appearance. Photograph taken by Mary Lewis with the kind permission of the Natural History Museum, London.

People with either sickle cell anemia or thalassemia have a resistance to malaria possibly because the infection cannot develop fast enough between the formation and death of the hemolytic red blood cells during their short life span (Cao and Vickers 2021). Malaria is carried from human to human through the bite of the infected female mosquito of the genus *Anopheles*, and the malaria parasites *Plasmodium vivax* and *falciparum* today are responsible for most cases and deaths (Cao and Vickers 2021). Angel (1966) felt that the porotic hyperostosis identified in skeletons from Cypriot, Greek, and Turkish contexts, deriving from marshy environments probably laden with malaria-carrying mosquitoes, was an adaptive response to malaria (through thalassemia development). Taylor et al. (1997) first reported aDNA analysis of *Plasmodium* (the malaria parasite's genus). Prior to this, Filon et al. (1995) had diagnosed beta-thalassemia using aDNA analysis, along with a mutated beta-thalasemia gene, in an 8-year-old child from Akhziv, Israel (16th–19th century). In Southeast Asia, Vlok et al. (2021) identified thalassemia in hunter-forgers from Man Bac, Vietnam (6200–6700 BCE), before agriculture and land clearances led to exposure of the population to malaria, suggesting a different driver for the development of that disease in that location. While porotic hyperostosis and cribra orbitalia may be an indirect indication of malaria, no specific (or pathognomonic) bone changes have been identified for malaria, and therefore aDNA analysis is the only method of directly diagnosing malaria in skeletal remains. Recognized as a distinct disease since antiquity because of the characteristic periodic fever, malaria and the history of its impact on various ancient populations has been reviewed by several authors (e.g., Aufderheide and Rodríguez-Martín 1998; Gowland and Western, 2012; Smith 2015; Sallares 2019; and see Chapter 6). In particular, Gowland and Western (2012) adopted a modeling approach to explore comorbidities, climate, environment, and infectious diseases with the frequency of cribra orbitalia.

The other type of inherited anemia is sickle cell anemia. Here, a genetic mutation at Position 6 on the gene that codes for the hemoglobin beta chain results in the substitution of the amino acid valine for glutamate (Williams and Thein 2018). Sickle cell disease occurs when both genes (one from each parent) are affected; a single gene substitution results in a carrier state. The disease causes the entire cell to collapse into a sickle shape, which is eventually destroyed as it circulates (hemolysis). Today, sub-Saharan African populations have high rates of sickle cell anemia, and it also affects people in India, the Middle East, and southern Europe (Piel et al. 2010), with 10–20% of these populations being carriers of the disease (Williams and Thein 2018). Sickle cell disease is now considered to have originated 7,300 years ago from a single origin in West Africa (Shriner and Rotimi 2018). Two reactions are precipitated in the skeleton. First, bone changes in the cranium (already described), vertebrae, pelvis, hand, and foot bones occur due to marrow overactivity and enlargement (hyperplasia) as the body produces more red blood cells and, second, painful ischemic necrosis (death) of bone develops due to blockage of the blood vessels by these abnormal cells (Williams and Thein 2018). Complications of this condition may include susceptibility to infections, chronic leg ulcers, chronic kidney disease, gallstones, and blindness (Murphy et al. 2002, 431). Apart from the macroscopic and radiographic features of sickle cell anemia, microscopy has also been used for diagnosis in the past. Maat and Baig (1991) identified fossilized sickle cells using scanning electron microscopy in bone from a 2,000-year-old skeleton, which supported the macroscopic bone lesions of anemia (Fig. 7.10); without this information, the diagnosis of this type of anemia would not have been possible. Faerman et al. (2000) isolated a ß-globin gene sequence for sickle cell anemia in a recent bone sample from

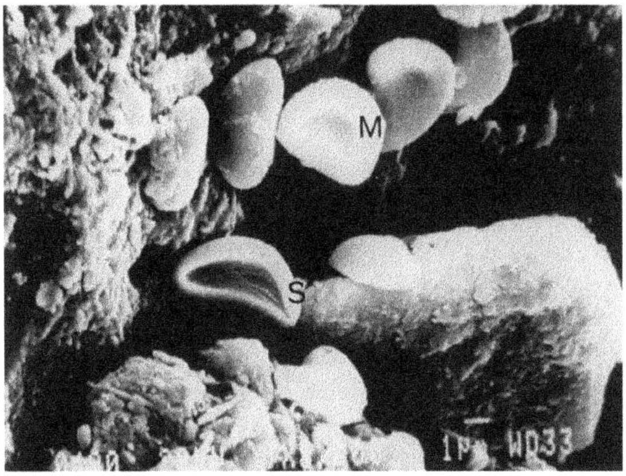

Figure 7.10. Scanning electron microscope image of a rib section from a 2,000-year-old individual with porotic hyperostosis, showing a sickle cell (S). Photograph courtesy of George Maat.

a male living in midwestern Africa, thought to be a descendant of enslaved Jamaicans. Possible evidence of sickle cell anemia was also described in a 7–12-year-old child who was buried in the Liberated African cemetery in Rupert's Valley, St. Helena, South Atlantic (ca. 1840 CE). The child had bilateral premature fusion of the proximal humeral epiphyses and flattening and elongation of the distal ends of the bone, which may have been the result of necrosis (Witkin, 2011).

The next section will concentrate on three conditions that are becoming more commonly identified in the archaeological record and undergoing a surge of interest in paleopathology: scurvy, rickets/osteomalacia, and osteoporosis. This is probably because of developments in their diagnosis since our last edition.

Scurvy (Vitamin C Deficiency)

Deficiencies of particular vitamins can produce more specific skeletal changes that allow them to be identified. When vitamin C is lacking for some time, scurvy develops. While rare today in high-middle-income countries (around 3–13%) except in particular circumstances (i.e., after gastrointestinal surgery) or in people with restrictive dietary habits (Deirawan et al. 2020), it might be assumed that in past hunter-forager and rural communities, access to vitamin C was easy and plentiful. This vitamin is found in fresh fruits and uncooked vegetables, with smaller amounts in milk and fish, all natural produce that probably contributed to the staple diet of many past human groups. Even on a purely carnivorous diet, there is enough vitamin C to prevent scurvy; for example, Inuit groups who eat a lot of uncooked meat do not develop scurvy (French 1993, 1000). The clinical features of scurvy and a specific plant-based antidote, called *anneda* (possibly an infusion of cedar), were known to the Indigenous people of present-day Quebec, and they offered it to French explorer Jacques Cartier and his crew who were suffering a grievous outbreak in the winter of 1535–1536 (Martini 2002). Today, scurvy is seen in infants fed boiled cow's milk instead of breastmilk (heat destroys the vitamin), and in older people, particularly older males living alone, who may not eat fresh fruit and vegetables (Elia 2002, 238). Scurvy is unlikely to develop in children of well-nourished, lactating mothers, in societies that have not adopted artificial feeding (Brickley et al. 2020), or where the older generation is well integrated into the community.

During the transition to agriculture, the availability of vitamin C may have been reduced. Cereals are totally lacking in the vitamin, while cooking and prolonged storage may destroy it. In urbanized communities, access to fresh produce would have been an additional potential risk factor for the development of the disease. Long sea voyages, military operations, and the California Gold Rush are all reported to have led to large numbers of people developing scurvy. These events provided observations that were used for the early recognition and treatment of scurvy. In 1497 CE, on a long voyage to India, Vasco da Gama's afflicted crew found relief with a supply of oranges (Rajakumar 2001). James Lind, an English physician in the eighteenth century, is probably the most famous observer and experimenter in the quest to conquer scurvy in sailors. In his 1747 clinical trial, he divided twelve scorbutic sailors into six groups of two and gave them various treatments; only the two sailors consuming fresh oranges and lemons recovered (Lind 1772, 149–150). His 1753 first edition served as an "authoritative argument . . . for the use of citrus fruits to prevent scurvy" (French 1993, 1002), although its impact was slow, and it was not until the end of the eighteenth century that lime juice was issued to sailors (Tröhler 2005). Buckley et al. (2023) used hospital files from the 1860s (case books, patient and death registers) to explore the frequency, duration, and factors related to adult scurvy in the goldfields of New Zealand. Their research showed that scurvy was only prevalent in the early years of the gold rush, ending when settlers were finally able to grow their own fresh food, and that it was the merchant sailors who were the main long-term victims of the disease. The records highlighted the previously invisible lives of these settlers, including discrimination against the Chinese, persistent rheumatic pain post-scurvy, and the subsequent burden on the family, as well as the psychosocial consequences of living in a mining community. The frequency of scurvy has also been examined in early settlement communities in seventeenth-century St. Croix Island, New France, Canada (Crist 2014) and in fifteenth-century North America (Tiesler et al. 2016), present-day Dominican Republic.

Vitamin C is necessary for combatting infections and for the absorption of iron, and it is essential for the normal formation of the body tissues, especially collagen (Deirawan et al. 2020). In addition to reducing the resistance to infection, vitamin C deficiency predisposes individuals to bleeding into the skin and beneath the periosteum. In addition to the faulty formation of the periosteum and the ligaments holding the teeth in their sockets, the cement substance in the blood vessels is faulty and predisposes the individual to hemorrhage in the form of bruising or petechiae into the soft tissues, bones (especially the jaws), and joints. The result is the formation of new bone on the skeleton as a response to bleeding. In adults, the most common symptom is swollen and bleeding gums, leading to periodontal disease (see Chapter 3), with weakness and muscle pain typical signs and symptoms (Elia 2002, 238). Generalized osteopenia, metaphyseal fractures, and fractured trabeculae have also been identified (Brickley et al. 2020, 66). Historical evidence for scurvy was considered in the examination of the skeletons of fifty Dutch whalers buried between 1642 CE and the late eighteenth century on an island called Zeeusche Uytkyck. Maat (1982, 2004) noted staining in the long bones, which was later proven to be the result of blood (i.e., hemorrhage) from sustained vitamin C deficiency (Maat and Uytterschaut 1984). In rapidly growing children, the effects of the disease produce severe lesions as new blood vessels and muscle tissue are being constantly laid down. Studies of nonadults have proven to be the most informative on the development and causes of this disease in past societies (Lewis 2018, 217–218).

Until the late 1990s, the paleopathological diagnosis of scurvy in children was often based on generalized new bone formation on long bones. However, Ortner and Ericksen (1997), in their detailed study, identified the lesions in more focused areas of the skull, notably porosity and new bone bilaterally on the greater wing of the sphenoid bone and on the temporal bone, as a result of hemorrhage from the deep blood vessels associated with the temporalis muscle, which is involved in chewing. New bone formation in the orbits, as a result of bleeding during eye movement, is particularly characteristic (Fig. 7.11), and ossified hematomas on the cranial vault can form on the occipital, parietal, and frontal bones, mimicking the porotic hyperostosis of anemia (Fig. 7.12). In later papers, Ortner et al. (1999, 2001) observed these changes in a series of non-adult crania from Peru and in North America. Since then, the diagnostic criteria for infantile scurvy have become well established, with characteristic skeletal and radiographic signs of scurvy recognized on the skull and long bones (see Brickley et al. 2020, 53). Because it is unlikely that a malnourished individual will be deficient in just one vitamin or mineral, individuals may also have lesions consistent with rickets (see next section) and iron-deficiency anemia (comorbidity), as well as deficiencies in many other nutrients that we are less adept at recognizing (Brickley and Morgan 2023).

Symptoms of what is now infantile scurvy have been recognized clinically since antiquity, but it was often combined with other nutritional diseases. It was not considered as a distinct childhood disease until the late nineteenth century when an infantile form appeared almost as an epidemic, owing, it is hypothesized, to the heating of milk and the use of proprietary products. Barlow (1883) observed the familiar sign of bleeding gums when the teeth began to erupt (Rajakumar 2001). Consequently, our understanding of the frequency of infantile scurvy in the past relies on studying skeletal remains. Large-scale studies carried out since the refinement of the diagnostic criteria have identified scurvy in children across wide geographical areas, from the prehistoric to postmedieval periods, and with prevalence rates between 0.8% and 68% (Lewis 2018, 217). The highest rates so far were found in the 545 children buried at Kilkenny Workhouse in Ireland during the Irish potato famine, with 28% ($n = 9/32$) of neonates and 32% ($n = 20/63$) of infants affected. As babies derived their vitamin C from maternal stores in the womb and in breastmilk, scurvy in such young children suggests scurvy would have also affected their mothers (Geber and Murphy 2012).

Rickets and Osteomalacia (Vitamin D Deficiency)

Vitamin D deficiency can also produce chronic abnormalities in the skeleton. This vitamin, more accurately termed a prohormone, is necessary for the

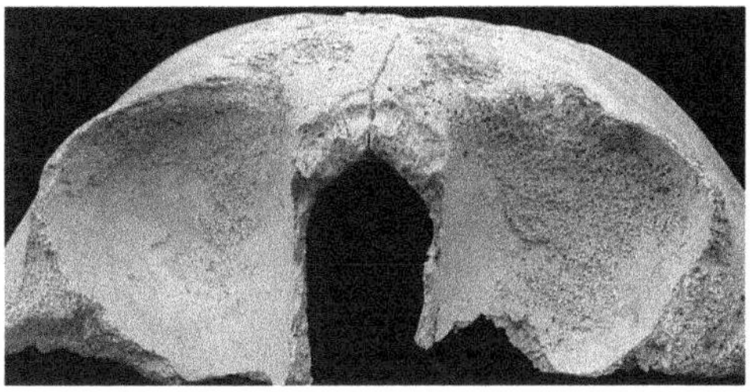

Figure 7.11. New bone formation in the orbits of a 1–2-year-old from Roman Poundbury Camp, Dorset, England (fifth century CE). Photograph by Mary Lewis taken with the kind permission of the Natural History Museum, London.

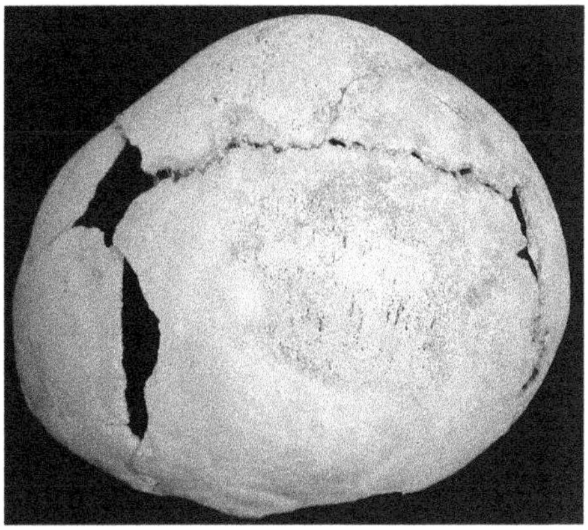

Figure 7.12. Scorbutic changes on the cranial vault as the result of ossified hematomas (or "Parrot's skull") in a 1–2-year-old child from Roman Poundbury Camp, Dorset, England (fifth century CE). Photograph taken by Mary Lewis with the kind permission of the Natural History Museum, London.

absorption and mobilization of calcium and phosphorus from previously formed bone and calcium through the intestine. It is also responsible for healthy bone growth through maturation and mineralization of the organic matrix (Resnick et al. 2024, 753). Ninety percent of the body's vitamin D requirement is obtained through exposure of the skin to sunlight (cholcalciferol, or vitamin D_3), which effects a chemical change in the skin, producing vitamin D from a chemical precursor, or 7-dehydrocholesterol (Levene 1991). Smaller amounts of vitamin D (ergocalciferol, or vitamin D_2) are present in foods such as fish, animal fat, and egg yolks (Fraser 1995). Vitamin D deficiency can result from a fault in vitamin D metabolism, lack of exposure to ultraviolet light, or dietary deficiency (Elia 2002). Data on vitamin D deficiency for the United States, Canada, and Europe put the current frequency at 5.9%, 7.4%, and 13%, respectively, with countries in northern Europe having higher rates than southern Europe, especially in the winter months when access to ultraviolet light is scarce (Cashman 2020). Factors such as clothing, age, outdoor activities, and skin pigmentation all have an impact on disease susceptibility/prevention, with darker-skinned individuals more susceptible, especially when living in temperate zones where UV light levels are typically low (Cashman et al. 2016). Vitamin D deficiency has been linked to a greater risk of developing cardiovascular diseases, and its effect on the immune system leaves sufferers susceptible to other infections (de la Guía-Galipienso et al. 2021; for more detailed information on vitamin D see Hewison et al. 2023).

Put simply, vitamin D deficiency leads to a "softening" of the bones. Inadequate or delayed mineralization of osteoid (unmineralized bone) in cortical and spongy bone under the periosteum is referred to as osteomalacia, while interruption in development and mineralization of the cartilage growth plates is rickets. Children suffer from both conditions (see below), as their bones need to grow both in length at the growth plates and in strength (appositional growth) under the periosteum (Pettifor 2003).

Since children are growing rapidly, vitamin D deficiency, like vitamin C deficiency, produces more severe changes in the young than in adults.

The clinical features of rickets have been known since antiquity. In 300 BCE, crooked legs and a "hunchback" were described in China (Steinbock 1993, 978), and Soranus of Ephesus of the second century CE is attributed with the first clear description in a child and possibly a parturient mother (*Gynaecology,* book II, 48 (112) and book IV, 5 (57); Aufderheide and Rodríguez-Martín 1998, 309). Soranus described how the weight-bearing bones of the legs became unnaturally bowed when walking commenced (Fig. 7.13a and b). The arm bones may also be affected when the child begins to crawl, and other bones of the body can deform under the influence of muscular contraction. The ends of the growing long bones expand and, in appearance, resemble the widened end of a trumpet; this reflects excessive unmineralized cartilage causing an increase in length and width in the growth plates of the bones. In addition, the costochondral areas of the ribs become nodular prominences ("rachitic rosary"), the pelvis is restricted in growth, dental development may be delayed or deficient, and the cranial bones may be thinned and flattened, usually in the area subject to pressure when the infant is resting (Brickley and Mays 2019). The skeletal and radiographic signs of active and healed rickets in children are now well documented (see Brickley et al. 2008), as are particular changes seen in adolescents (i.e., a curved sternum) and residual rickets in adults (excessive curvature of long bones, ribs, spine, sacrum). The identification of changes to the shape of the tooth pulp cavity seen on radiographs, due to defects in dentine mineralization, mean we now have the means to identify childhood rickets in adults with no other signs that they ever had the disease (D'Ortenzio et al. 2016, 2018a). Consideration of the syndemic relationship of rickets with other comorbidities is also beginning (Perry and Gowland 2022).

Clearly, the majority of children in antiquity spent their days outside and were unlikely to develop rickets, even during the northern winter months. However, Littleton (1998) argued that prolonged swaddling caused rickets in 10 (1.5%) children from Bahrain in the Middle East (1000 BCE–250 CE). In Europe prior to the Industrial Revolution, rickets was considered a disease of affluence, where wealthy children were expected to be fully clothed and to stay indoors, reducing their exposure to sunlight (O'Riordan and Bijvoet 2014; Pettifor and Daniels 1997). Indeed, Madonna and Child paintings produced in the Netherlands in the fifteenth–sixteenth centuries show the characteristic bowed legs and distorted chests of rickets (Fildes 1986). With increased urbanization and industrialization, both in the past and today, this all changed. The relationship of vitamin D deficiency to industrial England was cemented when Daniel Whistler titled his 1645 thesis "On the Children's Disease of the English, Which the Inhabitants Idiomatically Call the Rickets," citing the overcrowded streets and dense housing that blocked sunlight from penetrating the barrier of industrial smoke. Poor, often underfed children were compelled to work the daylight hours in the noise, danger, and shelter of the factory. In such circumstances rickets was prevalent, but it was not confined to England. In 1900, Morse reported rickets in 79.5% of infants born in Boston, Massachusetts, and, in

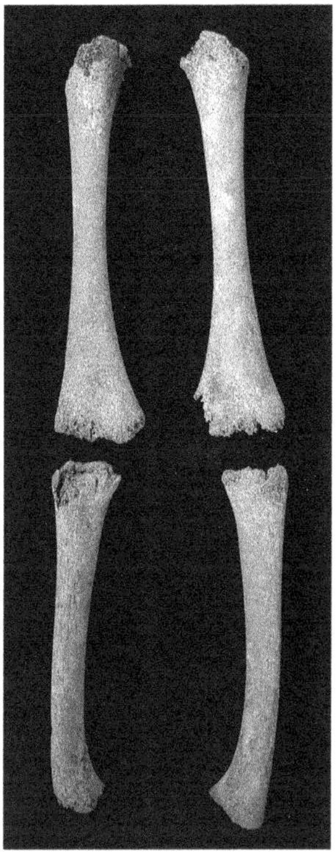

Figure 7.13A. Anterior view of bowing deformities of vitamin D deficiency in the tibiae in a 1–2-year-old from Redhill, Surrey, England (1750–1850 CE). Photograph by Mary Lewis.

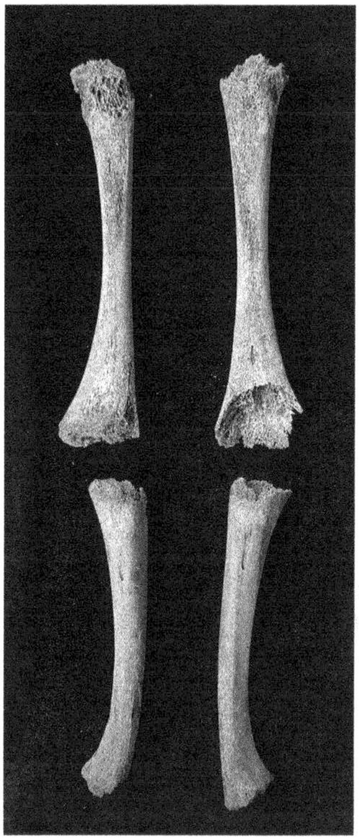

Figure 7.13B. Posterior view of bowing deformities of vitamin D deficiency in the tibiae in a 1–2-year-old from Redhill, Surrey, England (1750–1850 CE). Photograph by Mary Lewis.

Germany, 89% of Dresden children aged 2–4 years had the disease (Hardy 1992). Massage and splinting of affected limbs, and the wearing of special boots and long coats to hide deformities, were advocated, while the livers of birds and fish, and later (post-1780s) cod liver oil, were dietary recommendations (Fildes 1986, 128). The intimate relationship between vitamin D deficiency and industrialization is well illustrated in the archaeological record. Prevalence rates in these groups range from 7.1% in high-status children from early modern Germany (Pēterstone et al. 2013) to 34% from nineteenth-century Spring Street, New York. Here, Ellis (2010) highlighted the impact of a temperate climate on individuals with African ancestry. The inhibiting effects of melanin in their skin, in addition to air pollution, swaddling, and dietary practices, were suggested as contributory factors to high rates of the disease. Rickets has been seen in both high- and low-status children from nineteenth-century England and Renaissance Italy (Mays et al. 2009a; Giuffra et al. 2013, respectively), and even in rural areas (Veselka et al. 2015). Before the Industrial Revolution, the presence of vitamin D deficiency (sometimes with scurvy) in 11.2% of children from Romano-British Dorset, England, suggests urbanization had devastating effects during the Roman occupation too (Lewis 2010), a pattern also seen in the Italian provinces (Lockau et al. 2019).

Evidence for rickets outside urbanized areas is sporadic and often confined to a single individual. In these instances, it may be that the individuals had a genetic form of the disease that inhibits the processing of vitamin D, or that it occurred secondary to liver, endocrine, or intestinal conditions (although it is also worth noting that our ability to synthesize vitamin D diminishes with age) (Holick and Adams 1998). Pfeiffer and Crowder (2004) reported the earliest known evidence of rickets in a 3–5-year-old from "sun drenched" South Africa (4820 ± 90 BCE), and Formicola (1995) argued for a genetic anomaly causing rickets (X-linked hypophosphatasia) in an adult male from Upper Paleolithic Italy. Blondiaux et al. (2002) noted the association of rickets and caregiver violence in fourth-century Normandy, France, adding to a picture of overall neglect of the child. The discovery of rickets in eight children (2%) from rural later medieval Wharram Percy in Yorkshire, England, was unexpected. Ortner and Mays (1998) suggested that perhaps these children were already sick and remained indoors, resulting in rickets as a secondary insult (also see Ventades et al. 2020).

After a nonadult's bones have all fused, osteomalacia persists if vitamin D continues to be deficient. Prolonged suckling of infants and multiple pregnancies in rapid succession will deplete calcium stores in females, especially in areas with low levels of sunlight, or when the mothers spend the majority of their time indoors (Dawodu et al. 2015). The result of this bone demineralization in adults is collapse of the vertebrae under weight-bearing stress and changes to the morphology of the pelvis, which is of catastrophic obstetric significance. A woman in labor unable to give birth because of the obstruction of a constricted pelvis due to osteomalacia was a recognized hazard of past obstetric practice and led to some of the earliest Caesarean sections (Mörgeli and Schultz 1996). Pelvic dysplasia causing obstructed labor may have been responsible for intrapartum death of the fetus and their mother, or, if the mother survived, subsequent complications may have caused urinary incontinence and associated social exclusion. Bending and flaring of epiphyses in the long bones are rare in adults and may instead indicate residual childhood rickets. Pseudofractures, or "Looser zones" (lesions that mimic a fracture in bone), are also seen perpendicular to the cortices and bilaterally (Resnick et al. 2024, 759) and have been identified in adults living in past industrial societies (Ives and Brickley 2014; Fig. 7.14). The frequency of minor degrees of vertebral collapse in skeletal remains suggests that osteomalacia may have been a common feature of earlier people, but there are many other causes of vertebral collapse, such as tuberculosis, acute trauma, and osteoporosis.

Osteoporosis

Osteoporosis is the most common skeletal metabolic disease in the world today, with a global prevalence rate estimated to be 18.3% (23.1% of females and 11.7% of males; Salari et al. 2021). It brings with it a medical, social, and economic burden

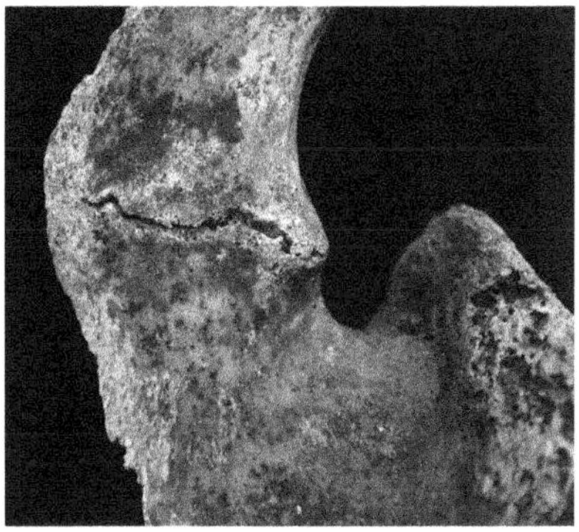

Figure 7.14. Pseudofracture (Looser zone) of osteomalacia on the spinous process of the right scapula from postmedieval Egham, England. Photograph courtesy of Rachel Ives with the kind permission of AOC Archaeology and St. John's Church, Egham, Surrey, England.

as the result of bone pain, fragility, pathological fractures, and elevated mortality rates, with 20% of females estimated to die within one year of a fracture (Salari et al. 2021). Osteoporosis is characterized by a loss of bone mass (or mineral density, BMD) and changes in bone quality resulting in a reduction in total bone volume (for more detailed information see Brickley et al. 2020). Osteopenia is defined as a general loss of bone mineral density between 1.0 and 2.5 standard deviations (SD) below the mean for an individual's biological sex, age, and ancestry. It is a warning sign and a precursor for osteoporosis. Osteoporosis is diagnosed when the BMD falls below 2.5 SD (Karaguzel and Holick et al. 2011). Osteopenia can occur secondary to other diseases such as osteomalacia or rheumatoid arthritis. A localized loss of bone mass is also evident in single bones of whole limbs as a result of long-term paralysis (or disuse atrophy). Osteoporosis refers to a systemic condition affecting all areas of the skeleton—although its impact is more readily seen in highly cancellous areas where continued loss of bone results in pathological fractures (wrist, hip, spine).

Osteoporosis is classified into two types: Type I is seen in postmenopausal females when there is a drop in protective estrogen, and in men and women over 70 years of age. Secondary (type II) osteoporosis is caused by other diseases (e.g., cancer and endocrine disease) or environmental and lifestyle choices, such as excessive alcohol or caffeine consumption, tobacco smoking, lack of exercise, or diet-related calcium deficiency (Salari et al. 2021). Although yet to be clearly defined, evidence suggests that some families may be genetically susceptible to osteoporosis, and an individual's immune status may also play a role (Brickley et al. 2020; Teerlink et al. 2021). Despite an understanding that bones could break due to fragility since the eighteenth century (Curate 2014), relatively little is known of the frequency of osteoporosis in the past, owing to problems in diagnosis. However, given its association with aging, diet, and inactivity, we should expect to see an increase in its occurrence in urbanized societies that promoted increased longevity.

Females naturally have a lower bone mass than males, a difference that becomes more pronounced during the adolescent growth spurt (Lewis 2022). The importance of optimum pubertal growth on peak bone mineral density is illustrated by the finding that females who experience delay in their first menstruation by as little as two years are more vulnerable to bone loss osteopenia before the age of 40 years and, potentially, early osteoporosis (Karapanou and Papadimitriou, 2010). Estrogen is a hormone that, among other functions, prevents excessive destruction of bone by osteoclasts; hence, with a decline in circulating estrogen postmenopausal females lose this protection. In 2018, the rate of osteoporosis in postmenopausal females in India was reported to be 10.3%, compared to 4.7% in premenopausal females (Salari et al., 2021). A study of twenty-four countries across six continents determined the overall mean menopausal age in modern populations is between 46 and 52 years (WHO 2011), although it appears to be slightly earlier for females living in the Middle East, compared to Europe, Australia, and the United States (Schoenaker et al. 2014). Historical accounts from classical Greece and Rome (Amundsen and Diers 1970) suggest the menopause occurred similarly around 40 to 50 years of age. This is a factor to bear in mind in the study of past human groups. If more females in the past died in their earlier years, perhaps as the result of childbirth, then menopause may not have been a significant factor in the development of osteoporosis. Obviously, longevity will also vary between groups from different periods and geographical locations.

Diet appears to be another major factor in influencing osteoporosis development (Burckhardt et al. 2004). Calcium is the most abundant mineral in the body, and it is crucial to the formation of teeth and bones. Disturbances in calcium intake alter the rate of mineralization of new bone matrix. A high intake of calcium throughout life is associated with higher bone mass, but the effects of calcium (and hormone) supplementation on osteoporosis development in postmenopausal females varies among studies. Vitamin D is also essential for the absorption of calcium (and phosphorus), while a high-protein diet leads to inhibition of calcium absorption and an increase in urinary calcium (Stini 1990). Overall, however, a balanced nutrient intake, achieved through the consumption of fruit, nuts, legumes, poultry, and dairy products, is required to maintain bone mass and reduce the risk of osteoporotic fractures (Muñoz-Garach et al. 2020). Finally, higher bone mass is seen in people who exercise regularly. Mechanical demands on the skeleton actively promote increased bone mass. We might expect then that osteoporosis would be greater in more sedentary groups when compared to hunter-forager societies. Diet and exercise would be considered (along with age) as relevant factors in osteoporosis development, and the analysis of other factors, such as early adult mortality, reduced stature, and the frequency of enamel hypoplasia, Harris lines, and cribra orbitalia, may allow us to read the complex etiological web that influenced the occurrence of osteoporosis in the past. In relation to osteoporosis, Salari et al. (2021) performed a global meta-analysis of publications (2000 to 2021) that reported osteoporosis-related fractures. Sixty-four studies were based in Asia, nine each were from Europe and the United States, three derived from Africa, and one from Australia. The sample size was 103,334,579 individuals aged 15–105 years. They found the African continent had the highest frequency, and that overall frequency of osteoporosis globally is very high, especially in Africa and Europe. In reporting their data, they identified the need to develop health systems to cope with this ever-increasing burden of osteoporosis. Osteoporosis is considered a silent disease that often is diagnosed only when a person sustains a fracture, especially in the most frequently affected areas of the body in this condition: the wrist (Colles fracture of the radius, Fig. 7.15), the hip (femoral neck or intertrochanteric area of the femur, which is more common in females, Fig. 7.16) and the spine (compression of the thoracic and lumbar vertebral bodies—"cod fish vertebrae"), leading to kyphotic collapse or "dowager's hump." These highly cancellous areas are susceptible because trabecular bone has a greater turnover than cortical bone, which also becomes thinner and more porous. In addition, the spine and femur are intricately designed to bear weight, a mechanical feature that is drastically undermined by the loss of the trabecular structure that sustains it. For the paleopathologist, as for the clinician, a fracture in one of these areas may be the first indication for osteoporosis in that individual. Osteological methods have been developed to explore this condition in the past, often by adapting clinical techniques. Clinical diagnosis uses dual-energy X-ray absorptiometry (DEXA) to assess bone mineral density. Because archaeological bone lacks bone marrow and other soft tissue, we cannot directly compare its BMD to that of living

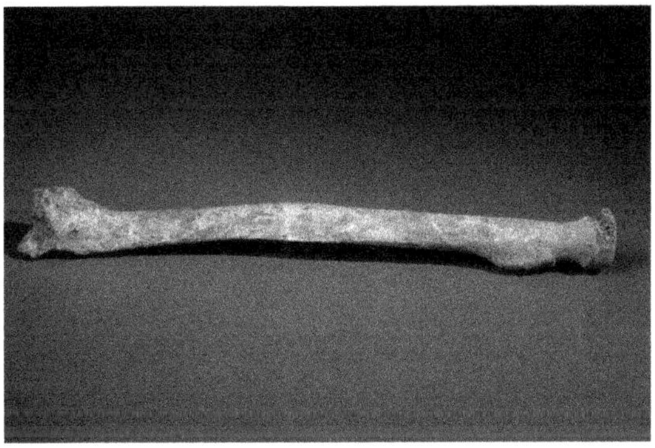

Figure 7.15. Healed Colles fracture in distal radius (early medieval Berinsfield, Oxfordshire, England); note the posterior displacement of the distal fragment ("dinner fork" deformity). Photograph by and courtesy of Jean Brown.

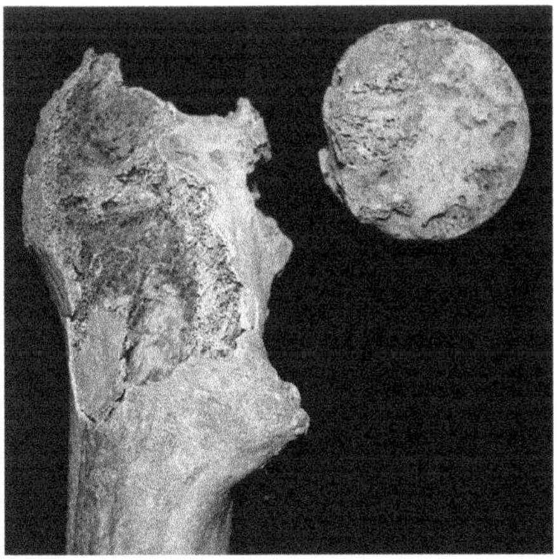

Figure 7.16A. Ununited fracture of the left femoral neck due to osteoporosis in an older female from St. Oswald's Priory, Gloucester, England (1250–1550 CE). Viewed from the front. Photography by Mary Lewis.

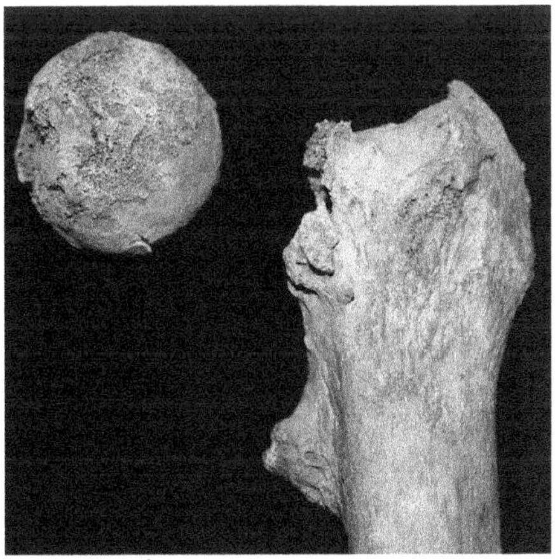

Figure 7.16B. Ununited fracture of the left femoral neck due to osteoporosis in an older female from St. Oswald's Priory, Gloucester, England (1250–1550 CE). Viewed from the back. Photography by Mary Lewis.

patients. However, a general assessment of reduced BMD can be made, using the World Health Organization's (2011) 2.5 SD model (Brickley and Mays 2019), provided diagenetic (environmental) alteration in the structure of the bone can be ruled out (using radiographs, microscopy, or chemical analyses).

Measuring cortical bone thickness using a digital radiograph (radiogrammetry) has also been employed by paleopathologists to provide a cortical index, usually focused on the second metacarpal, mimicking the clinical use of the second and fourth metacarpals (Mays 1996b; Ives and Brickley 2004). These methods are continually being developed (Schneider and Gilmour 2022). Work has also shown the value of scanning electron microscopy (SEM) in assessing osteoporotic changes in bones from archaeological populations (Roberts and Wakely 1992). SEM records the topographic features of bone, and excessive bone resorption with reduced formation may be identified in sections of bone (Fig. 7.17). The study of healing microfractures (see Fig. 1.11 in Chapter 1) in the trabeculae of vertebrae suggests that they increase with osteoporosis (Vernon-Roberts and Pirie 1973; Mosekilde 1990) and can be interpreted as a repair mechanism to preserve the bone's integrity. These features could be used to diagnose osteoporosis before any more significant changes in the skeleton occur, such as reduction in mineral density or structural collapse of bone. As imaging techniques have developed, paleopathologists have also turned to high-resolution CT scanning to provide 3D images of the cortical and trabecular architecture, evaluating the number, thickness, and connectivity of the trabecular bone, or porosity of the cortex (Agarwal et al. 2004; Agnew and Stout 2012). Phalangeal ultrasonometry (Rinaldo et al. 2018) and synchrotron Fourier-transform infrared microspectroscopy have also been employed to measure vascular canal densities in bone (Miszkiewicz et al. 2021). The use of ever more sophisticated technology in the absence of standardized terminology and operational protocols has led to some criticism, especially when diagnosis is carried out without consideration of the environmental and social factors that may have contributed to its apparent occurrence in the past (van Spelde et al. 2021). There is also a debate on what level of bone loss should be considered normal and what is pathological (Agarwal 2021).

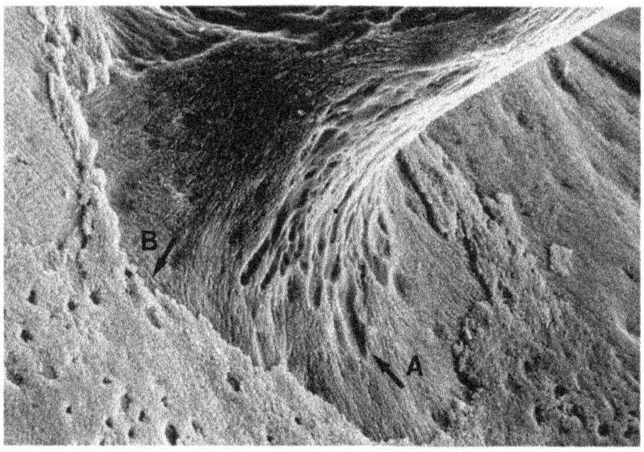

Figure 7.17. SEM image of rib section from 79-year-old female showing a Howship lacunae caused by osteoclast resorption (A) and new bone formed by osteoblasts (B). From the Terry Collection, National Museum of Natural History, Washington, DC. Originally reproduced with kind permission from Don Ortner.

Reports of osteoporosis in the archaeological record have shown that patterns of bone loss with age were also a feature of past populations. Curate (2014) provided an excellent summary of the history and paleopathology of the disease, but Dewey et al. (1969) were the first to demonstrate age-related bone loss in past populations across time in their study of individuals from the Meroitic to Christian periods in Nubia (350 BCE–1400 CE). Mays (1996b; Mays et al. 1998) explored bone loss using metacarpal radiographs and, later, DEXA scans, to measure bone density of eighty-three males and seventy-one females from the medieval rural site of Wharram Percy, England. Mays found significant bone loss in females but not males, and the magnitude of bone loss for the older females was similar to age-matched living individuals. The similarities between medieval and modern women were surprising considering the presumed more active lifestyle of people in the past compared to today. Mays (2015) also demonstrated that age-related cortical bone loss has occurred at the same rate for men for over 1,800 years. Lorkiewicz et al. (2019), by contrast, argued that bone loss in ancient males was accelerated compared to their modern counterparts, at least in the 267 Neolithic to early modern males they examined in north-central Poland. This was despite the fact that the Neolithic males had higher rates of BMD to begin with. White and Armelagos (1997) measured stable carbon and nitrogen isotopes ratios in both osteopenic and nonosteopenic males and females from the X-Group Sudanese Nubian population (fourth–sixth century CE). They found that females with osteopenia had elevated nitrogen isotope values, which may signify that processes involved in the development of bone loss also affect the isotope composition of the collagen. In their study of 1,032 individuals from within and outside London in the preindustrial and industrial periods, Western and Bekvalac (2020, 202) reported higher rates of osteoporosis in females compared to males, that frequency increased with age, and that Londoners had higher rates of osteoporosis then those living outside of London in both periods. It is clear that osteoporosis is a complex disease, and a mixture of biological and cultural factors, including diet, age at menarche and menopause, genetics, and possibly exposure to stress (suggested by increased nitrogen values) may have influenced the development of this disease in the past.

Reconstructing Ancient Diets

Understanding the diet of a population can help us to identify nutritional and social factors that may have contributed to poor health in the past. The study of past diets can be undertaken in several ways, such as the analysis of plant and animal remains from archaeological sites, including their containment within coprolites (ancient feces), and the study of artifacts associated with growing, processing, and eating food. These must be classed as indirect evidence because we cannot be sure that they represent the diet being consumed by every individual. Direct evidence for diet can be gleaned in other ways. If studies of mummified or other preserved remains are possible, then analysis of the contents of the intestines may help shed light on the last meal the person ate before death, bearing in mind that this may have been a "special ritual" rather than a normal meal. Analysis of pollen and larger plant remains, along with small bones from the consumption of meat or fish in intestinal contents, can be very helpful in highlighting actual food consumption. For example, Maixner et al. (2018) analyzed the contents of the intestines of the Tyrolean Iceman ("Ötzi") using aDNA analysis and concluded that his last meal was high in fat and contained a type of toxic plant (*Pteridum*, or bracken) whereas previously he had consumed ibex (wild goat) and cereals.

More direct evidence for the food people consumed can be gained from the analysis of dental calculus (see Chapter 3), but stable isotope analysis remains the most popular method to reconstruct diet in the past. Stable carbon and nitrogen isotope values in teeth and bone are derived from those of the food consumed by humans. Dietary signatures from dental tissues (enamel and dentine) reflect childhood food consumption because they do not remodel once the teeth are formed. Conversely, continuing bone turnover means isotopic signatures from the rest of the skeleton reflect average diet across an individual's life span (Larsen 2015, 301–332). Work in this field began in the 1970s, initially with the analysis of elemental concentrations in bone to reconstruct past diets. Methodological issues and especially increasing awareness of bone diagenesis by postmortem uptake of elements from external sources (especially soil), means that trace element analysis of bone is rarely applied today, although new analytical techniques may provide a way forward (e.g., see Maurer et al. 2019 and Rasmussen et al. 2020). In the meantime, stable isotope analysis has firmly established itself as a routine source of dietary information for paleopathologists.

The method is based on the principle that the isotope ratios of the food and drink consumed during life can be traced in the skeletal tissues of consumers. Carbon has two stable isotopes: carbon-12 (^{12}C) and the heavier isotope carbon-13 (^{13}C). Their relative natural abundance or ratio ($^{13}C/^{12}C$, usually referred to as $\delta^{13}C$ [delta-13-C] values) varies between different environments and organisms such as between C_3 and C_4 plants (Fig. 7.18). Differing in their chemical pathways for photosynthesis, C_4 plants originally come from hot and dry climates while C_3 plants are adapted to temperate areas. Relevant to isotopic analysis, C_4 plants (e.g., the cultigens maize, millet, and sorghum, which are all derived from tropical grasses) have higher carbon isotope ratios (i.e., contain more ^{13}C relative to ^{12}C) than C_3 plants, which include staples like wheat and rice. These differences are passed on to the tissues of the consumers of these plants (Katzenberg and Waters-Rist 2018). Marine organisms have $\delta^{13}C$ values between those of C_3 and C_4 plants, although their carbon isotope values often overlap with C_4 consumers (Larsen 2015, 302). Nitrogen stable isotope ratios ($^{15}N/^{14}N$, or $\delta^{15}N$) also vary in relation to diet. They increase by trophic level and therefore give insights into the proportions of plant and animal products consumed. Because of the higher number of trophic levels in marine food chains, they are also useful for distinguishing marine from terrestrial diets, although this may be complicated by the fact that terrestrial foods can present with high $\delta^{15}N$ values if they were grown in hot and arid environments, or due to anthropogenic input (e.g., manuring) (Katzenberg and Water-Rist 2018).

Although stable isotope data reflect only the main sources of dietary intake, usually averaged over a number of years, it can provide important contextual information for the archaeology of disease. It can, for example, trace large-scale subsistence shifts like the adoption of agriculture, or demonstrate dietary variation between males and females, or groups of different socioeconomic status, all of which may be linked to health and disease (Katzenberg 2012; Richards and Montgomery 2012).

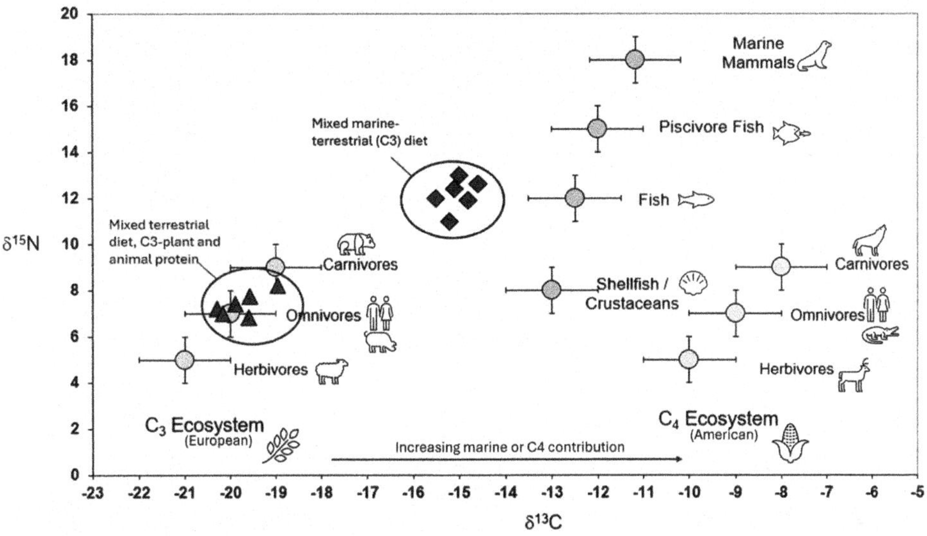

Figure 7.18. Average carbon and nitrogen stable isotope values derived from bone collagen for the reconstruction of diet. Redrawn with kind permission of Gundula Müldner, modified from Richards 2000, fig. 1.

For example, Papathanasiou (2003) suggested that a diet rich in pulses (but low in iron) that is indicated by isotope data from Neolithic Greece may have contributed to the high frequencies of anemia observed in these populations. In addition, isotope evidence from several medieval monastic sites suggests that individuals with DISH (see Chapter 5) on average consumed a higher proportion of animal protein than those without (Müldner and Richards 2007; Quintelier et al. 2014). Although similar studies in the Roman period did not see a similar pattern (Richards and Montgomery 2012; Castells Navarro and Buckberry 2022). A key difficulty in interpreting isotope data from pathological remains is that the disease process may affect bone isotope composition. Alternatively, newly formed bone may overemphasize short-term fluctuations in diet compared to more mature tissues (Katzenberg and Lovell 1999; Reitsema and Holder 2018).

Stable isotopic analysis has been used extensively in North America to explore the adoption of maize agriculture (e.g., Buikstra and Milner 1991; Katzenberg et al. 1995), indicating spatial differences in its timing and intensity. Stable isotope analysis has also been used to explore dietary differences between males and females, or people of different socioeconomic groups. In later medieval England, for example, some of the earliest research into the diet of people given high- or low-status burials was carried out on skeletons from Fishergate House, York, England. In general, in medieval Europe, high-status individuals appear to have had more animal protein, including fish, than lower-status individuals, and a review of published studies suggested that people who lived in religious orders had a consistently higher component of marine fish in their diet (Müldner et al. 2009). However, what people ate is not always about where they lived, as food can be imported and exported. While stable isotopes are helping us to develop a more nuanced understanding of what people ate in the past, differentiating between the consumption of freshwater rather than saltwater fish, the impact of manuring, or exactly which proteins and cuts of meat were being consumed is still a challenge (Müldner 2018).

Our knowledge of stable nitrogen isotope variation in infant remains has undergone a transition since the last edition of this book. Traditionally, nitrogen isotope values of bulk bone collagen have been used on a population level to identify the age at which weaning foods were introduced to an infant's diet and when breastfeeding was reduced. This is because the nursing infant is at a higher trophic level to their mother—that is, they are higher up in the food chain (Wright and Schwarcz 1998; Fuller et al. 2006). For example, Dupras et al. (2001) studied infants from the Roman period site of Dakhleh Oasis, Egypt (ca. 250 CE) and found that the weaning process began at 6 months and was completed by 3 years of age, whereas Richards et al. (2002) inferred that weaning was complete by the age of 2 years at Wharram Percy, England (950–1500 CE). The use of incremental dentine to map the entire development of a tooth has allowed us to explore early life stages in more detail and at an individual level. It has been demonstrated that nitrogen isotope values in infant tissue are not just dependent on diet, but are also impacted by physiological stress experienced by the child or the mother. Under stress, such as undernutrition, the body's tissues are recycled and reformed into ^{15}N-enriched tissue, thus documenting $\delta^{15}N$ values resembling a breastfeeding signature (Beaumont et al. 2013; D'Ortenzio et al. 2015). Elevated nitrogen isotope values later on in childhood would, in the same way, suggest nutritional stress and recycling of the body's tissues as a response, although rapid growth may have the opposite effect (Beaumont and Montgomery 2016; Reitsema 2013). What happens to carbon isotope signatures during stress episodes is less well understood. In a stress-free environment, carbon signatures should increase during growth as body fat is laid down, and they might be expected to decrease if the body becomes wasted (Kaupová et al. 2023). To date, only a few have attempted to correlate evidence for metabolic disease with direct evidence for diet using stable isotope analysis (e.g., Zariņa et al. 2016). No doubt this will be a focus for the future. A much more extensive and detailed account of specific metabolic disorders and how they are identified in archaeological skeletal remains is provided by Brickley et al. (2020).

Paget's Disease

Paget's disease of bone, or osteitis deformans, was first described by James Paget in 1877 and is currently classified as a noninflammatory metabolic disorder. After osteoporosis, it is the second most prevalent metabolic disease in the world. Paget's disease has a frequency of 1.5–8.3%, with the highest incidence in European populations, especially in the UK, followed by Australia, New Zealand, and North America (Cook and Wall 2021). The lowest occurrence is among Scandinavians, Africans, and Asians, and only isolated cases are reported in other areas. Paget's disease rarely occurs before 55 years of age and is more common in males than females

(Michou and Orcel 2019). People with the disease tend to be lethargic and withdrawn, and they have an increased heart rate and blood flow, leading to a very warm skin and heart problems.

The cause of this disease is complex, with environmental, viral, and genetic factors all thought to contribute to its occurrence. Environmental factors include exposure to heavy metals and tobacco smoke, which would have been risk factors in certain periods of our past. Viral infections carried by different animals (e.g., dogs, cattle, pigs) have also been implicated in triggering the disease (Gennari et al. 2022), with implications for One Health research. The genetic mutations associated with Paget's disease are multiple and include germline mutations affecting proteins encoded by specific genes (TNFRSF11A, ZNF687, PFN1), as well as more sporadic (epigenetic) modifications to genes involved in bone remodeling and regulation (e.g., RANKL, OPG, HDAC2, DNMT1, and SQSTM1). Such mutations increase an individual's susceptibility to, and the severity of, the condition (Banaganapalli et al. 2023).

Paget's disease is characterized by slow and progressive enlargement and distortion of a single (monostotic) or multiple (polyostotic) bones of the skeleton, most commonly the proximal femur, pelvis, spine, cranium, and tibia; 90% of people with Paget's disease have one or many of these areas affected (Gennari et al. 2019). Rapid bone turnover results in a "mosaic" patterning of the bone, both radiographically and histologically; this is the result of irregular and excessive fiber and lamellar bone formation. The normally demarcated cortex (compact bone) and medullary cavity become less precise as the cortex becomes thickened and spongy (Figs. 7.19 and 7.20). The head enlarges due to cranial thickening and is a startling feature of the person's appearance, and prominent meningeal vessel grooves are obvious on the endocranial surface, representing increased blood flow. There also may be spinal collapse (kyphosis). The whole picture of the bone changes is complicated by frequent spontaneous bone fractures, and by the occasional development of an osteosarcoma, osteoarthritis, or neurological symptoms (muscle weakness, paralysis) caused by pressure on the body systems from enlargement of bone.

The high incidence of the disease in England, and in the northwest in particular, seemed to be reflected in the archaeological record, with Mays (2010) reporting that of the 109 affected individuals reported from archaeological contexts in Europe, 93% were from England, peaking in the later medieval period, and 71% were males. Later research, using reports from non-English publications, suggests the disease may have actually originated in the Mediterranean (Menéndez-Bueyes and Fernández 2017). Further insight into the origin and evolution of Paget's disease came in 2019, when 4.6% (n = 6/130) of individuals from medieval Norton Priory in northern England demonstrated a widespread form of Paget's disease affecting 75% of the skeleton. Shaw et al. (2019) used ancient protein analysis (proteomics) to explore the presence of the protein mutation SQSTM1 in these people. As it was absent, they suggested that these individuals suffered from a more ancient and more severe form of the disease than is present today.

In 2022, Garnett and Lewis reassessed the high frequency of Paget's disease in the people buried in Redhill, Surrey (1843–1896 CE). The original macroscopic analysis

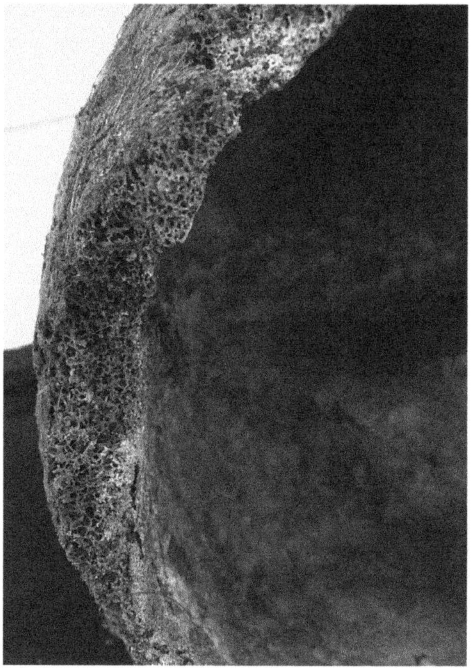

Figure 7.19. Paget's disease causing thickening of the vault of the cranium in a mature male from Redhill, Surrey, England (1750–1850 CE). Photograph by Mary Lewis.

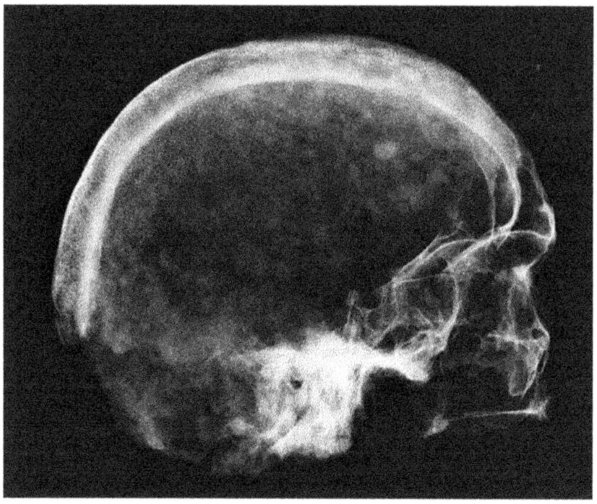

Figure 7.20. Radiograph of the same cranium as Fig. 7.19 showing characteristic mosaic patterning of bone. Photograph by Mary Lewis.

had suggested Paget's disease as the cause of bone enlargement in a staggering 15% of individuals (*n* = 8/53; Watts 2015). When radiographed, only two individuals showed the classic features of Paget's disease—"cotton wool" skull, ivory or picture frame vertebrae, thickened trabeculae, and radiolucent cutting zones in the long bones—while the systematic radiography of the rest of the group revealed additional skeletons showing Paget's disease: two males and one female, all over 45 years old. This analysis reduced the prevalence rate of Paget's disease at Redhill to a still high 5.7%. Histology supported the conclusions of the radiographic survey suggesting that, while macroscopic features alone are not sufficient for accurate identification, radiography can provide confirmation and the destructive and more time-consuming microscopic method used by clinicians may not be necessary to diagnose this disease in archaeological contexts.

Endocrine Disease

The endocrine system comprises a series of ductless glands whose cells secrete hormones into the blood. Hormones are chemical substances formed in a body organ or gland and carried by the blood to influence growth, function, and nutrition elsewhere in the body. Disfunction in the secretion of hormones, either too little or too much, causes endocrine diseases that affect the shape, size, and strength of the bones. The endocrine glands include the pituitary, thyroid, parathyroids, adrenals, ovaries, testes, and pancreas. In conjunction with the hypothalamus at the base of the brain, the pituitary gland is the principal organizer of the endocrine system (Hinson et al. 2010). The pituitary and thyroid glands are arguably the most relevant to paleopathology, as they control skeletal growth (pituitary) and maturation (thyroid), and so will be discussed here. The other glands, such as the parathyroids and adrenals, can all under- or overproduce hormones, and influence osteoblastic and osteoclastic activity and the release of calcium and phosphorus into the body. For example, hyperparathyroidism may result in a secondary form of rickets (discussed earlier). For further discussion of other endocrine disorders, see Lewis 2018 or 2019b.

Pituitary Disorders

Hyperpituitarism is characterized by overproduction of the growth hormone by the pituitary gland, often caused by the presence of a growth-hormone-secreting tumor (adenoma). Hyperpituitarism occurring during childhood produces gigantism, characterized by excessive growth and bone density. Onset or continuation of the condition, once the growth plates have fused and linear growth has halted, is referred to as acromegaly. Here, excessive bone turnover results in enlargement of bones, an increase in thickness of the cranial vault, enlarged frontal sinuses, spinal osteophytes, tufting of the distal phalanges (termed "arrow-heads"), and prominent tendon and ligament insertions. Adults who have had hyperpituitarism since childhood will also display extreme height (Resnick et al. 2024, 796). Gigantism is a rare condition, with only a few hundred people described with it globally today (Bogusławska et al. 2024). The majority of people with gigantism have genetic mutations on the *AIP* gene (Rostomyan et al. 2015), or somatic mutation of the *GNAS* gene. While gigantism has predominantly been reported in males, more recent studies have found an equal frequency in males and females (Bogusławska et al. 2024), and a new form of X-linked acrogigantism (X-LAG), caused by partial X-chromosome duplication inherited as a dominant gene has been discovered (Trivellin et al. 2014). There have been very few examples of acromegaly or gigantism reported in the paleopathological literature.

Gigantism and subsequent acromegaly was suggested by Mulhern (2005) for a male from the fifth dynasty in Egypt (ca. 2465–2325 BCE), with wedging of the lumbar vertebral bodies and a fractured femoral head. Thinned parietal bones were considered indicative of additional hypogonadism, and it was thought the individual may have been a eunuch (i.e., had been castrated). Based on the extreme size of the mandible, Viciano et al. (2015) argued for gigantism/acromegaly in a 20–30-year-old male from the Jewish necropolis of Ronda Sur in Lucena, Spain (eighth–twelfth century CE), but the poor preservation of this individual's skeleton hindered a conclusive diagnosis. A more modern example of the skeletal changes associated with gigantism is seen in the skeleton of Thomas Hasler, whose remains are curated in the Institute of Pathology at Munich University, Germany. Hasler developed a pituitary tumor at the age of 9, and by the age of 12, was 162 cm (63.8 inches) tall (Nerlich et al. 1991). Acromegaly is a more common condition than gigantism in the clinical literature, and this prevalence is also seen archaeologically. Seven male individuals with possible acromegaly have been reported in the paleopathological literature (see Lewis 2018). The most recently documented example of acromegaly is that seen in the mummified human remains of an adult male from Egypt, with an eroded sella turcica indicating the presence of a pituitary tumor (Panzer et al. 2019).

Hypopituitarism, or a deficiency in growth hormone during development, leads to short stature. Tumors, infection, or injury to the pituitary gland, as well as genetic factors such as mutations of genes *HESX1, LHX3, LHX4, PROP1*, and *PIT-1*, are potential causes, and 10% of cases are familial (Argyropoulou and Kiortsis 2005; Resnick et al. 2024, 805). It is the main cause of short stature today, and affects between 1 in 4,000 and 1 in 10,000 live births (Webb and Dattani 2015). Stunted growth, delayed development of the dentition, premature fusion of the secondary ossification centers, and a short, gracile, proportional skeleton results. Disproportionate short stature (e.g., achondroplasia) can be differentiated relatively easily from this condition (see Chapter 2). There are many causes of short, proportional stature, such as chronic infection or malnourishment during childhood. The distribution and character of bone changes seen in hypopituitarism should differentiate these conditions in skeletal remains, if not always in artistic representation. Five probable examples of affected individuals have been reported in skeletons in the literature (Roberts 1987; Ortner 2003, 424; Aristova et al. 2006; Molto and Kirkpatrick 2018; Halcrow et al. 2020), dating from precontact New Mexico, Romano-British England, Bronze Age Russia, Third Intermediate Period Egypt, and Neolithic China, respectively. Nevertheless, other endocrine disorders, such as Turner syndrome (a chromosomal disorder causing delayed growth and puberty in females) should be considered for these diagnoses (Arrieta et al. 2021). Interestingly, three of the five individuals where a biological sex was estimated were female. The individual described by Roberts (1987) was a proportionately short adult female skeleton, excavated from a fourth-century CE cemetery in Gloucester, England (Fig. 7.21). The diagnosis of hypopituitarism was based on delayed fusion of the secondary ossification centers, a gracile skeleton, abnormalities of the dentition, and a reduced stature (131 cm compared to the mean for females in that cemetery of 153 cm). The only possible cause of this disorder identified on the skeleton was in the form of long-standing plaques of new bone on the endocranial surface, suggesting an infection. This may indicate that the condition began later in childhood,

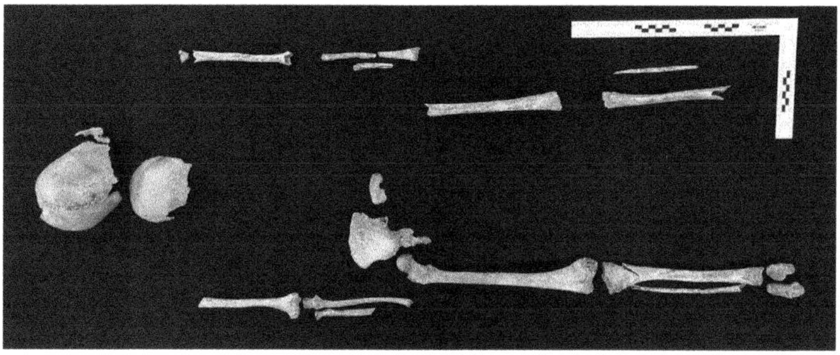

Figure 7.21. Individual with hypopituitarism from Romano-British Gambier-Parry Lodge, Gloucester, England (fourth century CE). A comparison of the size of the innominate with another individual of the same age can be seen in Roberts and Manchester 2005 (248). Photograph courtesy of Jo Buckberry and BARC, University of Bradford.

resulting in a slightly taller stature than that seen in people with a congenital cause for this disease (120 cm; Higham et al. 2016).

Microcephaly (see Chapter 2) can also cause the cranium to be much smaller than normal, and therefore, the postcranial skeleton is needed to make a diagnosis of hypopituitarism in the archaeological record (Lewis 2019b, 572). The identification of hypopituitarism in children is more challenging than in adults, as a child presenting with delayed growth and dental development may be interpreted as having faltering growth due to malnutrition (Waldron 2021, 267), or aged as much younger and remain "hidden." Halcrow et al. (2020) reviewed evidence of endocranial disorders and the differential diagnoses for short stature in their analysis of the skeleton of an adult female from Neolithic China. They concluded she suffered from either hypothyroidism (see later in the chapter) or hypopituitarism, and argued that secondary fractures to her neck as a result of osteopenia and potential cognitive issues would have impacted her quality of life. This female was also buried with her hands behind her back, a point of difference when compared to the other people in the cemetery, and Halcrow et al. (2020) suggested that, as an individual of short stature, she may have been considered an "outsider" in Chinese culture. By contrast, Molto and Kirkpatrick (2018) argued that individuals with dwarfism in ancient Egypt often occupied positions of high status and would not have been considered "disabled."

Hyperostosis Frontalis Interna

Related to the pituitary gland disorders is hyperostosis of the endocranial surface of the frontal bone (hyperostosis frontalis interna [HFI]; Alvarez et al. 2022). Prominent thickening and formation of nodules of new bone on the frontal bone occurs, most frequently, in postmenopausal females, but males over the age of 60 years can also have the condition (Fig. 7.22).

These changes are probably the result of altered pituitary gland secretion of hormones (May et al. 2011). Hershkovitz et al. (1999) developed a scheme to allow the

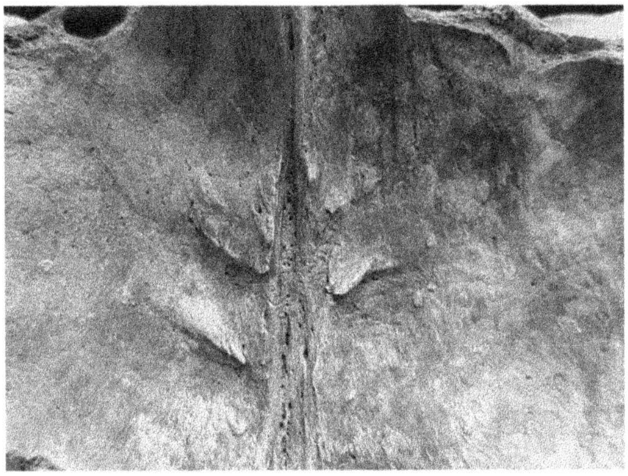

Figure 7.22. Hyperostosis frontalis interna in a mature female from St. Oswald's Priory, Gloucester, England (1100–1550 CE). Photograph by Mary Lewis.

different expressions of the lesions to be recorded, noting an increase in the severity of expression after 60 years, while milder forms occur more commonly in males (Wilczak and Mulhern 2012). Since the third edition of this book was published, research into HFI in archaeological populations has significantly increased, perhaps due to access to, and availability of, digital radiography and CT scanning that allow visualization of intact crania. Examples of the condition are now known from as early as 57,600 ± 4,600 years BCE in a Neanderthal individual from Charente, France (Garralda et al. 2014). The link between HFI and hypogonadism, resulting from surgical or chemical castration, has also been highlighted, with a fascinating study of HFI in the skeleton of the famous castrato "Farinelli" (Carlo Broschi), who underwent castration surgery as a prepubescent and died at age 78 in 1782 (Belcastro et al. 2011). Population-based studies have shown HFI appears to have increased in more recent populations, at least in Europe (Szeniczey et al. 2019). For example, research on a documented sample of fifteenth–nineteenth century Londoners showed HFI at a 16% frequency compared to 24% in individuals from known documented collections dating to the twentieth century (Western and Bekvalac 2017). This increase has been suggested to be the result of reduced exposure to estrogen over a female's lifetime due to a reduction in the number of pregnancies in industrialized societies (May et al. 2011; Western and Bekvalac 2017).

Thyroid Disorders

A normally functioning thyroid gland will secrete two main hormones when guided by the pituitary gland: thyroxin and triiodothyronine (Resnick et al. 2024, 806). Genetic factors that result in an autoimmune attack on the thyroid gland (Imani et al. 2017) can stimulate overproduction of thyroxine (thyrotoxicosis), resulting in toxic nodular goiter, characterized by a swelling in the neck. Increased bone resorption and osteoporosis, with cartilage calcification, characterize the disorder, with fatigue, nervousness, weight loss, and palpitations as some of the signs and symptoms. Pregnant females with untreated hyperthyroidism (as they would have been in the past) have an increased risk of complications, including miscarriages, premature births, low birth weight, and maternal heart failure (Turunen et al. 2020). The condition is rare in children but may occur in adolescents (Lewis 2018, 261) and may be evident even on radiograph through the presence of lytic lesions affecting the frontal bone, or premature osteoporosis (Resnick et al. 2024, 807–808). Its effects are most pronounced in soft tissue and, as noted earlier, the multiple other factors can lead to osteoporosis. Although there have been many representations of goiter in art, no examples of thyrotoxicosis have been reported from an archaeological context, except in a mummified individual from eighteenth-century Sicily, where an enlarged thyroid gland was found (Ciranni et al. 1999).

A deficiency in thyroxine or hypothyroidism may be endemic, due to a lack of naturally occurring iodine in the environment (e.g., water or soil), or sporadic, caused by a tumor or a genetic anomaly. Iodine is essential for the formation of thyroxine, as it contains several iodine atoms (Hinson et al. 2010). Iodine is found naturally in seawater and, hence, in the drinking water and plants of coastal areas around the world. Low levels of natural iodine are common in central regions of Asia, Africa, central and eastern Europe, and the central United States, as well as mountainous regions, such as the Alps, Andes, and Himalayas (Hatch-McChesney and Lieberman 2022). In 1998, it was estimated that 30% of the world's population was at risk for iodine deficiency, with 10% suffering from the disease (Dobson 1998; Cotran et al. 1989, 1227). Beginning in the 1920s, public health authorities in some countries added iodine to table salt for the prevention of goiter. However, resistance to the programs and a reduction in salt consumption in industrialized countries means this condition is on the rise. In the past, iodine would have been available in the diet through dairy, eggs, and fish (Hatch-McChesney and Lieberman 2022). As thyroxin stimulates skeletal maturation and feeds back to the pituitary gland to release the growth hormone, hypothyroidism (myxedema) causes a delay in both growth and maturation in children, along with irregular fragmentary ossification centers, prominent cranial sutures, and cranial ossicles, as well as generalized osteopenia. The symptoms of the disease are opposite to those of thyrotoxicosis: cognitive impairment, constipation, lethargy, slow heart rate, swelling (nontoxic goiter), decreased sweating, and weight gain. Although there are some differences in the skeletal changes compared to hypopituitarism, in archaeological populations, distinguishing between the two conditions may prove difficult (e.g., Halcrow et al. 2020). In fact, only one example of hypothyroidism has been reported in the paleopathological literature, in a 30-year-old mummified female from the Ica Valley, Peru (95 BCE), with a goiter and soft tissue calcifications in the aorta, that Gabrovsky et al. (2016) associated with atherosclerosis and heart disease.

Epilogue

Research into ancient diets and diseases of dietary deficiencies has advanced considerably since the third edition of this book. In particular, the study of rickets and scurvy in children has been transformed, and we now know much more about the complex alchemy of factors that contribute to their presence in the past. We now have a far more detailed understanding of the causes behind porotic lesions on the cranium and orbits, and we are beginning to find more evidence for the genetic anemias and what their presence tells us about migration and the spread of noncommunicable diseases in the past. Factors that cause food shortages and unequal access to adequate nutrition have resonance today, and form part of the UN's Sustainable Development Goals. Paleopathological research into Paget's disease and osteoporosis has been aided by new chemical, biomolecular, and imaging techniques, revealing both differences and similarities of these diseases in past and modern populations. Clearly, dietary deficiencies (often coupled with infections) were an ever-present danger in the past, as they are now.

8

Neoplastic Disease

> Environmental carcinogens undoubtedly have a long history, but both the number and the concentration of these agents have changed in recent human history, often to the disadvantage of human groups.
>
> —D. J. Ortner, *Identification of Pathological Conditions in Human Skeletal Remains*

In the high-income countries of the world today, everyone is familiar with the problem of cancer. In 2020, cancer was second only to heart disease as the leading cause of death worldwide, at 10.0 million deaths per year (WHO 2020). Globally, cancer treatment is estimated to cost around US$1.2 trillion annually, and people living in low- to middle-income countries carry 80% of the global cancer burden, and yet receive only 5% of global spending to help combat the disease. This situation means these countries will continue to fall behind others in their ability to provide effective cancer treatment for their citizens, threatening one of the UN's Sustainable Development Goal targets for 2030: (3) to ensure healthy lives and promote well-being for all at all ages, and to reduce death by noncommunicable disease, including cancer, by one-third compared to 2015. Delayed diagnosis, a lack of infrastructure, and limited access to the most up-to-date training, screening, and therapies exacerbate global challenges in cancer care (WHO 2020; Mao et al. 2021).

In females, breast cancer is the most commonly reported cancer worldwide, with an incidence of 46.8 per 100,000 new reports per year. In males, lung cancer has the highest incidence, at 32.5 per 100,000 cases, followed by cancer of the prostate gland at 30.7 per 100,000 cases (Ferlay et al. 2021). While breast cancer is the leading form of the disease today, developments in radiotherapy and chemotherapy have improved survival rates (WHO 2020). The risk factors for cancer are myriad and include biological sex, age, geographical location, socioeconomic status, ancestry, whether a person regularly smokes tobacco or consumes alcohol, a lack of fresh fruit and vegetables in the diet, being obese, and being exposed to air pollution. In low- and middle-income countries, chronic infections such as hepatitis B and C provide greater risks for cancer (Shen et al. 2022). Different cancers will also affect different age groups. Cancer is the second biggest killer (after accidents and injuries) of children aged 1–14 years, and in 2014 it affected 186.6 per one million children

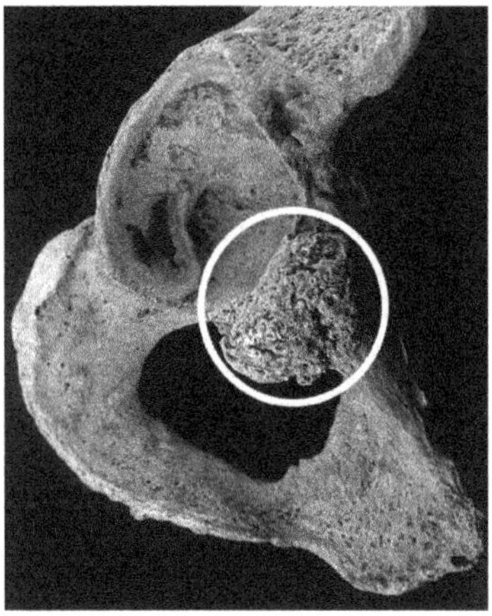

Figure 8.1. Bone tumor (osteochondroma) in the pelvic bone of an adult female from Lisht, Egypt, 1990–1786 BCE. With kind permission from the National Museum of Natural History, Washington, DC.

(Ward et al. 2014). The most common forms of neoplasm in children are malignant—leukemia, lymphoma, and tumors of the brain and central nervous system (i.e., neuroblastomas). However, in 75% to 90% of children with cancer the cause is unknown, making it one of the most poorly understood branches of medicine (Buka 2009), and prompting a global initiative to stimulate research (WHO 2020).

Today the word *tumor* is often considered synonymous with cancer, but this has not always been so. Until the early nineteenth century, inflammatory swellings, cysts, and new growths (both benign and malignant) were all considered tumors. Instead, it is "new growths"—literally, neoplasms—that signal neoplastic disease. Willis (1948) defined a neoplasm as an abnormal mass of tissue, the growth of which exceeds and is uncoordinated with that of the body's normal tissues (Fig. 8.1). Neoplasms may arise in any tissue of the body (bone, cartilage, fibrous tissue, or blood/marrow, and also fat and nerve cells), in any organ of the body, and in any individual. The frequency of specific neoplasms, however, may vary within groups of people.

Individual neoplasms may consist of differentiated cells characteristic of the original tissue; alternatively, the growth may comprise totally undifferentiated cells that divide rapidly and do not resemble any specific tissue of the body (anaplastic). In most cases, the tumors are considered to be monoclonal—that is, that all the cancerous cells can be traced back to a single parent cell. Neoplasms are considered either benign or malignant. Benign neoplasms are those that remain solely at their site of origin and tend to spread only locally. They occur more frequently than primary malignant neoplasms, although they are less common in bone than in other tissues of the body (Marques 2019, 639). The cells comprising benign neoplasms are generally well differentiated. They are clinically less significant when compared to malignant neoplasms unless their location impacts a vital structure, such as the eyes or brain. Instead, any symptoms from a benign neoplasm are due to the local effect of the growth on the surrounding body structures, and to the sheer size of the growth itself.

Malignant neoplasms are characterized by their propensity to spread to other tissues. For example, metastatic cancer is caused by the uncontrolled local spread of a primary malignant tumor into and onto other organs of the body, and by the secondary dissemination of cancer cells (metastases) to more distant organs, with the complete breakdown of that organ's function. They peak in young, actively growing individuals and in people aged over 60 years (Grimer et al. 2013). Their spread is achieved through the bloodstream and the lymphatic system, and by the direct implantation of cells in such areas as the pleural and peritoneal cavities (Marques

Table 8.1. Examples of neoplasms that affect bone

Cell source	Benign	Malignant
Hematopoietic (blood forming)		Myeloma Leukemia
Chondrogenic (cartilage producing)	Enchondroma Chondroblastoma Osteochondroma	Chondrosarcoma
Osteogenic (bone forming)	Osteoma Osteoid osteoma Osteoblastoma	Osteosarcoma
Osteogenic and osteoclastic (bone destroying)	Giant cell tumor	
Fibrogenic (fibrous tissue forming)	Nonossifying fibroma	Fibrosarcoma
Unknown		Ewing sarcoma

2019, 640). The signs/symptoms of cancer vary in their severity, but include pain, localized swelling, nerve damage, fractures, fever, weight loss, hypercalcemia, and fatigue (Anderson et al. 2020). The relentless unchecked growth of the primary malignant neoplasm and its metastases results ultimately in the death of the individual.

The classification of neoplasms is continually evolving, but they are currently ordered by the tissue the tumor arises from and the location on the body where it first develops. Tumors originating in bone have the prefix *osteo-*, while the suffix *-oma* identifies a swelling (or tumor) to the root of the tissue of origin. For example, the terms *chondroma*, *osteoma*, and *fibroma* refer to tumors originating in the cartilage, bone, and fibrous cells, respectively. *Adeno-* suggests the neoplasm forms in a gland, and *angiomas* arise in blood vessels. Some cancers show a greater propensity to metastasize to bone (known as osteotropism), with up to 80% of patients with prostate or breast cancer also showing skeletal lesions. In contrast, cancers of the gut are less likely to spread to bone (Marques 2019, 640). Table 8.1 lists the most common neoplasms found in archaeological remains, which are discussed in this chapter.

Cancers comprise many different diseases with different expressions, progression, underlying genetics, molecular characteristics, and outcomes, including individual reactions to each disease. For this reason, the diagnosis of neoplastic disease in skeletal remains can prove difficult. It relies on the identification of macroscopic and radiographic lesions affecting specific bones in particular age and biological sex groups. For example, the benign tumor called osteoid osteoma affects males twice as frequently as females, and more than 50% of people affected are in the 11–20-year-old age group; a quarter of osteoid osteomas affect the femur and a quarter affect the tibia. Extensive radiographic analysis should be undertaken to ensure that any lesions not visible externally on the bone are detected, but this ideal is rarely achieved in paleopathology, to the extent that we cannot be confident that all of the evidence for neoplastic disease in the group has been identified. At a minimum, surveys of the lumbar vertebrae, pelvis, femur, and cranium within a skeletal sample would be required to be sure any hidden lesions of cancer have been found.

For example, Western and Bekvalac (2020, 122–124) surveyed 1,373 middle-aged to mature adults from preindustrial and postindustrial London. They identified six individuals with metastatic cancer, three of whom (50%) were only identified using radiographs. Rothschild and Rothschild (1995), in their study of cancer in skeletons from the early twentieth century Hamann-Todd Osteological Collection curated in Cleveland, Ohio, identified cancer in eleven skeletons through macroscopic analysis alone, but diagnosed the condition in thirty-three more individuals using radiography. Marques et al. (2018) also demonstrated the difficulty in diagnosing cancer using the Coimbra and Lisbon Identified Skeletal Collections (nineteenth–twentieth-century Portugal). Although 131 individuals were known to have died from cancer in the collections, only 17.6% displayed skeletal lesions that were pathognomonic (diagnostic) for cancer, 45% had skeletal lesions that could not be directly attributed to cancer, and 37.4% of the individuals had no skeletal lesions at all. Fatula (2021) published useful guidelines on bone positioning during radiography to more easily visualize hidden cancerous lesions. They also recommended a three-tier system for radiographic skeletal surveys, starting with (1) the cranium, os coxae, and femora, moving on to (2) the humeri, clavicles, and thoracic and lumbar vertebrae, and finally, (3) the ribs, scapulae, sternum, and sacrum. The use of micro-CT scanning has also been shown to provide greater accuracy when examining neoplastic lesions (Mitchell et al. 2021), but access to these expensive scanners is not available to everyone. Indeed, not all paleopathologists have access to radiography.

How Common Was Cancer in the Past?

Cancer has afflicted all complex organisms since long before the evolution of *Homo sapiens*. Descriptions appear in most early medical texts; however, all that was once labeled "cancer" might not have been what we now consider it to be, and "tumor" can also be interpreted as a nonspecific swelling. The Edwin Smith papyrus, Egypt (1600 BCE), may hold the earliest reference to cancer, in its account of a bulging tumor of the breast for which there was no treatment (Breasted 1991, 403–406, case 45). Hippocrates (fifth century BCE) also described a female who died of breast cancer with a bleeding nipple (*Epidemics* 5, 101; *Epidemics* 7, 116; see Smith 1994, 215 and 407). He called the disease *καρκίνωμα* (karkinoma, "crab"), from which the word *cancer* originates—carcinoma. The Hippocratics also understood that cancer could spread widely and be occult (or hidden). The Sanskrit text *Sushruta Samhita* from ancient India (likely before 300 BCE) contains many references to tumors, the words for which seem to represent cancer: *granthi*, *gulma*, and *arvuda* (e.g., Bishagratna 1907–1916, 2, 16, 65–66, 75).

Despite multiple observations of the disease pervading ancient and medieval literature of Europe and Asia, the cause of cancer remained mysterious, just as it often is today. Nevertheless, numerous, sometimes durable, theories were expounded to explain it: excess black bile (one of the humors in Greek medicine), inflammation, blockage of lymph fluid, inheritance, contagion (infections like TB), trauma, mental illness, environmental factors, and occupations (Rather 1978; Wolff 1989).

Bernardino Ramazzini (1713) noticed the absence of cervical cancer and a high prevalence of breast cancer in nuns, concluding that both conditions resulted from their occupation-related sexual abstinence. In 1775, the prolific Percivall Pott in one short publication opined that soot induced cancer of the scrotum in chimney sweeps, thereby cementing his reputation as a founder of occupational health (Payne 2017). In 1845, making use of microscopy, Rudolf Virchow of Berlin published the first description of leukemia, and by 1858 he had elaborated cell theory to explain the origin and spread of cancer (Wolff 1989). This reorientation of the disease concept to cell theory allowed for the twentieth-century incorporation of genetics, virology, immunology, and later, molecular typing into the etiology of neoplasms.

As for treatment, bandages, poultices, heat, cold, painkillers, and herbal preparations were favored. Doctors acknowledged the dismal prognosis but could not resist trying to eradicate the painful, sometimes weeping tumors by cautery and surgery. The Hippocratic authors claimed success with cautery for a cancer of the pharynx (*Epidemics* 7, 111); however, for hidden cancer, he advised that it was better not to attempt treatment (*Aphorisms* VI, 38). The earliest mastectomy is said to have been performed by Leonidas of Alexandria (second century BCE), but we know of it only through later writers (Retief and Cilliers 2011). Special instruments and strategies were devised to excise cancers of the skin and the appendages, especially those of the breast, although the sixteenth-century French surgeon Ambroise Paré contended that operating on cancer only made matters worse. Clearly not daunted by this, the eighteenth-century *Encyclopédie* of René Diderot and Jean d'Alembert featured an illustration of an anxious but sentient female undergoing the horrific operation (Duffin 2021, 284). With the mid-nineteenth-century advent of anesthesia and antisepsis, operations became more tolerable but also more aggressive, as they responded to the advent of cell theory and aimed for cure by eliminating nearby sites of metastases, as well as the tumor itself. By 1900, shortly after their discovery, X-rays, radium, and other radioactive materials were found to destroy cancer even as they sometimes also caused it. Only in the mid-twentieth century did a wide array of chemical agents begin to appear that caused tumors to recede and sometimes disappear altogether.

Most histories of cancer concentrate on the last 150 years (Mukherjee 2010). Our understanding of rates in the prehistoric period can only be gleaned from the paleopathological record, but evidence is scarce. As life expectancy in the past may not have been as long as today, perhaps the number of individuals surviving to the age of higher cancer prevalence was not as great. Cancer is also a problem of the young, and therefore the presumed reduced longevity in antiquity cannot be the sole reason for the rarity of paleopathological evidence. If, as seems likely, there has been an increase in malignant disease in recent times, the reasons may be related to the changing environment throughout history (see Marques et al. 2022). Physical (e.g., ultraviolet light), chemical (e.g., asbestos, tobacco smoke, alcohol), and viral agents (e.g., hepatitis B virus can cause liver cancer) as well as diet (e.g., fatty foods) are all identified carcinogens that have their part to play today in the development of cancers. In particular, lack of fiber in the diet and excess fat and protein are believed to lead to colon cancer (Brennan and Davey-Smith 2022). The woodsmoke-filled cave environment, naturally occurring gases such as radon and uranium, and toxic fumes induced by metalworking in the past may all have contributed to the development of neoplastic disease. Since the eighteenth century, many agents have been found to stimulate malignant change. Most are the products of modern industrial development and would not have been encountered in the village or town life of preindustrial societies. The frequency of lung cancer in the West also rose steeply after the Second World War with an increase in the popularity of tobacco smoking (Huang et al. 2022). The relationship between lung cancer and cigarettes is well attested, but what of the cancers of the breast, prostate, stomach, and so on?

Whether cancers were rare in the past due to the lack of risk factors described here, or whether we lack the diagnostic capability to identify them, is still a matter of debate. It is more likely that a lack of standardization in recording and lack of large-scale radiographic surveys means we have only a snapshot of the disease through time. Importantly, while individual examples of metastatic cancer affecting people in the past may be published, the number of individuals within that sample who could be observed, but were not affected by cancer, is usually not reported (Marques et al. 2021). An example of this "snapshot" was illustrated by Hunt et al. (2018) in a meta-data study using their newly developed Cancer Research in Ancient Bodies (CRAB) database. They showed that the greatest number of individuals from archaeological contexts reported with cancer came from northern Europe and North Africa, a pattern that may be related more to the distribution of paleopathologists looking for them than a true distribution. They noted 272 published examples of malignant disease dating from 1.8 million years ago to 1900 CE. Perhaps due to their distinctive appearance, metastasizing cancer and multiple myeloma were the most common types of reported cancers, and 57% were in males.

The European Union defines a rare disease as one that occurs in 0.05% of the population, or 1 in 2,000 people (Genetic and Rare Diseases Information Centre, GARD). Taking this as a baseline, Marques et al. (2021) argued that with a crude prevalence rate of 1.2% (based on 151 individuals with cancer, where the total sample size was reported), cancer in the past exceeds this threshold. In order to progress our understanding of the archaeology of neoplasms, and contribute to modern debates on the causes of these diseases today, we need to provide the overall numbers of individuals with and without the disease in our study groups, and standardize the way in which we report the lesions that we identify. Ragsdale et al. (2018) suggested a diagnosis of "neoplastic disease" rather than a specific diagnosis may be the best we can hope for. The type of neoplasm might, however, be narrowed down using biological sex and age characteristics of the individual affected, and the nature and distribution of the lesions. A differential diagnosis is also essential, as conditions such as TB, treponemal disease, fungal infections, and even insect activity in the burial environment can produce similar lesions (Hunt et al. 2018). Hence, when describing neoplastic disease in individuals or in a group, high-quality photographs and, if possible, radiographs should accompany descriptions of lesions, alongside sociocultural and burial context (Marques et al. 2018;

Hunt et al. 2018; Ragsdale et al. 2018; Lewis 2018, 229). For each individual, information should include:

1. Details of the site (name, location, date/period)
2. The group from which the individual came (number of males/females/adults/children)
3. Methods used to screen the whole group, if appropriate
4. Environmental context (e.g., forager/farmer/urban/industrial)
5. Burial context (e.g., grave inclusions, body treatment, type of grave)
6. Identifier (skeleton number), level of preservation, biological sex, ancestry, and age of the affected individual(s)
7. Lesion type (destructive, bone forming, or both), number, and size
8. Appearance on a radiograph (e.g., evidence of sclerotic margin)
9. Periosteal reaction appearance (lamellar bone, onion skin, sunburst)
10. Type of bone matrix visible on a radiograph, if any
11. Nature of bone destruction (e.g., characteristics of margins, evidence of healing)
12. Location (e.g., for a long bone: metaphyseal, diaphyseal, epiphyseal involvement)

On a radiograph, a new bone matrix formed in the response to a tumor will appear as "nests" of dense bone, or as multiple opaque flecks, with osteosarcoma, osteoblastoma, chondrosarcoma, chondroblastoma, and enchondroma the only primary tumors that produce new bone; this allows diagnosis to be narrowed down (Edeiken et al. 1966). A well-defined and dense sclerotic margin around a lesion on a radiograph normally suggests a benign tumor. This appearance is characteristic of nonossifying fibromas, enchondromas, chondroblastomas, and chondrosarcomas (Ragsdale 1993). Conversely, malignant tumors spread so rapidly that the body usually has no time to produce a sclerotic (healed) bony margin. The amount of periosteal new bone formed is proportionate to the intensity, aggressiveness, and duration of the lesion and is more likely to occur on the long bones and in younger individuals (Ragsdale 1993). The following overview considers some of the most commonly reported benign and malignant neoplasms of bone, cartilage, fibrous tissue, and blood/marrow. It also includes Langerhans cell histiocytosis, a blood-borne disease once considered neoplastic, but which has a much-debated etiology.

Benign Neoplasms

The multitude of soft tissue benign neoplasms, the "warts and all" of the famous Oliver Cromwell portrait painted by Peter Levy in the seventeenth century CE, generally leave no evidence in skeletal remains. With few exceptions, only the benign neoplasms of the bone itself will be manifest in skeletal remains. These lesions, which remain discrete but vary in size, have been identified in many skeletal remains of antiquity. Cartilage is an essential component of developing bone, and neoplasms can originate from it. For the present discussion, only the more common benign neoplasms identified in adults and children in the past will be considered.

Osteochondroma

An osteochondroma (Fig. 8.2) is one of the most common benign bone tumors diagnosed in modern clinical practice. Osteochondromas are developmental aberrations caused by faulty ossification of the growth plate. They appear most often in long bones, with a 2:1 incidence in the lower limb, and they usually occur spontaneously or, more rarely, after trauma to the bone at the site (Resnick et al. 2024, 1146). Osteochondromas may be present at birth (and hence potentially seen in infant remains) but are not usually symptomatic until later in life (Steinbock 1976, 369). The tumor consists of bone marrow and trabeculae capped with a thick layer of cartilage, which may give rise to the malignant chondrosarcoma (Khurana and Unni 2003). On a radiograph there is a continuation of cancellous bone into the defect (Steinbock 1976, 369). Growth of the tumor ceases with the end of the bone's growing period. As these lesions develop out of the growth plate, the closer the lesion is to the end of the fused bone, the later in life the tumor arose. The morphology of these tumors may be broad and bulbous (sessile) or spurlike (pedunculated); the latter forms on a stalk of bone rising directly from the bone cortex (Lewis 2018, 231–233). By and large, the only sign of the tumour is the inconvenience of a localized swelling on a limb. The paleopathological literature includes a number of notable examples in adults (Buzon 2005; Čavka et al. 2022; Riccomi et al. 2023; Larentis et al. 2023) and in children (Nerlich and Zink 2000; Antikas and Grearkos 2010; Walker 2012; Lewis 2018:233). In one individual, an osteochondroma on the spine of an adolescent from Thebes, Egypt (1500–1000 BCE), is thought to have resulted in scoliosis (Nerlich and Zink 2000).

Osteochondromas are usually solitary tumors. Less commonly, they appear in many locations throughout the skeleton and are described as hereditary multiple osteochondromas (HMO; Fig. 8.3). HMO is an autosomal-dominant condition caused by a mutation of the exostosis in the genes on chromosome 8 (EXT1), 11 (EXT2) (Waldron 2021), and 19 (EXT3) (Vanhoenacker et al. 2001). Today it is known to have an incidence of 1 in 50,000, and when inherited, it normally passes from the father to the child, sometimes over several generations (Bovée 2008). HMO,

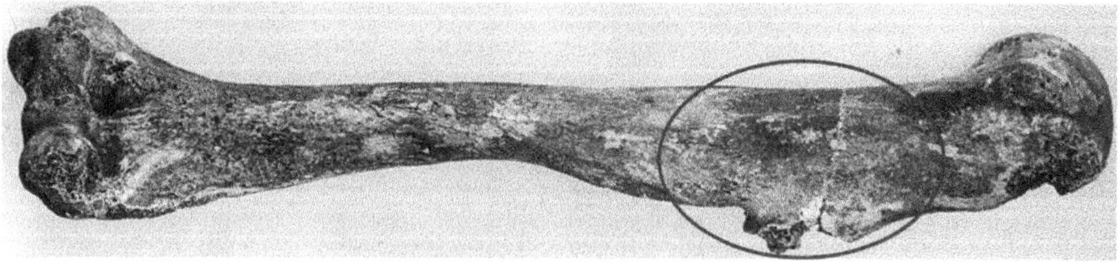

Figure 8.2. Osteochondroma in a left humerus of an unknown skeleton (Roman, Derby Racecourse cemetery, Derby, Derbyshire, England). Proximal end to the right. Photograph by and courtesy of Jean Brown.

however, also occurs spontaneously in 10% of individuals affected (Patil et al. 2012). As many as eighteen tumors have been identified across a single skeleton. They tend to be bilaterally symmetrical and are more common on the bones of the knee joint (70%) and on the humerus (50%) and fibula (30%) (Vanhoenacker et al. 2001; Patil et al. 2012). Just as with single osteochondromas, the lesions may become malignant (Waldron 2021). A particularly dramatic and fatal example of this condition was reported from a Danish medieval cemetery (Sjøvold et al. 1974). The person was a young pregnant female. Her multiple bony outgrowths were sufficiently large and ill-placed within her pelvis to prevent childbirth. The fetus contained within was at full term, but both mother and unborn child perished, probably because of the condition (seen in both individuals). A 4-year-old child from early medieval Winchester, England, has also been identified with the condition (Ortner 2003, 519), as have adolescents from Jericho (Lyall and Mann 1993) and Poland (Gladykowska-Rzeczycka and Urbanowicz 1970). Jackson et al. (2022) were the first to isolate a mutation in the second exon of EXT1 in two medieval males from the same cemetery in Ballyhanna, Ireland (1200–1650 CE), with HMO. It was expected that the men may have been related, explaining this cluster of the disease—but instead they demonstrated de novo (isolated) mutations, something rare in the modern clinical literature. Murphy and McKenzie (2010) provided a useful global survey of reported evidence, identifying 'clusters' of cases in Sweden (n = 3), Jordan (n = 3), England (n = 3), and Ireland (n = 4). Since this time, several new indviduals have been identified, including a mature male from Setúbal, Portugal (1531–1939 CE; Antunes-Ferreira et al. 2014); a child from the early Spanish contact site of La Falda (1460–1639 CE) in Argentina (Arrieta et al. 2018); and an adult male from Shandong province in China (1644–1911 CE) who also exhibited short stature, limb asymmetry, and deformities of the hip and ankle (Zhou et al. 2024). As more individuals are identified globally, our understanding about the extent of isolated and clustered evidence of this gene mutation in the past will undoubtedly increase.

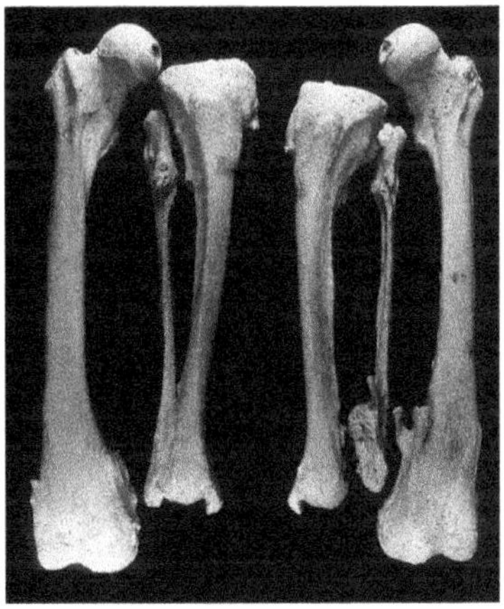

Figure 8.3. Hereditary multiple osteochondromas (HMOs) in the lower leg of an older female. From the Terry Collection, National Museum of Natural History, Washington, DC. Originally reproduced with kind permission from Don Ortner.

Osteoma

A particularly common finding in terms of neoplasms in skeletal remains is a small, round, smooth projection of mature organized lamellar bone with an unknown etiology. Osteomas seem to appear equally in males and females, arising in childhood and increasing with age (Siek 2020; Siek et al. 2021). There are three types that have been distinguished using histological analysis: (1) an "ivory" or "button" osteoma made up of dense lamellar bone without Haversian canals; (2) a cancellous osteoma containing trabecular bone, and (3) a mixture of the two (Marques 2019, 648). These lesions are sometimes no larger than a

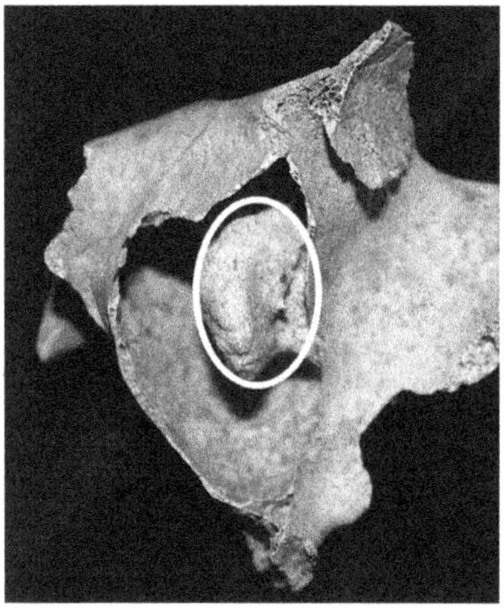

Figure 8.4. Large osteoma in the maxillary sinus of an adult male from St. Oswald's Priory, Gloucester, England (1250–1550 CE). Photography by Mary Lewis.

pinhead, but sometimes reach tennis-ball diameter. They are found most frequently on the outer surface of the frontal and parietal bones of the cranium and in the facial sinuses (Fig. 8.4; Siek 2020). In most cases, these neoplasia are symptomless, but if sizable they may cause facial pain, nerve compression, and, if located near the eyes, loss of vision (Marques 2019, 648). They have been reported in 0.42% of sinus radiographs, with Eshed et al. (2002) noting a prevalence rate of 37.6% in 585 skeletons in the Hamann-Todd Osteological Collection, Cleveland, Ohio, and in 41% of 233 archaeological skeletons, with no difference in frequency between biological sex or ancestry. In 590 individuals from medieval Poland (ninth to seventeenth century CE), Siek et al. (2021) reported an osteoma prevalence rate of 11%. While the lesion is usually solitary, some skeletal remains have multiple osteomas, which may be linked to Gardner syndrome, an autosomal-dominant disease (Resnick et al. 2024, 1051). For example, at the late medieval site of St. Andrew, Fishergate, York, England, of the seventeen individuals with an osteoma—including one with a very large lesion on the right mandibular ramus—6 (32%) had between two and six osteomas each, and one individual displayed twenty osteomas (Stroud and Kemp 1993, 224).

Osteoid Osteoma

An osteoid osteoma is a relatively rare, benign, and solitary tumor presenting, clinically, as an oval nest of activity (nidus) composed of osteoid (unmineralized bone) and an area of sclerotic reactive bone surrounding the lesion that is out of proportion to the size of the lesion itself (Steinbock 1976; Ortner 2003). The majority of osteoid osteomas occur three times more often in males than females, and in young people between the ages of 5 and 20 years (Isler and Turcotte 2003; Khurana and Unni 2003). These tumors are most common in the femur (25%) and tibia (25%), but may also be located in the humerus, spine, fibula, or foot bones (Jaffe 1958). In the long bones, they are normally less than 1.5 cm in length. Individuals experience persistent bone pain and, if the tumor is located in the spine

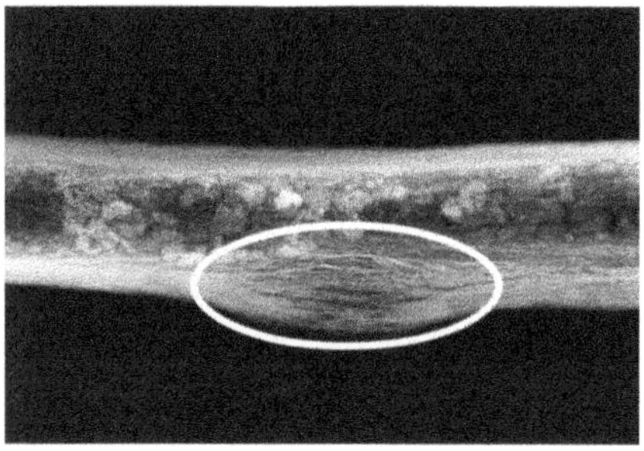

Figure 8.5. Radiograph of an osteoid osteoma on the tibia of a child, showing a radiolucent interior and laminated (layered) shell (late Roman Rhodas Town, Canterbury, England). Photograph courtesy of Louise Loe (Oxford Archaeology) and Canterbury Archaeological Trust.

or joint, it may cause scoliosis or joint flexion, respectively (Khurana and Unni 2003). As noted above, osteoid osteomas are identified on a radiograph by a well-defined radiolucent core where the nidus of osteoid was present in life (Fig. 8.5). This lesion may be confused with osteomyelitis, or other tumors such as an osteosarcoma or osteoblastoma. Such issues were highlighted in the case of a large benign tumor on the occipital bone of a young adult male from Muğla in Türkiye (second century BCE–third century CE). The tumor diagnosis was narrowed down to either an osteoid osteoma or an osteoblastoma based on its radiographic features (Bews et al. 2023).

Giant Cell Tumor

This benign tumor of bone is one of the most common primary bone tumors seen in adolescents and young adults, and is more frequent in females around 17 years of age (Isler and Turcotte 2003). The tumor is made up of stromal (connective tissue) cells and multinucleated giant cells similar to osteoclasts. It arises at the ends of the bones that have newly fused, usually at the knee, proximal humerus, and distal radius (Isler and Turcotte 2003). These tumors are painful and aggressive, breaking through the cortex of the bone and forming a hard tissue mass contained within a thin cortical shell. This fragile shell appears like a soap bubble on a radiograph. While these tumors may heal spontaneously, larger tumors may persist and cause disuse of the limb and atrophy (Resnick et al. 2024). Differential diagnoses should include a nonossifying fibroma, chondroblastoma, osteoblastoma, and osteosarcoma (Isler and Turcotte 2003). This tumor is rarely reported in paleopathology, perhaps due to the fragile nature of the characteristic shell that could be damaged during burial, or because it may heal completely in early adulthood. Nevertheless, a probable example was identified in the left distal femur of an adult from early medieval Finglesham in Kent (Brothwell 1967b), although at that time radiographs were not used to assess the internal characteristics of the tumor. Ventura et al. (2021) identified a giant cell tumor in the left femur, of a mummified female aged 40–49 years from sixteenth–eighteenth-century CE Modena, Italy. The atrophy of the affected femur suggested disuse of the left leg, with the individual having the condition for many years. The most common symptom is pain that worsens over time as the tumor increases in size.

Nonossifying Fibroma

A fairly common lesion in nonadult skeletal remains is the nonossifying fibroma (previously known as a fibrous cortical defect) at the metaphysis of the growing long bones. This relatively frequent finding reflects the modern incidence; the tumor occurs in 35% of individuals under the age of 20 years, and usually occurs in males between the ages of 4 and 8 years (Khurana and Unni 2003). The most commonly affected sites are the distal femur and tibia, and the proximal tibia and fibula. The defects are always longer than they are wide, symmetrical and multiple, and are positioned further away from the metaphyseal area as the bone increases in length (Fig. 8.6; Ortner 2003). The exact etiology of these lesions is not fully understood, and their

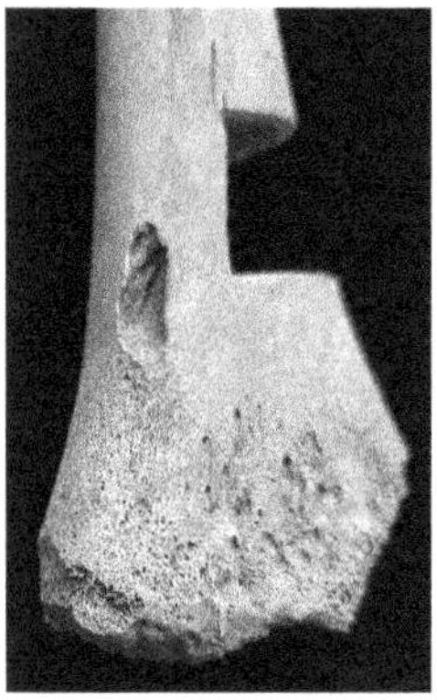

Figure 8.6. Nonossifying fibroma in the distal femur of a child from St. Oswald's Priory, Gloucester, England (1250–1550 CE). Photograph by Mary Lewis.

appearance as the child begins to walk has led to suggestions that they result from using the muscles. They heal spontaneously (Khurana and Unni 2003; Waldron 2021). Much evidence probably goes unpublished and it appears only in unpublished osteological reports, although Anderson (2001, 2002) has described these defects in several nonadults from medieval England (see Lewis 2018, 235).

Meningioma

Very rarely in paleopathology, a tumor of soft tissue may produce a bony reaction that itself resembles a neoplasm. Such reactions tend to occur in the cranium and are the cause of 15–20% of intracranial tumors (Waldron 1998, 213). One of the most frequently reported in the archaeological record is the meningioma, arising from the meninges (membranes) that cover the brain. This neoplasm may induce an alarming rate of growth of the ectocranium overlying the lesion, accompanied by destructive changes on the endocranial surface (Jónsdóttir et al. 2003; Cook and Dansforth 2022). Care must be taken to distinguish between porous lesions caused by porotic hyperostosis on the external surface of the cranium and a meningioma. The latter results in lesions that are described as a uniform mesh of new bone, containing macroscopically visible "whorls," or concentric circles (Rothschild 2022, 115).

Langerhans Cell Histiocytosis

Langerhans cell histiocytosis (LCH) is one of the most commonly cited conditions in nonadult archaeological human remains, but its status as a true neoplasm remains controversial (Auerbach and Aguilera 2023). LCH is a benign condition that occurs when the body produces too many histiocytes (Langerhans cells) in the medullary cavities of bones—these cells help regulate the immune system. These build up in the body and cause granulomatous destruction of bone and damage organs (Resnick et al. 2024, 906). LCH was originally described as three separate conditions: (1) Letterer-Siwe disease: multifocal, multisystem form, which is rare and sometimes fatal; (2) Hand-Schüller-Christian disease: chronic and often accompanied by diabetes; and (3) eosinophilic granuloma: mildest form and most common. Since the 1980s, they are now recognized as three different forms of disease severity rather than as separate diseases (Lampert 1998; Coppes-Zantinga and Egeler 2002; Lewis 2018, 237–238). LCH can occur anytime between the ages of 1 and 60 years, but it peaks in childhood between 5 and 10 years of age (Isler and Turcotte 2003). The incidence is 5–10 cases per million children per year and 1–2 individuals per million adults per year, with males affected more commonly than females (Gulati and Allen 2021). The disease can cause death in the very young due to multiple organ failure, with a 20% fatality rate; it can affect the pituitary gland system, causing severely

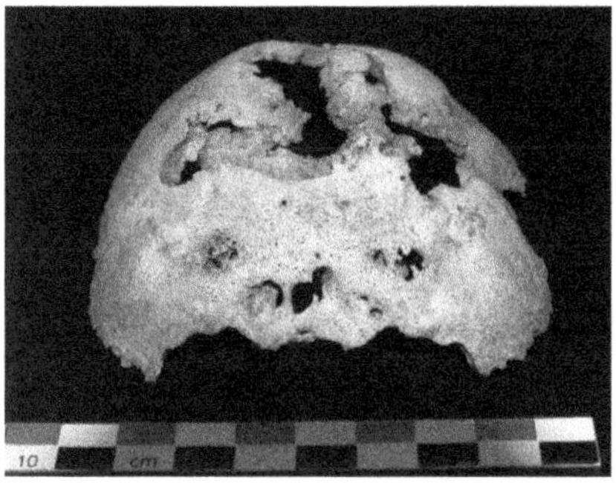

Figure 8.7A. Langerhans cell histiocytosis in a 1–2.5-year-old from medieval Oppidum de la Granède, Millau, France (tenth–eleventh century CE). Lytic lesions on the occipital bone are seen. TB was considered as a differential diagnosis. Photographs courtesy of Antony Colombo and Christophe Saint-Pierre.

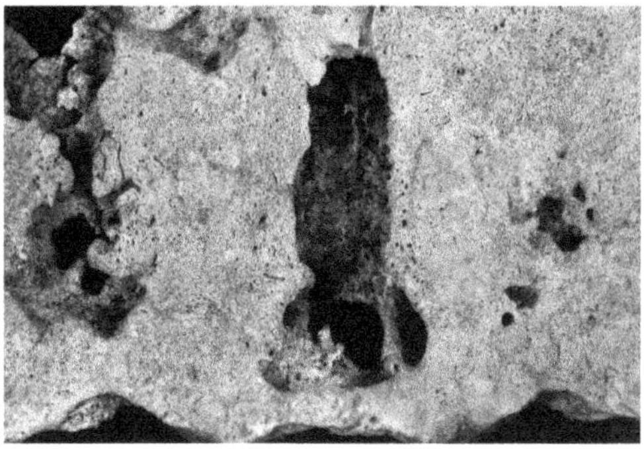

Figure 8.7B. Langerhans cell histiocytosis in a 1–2.5-year-old from medieval Oppidum de la Granède, Millau, France (tenth–eleventh century CE). Close-up of the lytic lesions on the endocranial surface.

retarded growth, or it may heal spontaneously (Broadbent et al. 1994; Resnick et al. 2024, 907). LCH is a "great imitator" of other bone tumors (Isler and Turcotte 2003, 739), especially in younger children who develop large punched-out lesions in the skull. Secondary periosteal new bone formation in reaction to the excess of Langerhans cells in the medullary cavity of a long bone may mimic Ewing sarcoma or osteomyelitis (Steinbock 1976, 360), and differential diagnoses include leukemia or tuberculosis (TB), where there is spinal involvement.

At least sixteen nonadult skeletons with LCH have been identified since 1976 (Lewis 2018, 239). Remarkable evidence was identified from medieval Oppidum de la Granède, Millau, France (tenth–eleventh century CE). Extensive lesions were found on the occipital and parietal bones of a child, as well as the ribs (Fig. 8.7). While the Hand-Schüller-Christian form of LCH was considered the most likely diagnosis, TB or the coexistence of TB in the child could not be ruled out (Colombo et al. 2015). The youngest individual that has been identified was a 36-week-old fetus from postmedieval Cross-Bones in London with large lytic lesions in the cranium and some reactive new bone formation, perhaps as the result of secondary hemorrhaging (Walker 2012, 262). Only the cranium survives. The extremely young age of this child makes the fatal Letterer-Siwe form the most likely.

Malignant Neoplasms

The malignant neoplasms of bone are of the greatest paleopathological interest, having the most terrifying clinical symptomatology and the most revealing epidemiological significance. Yet, in spite of their significance for modern cancer research, malignant neoplasms, both primary and secondary, are uncommon findings in paleopathology (Strouhal and Němečková 2009). As discussed, this rarity in the past may be more apparent than real owing to limited use of radiography to review skeletal remains, poor preservation, small sample sizes, or diagnostic difficulties (Marques 2019, 648). The most common malignant tumors are sarcomas, carcinomas, and neoplasms of the hemopoietic and lymphoid systems. Sarcomas develop in connective tissue (e.g., bone, muscle, cartilage). Carcinomas arise in the epithelial tissue present in the lining of many organs in the body, such as skin, glands, liver, and kidney. Both can spread to other places in the body—that is, they metastasize.

Osteosarcoma

It is a cruel twist of nature that the most deadly tumors of humans are the malignant neoplasms affecting the young. Osteosarcoma, one of the most common primary malignant neoplasms of bone, is no exception. This cancer, sometimes known as an osteogenic sarcoma, arises de novo from the cells constituting bone tissue (Marques 2019, 680). It has a bimodal age distribution, peaking at 18 years and again at 65 years of age. Second only to leukemia and lymphoma, it is the most common primary tumor seen in children and adolescents, with an incidence of 5.6 per 1 million children (Belayneh et al. 2021). A second peak in incidence, occurring in much older people, may be associated with Paget's disease (see Chapter 7). Males more than females are affected, and the humerus, distal femur, and proximal tibia are the usual sites. In children, the tumor develops at the metaphyseal areas of the growth plate and extends through the cortex into the soft tissues (Ortner 2003, 524). The new bone formed is woven in nature, radiating outward in a "sunburst" appearance on the surface of the affected bone. An osteosarcoma is so highly malignant that in the absence of treatment, early death results. No doubt such was the case in antiquity before the advent of surgery, radiotherapy, and chemotherapy. A constant, severe, boring pain, deep in the affected bone, is the presenting symptom. This may be followed by spontaneous bone fracture at the site of the neoplasm, a so-called pathological fracture. It is the spread of neoplastic cells to other parts of the body that leads to death.

Perhaps the earliest example of an osteosarcoma in paleopathology was found in the femur of a 14–17-year-old from the Dongxin cemetery in the Shanxi province of China, dated to the Northern Wei Dynasty (386–534 BCE; You et al. 2021). Interestingly, You et al. (2021) also documented several ancient Chinese medieval texts that refer to "hard masses of bone" that "may become larger." In fact, in a text from 752 CE a term (骨瘤/guliu) meaning "osteoma" or "tumor of bone" was used. A striking example was also described in a humerus of Iron Age date from Muensingen, Switzerland (Brothwell 1967b). The craggy disorganized growth, with spicules of bone developing at right angles to the original bone axis, is characteristic. A burst of frenzied and uncontrolled bone growth in this single humerus doubtless resulted in secondary spread, which was responsible for death. An enormous osteosarcoma measuring about 25 cm by 27 cm was also found at the right knee of an early medieval individual from Standlake, Oxfordshire, England (Brothwell 1967b). A pathological fracture had occurred, and the individual probably died bedridden and in excruciating pain. Di Ruffano and Waldron (2018) suggested osteosarcoma as a diagnosis for a large spherical mass found on the right humerus of a 45-plus-year-old female from early medieval Cherry Hinton,

England (ninth–tenth century CE), and the association of a secondary osteosarcoma as the result of Paget's disease was described by Henderson, et al. (2013) from the mid-nineteenth-century Sheen's burial ground in London.

Chondrosarcoma

The chondrosarcoma is also a common malignant tumor that occurs in the metaphysis of long bone extremities (Ortner 2003, 526). Both ends of the femur, proximal humerus, and pelvis are the sites most frequently affected. The malignant cartilage is nodular in appearance with destruction of the cancellous bone. If the tumor calcifies (where calcium salts replace tumor cells) or ossifies (where bone tissue replaces tumor cells), then it may be recognizable in skeletal remains. Possible evidence was identified on the tibia of a young adult from the pre-Hispanic Canary Islands, Spain (1600–1800 CE). Radiographic features of sharply defined osteolytic lesions with lobulated borders and "spotty" radiopacity provided strong evidence for this diagnosis (Arnay-de-la-Rosa et al. 2015; Marques 2019, 696).

Ewing Sarcoma

A primary bone neoplasm of similar type but differing in the involved cells and site of origin is Ewing sarcoma, the second most common malignant tumor of bone in children (Spector et al. 2021). Perhaps due to genetic factors, the tumor is more common today in individuals of European, North African, and Middle Eastern descent, and with a predominance in males (Spector et al. 2021). While an osteosarcoma develops from the bone cortex, Ewing sarcoma develops in immature mesenchymal round (stem) cells within the medullary cavity that turn into different blood cell types (Steinbock 1976, 371; Isler and Turcotte 2003). The result is a swelling, with the expanding tumor eventually breaking through the cortex. It is seen more frequently in young individuals (10–19 years) whose bones are full of predominantly red bone marrow, but it can occur at any age up to 49 years (Spector et al. 2021). Although these tumors appear in any bone, they are more often observed in the humerus, ribs, pelvis, and femur and tend to spare the epiphyses (Isler and Turcotte 2003). The tumor destroys the marrow spaces and may attack the cortex, spreading into the periosteum and producing new bone formation, either of "sunburst" appearance or as multiple layers of bone ("onion skin"). Osteomyelitis and an osteosarcoma should be considered in the differential diagnosis, although in Ewing sarcoma there is less bone destruction, but permeative (diffuse) lesions are evident as small radiolucent areas within the bone cortex (known as permeative intracortical resorption; Ortner 2003, 527). No definite diagnosis of this tumor in antiquity has yet been made, but a possible example exists in the pelvis of an individual from the Egyptian Roman period (Ruffer and Willmore 1914). Another potential example comes from medieval Barton-on-Humber, England, where the left tibia of a 13–15-year-old exhibits a thick layer of active new bone penetrated by a lytic lesion that passes through this new layer and penetrates the original cortical surface (Waldron 2007).

Cancers or Cancer-like Disorders of the Blood

Multiple Myeloma

Multiple myeloma is a malignant cancer originating in the plasma cells, plasma making up 50% volume of the blood; it is usually preceded by a premalignant and intermediate malignant stage—or "smouldering multiple myeloma"—without bone lesions (Rajkumar et al. 2014). Plasma cells originate from B lymphocyte cells in the blood-forming tissues of the bone marrow, which, in normal circumstances, secrete antibodies. Although solitary lesions can occur, the location of mutated plasma cells within the bone marrow causes multifocal and widespread tumors—hence "multiple myeloma." It is the most common of the primary malignant tumors of the adult skeleton and occurs in 1.8% of all malignant tumors and 15% of all cancers affecting the blood (Resnick et al. 2024, 877). It is a disease of older age, rarely being found in people below the age of 40 years, and 90% occur in individuals between the ages of 50 and 60 years. Males are marginally more affected than females, and some studies indicate it is twice as common in African Americans as other groups, perhaps as the result of genetic factors (Padala et al. 2021).

Multiple myeloma activates osteoclasts and results in a reduction of density in density of the bone, perforation of the cortex, and possible pathological fracture, in addition to clinical symptoms of hypercalcemia, kidney damage, and anemia (Padala et al. 2021). The most commonly involved sites in the skeleton are the cranium, spine, ribs, and pelvis (Resnick et al. 2024, 880). Since the cranium is relatively thin, perforation of the cranial bones may be a feature (Figs. 8.8 and 8.9), and at least in skeletal remains, it is the feature upon which the disease is first identified macroscopically. The multiple and exclusively destructive nature of these cranial perforations distinguishes them from the destruction of chronic infections such as venereal (acquired) syphilis and TB, and from sharp force trauma. What is more difficult in

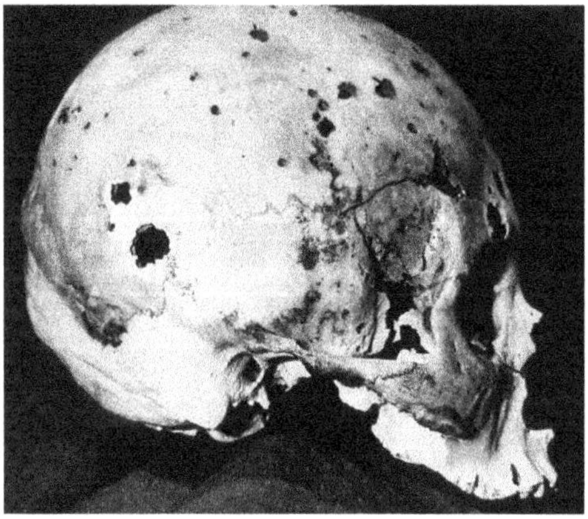

Figure 8.8. Multiple myeloma of the cranium of an adult female from Caudiville, Peru (500–1530 CE). Originally reproduced with kind permission from Don Ortner.

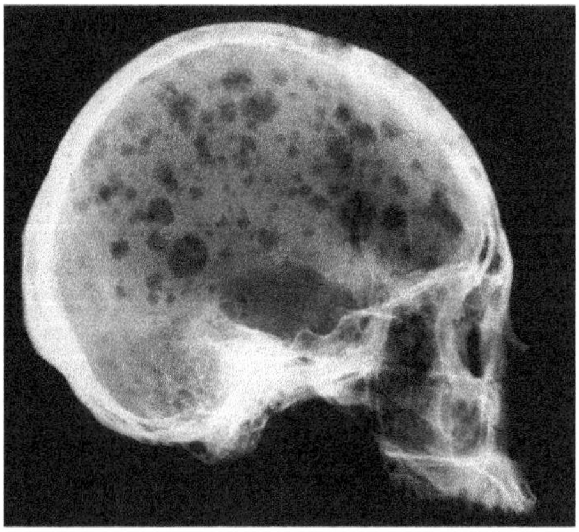

Figure 8.9. Radiograph of the same cranium as in Fig. 8.8, showing many more lytic lesions with the cranial bones.

paleopathological diagnosis is the separation of these lesions from the bone perforations of secondary cancers. Rothschild et al. (1998) provided a useful set of criteria for distinguishing between them. Lesions associated with multiple myeloma are described as spherical, sharply defined, and of uniform diameter, with no evidence of remodeling; on a radiograph they appear "punched out." Secondary metastatic cancers, on the other hand, have less widespread or localized perforations in the affected bone, which vary considerably in size. In the cranium, these perforations may coalesce and the limited size of area affected means that a lesion looks like the surface of a golf ball. In leukemia (see next section), the lesions are also numerous but more superficial (i.e., they do not penetrate the whole of the bone) and smaller (1–3 mm) with some periosteal reaction.

Riccomi et al. (2019) confirmed twenty-five individuals with multiple myeloma from prehistoric and historic sites from around the globe, assessing their geographical location, time period, biological sex, and age profile. The lack of images, detailed descriptions, or noncharacteristic lesions meant that thirty-two individuals were excluded from their survey. While global distributions may be the result of a paucity of paleopathological research in some areas, evidence of multiple myeloma appeared to increase in medieval Europe, while in the Americas there was more prehistoric evidence. Following their own review of multiple myeloma, Dittmar et al. (2020) also described the condition in an individual from Bronze Age Mogou, China (1750–1400 BCE).

Leukemia

The leukemias are a group of cancers resulting from the malignant transformation of the myeloid or lymphoid hemopoietic cells within the bone marrow that can occur in both adults and children (Marques 2019, 520). Global frequency is increasing today (Dong et al. 2020). In 2018, there were 437,000 new cases worldwide, with acute leukemia peaking between the ages of 2 to 5 years (Dong et al. 2020). The skeletal changes in adult leukemia are subtle and may include loss of bone mass and small destructive lesions in the cortex (Ortner 2003, 376). Children with acute leukemia are more likely to demonstrate more characteristic skeletal changes as the normal bone marrow cells are gradually replaced by tumor cells during the growth process (Willson 1959; Rothschild et al. 1997). Lesions—which may be in the form of lytic lesions and subperiosteal new bone formation—tend to arise in rapidly growing areas of the skeleton, such as the knee and wrist (Isler and Turcotte 2003; Sinigaglia et al. 2008). A differential diagnosis of tuberculosis should be considered where collapse of the spine due to lytic lesions has occurred. A small number of children may develop bilateral transverse fractures of the lower limbs due to diffuse osteopenia.

There are two radiographic features that could be used to identify the disease, but these do not consistently occur in every individual. The first is a narrow radiolucent band seen at the metaphyseal side of the growth plate in children, accompanied by an increase in the diameter of the blood vessel foramina and grooving and porosity of the cortex (Kobayashi et al. 2005). Rothschild et al. (1997) documented these and other changes in skeletons of two people diagnosed with leukemia from the Hamann-Todd Osteological Collection. These bands, however, can occur in individuals without leukemia, although they are present (perhaps unhelpfully) in between 10% and 89% of those with the disease (Willson 1959; Bolton-Maggs and Thomas 2008). The second feature is a series of large multiple discrete radiolucent lesions that extend down the long bone diaphysis as the disease progresses. These lesions were symmetrical and seen in 38% of people diagnosed with leukemia from the Johns Hopkins Hospital in Baltimore, Maryland (Willson 1959). Rothschild et al. (1997) concluded that lytic lesions and periosteal reactions on the cranium were more extensive in lymphocytic leukemia, while the ribs and vertebrae were involved only in myelocytic leukemia, which is more common in older individuals.

Klaus (2014a) proposed leukemia as a diagnosis for bone changes seen in a non-adult from Lambayeque Valley, Peru (1533–1620 CE). Porosity on the clavicles, scapulae, vertebral neural arches, and long bones, in addition to areas of finely deposited new bone, suggested a blood-borne condition, with leukemia considered the most likely diagnosis. Unfortunately, the lytic lesions and radiolucent bands seen in clinical medicine could not be assessed, as the long bones were not recovered. Other possible evidence, in an older male from Vaste, Lecce, in fourth–sixth-century CE Italy, was described by Tulumello et al. (2020) showing pits ranging in size from 1 to 3 mm on the marrow-rich areas of the skeleton: the vertebrae, ribs, scapulae, and metaphyseal ends of the long bones. The absence of healing, small and regular size of the lesions, plus the age of the individual led to a diagnosis of leukemia rather than metastatic carcinoma, Langerhans cell histiocytosis, or multiple myeloma.

Secondary Cancer

The prevalence of cancer suggested by the paleopathological record demonstrates an overall increase in malignant disease from the distant past until today. If, as seems likely, worsening environmental conditions due to air and water pollution, and changes in diet, have brought about an increase in cancer, this increase is unlikely to be of primary bone neoplasms arising anew in bone cells. It is surely in the cancers of bowel, breast, lung, skin, and stomach, among others, that the increase has occurred. These are primary soft tissue neoplasms that would potentially only be evident in archaeological individuals with soft tissue preservation. Furthermore, only a small percentage of cancers metastasize into the bone, and a person may die before the cancer has spread. Death may also ensue from intercurrent infection in the early stages of malignant disease. In modern practice, infections are treated, but in antiquity the individual may have died from an infection before the cancer had time to metastasize. A further problem in paleopathological recognition is the fact that secondary cancer commences in the marrow cavities deep inside the bones and only later destroys and perforates the cortex to the bone's exterior. Mere macroscopic inspection of bones may fail to reveal these deeper lesions, which may be demonstrated only by radiography. As discussed at the start of this chapter, wholesale radiography of entire skeletal collections is not usually a practical option for most paleopathologists.

Metastatic cancer from a primary neoplasm in another part of the body is the most common cause of tumors affecting the skeleton, with the majority being destructive of bone (Ortner 2003, 533). Metastases do not tend to be uniformly distributed throughout the whole skeleton. As was first recorded by Von Recklinghausen in 1891, the cranium, sternum, ribs, pelvis, vertebrae, and proximal ends of the femur and humerus are perhaps the most commonly affected bones. Notably, groups living in different environments today have different types of cancer. For example, forager societies seem to have fewer hormonally induced cancers, such as breast and prostate cancer. While genetic factors likely play a more important role in this pattern, risk factors for breast cancer may include age at menarche and menopause, multiparity, duration of lactation, the nature of the diet, and levels of physical activity (Ursin et al. 2005; Marques et al. 2021, 2022; Emons 2022). Exposure to burning biomass fuels in the home may mean there were more nasopharyngeal or lung cancers in the past than today, while smoking or salting foods, and higher levels of infection may have made people more vulnerable to liver, gastrointestinal, rectal, oropharyngeal, and cervical cancer (Ewald 2018). The problem for paleopathologists is that these types of cancer are less likely to produce bone lesions (Marques et al. 2021). Secondary spread to bone is more frequently seen in cancer of the breast, lung, and prostate gland; prostate cancer metastases predominantly form bone, while breast and lung metastases tend to be destructive (Fig. 8.10; Lipton and Vigorita 2016).

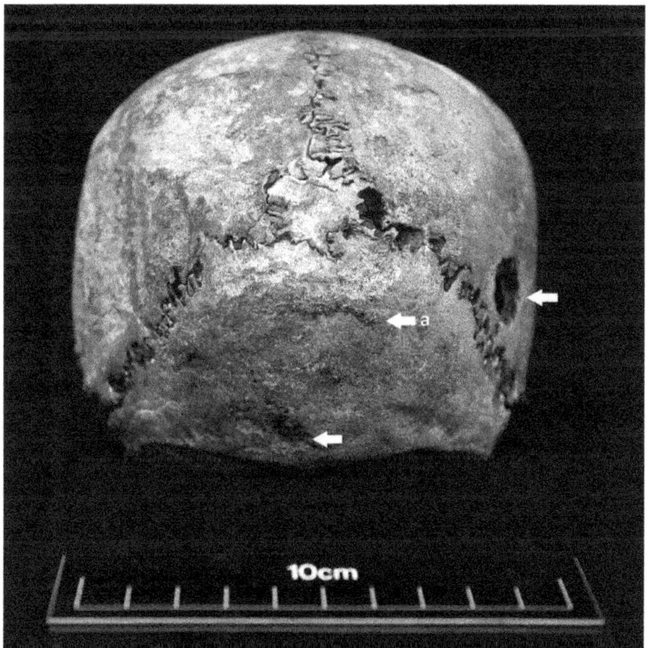

Figure 8.10. Cranium of a female with perforations of secondary cancer (arrows) and active new bone formation on the ectocranial surface (a). From Eccles, Kent, England, sixth–eighth century CE. Photograph courtesy of Jo Buckberry and BARC, University of Bradford.

Metastatic spread is hematogenous, whereby tumor cells (emboli) enter the circulatory system, travel through the capillaries, and bind to the inner lining of the blood vessels (endothelium), only to exit, form tumors, and develop their own blood supply (Klaus 2014b).

One of the first detailed studies of metastatic cancer in a skeleton from an archaeological context was that by Møller and Møller-Christensen (1952). Secondary lesions were noted in the cranium of a female from the medieval cemetery at Aebelholt, Denmark. Through analogy with modern studies, they suggested that the individual may have died of a primary cancer of the breast and its metastases. The earliest example known at present is from the European early Bronze Age, a 35–45-year-old male dated to 5200–4000 BP from the Cis-Baikal region of eastern Siberia (Lieverse et al. 2014). Large lytic perforations and mixed osteoblastic and lytic lesions on the cranium, scapulae, vertebrae, ribs, pelvis, and femur were evident macroscopically, with additional lesions identified radiographically. While the primary site of the cancer could not be identified, it was interesting to note that this individual, who would likely have been in tremendous pain, was buried in a tightly flexed position within a circular grave with rich grave goods—unusual for the time and perhaps signifying marked difference owing to extreme suffering.

In addition, Schultz et al. (2007) used biochemical analysis to identify prostate cancer from tumor tissue trapped within an osteoblastic lesion in the skeleton of a 2,700-year-old Scythian king from Siberia. Klaus (2018) further described four individuals from early Peru (900–1600 CE), showing a mix of profuse new bone formation and bone loss concentrated on the lumbar vertebrae and sacrum. A primary prostate tumor was the most likely diagnosis because of the location of the secondary lesions, and because the tumor emboli would probably have infiltrated the network of vessels that make up the paravertebral plexus of Baston, taking emboli directly to the lower part of the axial skeleton. These veins have no valves and connect the thoracic vessels and deep pelvic veins that drain the bladder and prostate gland. Klaus also described how modern research using bisphosphonate treatment has shown how many osteoblastic metastases begin with bone resorption before reverting to florid new bone formation. Biehler-Gomez et al. (2019) also investigated bone lesions associated with bladder cancer in thirteen individuals aged 56–86 years from the CAL Milano Cemetery Skeletal Collection in Italy (1910–2001 CE). Only three individuals (or 23% of the sample) had evidence of macroscopic bone lesions, which took the form of mixed "coral-like" layers of spiculated bone and osteolytic lesions. Antunes-Ferreira et al. (2023) considered the quality of life and potential social stigma experienced by a female of high social status found in the Chapel of the Holy Spirit in Loures, Portugal (sixteenth–nineteenth century CE). This female had a form of metastatic cancer that is rare today, affecting her extremities (elbow, knees, hand and foot bones, i.e., acrometastasis). This type of spread that appears to have been more common in the past, and making up around 2% of published evidence in paleopathology, compared to 0.1% of cases in the clinical literature. The female would most likely have been in considerable pain and would have been reliant on others for her care—something that perhaps her wealth allowed her to access.

Secondary cancer has been recognized in mummified remains too. For example, melanoma has been noted in pre-Columbian Incas from Peru (Urteaga and Pack 1966). This pigmented growth resulted in small, dark masses preserved within the mummified skin and in multiple pigmented lesions in the cranium. The mummified remains of the king of Naples, Italy (1431–1494 CE), displayed a pelvic tumor that appeared to be an adenocarcinoma, which was confirmed through microscopy; further biomolecular analysis identified a mutation in the K-*ras* gene, compatible with this type of tumor (Marchetti et al. 1996, in Aufderheide 2003). Nerlich (2018) has argued for the greater use of protein (proteomic) analysis in paleopathology to understand the genetics and evolution of tumors in the past, with a focus on preserved soft tissue remains, but stable isotope analysis may also have something to offer in our search for cancer. For example, D'Ortenzio et al. (2015) found higher $\delta^{15}N$ values in the hair of an 82-year-old female who died of lung cancer. This may have been because of cachexia (loss of muscle mass) and chronic weight loss associated with the disease. Building on this work, Drtikovolá Kaupová and colleagues (2021), using stable isotope analysis, found elevated nitrogen values in the ribs of people who died of cancer. They suggested multiple factors to explain the higher nitrogen values, such as the decay of nitrogen-rich cancer emboli or the use of protein-rich foods in caring for the sick.

The clinical manifestations of malignancy have probably not changed throughout history; only from the mid-twentieth century did therapy begin to alleviate the problem. The surgical treatment of cancer is not exclusively a modern phenomenon, however. A cranium of the twelfth century from Caen, France, exhibits an enormous fungating malignant tumor projecting from the right side of the facial skeleton that extended into the eye socket and the nasal cavity. An attempt, albeit unsuccessful, at surgical treatment had been made by cutting a hole in the adjacent bone (Dastugue 1965). Similarly, the cranium of an individual with metastatic cancer (perhaps a neuroblastoma) had resulted in large lytic lesions and "sunburst" new bone formation. It was also described with signs of what was described as a "scraping" operation, or pseudo-trepanation (Rubini et al. 2022: Vico nel Lazio, Italy, thirteenth–fifteenth century CE).

Epilogue

Cancer is one of the most common and fatal diseases of later life today, but also would probably have played a significant part in the past health of children too. Until relatively recently it was thought to be rare in the past—perhaps because people died too young of other diseases, or because cancer's fragile lesions failed to survive the burial environment, or even because the types of cancer suffered in the past had no predilection for bone. With greater emphasis on population-based systematic research in paleopathology and use of more sophisticated imaging techniques, stable isotope analysis, and even proteomics, we are beginning to better understand the nature of this disease in the past. Current prevalence rates show that it was not rare—and it affected the young and old. New databases are helping to track the evidence, while greater emphasis on anatomically and biochemically driven analyses is allowing us to unravel this elusive disease and the environmental, lifestyle, and genetic factors that predispose people to it, not only in the past but in the present too. This new understanding has the potential to contribute to current efforts in evaluating the causes of cancer around the globe, and potentially add a deep-time perspective to the UN Sustainable Development Goal of reducing deaths from non-communicable diseases.

Conclusion

The Next Ten Years?

> The intricate relationship between a people's way of life and the diseases they endure is the chief reason for the study of paleopathology.
>
> —C. Wells, *Bones, Bodies and Disease*

What Has Been Achieved Since 2005?

So much! In 2022, a landmark paper was published by Buikstra et al. on twenty-first-century bioarchaeology. They suggested there should be two key drivers for the discipline: (1) best practices for research (training, statistical approaches, contextualization, hypothesis testing) and (2) a focus on topics of contemporary and historical significance (including ethics, social inequality, identity, climate change, migration, violence, epidemic disease, and developmental origins of health and disease). Our volume has sought to address many of these suggestions, and we hope that scholars of paleopathology around the world will find the inspiration from these discussions to help keep this discipline relevant, exciting, and robust further into the twenty-first century and beyond.

In writing the conclusion for the 2005 edition, we noted that even though studies of individual skeletons or mummified remains were still common, population-based studies of health were increasing markedly. Although this desire to understand more about the social factors that impact health at a population level continues, we are more aware that within each population are groups of individuals whose life experiences differ from the rest of their community, perhaps due to their gender, ethnicity, religion, or migrant status, just as they do in the present. Rising interest in the complexity of life in the past has seen the development of detailed osteobiographies alongside population-based approaches to disease. This trend was prompted and endorsed by the Index of Care approach by Tilley and Cameron (2014), which encouraged careful consideration of a person's quality of life within their specific community—placing the importance of context up front and center. Similarly, early in the application of biomolecular (aDNA) analysis for the identification of diseases in the early 1990s, the focus was necessarily on single skeletons or mummified remains. Since 2005, the global ancient biomolecular infrastructure has increased and developed, data are being produced more rapidly, and there is much more of it, thanks partly to next-generation sequencing. More practitioners are being trained for work in this field, and greatly increased funding is available. Along with the aDNA "revolution" comes the opportunity to study larger numbers of individuals for exploring the origin, evolution, and spread of disease.

Scholars are more focused on hypothesis-led research, and they continue to emphasize contextualization of data, also termed a biocultural or bioarchaeological approach. We reiterate: no person working in paleopathology, from whatever educational background, can ignore the importance of integrating biological data on the pattern of a disease with the sociocultural context in which people with that disease existed. A plethora of peer-reviewed publications have also appeared in a much wider variety of outlets, along with "gray literature" reports on skeletal remains, particularly in commercial archaeology. Since our 2005 edition, two new journals have been launched that cater to our research: *International Journal of Paleopathology* (2011) and *Bioarchaeology International* (2017), while the older journal *Frontiers* has created a "Human Bioarchaeology and Paleopathology" (2023) section within *Frontiers of Environmental Archaeology*. Not only do journal papers feature prominently in communicating our work to academia, but edited books, research monographs, and textbooks all continue to be important in paleopathology. Many peer-review journals have moved toward open access (although many still exist behind paywalls) that allow for the publication of supplementary data and skeletal recording forms to share data and highlight best practices. Apart from many more publications, which may reflect the more numerous scholars in the field, the journals in which paleopathologists publish have become more diverse. These span the sciences, humanities, and social sciences, showing how paleopathology engages with disciplines beyond archaeology and anthropology. Multiauthored papers are also more frequent, especially in biomolecular analyses, reflecting the variety of collaborations that now go into the design and execution of paleopathological research: from the excavators and those who think up the research questions and acquire funding, to those caring for the human remains of interest (curators), and to the scientists performing the analyses and producing the results, interpretations, and publications.

During the compilation of the References for this edition we estimated that there has been a tenfold increase in multiauthored papers since the 2005 edition, along with a significant increase in female authors. As Buikstra et al. (2019b, 824) commented, "the advancement of our field is that our previous dilettante interest of medical men has become a specialty that requires a focus and collaborative efforts." This observation is played out in our references. It is far easier now to develop collaborations and build large teams, not only face to face at conferences and, following the COVID-19 pandemic, online, but also through a variety of communication modes and technology (e.g., video calling) that means distance is no longer a barrier to the exchange of ideas. It is worth considering the findings of Campbell and Simberloff (2020) here, in relation to their own discipline, invasion science, which is the transdisciplinary study of the causes and impacts of introducing non-native species into an environment. They analyzed 27,234 publications on invasion science published in 1,218 journals from 1980 to 2022. The number of authors of a paper was positively correlated with perceived research impact. Papers with two or more authors were more frequently cited compared to single-authored papers, and papers with five or more authors had annual citation rates almost double that of single-authored papers. We are not yet aware of anyone looking into this statistic for our discipline—but we suspect it is mirrored in paleopathological publications. Beyond publications, open access to research data is increasing, considerably aided by developments in digital technology. For example, websites host 3D images of pathological bones and teeth (e.g., Digitised Diseases 2024; Sketchfab 2024). Within an unpublished skeletal report produced by a commercial archaeological company (gray literature), considerable paleopathological data can also be waiting to be harnessed. In the UK, these reports can often be accessed through the Archaeology Data Service (2024). Large databases of pathological skeletal data are also available—for example, in museums, such as the Wellcome Osteological Research Database (Museum of London 2024), but also as a result of large research projects, including the Global History of Health, European module (2024) encompassing data on over 15,000 skeletons, from 101 sites from the premedieval (300–500 CE) to the Industrial era (1800–1900 CE), and the Cancer Research in Ancient Bodies (CRAB) project (Hunt et al. 2024). Finding and accessing relevant literature is, of course, key for scholars working in paleopathology, especially now that, relative to twenty years ago, much more is published in a greater range of outlets across the sciences, social sciences, and humanities. References on paleopathology are now easier to find using keyword searches in search engines such as Google Scholar and via institutional electronic libraries and libraries in general.

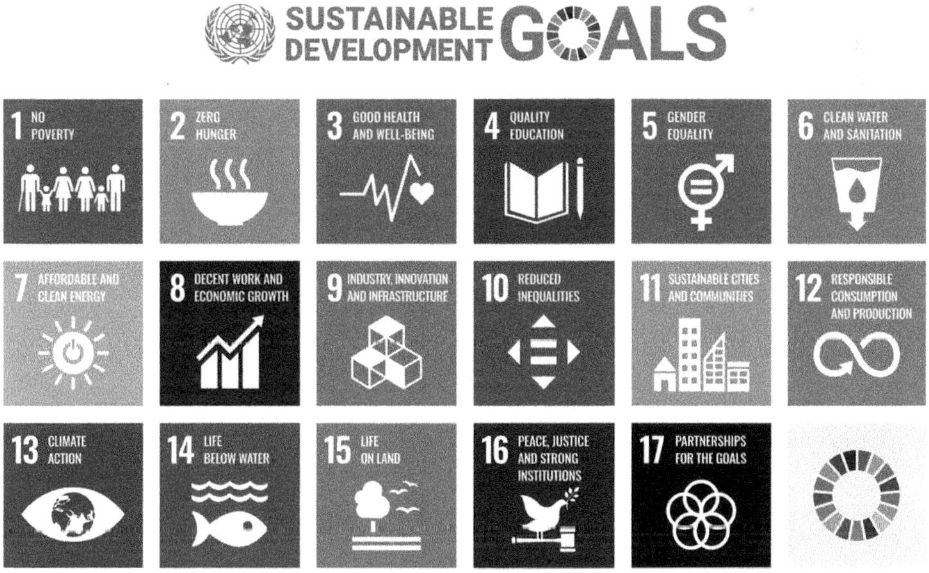

Figure 9.1. United Nations Sustainable Development Goals

Paleopathologists increasingly appreciate that what they have to say about health and well-being in the past has relevance for the present, and may also have implications for future plans for the health of humans, other animals, and the environment. They have also begun to focus their research on the 2015 United Nations Sustainable Development Goals (2023, 2024a and b; Fig. 9.1).

We acknowledge that these goals also have their dissenters, not least because they can be accused of oversimplifying the issues that face many of the countries with the greatest challenges in sustainable development, and the variability of data reporting makes measuring their success difficult (Orhan and Guajardo 2021; Ordonez-Ponce 2023). Notably too, many of these goals intersect, such as (1) no poverty; (2) good health and well-being; and (3) clean water and sanitation. We recall the motto of the now 50-year-old Paleopathology Association, *mortui viventes docente* (the dead teach the living), and we continue to revisit this mantra by using a deep-time perspective to explore the origins, evolution, and history of disease (Fig. 9.2).

That paleopathology is relevant and complementary to evolutionary medicine is well illustrated by the works of Nesse and Williams (1994) and Plomp et al. (2022b). Bentley et al. (2022, 350–351) emphasize that "there is much that each discipline can teach the other to the mutual benefit of both," although they noted that scholars of evolutionary medicine have yet to embrace paleopathology to the same extent. Some recommendations were made for more effective integration: for example, including chapters on paleopathology within evolutionary medicine texts

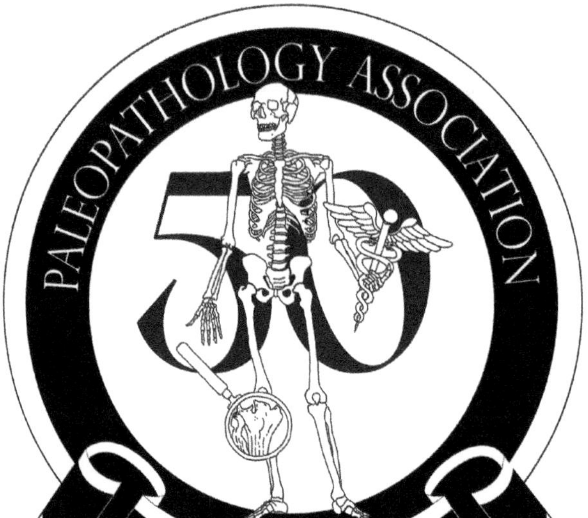

Figure 9.2. Paleopathology Association (PPA) logo at fifty years, designed by PPA student member Rebecca Pitt in 2023. With the kind permission of the PPA.

and within evolutionary medicine teaching; attendance at each other's conferences; collaboration in public engagement activities; and that journals and funding bodies could aid such collaboration by encouraging submissions from both disciplines. The last suggestion encourages further research focusing on One Health (2024 and Fig. 9.3), which is relevant to why people contract diseases and experience injuries, both past and present.

The One Health Initiative emphasizes the important links between humans, the natural environment, and other animals and considers health problems at the interface between them all. It recognizes that the health of humans, domestic and wild animals, plants, and the wider environment (including whole ecosystems) are closely linked and interdependent. Paleopathology is well placed to contribute to One Health perspectives. Along with studying evidence for disease, it incorporates archaeological and historical data in its interpretation, and it engages with environmental archaeology, a subfield of archaeology that provides a broad approach to understanding past ecosystems. Utilizing information from these paleoecosystems gives us clues to their potential impact on disease. Sources of information include soils and sediments, microscopic (diatoms, phytoliths, pollen, spores) and macroscopic (charcoal, seeds, wood) plant remains, coprolites, mollusks, insect remains, parasites, and animal bones and teeth (including bird and fish remains). They also include pathogenic organisms (bacteria, fungi, helminths, protozoa, and viruses). As Reitz and Shackley (2012, 1) explained: "To learn all that we can about the past, relationships among the record, people, cultural institutions, and ecosystems . . . must be examined."

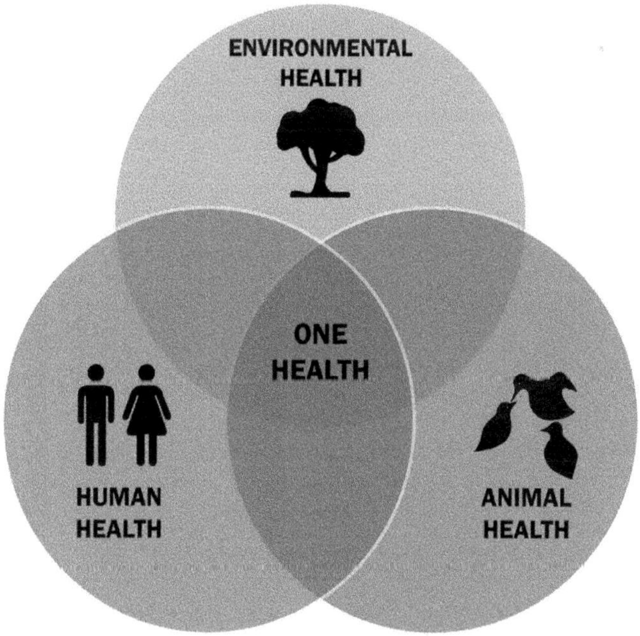

Figure 9.3. The One Health logo.

In the UK, at the time of our second edition (1995), people working in bioarchaeology, including paleopathology, came from a variety of backgrounds, and many were medically trained. In 2005, we noted that there were increasing numbers of archaeology and anthropology graduates (and other cognate disciplines) engaged with bioarchaeology, a trend that had started in the mid-1990s. Their presence continues to rise into the present day and has enhanced our discipline, not least in our adoption of social theory approaches. Graduate courses in bioarchaeology remain hugely popular, and they often include paleopathology and archaeological science (e.g., stable isotope, proteomics, and aDNA analyses). This shift has also led to an increasing number of PhD graduates in our field, and, in the UK at least, many more academic posts have been created over the past twenty years. In the UK, paleopathologists can often be found in archaeology departments, while in continental Europe they may reside in medical or biology departments, and in North America, within anthropology faculties. In the UK, commercial archaeology companies are also increasing the number of bioarchaeologists that they employ, both for excavation and post-excavation work. Some museums are now engaging qualified practitioners to curate human remains and conduct research too (e.g., in London: Museum of London, British Museum, Natural History Museum). We believe that these changes have resulted from increasing recognition of the value of research on human remains to a wide variety of other disciplines and communities. Paleopathology is more global than ever, with dedicated societies in many parts of the world, including South Korea, South America, and China.

What Might We Expect Over the Next Ten Years?

Just as chronicling the development of paleopathology is a matter of individual perspective and interests, considering where we go from here is also a subjective enterprise; none of us has a crystal ball. Exciting technological advances are moving at such a pace that it is almost impossible to imagine what will be achieved in the future; however, some things may be predicted based on the current direction of travel.

Since 2005, the call for paleopathologists to embrace theoretical concepts and frameworks employed in social medicine and other disciplines to understand health patterns (e.g., Gowland 2015) has given rise to new research and the development of several "indices." These include studies that focus on caregiving, frailty, the comorbidity, co-occurrence and syndemics of diseases, and the developmental origins of health and disease. These concerns describe a "paleopathology of the life course"—in that specific age or minority groups have become the focus. Improvements in osteological methods to estimate the age of individual skeletons beyond the ubiquitous 46-plus years, means we are beginning to consider aspects of health that affected those who lived into later life in the past (Appleby 2024), something that can be elucidated by advances in research on joint diseases and cancers we have touched on in this volume. The burgeoning interest in child health, evident in 2005, has extended into consideration of what it was like to be an adolescent in a particular community, the impact of social demands on their physical as well as mental wellbeing, and the use of ages of puberty maturation to measure health (Lewis et al. 2016; Lewis 2022). Research into child paleopathology has developed in other ways too—with a new focus on the diagnosis of trauma and disease in perinatal remains and on the intricate link between the (invisible) mothers and their children through a concentration on the health of newborns and children aged up to 3 years old (Hodson 2021). Providing more opportunities in the future, medical researchers are also concerned with paternal health and how that affects the next generation. Our ability to determine the biological sex of children—once considered a "golden chalice" of bioarchaeology—is now possible due to the development of sex-specific amelogenin protein analysis, meaning that we can start to explore the impact of biological sex and gender on child survival and health in the past. The results will contribute to modern discourse on this complex subject. Understanding how intersectional identities or racism influence health, combined with these osteological advances and stable isotope analysis that can trace the movement of people during their lifetime, allows us to consider the health of migrant populations, depending on their age, biological sex, ancestry, and health, and explore the motives for migration. Related to these endeavors is the use of paleoepidemiology and statistical methods to fully explore the impact of health transitions on population growth, morbidity, and mortality (McFadden 2021; Appleby 2024).

We anticipate that paleopathologists will continue to use methods and theory from other disciplines to enhance our understanding of the experience of disease in the past. As we saw during the COVID-19 pandemic, management of this viral infection relied on other fields of study beyond medicine, such as the behavioral sciences (Altieri et al. 2021). The British Academy (2024) also launched SHAPE (Social Sciences, Humanities and the Arts for People and the Economy), a tool that has been developed "to tell the story of these subjects, which help us make sense of the human world, to value and express the complexity of life and culture, and to understand and solve global issues . . . [with] research and skills [that] are . . . vital to the health, wellbeing and prosperity of the nation and to tackling grand challenges." STEM (science, technology, engineering, and mathematics) subjects cannot stand alone without appreciating the value of relevant research in the social sciences and humanities. While paleopathology increasingly relies heavily on science, we must also use information and methods from non-STEM subjects; after all, we are dealing with once-living people who had complex lives encompassed within a culture, which Whiten et al. (2011, 938) defined as being "all that individuals learn from others, that endures to generate customs and traditions, [and] shapes vast swathes of human lives." Bioarchaeologists have shown their worth in relation to contextualizing the COVID-19 pandemic too (e.g., DeWitte 2016), and publications increasingly address the need to engage with people and institutions beyond academia (e.g., Buikstra 2019a; Buikstra et al. 2022), but there is still work to do to place us "at the table" when decisions and policies are made to confront the health crises of today (Roberts 2024). We can provide the long view about disease over thousands of years as an "interesting insight" to life in the past; however, we could go further. By engaging with politicians and other policy makers, we can show how people managed disease in the past to inform how a disease may be managed in a population today. It is not just about engaging policy makers, though. Academic, commercial, and museum bioarchaeologists have many opportunities to talk to the general public about their work, work in which the public tends to be interested. We anticipate that this engagement will continue and hopefully increase in the future.

The rigor applied to the diagnosis of disease has advanced considerably since our first edition, but it still remains a challenge. Documented skeletal collections with known causes of death and with bone lesions linked to personal medical histories continue to help us understand the specific nature of the lesions that we associate with individual diseases (Henderson and Cardoso 2018). Indeed, these mostly pre-antibiotic populations are important because medications can affect the skeleton and cause additional signs (see examples in Márquez-Grant et al. 2022). Importantly, standardization of paleopathological data recording has been encouraged through a number of publications since 1994 and is described in Chapter 1. Previously established recording methods—for example, for cribra orbitalia, entheses, and visceral rib lesions—have been tested, extended, and improved. We hope that this refinement process continues for other pathological conditions and thus facilitates reliable comparisons of data in the future.

In our third edition, we noted the importance of ancient DNA analysis of microorganisms for future development, and our prediction was correct. For example, identifying genetic-related diseases has started (e.g., Maixner et al. 2021), and research on infections (genus, species, and strain) has markedly increased since 2005 (see Chapter 6). As we saw in Chapter 3, biomolecular study of ancient dental calculus has become key to unraveling the intricacies of ancient oral microbiomes. Exploring these oral microbiomes in living populations is also common (Deo and Deshmukh 2019; Sharma et al. 2018), the microbiome comprising mainly biomolecules from human microorganisms and less so organisms from the environment. Importantly, calculus analysis in bioarchaeology started some time ago with research on animals (Armitage 1975), and in the 1980s Dobney and Brothwell (1987, 1988) highlighted that calculus preserved a range of material inclusions. Over the past twenty years, many researchers have significantly extended the number of dental calculus studies, not only using microscopy, but also biomolecular analysis (e.g., Warinner et al. 2014; Warinner 2016; Wright et al. 2021). Health, diet, and overall lifestyle can clearly influence the composition of calculus. We are fortunate that a large proportion of excavated human remains preserve dental calculus from individuals representing a wide range of time periods, geographic locations, and cultures; compared to bone, calculus survives remarkably well. We would be surprised if this special interest did not continue, but we must be careful not to squander this valuable resource through (necessarily) destructive methods, and sample teeth only when robust, hypothesis-led research questions require it. These advances offer many exciting opportunities for the paleopathologist to explore ancient treatment, diet, and the oral and gut microbiomes.

Finally, we noted in the second and third editions that calcified tissues such as bladder, kidney, and gall stones had seen no advances in analysis and interpretation, and the study of parasitic infections through the eggs and larvae of parasites was rare. We are happy to report that both areas are now flourishing and on the radar of scholars. This change is the result of an increased awareness via recent conference presentations and publications, especially for parasitic infections. Remarkable research is being conducted, although the infrastructure and number of laboratories set up to work with parasite eggs remain limited, compared, for example, to the many stable isotope and aDNA laboratories that exist (see Chapter 6). Paleoparasitology not only shows the extent of human-parasite relationships, but it has also revealed previously unknown species (Reinhard and Camacho 2019). Finds of calcified tissues remain relatively rare, but greater awareness of their potential preservation is increasing their discoveries in funerary contexts. In their volume on the bioarchaeology of cardiovascular disease, Binder et al. (2023) considered the potential taphonomic factors that may preserve calcified blood vessels and the indirect evidence that may point to cardiovascular disease affecting individuals in the archaeological record, along with specific studies of cardiovascular disease in skeletons and mummified remains. We believe that our next edition will feature more of these so-called rare conditions in paleopathology.

We have only touched on other advances, such as micro-CT for detailed imaging of perinatal remains, CT scanning of skeletonized and mummified bodies in museum and medical collections, and the use of artificial intelligence to quantify large amounts of such data. They show much promise, however, and their future use will increase our ability to interrogate the assumptions we make regarding the etiology and mechanisms behind lesions associated with diseases in past human remains (for example, subperiosteal new bone formation, or the porosity associated with anemia, rickets, and scurvy; Megan Brickley, pers. comm.)

Chapter 1 explained the reasons for increasing concern about the ethical implications of studying archaeological human remains (including at the point of excavation and during their analysis, curation, and display), and we described what was being done to address these issues. A huge literature exists on this subject, which requires constant reflection as we move forward with our research. The concerns are not only about destructive analyses, but also about the ways in which we regard and treat human remains, the terminology we use, and how we conduct ourselves in the quest for knowledge about our past. Buikstra et al. (2022, 86) covered ethics extensively throughout their paper. In particular, they noted that effective formal training in ethics and human remains is generally lacking in university education, an area that urgently needs addressing: "Students need to be aware of how to be ethically responsible anthropologists who embrace the concept of 'do no harm,' within home institutions and field research settings." They also reflected on recent and increasing awareness that human remains were very much a part of colonization and taking those remains to other parts of the world for study. Much more attention needs to be paid to the sensitivities of descendant communities and their ancestors' remains too. The ethics of doing biomolecular research using samples of human remains has seen particular attention. Equal access to samples and data archiving are important goals, as is sharing data. At the same time, however, such research must be justified before destructive analysis takes place, and relevant communities should be consulted, especially in the case of ancestral remains of descendant groups. Transparency throughout the research should be the ultimate goal—for example, what samples have been taken, from which human remains, and for what reason; this should be regardless of whether the results were positive or negative.

In recent years, an excellent example of transparency was published by Sheridan et al. (2018) who summarized Scottish archaeological human remains that had been sampled and analyzed for aDNA up to January 2019. Even if it serves only one purpose—to prevent more samples for the same research being done on the same human remains—it is a practice that could be followed by all museums. Austin et al. (2019) also made recommendations for curating the biomolecular past in museum spaces, a past that is not finite. They focused on aDNA, but we should emphasize that stable isotopes and other biomolecules such as proteins should equally be part of conversations about destructive analysis. They noted issues that need addressing, including potential negative impacts of such analyses on descendant communities, competition among aDNA laboratories for samples, and hoarding of samples. As they said, museums are "stewards of collections that contain ancient biomolecules (e.g., isotopes, proteins, DNA, and metabolites), [and] museums play a critical role among stakeholders in biomolecular research and should be responsive to such concerns" (2019, 1472). They recommended that museums should be part of any discussions regarding sampling of remains from their collections for biomolecular research.

In relation to ethics, we also point to a "diversity bias" in what human remains have been studied globally, and therefore in what we know about our ancestors' lives. Much depends on what has been excavated when, where, and of what period, and that is often dictated by research programs led by universities, availability of funding, and modern developments that dictate what areas are surveyed for archaeological evidence and then excavated, as seen in commercial archaeology operations. Furthermore, for many reasons, biases occur in accessing human remains for study, including having no accessible information (e.g. on a museum's website) about where specific remains are curated (see Roberts and Mays 2010). Some parts of the world also see little or no bioarcheological research at all. Ultimately, these biases create gaps in knowledge of our past as seen through the lens of human remains.

We must also consider the origin of human remains curated in museum collections more closely. How did they get there? Who accessioned them to the museum? Were their descendants from marginalized communities, and are they still? For example, documented collections of skeletons are often of late nineteenth- to early twentieth-century date and comprise individuals who were poor, deprived, and older at the time of death. Thus, in addition to the risk of perpetuating the prejudices that were responsible for their creation, these collections do not necessarily reflect a true cross-section of society at the time that they were living. As they have frequently been used for developing osteological methods for biological sex and age estimation, for example, the resulting outcomes of such research are not necessarily applicable to other individuals from archaeological time periods, or even of their own (see de la Cova et al. 2024). As Buikstra et al. (2022, 60) explained, "bioarchaeologists should recognize, not only their privilege in having access to human remains, but also should work together with descendant groups and other communities of concern on the lawful, proper, and humane disposition of the remains of such individuals and their cultural heritage." We hope that readers of this volume agree.

Acknowledgments

As with any book, we have many people to thank. Charlotte thanks Stewart Gardner for his continuing support for the academic side of her retirement life during the production of this edition of *The Archaeology of Disease*. He is relieved that she now has more time for her other life, especially gardening! Charlotte dedicates this book to her late mum, Ann Hunter, for her support, encouragement, understanding, and tolerance; a midwife all her working life, Charlotte's mum was curious about the career path Charlotte took, but Charlotte's first career in nursing certainly prepared her well for palaeopathology! Charlotte also thanks all her friends in the Yorkshire Dales for gradually taking her away from academia into yoga, cycling, open-water swimming, running and hiking, floristry, the Women's Institute, Sustainable Swaledale, the Dales Community Pop Choir, and Reeth Community Centre—her book group is also brilliant at encouraging her to read nonfiction! Durham University is also thanked for supporting Charlotte as emerita professor, and enabling her access to Durham University Library, which has been so important for updating this book.

Keith thanks his late wife, Ann, for her unwavering devotion and commitment to him throughout his two careers, medicine and paleopathology, and in the four editions of *The Archaeology of Disease*. He also thanks lovingly their family, Giles, Sally, James, and Edward, for their patience and forbearance in both careers in all facets. Keith also thanks the University of Bradford for giving him the opportunity to introduce the subjects of human osteology and paleopathology into the undergraduate curriculum in 1978 and, with Charlotte, into the creation of the master's degree program in 1990, initially in association with Sheffield University, and subsequently alone. We are all grateful to Laura Csontos, MSc graduate in human osteology and paleopathology at Bradford University, for her dedication to Keith in his computer and software difficulties, and in keeping him encouraged in the development of this fourth edition.

Mary thanks her friends and colleagues in the Department of Archaeology, University of Reading, and Ceri Falys for their constant support and understanding during the writing of this book, and Andrew Codrai for his encouragement, laughs, gin, Lola, and gardening.

Jacalyn thanks Robert David Wolfe for his unflappable problem-solving, persistent bike riding, and good-natured interest in yet another book.

The authors are also indebted to the late Johs Andersen, Cecil Hackett, William Jopling, Freddie Wells, Arnold Aspinall, and Don Ortner for their guidance and encouragement for previous editions of this book. Thank you so much Anne Grauer (Loyola University Chicago, USA) for writing the Foreword. Like Charlotte, Anne was in at the get-go for the first edition of the book and the ones that succeeded it—so she has a good knowledge of how this book has developed. Equally we are grateful to Francisca Alves Cardoso (Centre for Research in Anthropology, Portugal), Linda Fibiger (University of Edinburgh, Scotland), Rachel Ives (Natural History Museum, London, England), Carina Marques (University of Texas, Rio Grande Valley, Texas, USA), Gundula Müldner (University of Reading, England), Greg Nelson (University of Oregon, Portland, USA), Ana Luisa Santos (University of Coimbra, Portugal), and Anne Titelbaum (University of Arizona College of Medicine, USA) for taking time out of their busy schedules to read the penultimate drafts of Chapters 2–8.

Many of the illustrations that have been retained in this book from previous editions were produced by Jean Brown (formerly of the University of Bradford, Department of Archaeological Sciences). Jean's enthusiasm, understanding of, and dedication to the photography of human remains is gratefully acknowledged. Jean remains fascinated by archaeology, and particularly paleopathology. Over her life she has known many of the graduates of the University of Bradford as friends and keeps in touch with many of them directly or indirectly. We also graciously thank the other friends and colleagues who have so generously contributed to the illustrations in this book, by providing us with permission to use their photographs or for creating line drawings. Thus, our thanks go to Francisca Alves Cardoso (Nova University, Lisbon, Portugal); Daniel Antoine (British Museum, London); the late Johs Andersen, Denmark; Yvonne Beadnell (formerly of Durham University); Jelena Bekvalac (Museum of London, UK); Silvia Bodoriková (Comenius University in Bratislava, Slovakia); Ben Brace (University of Bradford, UK); Tjasse Bruintjes (University of Leiden, The Netherlands); Jo Buckberry (University of Bradford, UK); Scott Burnett (Eckerd College, St. Petersburg, Florida, USA); Anwen Caffell (Durham University, UK) Aishling Caomhanach (Wellcome Collection, UK), Liang Chen (Northwest University, Xi'an, China) Cecilia Collins (Institute for Biomedical and Neural Engineering, University of Iceland, Reykjavik); Antony Colombo (Pennsylvania State University, USA); David Cooper (Manchester Metropolitan University, UK); Anna Davies-Barrett (University of Leicester, UK); Ceri Falys (Thames Valley Archaeological Services and University of Reading); Harriet Haugvik (Reading Museum, UK); Diane Hawkey (Arizona State University, Tempe, USA); Josh Horrocks (University of Bradford, UK); Javier Irurita (University of Granada, Spain); Rachel Ives (Natural History Museum, London, UK); Bronwen Kennedy (York Archaeology, UK); Fikri Kulakoğlu (Ankara University, Türkiye); Angela Lieverse (University of Saskatchewan, Saskatoon, Canada); Louise Loe (Oxford Archaeology, UK); George Maat (University of Leiden, The Netherlands); Patrick Mahoney (University of Kent, Canterbury, UK); Charles (Chuck) Merbs (Arizona

State University, Tempe, USA); Chessie Monks-Kelly (Historic Saranac Lake, New York, USA); Gundula Müldner (University of Reading, UK); Alan Ogden (formerly of the University of Bradford, UK); the late Don Ortner (formerly of the National Museum of Natural History, Smithsonian Institution, Washington, DC, USA); Raphael Panhuysen (Amsterdam Archaeological Centre, University of Amsterdam, The Netherlands); the late Juliet Rogers (formerly of the University of Bristol, UK); Christophe Saint-Pierre (Service Departmental d'Archeologie de l'Aveyron, France); Ana Luisa Santos (University of Coimbra, Portugal); Sarah Schrader (University of Leiden, The Netherlands); Doon Hoon Shin (Seoul National University, South Korea); Mario Šlaus (Croatian Academy of Sciences and Arts, Zagreb, Croatia); Mario Slovak (Institute for Anthropological Research, Zagreb, Croatia); Sam Tipper (Anglia Ruskin University, Cambridge, UK); Handan Üstündağ (Anadolu University, Eskişehir, Türkiye); Jeff Veitch (formerly of Durham University); John Verano (Tulane University, New Orleans, Louisiana, USA); Chiara Villa (University of Copenhagen, Denmark); the late Tony Waldron (University College, London, UK); Jo Walser III (National Museum of Iceland and Department of Archaeology, University of Iceland, Reykjavik); Trevor Woods (formerly Durham University, UK). Finally, Charlotte would like to acknowledge help with images and information for Chapters 4 and 6 from Kelly Blevins and Tina Jakob (Durham University, UK) and Sylvia (Mocen) Li (Beijing Normal University, China), and Sarah Semple for directing her to Wikipedia Commons for images.

Thanks also go to the organizations and institutions who have provided images and permission to use them: AOC Archaeology and St. John's Church, Egham, UK; Biological Anthropology Research Centre, University of Bradford, UK; the Trustees of the British Museum, London, UK; Canterbury Archaeological Trust, UK; the Natural History Museum, London, UK; National Museum of Natural History, Washington, DC, USA; Reading Museum, Berkshire, UK; Science Museum Group @The Board of Trustees of the Science Museum, London, UK; Thames Valley Archaeological Services (TVAS), UK; Historic Saranac Lake, New York; the UK's Wellcome Collection; Wikipedia Commons; and York Archaeology.

Finally, we would like to thank the numerous people at Cornell University Press who have brought this fourth edition to fruition, but particularly Bethany Wasik.

References

Aaron J.E., Rogers J., and Kanis J.A. 1992. Paleohistology of Paget's disease in 2 skeletons. Am J Phys Anthropol 89:325–331.

Abdul Rahman N. et al. 2022. Experiences of living with leprosy: a systematic review and qualitative evidence synthesis. PLoS Negl Trop Dis 16(10): e0010761. https://doi.org/10.1371/journal.pntd.0010761.

Abegg C., Dutour O., Desideri J., and Besse M. 2020. Cases of serpens endocrania symmetrica in young individuals from Neolithic Western Switzerland: description and interpretation. Int J Osteoarchaeol 30:401–409. https://doi.org/10.1002/oa.2863.

Abuseir S. 2021. Meat-borne parasites in the Arab world: a review in a One Health perspective. Parasitol Res 120:4153–4166. https://doi.org/10.1007/s00436-021-07149-0.

Adler C.J. et al. 2013. Sequencing ancient calcified dental plaque shows changes in oral microbiota with dietary shifts of the Neolithic and Industrial revolutions. Nat Genet 4:450–455.

Advisory Panel on the Archaeology of Burials in England. 2023. Science and the dead: a guideline for the destructive sampling of archaeological human remains for scientific analysis, 2nd ed. https://historicengland.org.uk/content/docs/advice/science-and-the-dead-2nd-ed.

Afshar Z., Roberts C.A., Millard A., and Gröcke D. 2019. The evolution of diet during the 5th to 2nd millennium BC for the population buried at Tepe Hissar, North-eastern Central Iranian Plateau: the stable isotope evidence. J Archaeol Sci: Rep 27:101983. https://doi.org/10.1016/j.jasrep.2019.101983.

Agarwal A. and Agarwal R. 2010. The practice and tradition of bonesetting. Educ Health 23(1): 225.

Agarwal S.C. 2021. What is normal bone health? A bioarchaeological perspective on meaningful measures and interpretations of bone strength, loss, and aging. Am J Hum Biol 33(5): e23647. https://doi.org/10.1002/ajhb.23647.

Agarwal S.C., Dumitriu M., Tomlinson G.A., and Grynpas M. 2004. Medieval trabecular bone architecture: the influence of age, sex, and lifestyle. Am J Phys Anthropol 124(1): 33–44.

Agarwal S.C. and Stout S.D. 2003. Bone loss and osteoporosis: an anthropological perspective. Kluwer Academic/Plenum Publishers.

Agarwal Y., Chopra R.K., Gupta D.K., and Sethi R.S. 2017. The tuberculosis timeline: of white plague, a birthday present, and vignettes of myriad hues. Astrocyte 4(10): 7. https://doi.org/10.4103/2349-0977.217662.

Agnew A.M. and Stout S.D. 2012. Brief communication: reevaluating osteoporosis in human ribs: the role of intracortical porosity. Am J Phys Anthropol 148(3): 462–466.

Ahmed A.U. 2011. An overview of inflammation: mechanism and consequences. Front Biol 6:274–281. https://doi.org/10.1007/s11515-011-1123-9.

Ahmed O. et al. 2022. Diffuse idiopathic skeletal hyperostosis prevalence, characteristics, and associated comorbidities: a cross-sectional study of 1815 whole spine CT scans. Glob Spine J 14(4): 1201–1209. https://doi.org/10.1177/21925682221136844.

Ahn E. et al. 2015. Neonatal clavicular fracture: recent 10-year study. Pediatr Int 57:60–63.

Aidonis A., Papavramidou N., Moraitis K., and Papageorgopoulou C. 2021. Trepanations in the ancient Greek colony of Akanthos: skull surgery in the light of Hippocratic medicine. Int J Paleopathol 35:8–21. https://doi.org/10.1016/j.ijpp.2021.07.008.

Al-Azzani W., Adam Maliq Mak D., Hodgson P., and Williams R. 2016. Epidemic of fractures during a period of snow and ice: has anything changed 33 years on? BMJ Open 6(9): e010582. https://doi.org/10.1136/bmjopen-2015-010582.

Alam M.S., Han B., Al-Mizan R., and Pichtel J. 2019. Assessment of soil and groundwater contamination at a former tannery district in Dhaka, Bangladesh. Environ Geochem Health 42:1905–1920. https://doi.org/10.1007/s10653-019-00457-6.

Albee M.E. 2023. A test of the New Coimbra method of recording entheseal changes as applied to the foot skeleton. Int J Osteoarchaeol 33(6): 1028–1041.

Alberto-Barroso V. et al. 2022. Perinatal burials at pre-Hispanic noncemetery sites in Gran Canaria: tophet, infanticide, or natural mortality? Int J Osteoarchaeol 32(1): 100–110.

Allen K.D. and Golightly Y.M. 2015. Epidemiology of osteoarthritis: state of the evidence. Curr Opin Rheumatol 27(3): 276–283.

Allen T. 2003. Perception is everything. New Scientist (1 March): 25.

Allison M.J., Gerszten E., Munizaga J., Santoro C., and Mendoza D. 1981. Tuberculosis in pre-Columbian Andean populations. In: Prehistoric tuberculosis in the Americas, ed. J.E. Buikstra, 49–51. Northwestern University.

Alpaslan-Roodenberg S. et al. 2021. Ethics of DNA research on human remains: five globally applicable guidelines. Nature 599:41–46. https://doi.org/10.1038/s41586-021-04008-x.

AlQahtani S.J., Hector M.P., and Liversidge H.M. 2010. Brief communication: the London atlas of human tooth development and eruption. Am J Phys Anthropol 142:481–490. https://doi.org/10.1002/ajpa.21258.

Altieri E. et al. 2021. Harnessing the power of behavioural science to improve health. Bull World Health Organ 99(11): 754.

Alum A., Rubino J.R., and Ijaz M.K. 2010. The global war against intestinal parasites—should we use a holistic approach? Int J Infect Dis. 14(9): e732–738. https://doi.org/10.1016/j.ijid.2009.11.036.

Alvarez L.A., Corrigan W, and Gardner S. 2022. A case report of hyperostosis frontalis interna. Cureus 14(5): e24967. https://doi.org/10.7759/cureus.24967.

Alves Cardoso F. 2008. A portrait of gender in two 19th and 20th century Portuguese populations: a palaeopathological perspective. PhD dissertation, Durham University, England.

Alves Cardoso F.A., and Henderson C. 2013. The categorisation of occupation in identified skeletal collections: a source of bias? Int J Osteoarchaeol 23(2): 186–196.

Alves Cardoso F. et al. 2022. Metagenomic research of infectious diseases in archaeological contexts: evidence from the Hospital Real de Todos-os-Santos (Portugal). Appl Sci 12(12): 6096. https://doi.org/10.3390/app12126096.

Alvrus A. 1999. Fracture patterns among the Nubians of Semna south, Sudanese Nubia. Int J Osteoarchaeol 9:417–429.

Ambrose C.T. 2018. The conquest of pus—a history of bitumen, creosote and carbolic acid. J Infect Dis Prev Med 6(2): 179. https://doi.org/10.4172/2329-8731.1000179.

Amicizia D. et al. 2019. Burden of typhoid fever and cholera: similarities and differences: prevention strategies for European travellers to endemic/epidemic areas. J Prev Med Hyg 60(4): E271–E285.

Amundsen D.A. and Diers C.J. 1970. The age of menopause in Classical Greece and Rome. Hum Biol 42:79–86.

Andahl R.O. 1978. The examination of saw marks. J Forensic Sci Soc 18:31–46.

Andersen J.G. 1969. Studies in the diagnosis of leprosy in Denmark: an osteological, historical and clinical study. Costers Bogtrykkeri.

Andersen J.G. and Manchester K. 1987. Grooving of the proximal phalanx in leprosy: a palaeopathological and radiological study. J Archaeol Sci 14:77–82.

Andersen J.G. and Manchester K. 1988. Dorsal tarsal exostoses in leprosy: a palaeopathological and radiological study. J Archaeol Sci 15:51–56.

Andersen J.G. and Manchester K. 1992. The rhinomaxillary syndrome in leprosy: a clinical, radiological and palaeopathological study. Int J Osteoarchaeol 2:121–129.

Andersen J.G., Manchester K., and Ali R.S. 1992. Diaphyseal remodelling in leprosy: a radiological and palaeopathological study. Int J Osteoarchaeol 2(3): 211–221.

Andersen J.G., Manchester K., and Roberts C. 1994. Septic bone changes in leprosy: a clinical, radiological and palaeopathological study. Int J Osteoarchaeol 4: 21–30.

Andersen, Johannes G. 1969. Studies in the diagnosis of leprosy in Denmark. Costers Bogtrykkeri.
Anderson A.S. and Loeser R.F. 2010. Why is osteoarthritis an age-related disease? Best Pract Res Clin Rheumatol 24:15–26.
Anderson M., DuBois S., and Gebhardt M. 2020. Sarcomas of bone. In: Abeloff's clinical oncology, ed. J. Niederhuber, J. Armitage, M. Kastan, J. Doroshow, and J. Tepper, 1604–1654. Elsevier.
Anderson T. 1994. Example of cleft lip and palate from St Gregory's Priory, Canterbury. Cleft Palate-Craniofacial Journal 31(6): 466–472.
Anderson T. 2000. An Italian child with osteochondritis dissecans of the cuboid. The Foot 10(4): 216–218. https://doi.org/10.1054/foot.2000.0620.
Anderson T. 2001. The human remains. In: St Gregory's Priory, Northgate, Canterbury Excavations 1988–1991, ed. M. Hicks and A. Hicks, 338–370. Canterbury Archaeological Trust.
Anderson T. 2002. Metaphyseal fibrous defects in juveniles from Norwich. Int J Osteoarchaeol 12:144–148.
Anderson T. and Carter A.R. 1995. The first archaeological case of Madelung's deformity? Int J Osteoarchaeol 5:168–173.
Anderson T. and Thomas T.G. 1997. A possible case of arthrogryposis multiplex from Canterbury. Int J Osteoarchaeol 7:171–185.
Angel J.L. 1966. Porotic hyperostosis, anaemias, malarias, and marshes in the prehistoric eastern Mediterranean. Science 153(3737): 760–763.
Angel J.L. 1969. Human skeletal remains at Karataş. In: Excavations at Karataş-Semayük and Elmali, Lycia, ed. M.J. Mellink, 253–258. Am J Archaeol 74:245–259.
Anil S. and Anand P.S. 2017. Early childhood caries: prevalence, risk factors, and prevention. Front Pediatr 5:157. https://doi.org/10.3389/fped.2017.00157.
Anselmo D., Capela e Silva F., and Fernandes T. 2016. Characterization of hypertrophic osteoarthropathy in an identified skeleton from Évora, Portugal, using combined and comparative morphology and microscopy. Int J Paleopathol 12:11–16. https://doi.org/10.1016/j.ijpp.2015.11.001.
Antikas T., and Graeaekos I. 2010. Scapular lesions on a juvenile of the 3rd Century CE from Northern Greece. Paleopathology Newsletter 149:19–20.
Antoine D., Hillson S., and Dean M.C. 2009. The developmental clock of dental enamel: a test for the periodicity of prism cross-striations in modern humans and an evaluation of the most likely sources of error in histological studies of this kind. J Anat 214:45–55. https://doi.org/10.1111/j.1469-7580.2008.01010.x.
Antoine D., Vandenbeusch M., Whiting R., and Moreno B. 2023. Cardiovascular disease in Nile Valley mummies. In: The bioarchaeology of cardiovascular disease, ed. M. Binder, C.A. Roberts, and D. Antoine, 91–98. Cambridge University Press.
Antunes-Ferreira M., Cunha E., and Marques C. 2014. Multiple osteochondromas in a 16th–19th century individual from Setúbal (Portugal). Anthropol Sci 122(3): 157–163.
Antunes-Ferreira N., Matos V.M.J., and Santos A.L. 2013. Leprosy in individuals unearthed near the Ermida de Santo André and leprosarium of Beja, Portugal. Anthropol Sci 121:149–159.
Antunes-Ferreira N., Prates C., and Curate F. 2021. Interpreting injury recidivism in a rural post-male individual from Bucelas, Portugal. Int J Osteoarchaeol 31:243–251.
Antunes-Ferreira M., D'Ambrosi S., Arkani M., Post E. et al. 2023. Tumor-educated platelet blood tests for non-small cell lung cancer detection and management. Scientific Reports 13(1). https://doi.org/10.1038/s41598-023-35818-w.
Appleby J. 2008. The social role of the elderly in the early Bronze Age of central Europe. PhD dissertation, Newnham College, University of Cambridge.
Appleby J. 2010. Why we need an archaeology of old age, and a suggested approach. Norw Archaeol Rev 43(2): 145–168.
Appleby J. 2018. Ageing and the body in archaeology. Cambridge Archaeol J 28(1): 145–163. https://doi.org/10.1017/S0959774317000610.
Appleby J. 2023. Differential diagnosis and rigor in paleopathology. In: The Routledge handbook of paleopathology, ed. A.L. Grauer, 43–63. Routledge.
Appleby J., 2024. Ageing and disease risk factors: a new paleoepidemiological methodology for understanding disease in the past. Int J Paleopathol 44:33–45.
Appleby J., Thomas R., and Buikstra J.E. 2015. Increasing confidence in paleopathological diagnosis—application of the Istanbul terminological framework. Int J Paleopathol 8:19–21.
Appleby J. et al. 2015. Perimortem trauma in King Richard III: a skeletal analysis. Lancet 385(9964): 253–259. https://doi.org/10.1016/S0140-6736(14)60804-7.

Archaeology Data Service. 2024. The digital repository for archeology and heritage. https://archaeologydataservice.ac.uk/. Accessed 30 May 2024.
Archibald E. 2001. Incest and the medieval imagination. Oxford University Press.
Arcini C. and Artelius T. 1993. Äldsta fallet av spetälska i Norden [Oldest case of leprosy in Norway]. Arkeologi i Sverige 2:55–71.
Ardagna Y., Richier A., Vernet G., and Dutour O. 2005. A case of beheading dating from the Celtic period (la Tène B, Sarliève-Grande Halle, France). Int J Osteoarchaeol 15:73–76. https://doi.org/10.1002/oa.776.
Arends C.M. et al. 2020. Clonal hematopoiesis in patients with anti-neutrophil cytoplasmic antibody-associated vasculitis. Haematologica 105(6): e264–e267. https://doi.org/10.3324%2Fhaematol.2019.223305.
Argyropoulou M.I. and Kiortsis D.N. 2005. MRI of the hypothalamic-pituitary axis in children. Pediatr Radiol 35(11): 1045–1055.
Ariès P. 1962. Centuries of childhood: a social history of family life. Translated by Robert Baldick. J. Cape.
Aristova E., Chikisheva T., Seidman A., Mashak A., and Khoroshevskaya Y. 2006. Pituitary dwarfism in an early Bronze Age individual from Tuva. Archaeology, Ethnology and Anthropology of Eurasia 27(1):139–147.
Armelagos G.J. 1990. Health and disease in prehistoric populations in transition. In: Disease in populations in transition: anthropological and epidemiological perspectives, ed. A.C. Swedlund and G.J. Armelagos, 127–146. Bergin and Garvey.
Armelagos G., Meilke J., and Winter J. 1971. Bibliography of human paleopathology EH. Medizinische Klinik 27:172–174.
Armentano N., Malgosa A., and Campillo D. 1999. A case of frontal sinusitis from the Bronze Age site of Can Filuà (Barcelona). Int J Osteoarchaeol 9:438–442.
Armitage P.L. 1975. The extraction and identification of opal phytoliths from the teeth of ungulates. J Archaeol Sci 2:187–197.
Arnay-de-la-Rosa M. et al. 2015. Cartilage-derived tumor in a prehispanic individual from La Gomera (Canary Islands). Int J Paleopathol 11:66–69.
Arnott R., Finger S., and Smith C.U.M, eds. 2003. Trepanation: history, discovery, theory. Swets and Zeitlinger.
Arrieta M.A., Mendonça O.J., and Bordach M.A. 2018. Differential diagnosis of a neoplastic condition in a prehistoric juvenile individual from La Falda site, northwest Argentina. Int J Paleopathol 21:111–120.
Arrieta M., Ramos Gaspar R., and Santos A.L. 2021. Paleopathological diagnosis of a proportionate short stature on a female skeleton from the Coimbra collection: Turner syndrome versus other causes. Int J Paleopathol 33:234–244.
Arrizabalaga J. 2018. At the intersection of medical geography and disease ecology: Mirko Grmek, Jacques May and the concept of pathocenosis. Hist Philos Life Sci 40(4): 71. https://doi.org/10.1007/s40656-018-0236-8.
Arrizabalaga J., Henderson J., and French R. 1997. The great pox: the French disease in Renaissance Europe. Yale University Press.
Assis S. and De Boer H.H. 2023. Paleohistopathology, history, technical aspects, and diagnostic challenges. In: The Routledge handbook of paleopathology, ed. A.L. Grauer, 82–104. Routledge.
Assis S. and Keenleyside A. 2019. The macroscopic and histomorphological properties of periosteal rib lesions and its relation with disease duration: evidence from the Luis Lopes Skeletal Collection (Lisbon, Portugal). J Anat. 234(4): 480–501. https://doi.org/10.1111/joa.12936.
Assis S., Keenleyside A., Santos A.L., and Cardoso F.A. 2015. Bone diagenesis and its implication for disease diagnosis: the relevance of bone microstructure analysis for the study of past human remains. Microsc Microanal 21:805–825.
Assis S., Santos A.L., and Roberts C.A. 2011. Evidence of hypertrophic osteoarthropathy in individuals from the Coimbra Skeletal Identified Collection (Portugal). Int J Palaeopathol 1:155–163.
Åström M.E. and Roos P.M. 2022. Geochemistry of multiple sclerosis in Finland. Sci Total Environ 841:156672. https://doi.org/10.1016/j.scitotenv.2022.156672.
Atiyeh B. and Habal M. 2023. Origins of maxillofacial surgery in Mediterranean medical history. J Craniofac Surg 34(3): 1137–1139. https://doi.org/10.1097/SCS.0000000000009159.

Atkins P.J. 1992. White poison? The social consequences of milk consumption, 1850–1930. Soc Hist Med 15(2): 207–226.

Auerbach A. and Aguilera N.S. 2023. The changing landscape of pediatric histiocytoses: birth, life, and transdifferentiation of pediatric histiocytes. Semin Diagn Pathol 40(6): 420–428. https://dx.doi.org/10.1053/j.semdp.2023.05.003.

Aufderheide A.C. 2003. The scientific study of mummies. Cambridge University Press.

Aufderheide A.C., and Rodríguez-Martín C. 1998. The Cambridge encyclopaedia of human palaeopathology. Cambridge University Press.

Austin R.M., Sholts S.B., Williams L., Kistler L., Hofman C.A. 2019. To curate the molecular past, museums need a carefully considered set of best practices. Proc Nat Acad Sci USA 116:1471–1474.

Ayorinde A. et al. 2023. Health inequalities in infectious diseases: a systematic overview of reviews. BMJ Open 13:e067429. https://doi.org/10.1136/bmjopen-2022-067429.

Azad A.D., Charles A.G., Ding Q., Trickey A.W., and Wren S. 2020. The gender gap and healthcare: associations between gender roles and factors affecting healthcare access in central Malawi, June–August 2017. Arch Public Health 78:119. https://doi.org/10.1186/s13690-020-00497-w.

Badger L. 1964. Epidemiology. In: Leprosy in theory and practice, ed. R. Cochrane and T. Davey, 69–97. Wright.

Bahn P. 1989. Early teething troubles. Nature 337:693.

Bai Y. et al. 2021. Archaeobotanical evidence of the use of medicinal cannabis in a secular context unearthed from south China. J Ethnopharmacol 275:114114. https://doi.org/10.1016/j.jep.2021.114114.

Baker B. 1999. Early manifestations of tuberculosis in the skeleton. In: Tuberculosis: past and present, ed. G. Pálfi, O. Dutour, J. Deák, and I. Hutás, 301–307. Golden Book Publishers and Tuberculosis Foundation.

Baker B. and Armelagos G.J. 1988. Origin and antiquity of syphilis: a paleopathological diagnosis and interpretation. Curr Anthrop 29(5): 703–737.

Baker B.J. 2023. Treponemal infection. In: The Routledge handbook of paleopathology, ed. A.L. Grauer, 292–305. Routledge.

Baker B.J. et al. 2020. Advancing the understanding of treponemal disease in the past and present. Yearbook of Physical Anthropology 171:5–41.

Baker B.J. and Bolhofner K.L. 2014. Biological and social implications of a burial from Cyprus for understanding leprosy in the past. Int J Paleopathol 4:17–24. https://doi.org/10.1016/j.ijpp.2013.08.006.

Baker P. 2013. The archaeology of medicine in the Graeco-Roman world. Cambridge University Press.

Baker R.E. et al. 2022. Infectious disease in an era of global change. Nat Rev Microbiol 20:193–205. https://doi.org/10.1038/s41579-021-00639-z.

Bălă G.P., Râjnoveanu, R.M., Tudorache E. et al. 2021. Air pollution exposure—the (in)visible risk factor for respiratory diseases. Environ Sci Pollut Res 28:19615–19628. https://doi.org/10.1007/s11356-021-13208-x.

Balato G. et al. 2021. Management of septic arthritis of the hip joint in adults: a systematic review of the literature. BMC Musculoskelet Disord 22:1–13.

Banaganapalli B. et al. 2023. Paget's disease: a review of the epidemiology, etiology, genetics, and treatment. Front Genet 14:1131182. https://doi.org/10.3389/fgene.2023.1131182.

Bang P.F. and Scheidel W. 2013. The Oxford handbook of the state in the Ancient Near East and Mediterranean. Oxford University Press.

Bansal M. 2016. Prevalence and diagnostic features of osteoarthrosis of the temporomandibular joint: a review. Int J Res Orthop 2(1): 1–4. http://dx.doi.org/10.18203/issn.2455-4510.IntJResOrthop20160708.

Bao Y., Xu Y., Li Z., and Wu Q. 2023. Racial and ethnic difference in the risk of fractures in the United States: a systematic review and meta-analysis. Sci Rep 13:9481. https://doi.org/10.1038/s41598-023-32776-1.

Barbera A.R., Camacho M., and Reinhard K. 2023. Parasitology and paleopathology. In: The Routledge handbook of paleopathology, ed. A.L. Grauer, 158–179. Routledge.

Barbian L.T. and Sledzik P.S. 2008. Healing following cranial trauma. J Forensic Sci. 53(2): 263–268. https://doi.org/10.1111/j.1556-4029.2007.

Barbieri R. et al. 2017. Paleoproteomics of the dental pulp: the plague paradigm. PLoS One 12(7): e0180552. https://doi.org/10.1371/journal.pone.0180552.

Barbieri R. et al. 2021. *Yersinia pestis*: the natural history of plague. Clin Microbiol Rev 34(1): e00044–19. https://doi.org/10.1128/CMR.00044-19.

Barker G. and Goucher C., eds. 2015. The Cambridge world history. Vol. 2: A world with agriculture, 12,000 BCE–500 CE. Cambridge University Press.

Barker G., Roberts C.A., Gosden C., Horning A., and Welham K. 2016. Reflections on archaeology. British Academy.

Barlow T. 1883. On cases described as 'acute rickets' which are probably a combination of scurvy and rickets, the scurvy being an essential, and the rickets a variable, element. Medico-Chirurical Transactions 66:159–219.

Barlow G., Irving W.L., and Moss P.J. 2021. Infectious disease. In: Kumar and Clark's clinical medicine, ed. A. Feather, D. Randall, and M. Waterhouse, 487–582. Elsevier.

Barnes E. 1994. Developmental defects of the axial skeleton in palaeopathology. University Press of Colorado.

Barnes E. 2012. Atlas of developmental field anomalies of the human skeleton: a paleopathology perspective. Wiley.

Barnes I. and Thomas M.G. 2006. Evaluating bacterial pathogen DNA preservation in museum osteological collections. Proc Biol Sci 273(1587): 645–653. https://doi.org/10.1098/rspb.2005.3339.

Barnett, R. 2017. The smile stealers: the fine and foul art of dentistry. Thames and Hudson.

Barrett R., Kuzawa C.W., McDade T., and Armelagos G.J. 1998. Emerging and re-emerging infectious diseases: the third epidemiologic transition. Ann Rev Anthrop 27:247–271.

Barton M. 2023. Canaries in the coal mine. British Trust for Ornithology News (Summer).

Bartosiewicz L. and Mansouri K. 2023. Zooarchaeology and the paleopathological record. In: The Routledge handbook of paleopathology, ed. A.L. Grauer, 557–575. Routledge.

Basal D. and Steiner R. 2009. Osteogenesis imperfecta: recent findings shed new light on this once well-understood condition. Genet Med 11(6): 375–385.

Bastone E.B., Freer T.J., and McNamara J.R. 2000. Epidemiology of dental trauma: a review of the literature. Aust Dent J 45(1): 2–9. https://doi.org/10.1111/j.1834-7819.2000.tb00234.x.

Baten J., Benati G., and Sołtysiak A. 2023. Violence trends in the ancient Middle East between 12,000 and 400 BCE. Nat Hum Behav 7:2064–2073. https://doi.org/10.1038/s41562-023-01700-y.

Baten J., and Steckel R.H. 2019. The history of violence in Europe: evidence from cranial and postcranial trauma. In: The backbone of Europe: health, diet, work and violence over two millennia, ed. R.H. Steckel, C.S. Larsen, C.A. Roberts, and J. Baten, 300–324. Cambridge University Press.

Baten J., Steckel R.H., Larsen C.S., and Roberts C.A. 2019. Multidimensional patterns of European health, work, and violence over the last two millennia. In: The backbone of Europe: health, diet, work and violence over two millennia, ed. R.H. Steckel, C.S. Larsen, C.A. Roberts, and J. Baten, 381–396. Cambridge University Press.

Bause G.S. 2009. How American dentists helped pioneer oxygenation of general anaesthetics worldwide. J Hist Dent 57(3): 123–133.

Bayliss A., Shepherd Popescu E.S., Beavan-Athfield N., Bronk Ramsay C., Cook G.T., and Locker A. 2004. The potential significance of dietary offsets for the interpretation of radiocarbon dates: an archaeologically significant example from Norwich. J Archaeol Sci 31:563–575.

Beale M. et al. 2019. Genomic epidemiology of syphilis reveals independent emergence of macrolide resistance across multiple circulating lineages. Nat Commun 10(3255): 1–9. https://doi.org/10.1038/s41467-019-11216-7.

Beaumont J. and Montgomery J. 2016. The Great Irish Famine: identifying starvation in the tissues of victims using stable isotope analysis of bone and incremental dentine collagen. PLoS One 11:e0160065. https://doi.org/10.1371/journal.pone.0160065.

Beaumont J. et al. 2013. Victims and survivors: stable isotopes used to identify migrants from the Great Irish Famine to 19th century London. Am J Phys Anthropol 150(1): 87–98.

Becker M.J. 1994. Etruscan dental appliances: origins and functions as indicated by an example from Orvieto, Italy in the Danish national museum. Dent Anthrop Newsl 8(3): 2–8.

Becker S.K. 2019. Evaluating elbow osteoarthritis within the prehistoric Tiwanaku state using generalized estimating equations (GEE). Am J Phys Anthropol 169(1): 186–196.

Becker S.K. 2020. Osteoarthritis, entheses, and long bone cross-sectional geometry in the Andes: usage, history, and future directions. Int J Paleopathol 29:45–53.

Bedić Z., Šlaus M., and Donoghue H.D. 2019. The earliest recorded case of lepromatous leprosy in continental Croatia. J Archaeol Sci: Rep 25:47–55.

Bedić Ž., Bebek A.A., Čavka M., and Šlaus M. 2019. A case of hydrocephalus in a child from early modern period Žumberak, Croatia. Int J Paleopathol 26:1–7.

Been E., Barash A., Pessah H., and Peleg S. 2010. A new look at the geometry of the lumbar spine. Spine 35(20): e1014–e1017.

Beier J., Anthes N., Wahl J., and Harvati K. 2018. Similar cranial trauma prevalence among Neanderthals and Upper Palaeolithic modern humans. Nature 563:686–690.

Beier J., Anthes N., Wahl J., and Harvati K. 2021. Prevalence of cranial trauma in Eurasian Upper Paleolithic humans. Am J Phys Anthropol 174:268–284. https://doi.org/10.1002/ajpa.24163.

Belayneh R., Fourman M.S., Bhogal S., and Weiss K.R. 2021. Update on osteosarcoma. Curr Oncol Rep 23(6): 1–8. https://doi.org/10.1007/s11912-021-01053-7.

Belcastro M.G., Todero A., Fornaciari G., and Mariotti V. 2011. Hyperostosis frontalis interna (HFI) and castration: the case of the famous singer Farinelli (1705–1782). J Anat 219(5): 632–637.

Bendrey R. et al. 2020. Approaching ancient disease from a One Health perspective: interdisciplinary review for the investigation of zoonotic brucellosis. Int J Osteoarchaeol 30:99–108. https://doi.org/10.1002/oa.2837.

Bendrey R., and Martin D. 2022. Zoonotic diseases: new directions in human–animal pathology. International Journal of Osteoarchaeology 32(3): 548–552. https://doi.org/10.1002/oa.2975.

Benedek T.G. 2014. 'Case Neisser': experimental design, the beginnings of immunology, and informed consent. Perspect Biol Med 57(2): 249–267. https://doi.org/10.1353/pbm.2014.0018.

Bengtson J. and O'Gorman J. 2017. Women's participation in prehistoric warfare: a central Illinois River valley case study. Int J Osteoarchaeol 27:230–244. https://doi.org/10.1002/oa.2532.

Benítez J.T. 1988. Otopathology of Egyptian mummy PUM II: final report. J Laryngol Otol 102:485–490.

Benjamin N., Rawlins M., and Vale J.A. 2002. Drug therapy and poisoning. In: Clinical medicine, 5th edition, ed. P. Kumar and M. Clark, 957–990. W.B. Saunders.

Benmoussa N., Hansen K., and Charlier P. 2018. Hippocrates the otolaryngologist: an epidemiological analysis of ear–throat–nose diseases in the Corpus Hippocraticum. Acta Oto-Laryngologica 138(3): 194–197. https://doi.org/10.1080/00016489.2018.1429654.

Bennike P. 1985. Palaeopathology of Danish skeletons: a comparative study of demography, disease and injury. Akademisk Forlag.

Bennike P. 2002. Vilhelm Møller-Christensen: his work and legacy. In: The past and present of leprosy: archaeological, historical, palaeopathological and clinical approaches, ed. C.A. Roberts, M.E. Lewis, and K. Manchester, 135–144. British Archaeological Reports International Series 1054. Archaeopress.

Bennike P. and Fredebo L. 1986. Dental treatment in the Stone Age. Bull Hist Dent 34(2): 81–87.

Bentley G.R., Roberts C.A., Elton S., and Plomp K.A. 2022. Now that you have read the book, what next? In: Palaeopathology and evolutionary medicine: an integrated approach, ed. K. Plomp, C.A. Roberts, S. Elton, and G. Bentley, 350–351. Oxford University Press.

Bereczki Z., Teschler-Nicola M., Marcsik A., Meinzer N.J., and Baten J. 2019. Growth disruption in children: linear enamel hypoplasia. In: The backbone of Europe: health, diet, work and violence over two millennia, ed. R.H. Steckel, C.S. Larsen, C.A. Roberts, and J. Baten, 175–197. Cambridge University Press.

Berezina N. and Buzhilova A. 2021. Rare cases of rare diseases: re-examining early 20th century cases of anencephaly from the collection of the Moscow State University, Russia. Int J Paleopathol 34:12–19.

Berger E., Yang L., and Ye W. 2019. Foot binding in a Ming dynasty cemetery near Xi'an, China. Int J Paleopathol 24:79–88. https://doi.org/10.1016/j.

Berger T.D. and Trinkaus E. 1995. Patterns of trauma among Neandertals. J Archaeol Sci 22:841–852.

Bergh C., Wennergren D., Möller M., and Brisby H. 2020. Fracture incidence in adults in relation to age and gender: a study of 27,169 fractures in the Swedish Fracture Register in a well-defined catchment area. PLoS One 15(12): e0244291. https://doi.org/10.1371/journal.pone.0244291.

Bergström A. et al. 2021. Origins and genetic legacy of prehistoric dogs. Science 370(6516): 557–564. https://doi.org/10.1126/science.aba9572.

Bernard M-C. 2003. Tuberculosis: a demographic analysis and social study of admissions to a children's sanatorium (1936–1954) in Stannington, Northumberland. PhD dissertation, Durham University, England.

Bernardini F. et al. 2012. Beeswax as dental filling on a Neolithic human tooth. PLoS One 7(9): e44904. https://doi.org/10.1371/journal.pone.0044904.

Bernofsky K.S. 2010. *Respiratory health in the past: a bioarchaeological study of chronic maxillary sinusitis and rib periostitis from the Iron Age to the post period in southern England.* PhD dissertation, Durham University, England. http://etheses.dur.ac.uk/614/.

Berrang-Ford L. et al. 2021. A systematic global stocktake of evidence on human adaptation to climate change. Nat Clim Chang 11:989–1000: https://doi.org/10.1038/s41558-021-01170-y.

Berryman H.E. and Haun S.J. 1996. Applying forensic techniques to interpret cranial fracture patterns in an archaeological specimen. Int J Osteoarchaeol 6:2–9.

Bertoloni Meli D. 2018. Visualizing disease: the art and history of pathological illustrations. University of Chicago Press.

Betsinger T.K. 2023. Trauma and violence in Poland. Bioarchaeol Int 7:265–281.

Betsinger T.K. and DeWitte S., eds. 2020. The bioarchaeology of urbanization: the biological, demographic, and social consequences of living in cities. Springer Nature.

Betsinger T.K. and Scott A.B. 2023. Back-to-back: the co-occurrence of DISH and ankylosing spondylitis from early modern Poland. Int J Paleopathol 40:1–6.

Bews E.A. et al. 2023. Differential diagnosis of an osseous cranial tumor from Hellenistic Muğla, Turkey. Int J Paleopathol 40:103–108.

Biehler-Gomez L. et al. 2023. Multiple injuries and injury recidivism in Milan over 2,000 years. J Archaeol Sci: Rep 49:103945. https://doi.org/10.1016/j.jasrep.2023.103945.

Biehler-Gomez L., Giordano G., and Cattaneo C. 2019. The overlooked primary: bladder cancer metastases on dry bone. A study of the 20th century CAL Milano Cemetery Skeletal Collection. Int J Paleopathol 24:130–140.

Biehler-Gomez L., Indra L., Martino F., Pietro Campobasso C.P., and Cattaneo C. 2020. Observer error in bone disease description: a cautionary note. Int J Osteoarchaeol 30:607–615.

Bifulco M. et al. 2016. Dental care and dentistry practice in the medical school of Salerno. Br Dent J 221(2): 87–89.

Binder M. and Quade L. 2018. Death on a Napoleonic battlefield—peri-mortem trauma in soldiers from the Battle of Aspern 1809. Int J Paleopathol 22:66–77.

Binder M. and Roberts C.A. 2014. Calcified structures associated with human skeletal remains: possible atherosclerosis affecting the population buried at Amara West, Sudan (1300–800 BC). Int J Paleopathol 6:20–29.

Binder M., Roberts C.A., and Antoine D., eds. 2023. The bioarchaeology of cardiovascular disease. Cambridge University Press.

Binder M., and Saad M. 2017. Hypertrophic osteoarthropathy in a young adult male from Berber, Sudan (2nd–3rd century CE). Int J Paleopathol 18:52–62. https://doi.org/10.1016/j.ijpp.2017.05.006.

Binder M. et al. 2016. Prosthetics in antiquity: an early wearer of a foot prosthesis (6th century AD) from Hemmaberg/Austria. Int J Paleopathol 12:29–40. https://doi.org/10.1016/j.ijpp.2015.11.003.

Bishagratna K.K.L. 1907–1916, trans. An English translation of the Susruta Samhita. 3 vols. Calcutta: by the author.

Biswas T.K., Chakrabarti S., Pandit S., and Mani R. 2023. Medicinal plants and products from traditional medicine systems contribute to clinical wound management. In: Chronic wound management, ed. R. Mani, 117–140. Springer. https://doi.org/10.1007/978-3-031-26110-7_7.

Black S. 2020. Written in bone: hidden stories we leave behind. Doubleday.

Blakey M.L., Leslie T.E., and Reidy J.P. 1994. Frequency and chronological distribution of dental enamel hypoplasia in enslaved African Americans: a test of the weaning hypothesis. Am J Phys Anthropol 95:371–383.

Blau S. and Yagodin V. 2005. Osteoarchaeological evidence for leprosy from central Asia. Am J Phys Anthropol 126:150–158.

Blažina Tomić Z. and Blažina V. 2015. Expelling the plague: the health office and the implementation of quarantine in Dubrovnik, 1377–1533. McGill-Queen's University Press.

Bleasdale M. et al. 2021. Ancient proteins provide evidence of dairy consumption in eastern Africa. Nat Commun 12(1): 632. https://doi.org/10.1038/s41467-020-20682-3.

Blevins K.E., McGrane M., Lory J.M., Arroyo S.G., and Buikstra J.E. 2023. Structural violence and physical death at Tlatelolco: selecting the chronically malnourished for sacrifice at a late postclassic Mesoamerican city (1300–1521 CE). Bioarchaeol Int 7:1–31.

Blickman J., Van Die C., and De Rooy J. 2004. Current imaging concepts in pediatric osteomyelitis. Eur Radio Suppl 14(4): L55–L64.

Blondiaux G. et al. 2002. Rickets and child abuse: the case of a two-year-old girl from the 4th century in Lisieux (Normandy). Int J Osteoarchaeol 12:209–215.

Blondiaux J. et al. 2012. Bilateral fractures of the scapula: possible archeological examples of beatings from Europe, Africa and America. Int J Paleopathol 2(4): 223–230. https://doi.org/10.1016/j.ijpp.

Blondiaux J. et al. 2016. The leprosarium of Saint-Thomas d'Aizier: the cementochronological proof of the decline of Hansen disease in Europe. Int J Paleopathol 15:140–151.

Bloom A.I., Bloom R.A., Kahila G., Eisenberg E., and Smith P. 1995. Amputation of the hand in the 3600-year-old skeletal remains of an adult male: the first case reported from Israel. Int J Osteoarchaeol 5:188–191.

Bodoriková S. et al. 2022. A unique find of juvenile cleft lip and palate in the post-mediaeval impious burial of two males in Dunajská Streda, Slovakia. Archaeol Anthropol Sci 14(4): 68. https://doi.org/10.1007/s12520-022-01546-x.

Boer C.G. et al. 2021. Deciphering osteoarthritis genetics across 826,690 individuals from 9 populations. Cell 184(18): 4784–4718.

Boer L.L., Naue J., De Rooy L. and Oostra R.J., 2017. Detection of G1138A mutation of the FGFR3 gene in tooth material from a 180-year-old museological achondroplastic skeleton. Genes 8(9): 214. https://doi.org/10.3390/genes8090214.

Bogusławska A. et al. 2024. Tall stature and gigantism in adult patients with acromegaly. Eur J Endocrinol 190(3): 193–200.

Boldsen J.L. 2001. Epidemiological approach to the paleopathological diagnosis of leprosy. Am J Phys Anthropol 115(4): 380–387. https://doi.org/10.1002/ajpa.1094.

Boldsen J.L. and Milner G.R. 2012. An epidemiological approach to paleopathology. In: A companion to paleopathology, ed. A.L. Grauer, 114–132. Wiley-Blackwell.

Boldsen J.L. and Mollerup L. 2006. Outside St. Jørgen: leprosy in the medieval Danish city of Odense. Am J Phys Anthropol 130:344–351. https://doi.org/10.1002/ajpa.20363.

Boldsen J.L., Milner G.R., and Ousley S.D. 2022. Paleodemography: from archaeology and skeletal age estimation to life in the past. Am J Biol Anthropol 178:115–150.

Bolk L. 1915. On the premature obliteration of sutures in the human skull. Am J Anat 17(4): 495–523.

Bolton-Maggs P. and Thomas A. 2008. Disorders of the blood and bone marrow. In: Forfar and Arneil's textbook of pediatrics, ed. N. McIntosh, P. Helms, R. Smyth, and S. Logan, 959–990. Churchill Livingstone.

Bonczarowska J.H. et al. 2022. Pathogen genomics study of an early medieval community in Germany reveals extensive co-infections. Genome Biol 23:250. https://doi.org/10.1186/s13059-022-02806-8.

Bonsall L., Ogden A.R., and Mays S. 2016. A case of early childhood caries from Late Roman Ancaster, England. Int J Osteoarchaeol 26:555–560. https://doi.org/10.1002/oa.2441.

Boocock P., Roberts C.A., and Manchester K. 1995. Maxillary sinusitis in medieval Chichester, England. Am J Phys Anthropol 98(4): 483–495.

Bor A., Jørgensen F., and Petersen M.B. 2023. Discriminatory attitudes against unvaccinated people during the pandemic. Nature 613:704–711. https://doi.org/10.1038/s41586-022-05607-y.

Bos K.I. and DeWitte S.N. 2022. Human resistance and the evolution of the plague in medieval Europe. In Palaeopathology and evolutionary medicine: an integrated approach, edited by K. Plomp, C.A. Roberts, S. Elton, and G. Bentley, 138–154. Oxford University Press.

Bos K.I. et al. 2011. A draft genome of Yersinia pestis from victims of the Black Death. Nature 478:506–510.

Bos K.I. et al. 2014. Pre-Columbian mycobacterial genomes reveal seals as a source of New World human tuberculosis. Nature 514:494–497.

Botelho J. et al. 2022. An umbrella review of the evidence linking oral health and systemic noncommunicable diseases. Nat Commun 13(1): 7614. https://doi.org/10.1038/s41467-022-35337-8.

Botha D., Masiu R., and Steyn M. 2024. Assessing tuberculosis in the skeleton with the use of decision tree analysis. Anthropologischer Anzeiger 81(2): 233–239. https://doi.org/10.1127/anthranz/2023/1737.

Botting B. and Abrahams C. 2000. Linking congenital anomaly and birth records. Health Stat Q 8:36–40.

Boucherie A., Castex D., Polet C., and Kacki S. 2016. Normal growth, altered growth? Study of the relationship between Harris lines and bone form within a post-medieval plague cemetery (Dendermonde, Belgium, 16th Century). Am J Hum Biol 29(1): e22885. https://doi.org/10.1002/ajhb.22885.

Boucherie A., Jørkov SML, and Smith M. 2017. Wounded to the bone: digital microscopic analysis of traumas in a medieval mass grave assemblage (Sandbjerget, Denmark, AD 1300–1350). Int J Paleopathol 19:66–79. https://doi.org/10.1016/j.ijpp.

Bouchet F. et al. 1996. Palaeoparasitology in a Pleistocene context: initial observations in the Grande Grotte at Arcy-sur-Cure (Department of the Yonne, France). CR Acad Sci Sér III 319:147–151.

Boulestin B. and Gomez de Soto J. 1995. Le cannibalisme au Néolithique: réalité et sens [Cannibalism in the Neolithic: reality and meaning]. In: 'La Mort': Passé, Présent, Conditionel, ed. J.M. Large, 59–68. Groupe Vendéen d'Études Préhistoriques.

Boutin A.T. 2016. Exploring the social construction of disability: an application of the bioarchaeology of personhood model to a pathological skeleton from ancient Bahrain. Int J Paleopathol 12:17–28.

Bouwman A.S. and Brown T.A. 2005. The limits of biomolecular palaeopathology: ancient DNA cannot be used to study venereal syphilis. J Archaeol Sci 32:703–713. https://doi.org/10.1016/j.jas.2004.11.014.

Bovée J. 2008. Multiple osteochondromas. Orphanet J Rare Dis 3(3): 1–7. https://doi.org/10.1186/1750-1172-3-3.

Boyce W.T. et al. 2010. Social inequalities in childhood dental caries: the convergent roles of stress, bacteria and disadvantage. Soc Sci Med 71(9): 1644–1652. https://doi.org/10.1016/j.socscimed.2010.07.045.

Boylston A. 2000. Evidence for weapon-related trauma in British archaeological samples. In: Human osteology in archaeology and forensic science, ed. M. Cox and S. Mays, 357–380. Greenwich Medical Media.

Boylston A. 2001. Physical anthropology. In: Blood red roses: the archaeology of a mass grave from the Battle of Towton AD 1461, ed. V. Fiorato, A. Boylston, and C. Knüsel, 45–49. Oxbow Books.

Boylston A., Knüsel C.J., and Roberts C.A. 2000. Investigation of a Romano-British rural ritual in Bedford, England. J Archaeol Sci 27:241–254.

Breasted J.H. 1991. The Edwin Smith surgical papyrus. University of Chicago Press.

Brenna C.T.A. 2022. Bygone theatres of events: a history of human anatomy and dissection. Anat Rec 305(4): 788–802. https://doi.org/10.1002/ar.24764.

Brennan P. and Davey-Smith G. 2022. Identifying novel causes of cancers to enhance cancer prevention: new strategies are needed. JNCI: Journal of the National Cancer Institute 114(3): 353–360.

Brenner E. and Touati F-O. 2021. Leprosy and identity in the Middle Ages. Manchester University Press.

Brickley M.B. 2024. Perspectives on anemia: factors confounding understanding of past occurrence. Int J Paleopathol 44:90–104.

Brickley M.B. and Morgan B. 2023. Assessing diagnostic certainty for scurvy and rickets in human skeletal remains. Am J Biol Anthropol 181(4): 637–645.

Brickley M., Ives R., and Mays S. 2020. The bioarchaeology of metabolic bone disease. Academic Press.

Brickley M., Mays S., and Ives R. 2008. Evaluation and interpretation of residual rickets deformities in adults. In J Osteoarchaeol 20:54–66.
Brickley M.B. 2006. Rib fractures in the archaeological record: a useful source of sociocultural information? Int J Osteoarchaeol 16:61–75.
Brickley M.B. 2018. Cribra orbitalia and porotic hyperostosis: a biological approach to diagnosis. Am J Phys Anthropol 167(4): 896–902.
Brickley M.B., Ives R., and Mays S. 2020. The bioarchaeology of metabolic bone disease. Academic Press.
Brickley M.B. and Mays S. 2019. Metabolic disease. In: Ortner's identification of pathological conditions in human skeletal remains, ed. J.E. Buikstra, 531–566. Academic Press.
Brickley M.B., and McKinley J.I., eds. 2004. Guidelines to the standards for recording human remains. Institute of Field Archaeologists Paper 7. Institute of Field Archaeologists.
Bridges P.S. 1994. Vertebral arthritis and physical activities in the prehistoric United States. Am J Phys Anthropol 93:83–93.
Bridges P.S., Blitz J.H., and Solano M.C. 2000. Changes in long bone diaphyseal strength with horticulture intensification in west-central Illinois. Am J Phys Anthropol 112:217–238.
Bridson E. 2001. The English 'Sweate' (Sudor Anglicus) and hantavirus pulmonary syndrome. Br J Biomed Sci 58(1): 1–6.
Brien T.G., Peters L.R., Hines M.E. 2013. Artificial cranial deformation: potential implications for affected brain function. Anthropology 1:107. doi:10.4172/2332-0915.1000107.
British Academy. 2024. This is SHAPE. https://www.thebritishacademy.ac.uk/this-is-shape/.
British Antarctic Survey. 2024. Penguins test positive for avian flu on South Georgia. https://www.bas.ac.uk/media-post/penguins-test-positive-for-avian-flu-on-south-georgia/.
British Association of Biological Anthropology and Osteoarchaeology. 2024. Guidelines and codes. https://babao.org.uk/resources/guidelines-codes/.
Britton W.J. and Lockwood D.N. 2004. Leprosy. Lancet 363:1209–1219.
Broadbent V., Egeler R.M., and Nesbit M.E. Jr. 1994. Langerhans cell histiocytosis—clinical and epidemiological aspects.Br J Cancer Suppl. 23:S11–S16.
Brødholt E.T. 2007. Skjelettene fra Mariakirken: Nytt Lys på Kongskirken Gjennom en Undersøkelse av Skjelettmaterialet [Skeletons from Mariakirken: new light on the King's Church through examination of the skeletal material] Antropologiske skrifter nr. 7. Oslo: Avdeling for anatomi, Institutt for medisinske basalfag, Universitetet i Oslo.
Brødholt E.T. and Holck P. 2012. Skeletal trauma in the burials from the royal church of St. Mary in medieval Oslo. Int J Osteoarchaeol 22:201–218. https://doi.org/10.1002/oa.1198.
Brook I. 2011. Microbiology of sinusitis. Proc Am Thorac Soc. 8(1): 90–100. https://doi.org/10.1513/pats.
Brooks D.R., Hoberg E.P., and Boeger W.A. 2019. *The Stockholm paradigm: climate change and emerging disease*. University of Chicago Press.
Brooks S.T. and Hohenthal W.D. 1963. Archeological defective palate crania from California. Am J Phys Anthropol 21(1): 25–32.
Brorson S. 2009. Management of fractures of the humerus in Ancient Egypt, Greece, and Rome: an historical review. Clin Orthop Relat Res 467(7): 1907–1914.
Brosch R. et al. 2002. A new evolutionary sequence for the *Mycobacterium tuberculosis* complex. Proc Nat Acad Sci 99(6): 3684–3689.
Brothwell D. 1960. A possible case of mongolism in a Saxon population. Ann Hum Genet 24: 141–150.
Brothwell D. 1967a. Major congenital anomalies of the skeleton: evidence from earlier populations. In: Diseases in antiquity, ed. D. Brothwell and A.T. Sandison, 423–444. Charles C. Thomas.
Brothwell D. 1967b. The evidence for neoplasms. In: Diseases in antiquity: a survey of the diseases, injuries and surgery of early populations, ed. D. Brothwell and A.T. Sandison, 320–345. Charles C. Thomas.
Brothwell D. 1981. Digging up bones. British Museum (Natural History).
Brothwell D. and Brothwell P. 1969. Food in antiquity: a survey of the diet of early peoples. Expanded edition. Johns Hopkins University Press.
Brothwell D. and Møller-Christensen V. 1963. Medico-historical aspects of an early case of mutilation. Danish Med Bull 10:21–27.

Brothwell D. and Powers R. 1968. Congenital malformations of the skeleton in earlier man. In: Skeletal biology of earlier human populations (Symposia of the Society for the Study of Human Biology, Volume 8), ed. D.R. Brothwell, 173–203. Pergamon Press.

Brown T.A. 2023. Archaeogenetics. In: Handbook of archaeological sciences. Vol. 1. 2nd edition, ed. M. Pollard, R.A. Armitage, and C. Makarewicz, 607–612. Wiley.

Brozou A. et al. 2021. Leprosy in medieval Denmark: exploring life histories through a multi-tissue and multi-isotopic approach. Am J Phys Anthropol 176(1): 36–53. https://doi.org/10.1002/ajpa.24339.

Bruintjes T. 1990. The auditory ossicles in human skeletal remains from a leper cemetery in Chichester, England. J Archaeol Sci 17:627–633.

Bryan C.P., trans. 1974. Ancient Egyptian medicine: the Papyrus Ebers. ARES.

Bryson B. 2019. The body: a guide for occupants. Penguin Books.

Bubb C. 2022. Dissection in classical antiquity: a social and medical history. Cambridge University Press.

Buchanan W.W, Kean W., and Kean R. 2003. History and current status of osteoarthritis in the population. Inflammopharmacology 11(4): 301–316. https://doi.org/10.1163/156856003322699483.

Buchanan W.W. and Laurent R.M. 1990. Rheumatoid arthritis: an example of ecological succession. Can Bull Med Hist 7:77–91.

Buckberry J. and Crane-Kramer G. 2022. The dark satanic mills: evaluating patterns of health in England during the industrial revolution. Int J Paleopathol 39:93–108.

Buckley H. 2011. Epidemiology of gout: perspectives from the past. Curr Rheumatol Rev 7(2): 106–113.

Buckley H.R., Vlok M., Petchey P., and Ritchie N. 2023. 'A long want': an archival exploration of scurvy in the Otago goldfields of New Zealand. J R Soc N Z 54(3): 368–389.

Buckley S., Usai D., Jakob T., Radini A., and Hardy K. 2014. Dental calculus reveals unique insights into food items, cooking and plant processing in prehistoric Sudan. PLoS One 9(7): e100808.

Bueschgen W.D. and Case D.T. 1996. Evidence of prehistoric scalping at Vosberg, central Arizona. Int J Osteoarchaeol 6:230–248.

Buhr A.J. and Cooke A.M. 1959. Fracture patterns. Lancet 1:531–536.

Buikstra J.E. 1981. Prehistoric tuberculosis in the Americas. Northwestern University Archaeological Program.

Buikstra J.E. 2016. Repatriation and bioarchaeology: challenges and opportunities. In: Bioarchaeology. the contextual analysis of human remains, ed. J.E. Buikstra and L.A. Beck, 289–415. Academic Press.

Buikstra J.E., ed. 2019a. Ortner's identification of pathological conditions in human skeletal remains. Academic Press.

Buikstra J.E., ed. 2019b. Bioarchaeologists speak out: deep time perspectives on contemporary issues. Springer.

Buikstra J.E. 2023. Paleopathology: a twenty-first century perspective. In: A companion to biological anthropology, ed. C.S. Larsen, 474–493. Wiley-Blackwell.

Buikstra J., Uhl E., and Robbins Schug G. 2025. One Paleopathology and lessons from the past. BioScience. https://doi.org/10.1093/biosci/biaf115.

Buikstra J. E. and Milner G.R. 1991. Isotopic and archaeological interpretations of diet in the central Mississippi valley. J Archaeol Sci 18:319–329.

Buikstra J.E., Poznanski A., Cerna M., Goldstein P., and Hioshower L. 1990. A case of juvenile rheumatoid arthritis from pre-Colombian Peru. In: A life in science. Papers in honour of J. Lawrence Angel (Scientific Papers, Vol. 6), ed. J. Buikstra, 99–137. Central American Archaeology.

Buikstra J.E. and Roberts C.A., eds. 2012. *The global history of paleopathology: pioneers and prospects*. Academic Press.

Buikstra J. E. and Ubelaker D. 1994. Standards for data collection from human skeletal remains. Arkansas Archeological Survey Research Series, no. 44.

Buikstra J.E., Uhl E.W., and Wissler A. 2023. Big pictures in 21st century paleopathology. Interdisciplinarity and transdisciplinarity. In The Routledge handbook of paleopathology, edited by A.L. Grauer, 625–635. Routledge.

Buikstra J.E. et al. 2022. 21st-century bioarchaeology: taking stock and moving forward. Yearbook Biological Anthropology 178(Suppl. 74): 54–114. https://doi.org/10.1002/ajpa.24494.
Builders P.F. and Builders M.I. 2016. Wound care: traditional African medicine approach. In: World-wide wound healing—innovation in natural and conventional methods, ed. C.J.V. da Fonseca. InTech. https://doi.org/10.5772/62668.
Buka I. 2009. Children and cancer. In: WHO training package for the health sector, ed. World Health Organization. https://www.who.int/publications/i/item/WHO-HSE-PHE-AMR-09.01.01.
Bullock J. et al. 2019. Rheumatoid arthritis: a brief overview of the treatment. Med Princ Pract 27(6): 501–507.
Bupp M.R.G. 2015. Sex, the aging immune system, and chronic disease. Cell Immunol 294(2): 102–110.
Burckhardt P., Dawson-Hughes B., and Heaney R.P., eds. 2004. Nutritional aspects of osteoporosis. Elsevier.
Burnett S.E. and Irish J.D, eds. 2017. A world view of bioculturally modified teeth. University Press of Florida.
Burt N.M., Semple D., Waterhouse K., and Lovell N. 2013. Identification and interpretation of joint disease in paleopathology and forensic anthropology. Charles C. Thomas.
Butlin C.R. and Peters R.M.H. 2022. Ethical considerations for leprosy researchers. Lepr Rev 93:2–11.
Buzon M.R. 2005. Two cases of pelvic osteochondroma in New Kingdom Nubia. Int J Osteoarchaeol 15(5): 377–382.
Buzon M.R., and Richman R. 2007. Traumatic injuries and imperialism: the effects of Egyptian colonial strategies at Tombos in upper Nubia. Am J Phys Anthropol 133:783–791. https://doi.org/10.1002/ajpa.20585.
Byl S. 1988. Rheumatism and gout in the Corpus Hippocraticum. L'antiquité classique 57:89–102.
Byrnes J.F. and Gaddis K. 2023. Sticks and stones may break my bones: traumatic injuries in palaeo-pathology. In: The Routledge handbook of paleopathology, ed. A.L. Grauer, 231–249. Routledge.
Caffell A.C., Roberts C.A., Janaway R.C., and Wilson A.S. 2001. Pressures on osteological collections—the importance of damage limitation. In: Human remains: conservation, retrieval and analysis. Proceedings of a conference held in Williamsburg, VA, 7–11 November 1999, ed. E. Williams, 187–197. British Archaeological Reports International Series 934. Archaeopress.
Cameron M. and Stock J. 2018. Ecological variation in later stone age southern African biomechani-cal properties. J Archaeol Sci: Rep 17:125–136.
Campbell S.E. and Simberloff D. 2022. Forty years of invasion research: more papers, more collaboration . . . bigger impact? Neobiota 75:57–77.
Campillo D. 1990. Etude des restes squelettiques d'un individu de l'époque tardi-romaine, atteint de polyarthrite rhumatoïde [Study of the skeletal remains of an individual from the late Roman period suffering with rheumatoid arthritis]. Anthropologie et préhistoire 101:71–83.
Cantini F. et al. 2010. Psoriatic arthritis: a systematic review. Int J Rheum Dis 13(4): 300–317.
Cao H. and Vickers M.A. 2021. Oxidative stress, malaria, sickle cell disease, and innate immu-nity. Trends Immunol 42(10): 849–851.
Capasso L. 1998. Lice buried under the ashes of Herculaneum. Lancet 351(9107): 992.
Cappella A. et al. 2014. The difficult task of assessing perimortem and postmortem fractures on the skeleton: a blind text on 210 fractures of known origin. J Forensic Sci 59:1598–1601.
Cappellini M.D., Musallam K.M., and Taher A.T. 2020. Iron deficiency anaemia revisited. J Intern Med 287(2): 153–170.
Cardy A. 1997. The environmental material: the human bones. In: Whithorn and St Ninian: the exca-vation of a monastic town 1984–91, ed. P. Hill, 519–562. Sutton Publishing.
Carroll G.A. 1972. Traditional medical cures along the Yukon. Alaska Med 14:50–53.
Carstairs C. 2022. The smile gap: a history of oral health and social inequality. McGill-Queen's University Press.
Case D., Hill R., Merbs C., and Fong M. 2006. Polydactyly in the prehistoric American Southwest. Int J Osteoarchaeol 16:221–235.
Cashman K.D. 2020. Vitamin D deficiency: defining, prevalence, causes, and strategies of addressing. Calcif Tissue Int 106(1): 14–29.

Cashman K.D. et al. 2016. Vitamin D deficiency in Europe—pandemic? Am J Clin Nutr 103:1033–1044.
Casna M., Burrell C.L., Schats R., Hoogland M.L.P., and Schrader S.A. 2021. Urbanization and respiratory stress in the northern Low Countries: a comparative study of chronic maxillary sinusitis in two early modern sites from the Netherlands (AD 1626–1866). Int J Osteoarchaeol 31(5): 891–901. https://doi.org/10.1002/oa.3006.
Cassano P., Ciprandi G., and Passali D. 2020. Acute mastoiditis in children. Acta Bio Medica: Atenei Parmensis 91 (1): 54–59.
Cassidy L.M. et al. 2020. A dynastic elite in monumental Neolithic society. Nature 582:384–388.
Cassman V., Odegaard N., and Powell J., eds. 2007. Human remains: guide for museums and academic institutions. Altamira Press.
Castells Navarro L., Buckberry J., and Beaumont J. 2022. An isotope signature for diffuse idiopathic skeletal hyperostosis? Am J Biol Anthropol 178(2): 312–327.
Castells Navaro L., Southwell-Wright W., Manchester K., and Buckberry J. 2017. Interpretation of a probable case of poliomyelitis in the Romano-British social context. Arch Rev Camb 32(1): 34–52.
Castex D. and Kacki S. 2016. Demographic patterns distinctive of epidemic cemeteries in archaeological samples. In: Paleomicrobiology of Humans, ed. M. Crancourt and D. Raoult, 1–11. Wiley.
Castilho S.D. and Rocha M.A. 2009. Pacifier habit: history and multidisciplinary view. J Pediatr (Rio J) 85(6): 480–489.
Castillo Aleman Y.M. 2021. Medical eponyms: redeeming or not the long-standing tradition. Postgrad Med J 97(1150): 498–500.
Castro de la Mata R. and Bonavia D. 1980. Lumbosacral malformations and spina bifida in a Peruvian preceramic child. Current Anthropology 21(4): 515–516.
Castro M., Pacheco A., Kuzmanic I., Clarot A., and Díaz P. 2020. Treponematosis in a pre-Columbian hunter-gatherer male from Antofagasta (1830 ± 20 BP, Northern Coast of Chile). Int J Paleopathol 30:10–16. https://doi.org/10.1016/j.ijpp.2020.01.004.
Castro M. et al. 2016. Thoracic aortic aneurysm in a pre-Columbian (210 BC) inhabitant of northern Chile: implications for the origins of syphilis. Int J Paleopathol 13:20–26. https://doi.org/10.1016/j.ijpp.2016.01.002.
Čavka M. et al. 2022. A case of a large pedunculated-type osteochondroma from late medieval Ilok, eastern Croatia: bioarchaeological, paleoradiological and histological study. J Archaeol Sci: Rep 45:103574. https://doi.org/10.1016/j.jasrep.2022.103574.
Cawley W. and Paine R. 2015. Skeletal indicators of reactive arthritis: a case study comparison to other skeletal conditions, such as rheumatoid arthritis, ankylosing spondylitis, ankylosing seronegative SpA, and DISH. Int J Paleopathol 11:70–74.
Celsus A.C. 1935 (1st C AD). De medicina. 3 vols. Translated by W.G. Spencer. Harvard University Press.
Chan J.Z. et al. 2013. Metagenomic analysis of tuberculosis in a mummy. N Engl J Med. 369(3): 289–290. https://doi.org/10.1056/NEJMc1302295.
Chandra P. and Adlakha V. 2015. Infant oral health. In: Emerging trends in oral health sciences and dentistry, ed. M. Virdi, 151–164. InTech. https://doi.org/10.5772/59245.
Charlier P. 2008. The value of palaeoteratology and forensic pathology for the understanding of atypical burials: two Mediterranean examples from the field. In: Deviant burial in the archaeological record, ed. E. Murphy, 57–70. Oxbow Books.
Charon P. 2004. Contribution to osteo-archaeological knowledge of anencephaly. J Paleopathol 16(1): 5–13.
Chau M.M. et al. 2021. Osteochondritis dissecans: current understanding of epidemiology, etiology, management, and outcomes. J Bone Joint Surg Am 103(12): 1132–1151. https://doi.org/10.2106/JBJS.20.01399.
Chaussinand R. 1953. Tuberculosis and leprosy: mutually antagonistic diseases. Leprosy Review 24:90–94.
Chen L. et al. 2022. A global meta-analysis of heavy metal(loid)s pollution in soils near copper mines: evaluation of pollution level and probabilistic health risks. Sci Total Environ 835:155441. https://doi.org/10.1016/j.scitotenv.2022.155441.
Cheng J., Ying S., and Lam P. 1999. A 10-year study of the changes in the pattern and treatment of 6,493 fractures. J Pediatr Orthop 19:344–50.

Cherniack M. 1992. Diseases of unusual occupations: an historical perspective. Occup Med 7(3): 369–384.
Cheung C., Zhang H., Hepburn J.C., Yang D.Y., and Richards M.P. 2019. Stable isotope and dental caries data reveal abrupt changes in subsistence economy in ancient China in response to global climate change. PLoS One 14(7): e0218943. https://doi.org/10-1371/journal.pone.0218943.
Chhabra BN et al. 2023. Pediatric hand and wrist fractures in osteogenesis imperfecta: an analysis of incidence, patient-specific risk factors, and fracture-specific characteristics. J Pediatr Orthop 43(8): e680–e685, https://doi.org/ 10.1097/BPO.0000000000002449.
Chi-Keb J.R., Albertos-Gonzalez V.M., Ortega-Munoz A., and Tiesler V.G. 2013. A new reference collection of documented human skeletons from Merida, Yucatan, Mexico. Homo 64(5): 366–376.
Chiara C., Frohlich B., and Lynnerup N. 2019. The role of imaging in paleopathology. In: Ortner's identification of pathological conditions in human skeletal remains, ed. J.E. Buikstra, 169–182. Elsevier.
Choi J.H. et al. 2022. Management of lumbar spondylolysis in the adolescent athlete: a review of over 200 cases. Spine J 22(10): 1628–1633. https://doi.org/10.1016/j.spinee.2022.04.011.
Choudhury S.M. 2021. Experience in receiving and practicing self-care as a person affected by leprosy. Leprosy Review 92(4): 379–384. https://doi.org/10.47276/lr.92.4.379.
Christen A.G. and Christen J.A. 2003. A historical glimpse of toothpick use: etiquette, oral and medical conditions. J Hist Dent 51(2): 61–69.
Chuma I.S. et al. 2018. Widespread *Treponema pallidum* infection in nonhuman primates, Tanzania. Emerg Infect Dis 24(6): 1002–1009. https://doi.org/10.3201/eid2406.180037.
Cilliers L. 2019. Roman North Africa: environment, society and medicine. University of Amsterdam Press.
Ciranni R., Castagna M., and Fornaciari G. 1999. Goiter in an 18th century Sicilian mummy. Am J Phys Anthropol 108:427–432.
Clark G. 2007. A farewell to alms: a brief economic history of the world. Princeton University Press.
Clarke N.G. and Hirsch R.S. 1991. Physiological, pulpal and periodontal factors influencing alveolar bone. In: Advances in dental anthropology, ed. M. Kelley and C.S. Larsen, 241–266. Alan Liss.
Clark G. et al. 1986. Poor growth prior to early childhood: decreased health and life-span in the adult. Am J Phys Anthropol 70:145–60.
Cobb M. 2020. The idea of the brain: the past and future of neuroscience. Basic Books.
Cogbill T.H., Steenlage E.S., Landercasper J., and Strutt P.J. 1991. Death and disability from agricultural injuries in Wisconsin: a 12-year experience with 739 patients. J Trauma 31(12): 1632–1637.
Cogulu D. and Saglam C. 2022. Genetic aspects of dental caries. Front Dent Med 3:1060177. https://doi.org/10.3389/fdmed. 2022.1060177.
Cohen H. et al. 2014. Trauma to the skull: a historical perspective from the southern Levant (4300BCE–1917CE). Int J Osteoarchaeol 24:722–736. https://doi.org/10.1002/oa.2258.
Cohen M. 2005. Perspectives on craniosynostosis. Am J Med Genet 136A:313–326.
Cohen M.N. and Armelagos G.J., eds. 1984. Paleopathology at the origins of agriculture. Academic Press.
Cohen M.N. and Crane-Kramer K., eds. 2007. Ancient health: skeletal indicators of economic and political intensification. University Press of Florida.
Cole G. and Waldron T. 2011. Apple Down 152: A putative case of syphilis from the sixth century AD Anglo-Saxon England. Amer J Phys Anthrop 144:72–79.
Cole G., and Waldron T. 2012. Letter to the editor: syphilis revisited. Am J Phys Anthropol 149:149–150.
Cole G. and Waldron T. 2015. Letter to the editor: Apple Down 152 putative syphilis: pre-Columbian date confirmed. Am J Phys Anthropol 156:489.
Cole P.A., Freeman G., and Dubin J.R. 2013. Scapula fractures. Curr Rev Musculoskelet Med 6:79–87. https://doi.org/10.1007/s12178-012-9151-x.
Cole S.T. et al. 1998. Deciphering the biology of *Mycobacterium tuberculosis* from the complete genome sequence. Nature 396(6707): 537–544.

Cole S.T. et al. 2001. Massive gene decay in leprosy bacillus. Nature 409:1007–1011.

Collado Z.C. 2019. Challenges in public health facilities and services: evidence from a geographically isolated and disadvantaged area in the Philippines. J Glob Health Rep 3:e2019059. https://doi.org/10.29392/joghr.3.e2019059.

Colleter R. et al. 2023. Dental care of Anne d'Alègre (1565–1619, Laval, France): between therapeutic reason and aesthetic evidence, the place of the social and the medical in the care in modern period. J Archaeol Sci: Rep 48:103794. https://doi.org/10.1016/j.jasrep.2022.103794.

Collier L. and Primeau C. 2019. A tale of two cities: a comparison of urban and rural trauma in medieval Denmark. Int J Paleopathol 24:175–184. https://doi.org/10.1016/j.ijpp.2018.10.002.

Collin S.M. et al. 2023a. Systematic review of Hansen disease attributed to *Mycobacterium lepromatosis*. Emerg Infect Dis 29(7): 1376–1385. https://doi.org/10.3201/eid2907.230024.

Collin S.M., Pettan-Brewer C., Rabinowitz P., and Deps P.D. 2023b. Hansen's disease and One Health. In: Hansen's disease—a complete clinical guide, ed. P. Deps, 65–70. Springer Nature.

Collins C. 2019. The palaeopathology of maxillary sinusitis, otitis media and mastoiditis in medieval Iceland: assessing the prevalence and aetiology of chronic upper respiratory disease and the presence of tuberculosis using microscopy, endoscopy and CT. Ph.D. dissertation, University of Reading, Berkshire, England. https://centaur.reading.ac.uk/84764/.

Collins P.H. and Bilge S. 2020. Intersectionality, 2nd ed. Polity Press.

Colombo A. et al. 2015. Langerhans cell histiocytosis or tuberculosis on a medieval child (Oppidum de la Granède, Millau, France–10th–11th centuries AD). Tuberculosis 95(Suppl. 1): S42–S50.

Connell B., Gray Jones A., Redfern R., and Walker D. 2012. A bioarchaeological study of the medieval burials on the site of St Mary Spital. Excavations at Spitalfields Market, London E1, 1991–2007. Museum of London Archaeology Monograph 60. Museum of London.

Connolly C., Keil R., and Ali S.H. 2021. Extended urbanisation and the spatialities of infectious disease: demographic change, infrastructure and governance. Urban Stud 58(2): 245–263. https://doi.org/10.1177/0042098020910873.

Conrad P. and Barker K.K. 2010. The social construction of illness: key insights and policy implications. J Health Soc Behav 51:S67–79. https://doi.org/10.1177/0022146510383495.

Cook D.C. and Danforth M.E. 2022. Meningiomas in ancient human populations. Cancers 14(4): 1058. https://doi.org/10.3390/cancers14041058.

Cook D.C., Bastos M.Q.R., Lopes C., Mendonça de Souza S., and Santos R.V. 2015. Pretos Novos: evidence for African oral hygiene practices in Brazil, 1769–1830. Int J Osteoarchaeol 25:238–244. https://doi.org/ 10.1002/oa.2278.

Cook S.J. and Wall C. 2021. Paget's disease of the bone: a clinical update. Aust J Gen Pract 50(1–2): 23–29.

Cooke R. et al. 2023. Catch-up growth in infants and young children with faltering growth: expert opinion to guide general clinicians. J Pediatr Gastroenterol Nutr 77(1): 7–15. https://doi.org/10.1097/MPG.0000000000003784.

Cooper A. and Poinar H.N. 2000. Ancient DNA: do it right or not at all. Science 289(5482): 1139. https://doi.org/10.1126/science.289.5482.1139b.

Cope D. and Dupras T. 2011. Osteogenesis imperfecta in the archaeological record: an example from the Dakhleh Oasis, Egypt. Int J Paleopathol 1:188–199.

Coppes-Zantinga A. and Egeler R.M. 2002. The Langerhans-cell histiocytosis X files revealed. Br J Haematol 116(1): 3–9. https://dx.doi.org/10.1046/j.1365-2141.2002.03232.x.

Coppola M. et al. 2018. Vaccines for leprosy and tuberculosis: opportunities for shared research, development, and application. Front Immunol 9:308. https://doi.org/10.3389/fimmu.2018.00308.

Corron L.K., Wolfe C.A., and Stull K.E. 2023. A multifaceted exploration of ontogenetic variation in vertebral neural canal size across contemporary populations. Am J Biol Anthropol 180(2): 328–351.

Corruccini R.S., Handler J.S., and Jacobs K.P. 1985. Chronological distribution of enamel hypoplasias and weaning in a Caribbean slave population. Hum Biol 57(4): 699–711.

Corthals A. et al. 2012. Detecting the immune system response of a 500 year-old Inca mummy. PLoS One 7(7): e41244. https://doi.org/10.1371/journal.pone.0041244.

Cosford K.L. 2018. Brucella canis: an update on research and clinical management. Can Vet J 59(1): 74–81.

Cotran R.S., Kumar V., and Robbins S.L. 1989. Robbins pathologic basis of disease, 4th ed. W.B. Saunders.
Coughlan J. and Holst M. 2001. Health status. In: Blood red roses: the archaeology of a mass grave from the Battle of Towton AD 1461, ed. V. Fiorato, A. Boylston, and C. Knüsel, 60–76. Oxbow Books.
Court-Brown C.M. and Caesar B. 2006. Epidemiology of adult fractures: a review. Injury 37(8): 691–697. https://doi.org/10.1016/j.injury.2006.04.130.
Courville C.B. 1965. War wounds of the cranium in the Middle Ages: 1. As disclosed in the skeletal material from the Battle of Wisby (1361 AD). Bull Los Angeles Neurolog Soc 30:27–33.
Cox S.L. et al. 2023. Socio-cultural practices may have affected sex differences in stature in Early Neolithic Europe. Nat Hum Behav 8:243–255. https://doi.org/10.1038/s41562-023-01756-w.
Craig M. 2004. Perinatal risk factors for neonaticide and infant homicide: can we identify those at risk? J R Soc Med 97(2): 57–61. https://doi.org/10.1177/014107680409700203.
Crane-Kramer G.M.M. 2002. Was there a medieval diagnostic confusion between leprosy and syphilis? An examination of the skeletal evidence. In: The past and present of leprosy: archaeological, historical, palaeopathological and clinical approaches, ed. C.A. Roberts, M.E. Lewis, and K. Manchester, 111–119. British Archaeological Reports International Series 1054. Archaeopress.
Craps D. and Gowland R. 2015. The proximal ulna as an additional diagnostic feature of advanced rheumatoid arthritis. Int J Paleopathol 10:26–30.
Crawford R.R., Hodson C.M., and Errickson D. 2024. Guidance for the identification of bony lesions related to smallpox. Int J Paleopathol 44:65–77. https://doi.org/10.1016/j.ijpp.2023.12.002.
Crawford-Adams J. 1983. Outline of fractures. 8th ed. Churchill Livingstone.
Crenshaw K. 1991. Mapping the margins: intersectionality, identity politics, and violence against women of color. Stanford Law Rev 43:1241–1299.
Crespo F., White J., and Roberts C.A. 2019. Revisiting the tuberculosis and leprosy cross-immunity hypothesis: expanding the dialogue between immunology and paleopathology. Int J Paleopathol 26:37–47.
Crews D.E. and Bogin B. 2010. Growth, development, senescence, and aging: a life history perspective. In: A companion to biological anthropology, ed. C.S. Larsen, 124–152. Blackwell.
Cristiani E., Radini A., Edinborough M., and Borić D. 2016. Dental calculus reveals Mesolithic foragers in the Balkans consumed domesticated plant foods. Proc Natl Acad Sci USA 113(37): 10298–10303.
Crist T.A. 2014. "That class of person who cannot afford a pew": analysis of the human remains from the Spring Street Presbyterian Church burial vaults. Northeast Hist Archaeology 39(1): 5. https://orb.binghamton.edu/neha/vol39/iss1/5/.
Cronk C.E. 1993. Down's syndrome. In: The Cambridge world history of human disease, ed. K. Kiple, 683–686. Cambridge University Press.
Crosby A.W. 2003. The Columbian exchange, biological and cultural consequences, 30th anniversary edition. Praeger.
Crubézy E. and Trinkhaus E. 1992. Shanidar 1: a case of hyperostotic disease (DIsH) in the Middle Paleolithic. Am J Phys Anthropol 89:411–420.
Cucina A. and Tiesler V. 2003. Dental caries and ante-mortem tooth loss in the northern Peten area, Mexico: a biocultural perspective on social status differences among the Classic Maya. Am J Phys Anthropol 122:1–10.
Cucina A., Cantillo C.P., Sosa T.S., and Tiesler V. 2011. Carious lesions and maize consumption among the prehispanic Maya: an analysis of a coastal community in northern Yucatan. Am J Phys Anthropol 145(4): 560–567. https://doi.org/10.1002/ajpa.21534.
Cui A. et al. 2023. Global and regional prevalence of vitamin D deficiency in population-based studies from 2000 to 2022: a pooled analysis of 7.9 million participants. Front Nutr 10:1070808. https://doi.org/10.3389/fnut.2023.1070808.
Cullamar E.K. and Lutwick L.I. 2002. Inhalational anthrax. Curr Infect Dis Rep 4(3): 238–243.
Cunha E. and Wasterlain S. 2007. The Coimbra identified osteological collections. Documenta Archaeobiologiae 5:23–33.
Cunningham C., Schuer L., and Black S. 2016. Developmental juvenile osteology. Academic Press.
Curate F. 2014. Osteoporosis and paleopathology: a review. J Anthropol Sci 92:119–146.

Curtis D.R. and Roosen J. 2017. The sex-selective impact of the Black Death and recurring plagues in the southern Netherlands, 1349–1450. Am J Phys Anthropol 164:246–259. https://doi.org/10.1002/ajpa.23266.

Curto A., and Fernandes T. 2022. Clubfoot and its implications for the locomotion of a medieval skeleton from Estremoz, Portugal. Int J Paleopathol 38:13–17.

Czarnetzki A. 1980. A possible trisomy 21 from the Late Hallstatt Period. In: Proceedings of the 3rd European Paleopathology Association Meeting, Caen, France, 1980. Paleopathology Association.

D'Angelo del Campo M.D., Suby J.A., García-Laborde P., and Guichón R.A. 2017. Spondylolysis in the past: a case study of hunter-gatherers from southern Patagonia. Int J Paleopathol 19:1–17. https://doi.org/10.1016/j.ijpp.2017.07.001.

D'Ortenzio L., Brickley M., Schwarcz H., and Prowse T. 2015. You are not what you eat during physiological stress: isotopic evaluation of human hair. Am J Phys Anthropol 157:374–388.

D'Ortenzio L., Kahlon B., Peacock T., Salahuddin H., and Brickley M. 2018a. The rachitic tooth: refining the use of interglobular dentine in diagnosing vitamin D deficiency. Int J Paleopathol 22:101–108.

D'Ortenzio L., Inskip M., Manton W., and Mays S. 2018b. The Franklin expedition: what sequential analysis of hair reveals about lead exposure prior to death. J Archaeol Sci: Rep 21:401–405.

D'Ortenzio L. et al. 2016. The rachitic tooth: a histological examination. J Archaeol Sci 74:152–163.

Dalal V., Pasupuleti N., Chaubey G., Rai N., and Shinde V. 2023. Advancements and challenges in ancient DNA research: bridging the global north-south divide. Genes (Basel) 14(2): 479. https://doi.org/10.3390/genes14020479.

Dalby G. 1994. Middle ear disease in antiquity. PhD dissertation, University of Bradford, Bradford, West Yorkshire, UK.

Dalby G., Manchester K., and Roberts C.A. 1993. Otosclerosis and stapedial footplate fixation in archaeological material. Int J Osteoarchaeol 3:207–212.

Dalmas F., Pech-Gourg G., Gallucci A., Denis D., and Scavarda D. 2020. Craniosynostosis and oculomotor disorders. Neurochirurgie 66(2): 91–96.

Dancer S.J., Bluyssen P.M., Li Y., and Tang J.W. 2021a. Why don't we just open the windows? Br Med J 375:n2895. https://doi.org/10.1136/bmj.n2895.

Dancer S.J., Li Y., Hart A., Tang J.W., and Jones D.L. 2021b. What is the risk of acquiring SARS-CoV-2 from the use of public toilets? Sci Total Environ 792:148341. https://doi.org/10.1016/j.scitotenv.2021.148341.

Danielsen K. 1970. *Odontodysplasia leprosa* in Danish mediaeval skeletons. Særtryk af Tandlægebladet 74:603–625.

Dasen V. 1988. Dwarfism in Egypt and classical antiquity: iconography and medical history. Med Hist 32:253–276.

Dastugue J. 1965. Tumeur maxillaire sur un crâne du moyen-âge [Maxillary tumor on a medieval skull]. Bull du Cancer 52 (1): 69–72.

Dauvergne E. and Mullié C. 2021. Brass alloys: copper-bottomed solutions against hospital-acquired infections? *Antibiotics* 10(3): 286. https://doi.org/10.3390/antibiotics10030286.

Davidson J., Cleary A., and Bruce C. 2008. Disorders of bones, joints and connective tissues. In: Forfar and Arneil's textbook of pediatrics, ed. N. McIntosh, P. Helms, R. Smyth, and S. Logan, 1385–1447. Elsevier.

Davies D.M., Picton D.C.A., and Alexander A.G. 1969. An objective method of assessing the periodontal condition in human skulls. J. Periodontal Res 4:74–77.

Davies J.H., Child J., Freer J., and Storr H.L. 2023. Inequalities in the assessment of childhood short stature. Br J Gen Pract 73(729): 150–151. https://doi.org/10.3399/bjgp23X732309.

Davies-Barrett A.M. 2018. *Respiratory disease in the Middle Nile Valley: a bioarchaeological analysis of the impact of environmental and sociocultural change from the Neolithic to medieval periods. PhD dissertation*, Durham University, England. http://etheses.dur.ac.uk/13095/.

Davies-Barrett A.M., Antoine D., and Roberts C.A. 2019. Inflammatory periosteal reaction on ribs associated with lower respiratory disease: a method for recording prevalence from sites with differing preservation. Am J Phys Anthropol 168(3): 530–542. https://doi.org/10.1002/ajpa.23769.

Davies-Barrett A.M., Antoine D., and Roberts C.A. 2021a. Time to be nosy: evaluating the impact of environmental and sociocultural changes on maxillary sinusitis in the Middle Nile Valley (Neolithic to medieval periods). Int J Paleopathol 34:182–196.
Davies-Barrett A.M., Antoine D., and Roberts C.A. 2023. Desert dust and city smoke: investigating the impact of urbanization and aridification on the prevalence of pulmonary/pleural inflammation in the Middle Nile Valley (2500 B.C. to 1500 A.D.). Bioarchaeol Int (May 17 early view). https://doi.org/10.5744/bi.2022.0037.
Davies-Barrett A.M., Owens LS, Eeckhout PA. 2021b. Paleopathology of the Ychsma: evidence of respiratory disease during the Late Intermediate Period (AD 1000–1476) at the central coastal site of Pachacamac, Peru. Int J Paleopathol 34:63–75. https://doi.org/10.1016/j.ijpp.2021.06.001.
Davis H.E. 2019. Leaf-cutter ants in wound closure. Wildern Environ Med 30(4): 469–470.
Dawes J.D. and Magilton J.R. 1980. The cemetery of St Helen-on-the-Walls, Aldwark. The archaeology of York. The medieval cemeteries 12/1. Council for British Archaeology for York Archaeological trust.
Dawodu A. et al. 2015. Sun exposure and vitamin D supplementation in relation to vitamin D status of breastfeeding mothers and infants in the global exploration of human milk study. Nutrients 7(2): 1081–1093.
Day C.A. 2017. Consumptive chic: a history of beauty, fashion, and disease. Bloomsbury.
Dayal M.R., Kegley A.D.T., Strkalj G., Bidmos M.A., and Kuykendall K.L. 2009. The history and composition of the Raymond A Dart Collection of human skeletons at the University of Witwatersrand, Johannesburg, South Africa. Am J Phys Anthrop 140:324–335.
De Araújo T.V.B. et al. 2018. Association between microcephaly, Zika virus infection, and other risk factors in Brazil: final report of a case-control study. Lancet Infect Dis 18(3): 328–336.
De Armas Y.C., Mavridou A.-M., Domínguez J.G., Hanson K., and Laffoon J. 2022. Tracking breastfeeding and weaning practices in ancient populations by combining carbon, nitrogen and oxygen stable isotopes from multiple non-adult tissues. PLoS One. https://doi.org/10.1371/journal.pone.0262435.
De Boer H.H., Van der Merwe A.E., and Maat G.J.R. 2013. The diagnostic value of microscopy in dry bone palaeopathology: a review. Int J Paleopathol 3(2): 113–121. https://doi.org/10.1016/j.ijpp.2013.03.004.
De Boer H.H., Van der Merwe A.E., Hammer S., Steyn M., and Maat G.J.R. 2015. Assessing post-traumatic time interval in human dry bone. Int J Osteoarchaeol 25:98–109. https://doi.org/ 10.1002/oa.2267.
De Groote I. and Humphrey L.T. 2015. Characterizing evulsion in the Later Stone Age Maghreb: Age, sex and effects on mastication. Quat Int 413(Part A): 50–61. https://doi.org/10.1016/j.quaint.2015.08.082.
De la Cova C. 2011. Race, health, and disease in 19th-century-born males. Am J Phys Anthropol 144:526–537.
De la Cova C. 2012. Patterns of trauma and violence in 19th-century-born African American and Euro-American females. Int J Paleopathol 2(2–3):61–68. https://doi.org/10.1016/j.ijpp.2012.09.009.
De la Cova C. 2017. Fractured lives: structural violence, trauma, and recidivism in urban and institutionalized 19th-century-born African Americans and Euro-Americans. In: Broken bones, broken bodies: bioarchaeological and forensic approaches for accumulative trauma and violence, ed. C. Tegemeyer and D. Martin, 153–180. Lexington Press.
De la Cova C. 2023. Ethical considerations for paleopathology. In: The Routledge handbook of paleopathology, ed. A.L. Grauer, 382–396. Routledge.
De la Cova C. et al. 2024. Ethical futures in biological anthropology: research, teaching, community engagement, and curation involving deceased individuals. Am J Bio Anthropol e24980. https://doi.org/10.1002/ajpa.24980.
De la Fuente M.F., Souto A., Albuquerque U.P., and Schiel N. 2022. Self-medication in nonhuman primates: a systematic evaluation of the possible function of the use of medicinal plants. Am J Primatol 84(11): e23438. https://doi.org/10.1002/ajp.23438.
De la Guía-Galipienso F. et al. 2021. Vitamin D and cardiovascular health. Clin Nutr 40(5): 2946–2957.

De Melo F.L., Moreira de Mello J.C., Fraga A.M., Nunes K., and Eggers S. 2010. Syphilis at the crossroad of phylogenetics and paleopathology. PLoS Negl Trop Dis 4(1): e575. https://doi.org/10.1371/journal.pntd.0000575.

De Miguel Ibáñez M.P., Ballesteros Herrái J.M., Unzu Urmeneta M., Faro Carballa J.A., and García-Barberena Unzu M. 2011. Tres posibles casos de lepra en La Plaza del Castillo, Pamplona, Navarra [Three possible cases of leprosy in La Plaza del Castillo]. In: Paleopatología: ciencia multidisciplinar. Proceedings of the 10th Meeting of the Spanish Society of Paleopathology, ed. A. González Martín O. et al., 355–365. Universidad Autónoma de Madrid.

Dean A.S. et al. 2012. Clinical manifestations of human brucellosis: a systematic review and meta-analysis. PLoS Negl Trop Dis 6:e1929. https://doi.org/10.1371/journal.pntd.0001929.

Dean V.L. 2004. Effects of different kinds of cranial deformation on the incidence of Wormian bones. Am J Phys Anthropol 123:146–155.

Dedmon L.E. 2020. The genetics of rheumatoid arthritis. Rheumatology 59(10): 2661–270.

DeGusta D. 1999. Fijian cannibalism: osteological evidence from Navatu. Am J Phys Anthropol 110:215–241.

DeGusta D. 2000. Fijian cannibalism and mortuary ritual: bioarchaeological evidence from Vunda. Int J Osteoarchaeol 10:76–92.

Deirawan H., Fakhoury J.W., Zarka M., Bluth M.H., and Moossavi M. 2020. Revisiting the pathobiology of scurvy: a review of the literature in the context of a challenging case. Int J Dermatol 59(12): 1450–1457.

Demaitre L. 2007. Leprosy in premodern medicine: a malady of the whole body. Johns Hopkins University Press.

Dendle P. and Touwaide A., eds. 2008. Health and healing from the medieval garden. Boydell and Brewer. https://doi.org/10.2307/j.ctvc16gkc.

Deo P.N. and Deshmukh R. 2019. Oral microbiome: unveiling the fundamentals. J Oral Maxillofac Pathol 23(1): 122–128. https://doi.org/10.4103/jomfp.JOMFP_304_18.

Depaermentier M.L.C., Kemp M., Bánffy E., and Alt K.W. 2020. Tracing mobility patterns through the 6th-5th millennia BC in the Carpathian Basin with strontium and oxygen stable isotope analyses. PLoS One 15(12): e0242745. https://doi.org/10.1371/journal.pone.0242745.

Department for Communities and Local Government. 2010. PPS 5: Planning for the historic environment impact assessment. Communities and Local Government.

Department of the Environment. 1990. Planning policy guidance 16: archaeology and planning. HMSO Books.

Deps P. and Cruz A. 2020. Why we should stop using the word leprosy. Lancet Infect Dis 20:E75–E78.

Deps P., ed. 2023. Hansen's disease—a complete clinical guide. Springer Nature.

Dequeker J. and Rico H. 1992. Rheumatoid arthritis-like deformities in an early 16th-century painting of the Flemish-Dutch school. J Am Med Assoc 268(2): 249–251.

Derry D.E. 1913. A case of hydrocephalus in an Egyptian of the Roman Period. J Anat (London) 48:436–458.

Derums V.J. 1979. Extensive trepanation of the skull in ancient Latvia. Bull Hist Med 53:459–464.

Dewey J.R., Armelagos G.J., and Bartley M.H. 1969. Femoral cortical involution in three Nubian archaeological populations. Hum Biol 41(1): 13–28.

DeWitte S.N. 2009. The effect of sex on risk of mortality during the Black Death in London, AD 1339–1350. Am J Phys Anthropol 139:222–234.

DeWitte S.N. 2010. Sex differentials in frailty in medieval England. Am J Phys Anthropol 143:285–297. https://doi.org/10.1002/ajpa.21316.

DeWitte S.N. 2012. Sex differences in periodontal disease in catastrophic and attritional assemblages from medieval London. Am J Phys Anthropol 149:405–416. https://doi-org.ezphost.dur.ac.uk/10.1002/ajpa.22138.

DeWitte S.N. 2015. Setting the stage for medieval plague: pre-Black Death trends in survival and mortality. Am J Phys Anthropol 158:441–451. https://doi.org/10.1002/ajpa.22806.

DeWitte S.N. 2016. Archaeological evidence of epidemics can inform future epidemics. Annu Rev Anthropol 45:63–77. https://doi.org/10.1146/annurev-anthro-102215–095929.

DeWitte S.N. 2018. Stress, sex, and plague: patterns of developmental stress and survival in pre- and post–Black Death London. Am J Hum Biol 30:e23073. https://doi.org/10.1002/ajhb.23073.
Dewitte S.N. and Bekvalac J. 2010. Oral health and frailty in the medieval English cemetery of St Mary Graces. Am J Phys Anthropol 142:341–354.
DeWitte S.N. and Bekvalac J. 2011. The association between periodontal disease and periosteal lesions in the St. Mary Graces cemetery, London, England A.D. 1350–1538. Am J Phys Anthropol 146:609–618. https://doi.org/10.1002/ajpa.21622.
DeWitte S.N. and Hughes-Morey G. 2012. Stature and frailty during the Black Death: the effect of stature on risks of epidemic mortality in London A.D. 1348–1350. J Archaeol Sci 39:1412–1419. https://doi.org/10.1016/j.jas.2012.01.019.
DeWitte S.N. and Stojanowski C. 2015. The osteological paradox 20 years later: past perspectives, future directions. J Archaeol Res 23(4): 397–450.
Di Ruffano L.F. and Waldron T. 2018. On the importance of considering disease subtypes: earliest detection of a parosteal osteosarcoma? Differential diagnosis of an osteosarcoma in an Anglo-Saxon female. Int J Paleopathol 21:128–137.
Diamond J. 1997. Guns, germs and steel: the fates of human societies. Norton.
Dias G. and Tayles N. 1997. 'Abscess cavity'—a misnomer. Int J Osteoarchaeol 7:548–554.
Dias G.J., Prasad K., and Santos A.L. 2007. Pathogenesis of apical periodontal cysts: guidelines for diagnosis in palaeopathology. Int J Osteoarchaeol 17:619–626.
Dickel D.N. and Doran G.H. 1989. Severe neural tube defect syndrome from early archaic Florida. Am J Phys Anthropol 80:325–334.
Dickson-Lowe, R., Buitendag J.J.P., Graham-Brown M.P.M., and Oosthuizen G.V.E. 2021. Falanga: the clinical correlates of surgical outcomes as a result of foot whipping in a resource poor setting. Injury 52:3139–3142.
DiGangi E.A. and Sirianni J.E. 2017. Maxillary sinus infection in a 19th-century almshouse skeletal sample. Int J Osteoarchaeol 27:155–166. https://doi.org/10.1002/oa.2526.
Digitised Diseases. 2024. http://www.digitiseddiseases.org/alpha/.
Dimopoulos K. et al. 2023. Cardiovascular complications of Down syndrome: scoping review and expert consensus. Circulation 147(5): 425–441.
Dittmar J.M., Berger E.S., Mao R., Wang H., and Yeh H.Y. 2020. A probable case of multiple myeloma from Bronze Age China. Int J Paleopathol 31:64–70.
Dittmar J.M. and Mitchell P.D. 2015. A new method for identifying and differentiating human dissection and autopsy in archaeological human skeletal remains. J Archaeol Sci: Rep 3:73–79. https://doi.org/10.1016/j.
Dittmar J.M., Mitchell P.D., Cessford C., Inskip S.A., and Robb J.E. 2021a. Fancy shoes and painful feet: *Hallux valgus* and fracture risk in medieval Cambridge, England. Int J Paleopathol 35:90–100. https://doi.org/10.1016/j.ijpp.2021.04.012.
Dittmar J.M., Mitchell P.D., Cessford C., Inskip S.A., Robb J.E. 2021b. Medieval injuries: skeletal trauma as an indicator of past living conditions and hazard risk in Cambridge, England. Am J Phys Anthropol. 175:626–645. https://doi.org/10.1002/ajpa.24225.
Dittmar J.M. et al. 2021c. Gout and 'podagra' in medieval Cambridge, England. Int J Paleopathol 33:170–181.
Dittmar J.M., Nagar Y., Arbiv K., Lieberman T., and Mitchell P.D. 2022. Violence in Hasmonean Judea: skeletal evidence of a massacre from 2nd–1st century BCE Jerusalem. Int J Osteoarchaeol 32(4): 731–745. https://doi.org/10.1002/oa.3084.
Dittmar J.M. et al. 2023. Caring for the injured: exploring the immediate and long-term consequences of injury in medieval Cambridge, England. Int J Paleopathol 40:7–19. https://doi.org/10.1016/j.ijpp.2022.07.004.
Dobbs M. and Gurnett C. 2009. Update on clubfoot: etiology and treatment. Clin Orthop Relat Res 467(5): 1146–1153.
Dobney K. and Brothwell D. 1987. A method for evaluating the amount of dental calculus on teeth from archaeological sites. J Archaeol Sci 14:343–351.
Dobney K. and Brothwell D. 1988. A scanning electron microscope study of archaeological dental calculus. In: Scanning electron microscopy in archaeology. British Archaeological Reports International Series 452, ed. S. Olsen, 372–385. Tempus Reparatum.

Dobson J. E. 1998. The iodine factor in health and evolution. Geogr Rev 88(1): 1–28.
Domett K., Colbert A., Chang N. 2022. The impact of clubfoot: a holistic paleopathological case study from Bronze Age Thailand using the bioarchaeology of care framework. Bioarchaeology International 6(4). https://doi.org/10.5744/bi.2021.0022.
Domett K., Evans C., Chang N., Tayles N., and Newton J. 2017. Interpreting osteoarthritis in bioarchaeology: highlighting the importance of a clinical approach through case studies from prehistoric Thailand. J Archaeol Sci: Rep 11:762–773.
Domett K.M. and Tayles N. 2006. Adult fracture patterns in prehistoric Thailand: a biocultural interpretation. Int J Osteoarcheol 16:185–199.
Domingo N.G.G. et al. 2021. Air quality-related health damages of food. Proc Natl Acad Sci USA 118(20): e2013637118. https://doi.org/10.1073/pnas.2013637118.
Dong Y. et al. 2020. Leukemia incidence trends at the global, regional, and national level between 1990 and 2017. Exp Hematol Oncol 9:14. https://doi.org/10.1186/s40164-020-00170-6.
Donoghue H.D. et al. 2005. Co-infection of *Mycobacterium tuberculosis* and *Mycobacterium leprae* in human archaeological samples: a possible explanation for the historical decline of leprosy. Proc R Soc Lond B Biol Sci 272:389–394.
Donoghue H.D. et al. 2015. A migration-driven model for the historical spread of leprosy in medieval eastern and central Europe. Infect Genet Evol 31:250–256.
Dorado-Fernández E., Herrerín J., Cáceres-Mollor D., and Botella M. 2021. An amputated leg in 18th–19th centuries central Spain. Int J Osteoarchaeol 31(2): 146–153. https://doi.org/10.1002/oa.2933.
Doughty C.E. 2010. The development of agriculture in the Americas: an ecological perspective. Ecosphere 1(6): 1–11. https://doi.org/10.1890/ES10-00098.1.
Downing M. and Fibiger L. 2017. An experimental investigation of sharp force skeletal trauma with replica Bronze Age weapons. J Archaeol Sci: Rep 11:546–554. https://doi.org/10.1016/j.jasrep.2016.12.034.
Drancourt M., Aboudhaaram G., Signoli M., Dutour O., and Raolut D. 1998. Detection of 400-year-old *Yersinia pestis* DNA in human dental pulp: an approach to the diagnosis of ancient septicemia. Proc Nat Acad Sci USA 95:12637–12640.
Dreizen S., Currie C., Gilley E.J., and Spies T.D. 1959. Observations on the association between nutritive failure, skeletal maturation rate and radiopaque transverse lines in the radius in children. Am J Roentgenol 76(3): 482–487.
Drinkall G. and Foreman M. 1998. The Anglo-Saxon cemetery at Castledyke South, Barton-on-Humber. Academic Press.
Drtikolová Kaupová S. et al. 2021. The impact of pathological conditions on carbon and nitrogen isotopic values in the bone collagen of individuals with known biographic data and medical history. Int J Osteoarchaeol 31(6): 1105–1124.
Duchêne S., Ho S.Y.W., Carmichael A.G., Holmes E.C., and Poinar H. 2020. The recovery, interpretation and use of ancient pathogen genomes. Curr Biol 30(19): R1215–R1231. https://doi.org/10.1016/j.cub.2020.08.081.
Dudar J. 2010. Qualitative and quantitative diagnosis of lethal cranial neural tube defects from the fetal and neonatal human skeleton, with a case study involving taphonomically altered remains. J Forensic Sci 55(4): 877–883.
Dudgeon J.V. and Tromp M. 2014. Diet, geography and drinking water in Polynesia: microfossil research from archaeological human dental calculus, Rapa Nui (Easter Island). Int J Osteoarchaeol 24:634–648.
Duffin J. 2021. History of medicine: a scandalously short introduction, 3rd ed. University of Toronto Press.
Dunnavant J., Justinvil D., and Colwell C. 2021. Craft an African American Graves Protection and Repatriation Act. Nature 593(7859):337–340. https://doi.org/10.1038/d41586-021-01320-4.
Dupras T.L. et al. 2010. Evidence of amputation as medical treatment in ancient Egypt. Int J Osteoarchaeol 20:405–423. https://doi.org/10.1002/oa.1061.
Dupras T.L., Schwarcz H.P., and Fairgrieve S.I. 2001. Infant feeding and weaning practices in Roman Egypt. Am J Phys Anthropol 115:204–212.
Duray S. 1990. Deciduous enamel defects and caries susceptibility in a prehistoric Ohio population. Am J Phys Anthropol 81:27–34.

Duray S. 1996. Dental indicators of stress and reduced age at death in prehistoric native Indians. Am J Phys Anthrop 99:275–86.

Durband A.C., Littleton J., and Walshe K. 2014. Patterns in ritual tooth avulsion at Roonka. Am J Phys Anthropol 154(4): 479–485. https://doi.org/10.1002/ajpa.22531.

Dutour O. 2013. Paleoparasitology and paleopathology: synergies for reconstructing the past of human infectious diseases and their pathocenosis. Int J Paleopathol 3(3): 145–149. https://doi.org/10.1016/j.ijpp.2013.09.008.

Dutour O. 2023a. Paleopathology of infectious disease. In: The Routledge handbook of paleopathology, ed. A.L. Grauer, chap. 18. Routledge. https://doi.org/10.4324/9781003130994.

Dutour O. 2023b. The paleopathology and paleoepidemiology of Upper Paleolithic tuberculosis: review of evidence and hypotheses. Tuberculosis (Edinb.) 143S:102348. https://doi.org/10.1016/j.tube.2023.102348.

Dutour O., Pálfi G., Bérato J., and Brun J.-P., eds. 1994. L'origine de la syphilis en Europe: avant ou après 1493? Toulon: Centre Archéologique du Var, Éditions Errance.

Dyer C. 1989. Standards of living in the Middle Ages: social change in England c. 1200–1520. Cambridge University Press.

Dyer M. and Fibiger L. 2017. Understanding blunt force trauma and violence in Neolithic Europe: the first experiments using a skin-skull-brain model and the Thames Beater. Antiquity 91(360): 1515–1528. https://doi.org/10.15184/aqy.2017.189.

Dzierzykray-Rogalski T. 1980. Palaeopathology of the Ptolemaic inhabitants of Dahkleh Oasis (Egypt). J Hum Evol 9:71–74.

Eaton K. et al. 2023. Emergence, continuity, and evolution of *Yersinia pestis* throughout medieval and early modern Denmark. Curr Biol 33(6): 1147–1152.e5 https://doi.org/10.1016/j.cub.2023.01.064.

Edeiken J., Hodes P.J., and Caplan L.H. 1966. New bone production and periosteal reaction. Am J Roentgenol 97(3): 708–718.

Eerkens J.W. et al. 2018. A probable prehistoric case of meningococcal disease from San Francisco Bay: next generation sequencing of Neisseria meningitidis from dental calculus and osteological evidence. Int J Paleopathol 22:173–180. https://doi.org/10.1016/j.ijpp.2018.05.001.

Efthymia N. 2017. Osteoarchaeology: a guide to the macroscopic study of human skeletal remains. Academic Press.

Eger E.I., II, Saidman L., and Westhorpe R.N. 2014. The wondrous story of anesthesia. Springer.

Eisenberg M. and Mordechai L. 2020. The Justinianic plague and global pandemics: the making of the plague concept. Am Hist Rev 125(5): 1632–1667.

El-Najjar M.Y. and Mulinski T.M.J. 1980. Mummies and mummification practices in the southwestern and southern United states. In: Mummies, disease and ancient cultures, ed. A. Cockburn and E. Cockburn, 103–117. Cambridge University Press.

Elia M. 2002. Nutrition. In: Clinical medicine. 5th edition, ed. P. Kumar and M. Clark, 221–225. W.B. Saunders.

Eliopoulos C., Lagia A., and Manolis S. 2006. A modern, documented human skeletal collection from Greece. Homo 58(3): 221–228. https://doi.org/10.1016/j.jchb.2006.10.003.

Elliot-Smith G. and Dawson W.R. 1924. Egyptian mummies. Dial Press.

Ellis H. 2009. Cambridge illustrated history of surgery, 2nd ed. Cambridge University Press.

Ellis M.A. 2010. The children of Spring Street: rickets in an early nineteenth-century urban congregation. Northeast Historical Archaeology 39:120–133.

Elmahi A.T. 2000. Prehistoric population controls in the Sudanese Nile Valley: a consideration of infanticide. Beiträge zur Sudanforschug 7:103–118.

Eman A. and Mahsa S. 2019. Data marketplace: an analysis of the ethical concerns regarding the participation of the individuals. Front Genet 10:1107. https://doi.org/10.3389/fgene.2019.01107.

Emons G. 2022. Hormone-dependent cancers: molecular mechanisms and therapeutical implications. Cells 12(1): 110. https://doi.org/10.3390/cells12010110.

Enderle A., Meyerhofer D., and Unverfehrt G. 1994. Small people—great art: restricted growth from an artistic and medical viewpoint. Artcolor Verlag.

Eng J.T. 2016. A bioarchaeological study of osteoarthritis among populations of northern China and Mongolia during the Bronze Age to Iron Age transition to nomadic pastoralism. Quat Int 405:172–185.

Eng J.T., Szocs P., and Hagen C. 2009. Developmental dysplasia of the hip in a post-medieval Transylvanian population: case study and diagnosis. Paleopathol Newsl 148:25–32.

Engelhardt H.K. 1959. A study of yaws (does congenital yaws occur?). J Trop Med Hyg 62:238–240.

Entezami P., Fox D.A., Clapham P.J., and Chung K.C. 2011. Historical perspective on the etiology of rheumatoid arthritis. Hand Clin 27(1): 1–10. https://doi.org/ 10.1016/j.hcl.2010.09.006.

Erkilinc M., Gilmore A., Weber M., and Mistovich R.J. 2021. Current concepts in pediatric septic arthritis. J Am Acad Orthop Surg 29(5): 196–206.

Errickson D. and Thompson T.J.U. 2019. Sharing is not always caring: social media and the dead. In: Ethical challenges in the analysis of human remains, ed. K. Squires, D. Errickson, and N. Márquez-Grant, 299–313. Elsevier.

Eshed V. et al. 2002. Button osteoma: its etiology and pathophysiology. Am J Phys Anthropol 118:217–230.

Esmaeilnejad-Ganji S.M. and Esmaeilnejad-Ganji S.M.R. 2019. Osteoarticular manifestations of human brucellosis: a review. World J Orthop. 10(2): 54–62. https://doi.org/10.5312/wjo.v10.i2.54.

Esper J.F. 1774. Ausführlich Nachricht von neuentdeckten Zooolithen unbekannte vierfüssiger Thiere [Detailed information on newly discovered zooliths of unknown four-footed animals]. Georg Wolfgang Knorr, pp. 74–74.

Espinosa R., Tago D., and Treich N. 2020. Infectious diseases and meat production. Environ Resour Econ (Dordr) 76(4): 1019–1044. https://doi.org/10.1007/s10640-020-00484-3.

Estalrrich A., Alarcon J.A., and Rosas A. 2017. Evidence of toothpick groove formation in Neandertal anterior and posterior teeth. Am J Phys Anthropol 162(4): 747–756.

European Commission. 2024. European surveillance of congenital anomalies. https://eu-rd-platform.jrc.ec.europa.eu/eurocat/eurocat-data/prevalence_en. Accessed 8 July 2024.

Evans C.C. 1998. Historical background. In: Tuberculosis, 2nd edition, ed. P.D.O. Davies, 1–19. Chapman and Hall Medical.

Everett N. 2012. The alphabet of Galen: pharmacy from antiquity to the Middle Ages. University of Toronto Press.

Evershed R.P. et al. 2022. Dairying, diseases and the evolution of lactase persistence in Europe. Nature 608:336–345. https://doi.org/10.1038/s41586-022-05010-7.

Ewald P.W. 2018. Ancient cancers and infection-induced oncogenesis. Int J Paleopathol 21:178–185.

Eyler W.R. et al. 1996. Rib enlargement in patients with chronic pleural disease. Am J Roentgenol 167:921–926. 10.2214/ajr.167.4.8819384.

Ezeanya-Esiobu C. 2019. Indigenous knowledge and education in Africa. Springer.

Fabra M. and Salega S. 2016. Developmental defects in the spine: initial findings in archaeological cases from Cordoba highlands (Argentina). Int J Osteoarchaeol 26(3): 397–407.

Faccia K.J. and Williams R.C. 2008. Schmorl's nodes: clinical significance and implications for the bioarchaeological record. Int J Osteoarchaeol 18(1): 28–44.

Faerman M. et al. 1997. DNA analysis reveals the sex of infanticide victims. Nature 385:212–213.

Faerman M. et al. 2000. From a dry bone to a genetic portrait: a case study of sickle cell anaemia. Am J Phys Anthropol 111(2): 153–163.

Farmer P.E., Nizeye B., Stulac S., and Keshavjee S. 2006. Structural violence and clinical medicine. PLoS Med. 3(10): e449. https://doi.org/10.1371/journal.pmed.0030449.

Farrer K. 1993. Lead and the last Franklin expedition. J Archaeol Sci 20(4): 399–409.

Fatula S. 2021. Detection of cancerous lesions in skeletal remains using visual methods and radiographs. Int J Osteoarchaeol 31(5): 916–925.

Ferlay J. et al. 2021. Cancer statistics for the year 2020: an overview. Int J Cancer 149(4): 778–789.

Fernandes D. et al. 2019. Cranial deformation and genetic diversity in three adolescent male individuals from the Great Migration period from Osijek, eastern Croatia. PLoS One 14(8): e0216366. https://doi.org/10.1371/journal.pone.0216366.

Fernandez-Dominguez F. 2023. Human populations—origins and movement. In: Handbook of archaeological sciences, Vol. 1. 2nd edition, ed. M. Pollard, R.A. Armitage, and C. Makarewicz, 629–645. Wiley.

Fernando-Jalvo Y., Carlos Díez J., Cáceres I., and Rosell J. 1999. Human cannibalism in the early Pleistocene of Europe (Gran Dolina, Sierra de Atapuerca, Burgos, Spain). J Hum Evol 37:591–622.

Fess E.E. 2002. History of splinting. J Hand Ther 15(2): 97–132.
Fibiger L., Ahlström T., Bennike P., and Schulting R.J. 2013. Patterns of violence-related skull trauma in neolithic southern Scandinavia. Am J Phys Anthropol 150:190–202. https://doi.org/10.1002/ajpa.22192.
Fibiger L., Ahlström T., Meyer C., and Smith M. 2023. Conflict, violence, and warfare among early farmers in northwestern Europe. Proc Natl Acad Sci USA 120(4): e2209481119.
Fife D. and Barancik J.I. 1985. Northeastern Ohio trauma study III: incidence of fractures. Ann Emerg Med 14(3): 244–248.
Fildes V.A. 1986. 'The English Disease': infantile rickets and scurvy in pre-Industrial England. In: Child care through the centuries, ed. J. Cule and T. Turner, 121–134. British Society for the History of Medicine.
Filipek K.L. et al. 2022. Creating communities of care: sex estimation and mobility histories of adolescents buried in the cemetery of St. Mary Magdalen Leprosarium (Winchester, England). Am J Biol Anthropol 178(1): 108–123. https://doi.org/10.1002/ajpa.24498.
Fillingim R.B. 2023. Sex, gender, and pain. In: Principles of gender-specific medicine, 4th edition, ed. M.J. Legato, 769–792. Academic Press.
Filon D., Faerman M., Smith P., and Oppenheim A. 1995. Sequence analysis reveals a ß-thalassaemia mutation in the DNA of skeletal remains from the archaeological site of Akhziv, Israel. Nat Genet 9:365–368.
Finckh A. et al. 2022. Global epidemiology of rheumatoid arthritis. Nat Rev Rheumatol 18(10): 591–602.
Findlen P. 1996. Possessing nature: museums, collecting, and scientific culture in early modern Italy. University of California Press.
Fiorato V., Boylston A., and Knüsel C., eds. 2001. Blood red roses: the archaeology of a mass grave from the Battle of Towton AD 1461. Oxbow Books.
Fiorin E. et al. 2024. First archaeological evidence for ginger consumption as a potential medicinal ingredient in a late medieval leprosarium at St Leonard, Peterborough, England. Sci Rep 14:2452. https://doi.org/10.1038/s41598-024-52422-8.
Fiorin E., Cristiani E., and Roberts C.A. 2023. Knowledge and perception of leprosy amongst high school students in Italy: a survey. Lepr Rev 94(4): 341–349. https://doi.org/10.47276/lr.94.4.341.
Fiorin E., Sáez L., and Malgosa A. 2019. Ferns as healing plants in medieval Mallorca, Spain? Evidence from human dental calculus. Int J Osteoarchaeol 29(1): 82–90. https://doi.org/10.1002/oa.2718.
FitzGerald O. et al. 2021. Psoriatic arthritis. Nat Rev Dis Primers 7(1): 59. https://doi.org/10.1038/s41572-021-00293-y.
Flammer P.G. and Smith A.L. 2020. Intestinal helminths as a biomolecular complex in archaeological research. Philos Trans R Soc Lond B Biol Sci 375(1812): 20190570. https://doi.org/10.1098/rstb.2019.0570.
Fleming T.G. 2011. Inventoried monsters: dwarves and hirsutes at court. Journal of the History of Collections / Ashmolean Museum Oxford, 23:267–81.
Fletcher A., Pearson J., and Ambers J. 2008. The manipulation of social and physical identity in the pre-pottery Neolithic: radiographic evidence for cranial modification at Jericho and its implications for the plastering of skulls. Cambridge Archaeol J 18(3): 309–325. https://doi.org/10.1017/S0959774308000383.
Flies M.J., Winther S.D., and Lynnerup N. 2017. Skeletal material from the cemetery of the 19th-century Copenhagen Hospital for the Poor: autopsies, surgical training and anatomical specimens. Int J Osteoarchaeol 27:1012–1021. https://doi.org/ 10.1002/oa.2612.
Flohr S. et al. 2015. Flint arrowhead embedded in a human humerus from the Bronze Age site in the Tollense valley, Germany—A high-resolution micro-CT study to distinguish antemortem from perimortem projectile trauma to bone. Int J Paleopathol 9:76–81. https://doi.org/10.1016/j.ijpp.2015.02.004.
Floreanova K., Gilat E., Koren I., and May H. 2020. Ear infection prevalence in prehistoric and historic populations of the southern Levant: a new diagnostic method. Int J Osteoarchaeol 30:449–457. https://doi.org/10.1002/oa.2873.
Fogl Á., Pálfi G., Molnár E., Just Z., Balázs J., and Maák I.E. 2023. Development of bilateral asymmetry of the upper limb in children from a medieval population in central Europe, Hungary. Anthropologischer Anzeiger 80(1): 49–56.

Foley A.J. 2020. The daily grind: assessing bruxism as a potential indicator of stress in archaeological human remains. J Archaeol Sci 117:105117. https://doi.org/10.1016/j.jas.2020.105117.

Foley M. and Akers H.F. 2018. Does poverty cause caries? Aust Dent J 64:96–102.

Foreman P.K. et al. 2020. Birth prevalence of achondroplasia: a systematic literature review and meta-analysis. Am J Med Genet 182(10): 2297–2316.

Formicola V. 1995. X-linked hypophosphotemic rickets: a probable case from Upper Paleolithic. Am J Phys Anthropol 98(4): 403–409.

Fornaciari G. et al. 2019. A remarkable case of gout in the Imperial Rome: surgery and diseases in antiquity by osteoarchaeological, paleopathological, and historical perspectives. Int J Osteoarchaeol 29(5):797–807.

Forsom E. and Smith M.J. 2017. Getting to the point: an experimental approach to improving the identification of penetrating projectile trauma to bone caused by medieval arrows. J Archaeol Sci: Rep 11:274–286. https://doi.org/10.1016/j.jasrep.2016.12.013.

Fortuine R. 1984. Traditional surgery among the Alaska natives. Alaska Med 26(1): 22–25.

Foster A. et al. 2018. Possible diffuse idiopathic skeletal hyperostosis (DISH) in a 3000-year-old Pacific Island skeletal assemblage. J Archaeol Sci: Rep 18:408–419.

Fracasso T., Schmidt S., and Schmeling A. 2011. Commentary [on Kremer et al. 2008]. J Forensic Sci 56(6): 1662; author reply 1663. https://doi.org/10.1111/j.1556-4029.2011.01929.x.

Franco G. 2020. Revisiting the past strengthens the present: Bernardino Ramazzini and the new occupational health. Public Health 181:180–181.

Franco G. 2021. Bernardino Ramazzini's De morbis artificum diatriba on workers' health: the birth of a new discipline. Journal of the University of Occupational Health, Japan 43(3): 341–348. https://doi.org/10.7888/juoeh.43.341.

Franco N.H. 2013. Animal experiments in biomedical research: a historical perspective. Animals (Basel) 3(1): 238–273. https://doi.org/10.3390/ani3010238.

Frangos C.C., Lavranos G.M., and Frangos C.C. 2011. Higoumenakis' sign in the diagnosis of congenital syphilis in anthropological specimens. Med Hypotheses 77(1): 128–131. https://doi.org/10.1016/j.mehy.2011.03.044.

Fraser C.M. et al. 1998. Complete genome sequence of *Treponema pallidum*, the syphilis spirochete. Science 281(5375): 375–388. https://doi.org/10.1126/science.281.5375.375.

Fraser D.R. 1995. Vitamin D. Lancet 345(8942): 104–105.

Frayer D. et al. 2020. Evidence for labret use in prehistory. Bull Int Assoc Paleodontol 14:1–23.

Frayer D.W., Horton W.A., Macchiarelli R., and Mussi M. 1987. Dwarfism in an adolescent from the Italian late Upper Palaeolithic. Nature 330:60–61.

French J.C., Riris P., Fernandéz-López de Pablo J., Lozano S., and Silva F. 2021. A manifesto for palaeodemography in the twenty-first century. Philos Trans R Soc Lond B Biol Sci 376:20190707. https://doi.org/10.1098/rstb.2019.0707.

French R. 1993. Scurvy. In: The Cambridge world history of human disease, ed. K. Kiple, 1000–1005. Cambridge University Press.

Fried L.P. et al. 2009. Nonlinear multisystem physiological dysregulation associated with frailty in older women: implications for etiology and treatment. J Gerontol A Biol Sci Med Sci 64(10): 1049–1057.

Frima H. et al. 2020. Clavicle fractures in adults; current concepts. Eur J Trauma Emerg Surg 46: 519–529. https://doi.org/10.1007/s00068-019-01122-4.

Fu J. et al. 2023. Influence of living environments on maxillary sinusitis for the Chinese Loess Plateau residents during Shang and Western Zhou dynasties: evidence from Zaoshugounao site, Chunhua County, Shaanxi Province[J]. Quat Sci 43(5): 1460–1470. https://doi.org/10.11928/j.issn.1001-7410.2023.05.23.

Fuller B., Molleson T.I., Harris D., Gilmore L., and Hedges R. 2006. Isotopic evidence for breastfeeding and possible adult dietary differences from late/sub Roman Britain. Am J Phys Anthropol 129:45–54.

Fuller G. 2018. The invisible killer: the rising global threat of air pollution—and how we can fight back. Melville House.

Funkhauser W.K. Jr. 2018. Pathology: the clinical description of human disease. In: Molecular Pathology, 2nd edition, ed. W.B. Coleman and G.J. Tsongalis, 217–229. Elsevier.

Gabrovsky A.N., O'Neill K.D., and Gerszten E. 2016. Paleopathology of cardiovascular diseases in South American mummies. Int J Cardiol 223:101–107.

Gagnet P., Kern K., Andrews K., Elgafy H., and Ebraheim N. 2018. Spondylolysis and spondylolisthesis: a review of the literature. J Orthop 15:404–407. https://doi.org/10.1016/j.jor.

Gagneux S. 2018. Ecology and evolution of *Mycobacterium tuberculosis*. Nat Rev Microbiol 16:202–213. https://doi.org/10.1038/nrmicro.2018.8.

Gagnon C.M. 2020. Exploring oral paleopathology in the central Andes: a review. Int J Paleopathol 29:24–34.

Gaither C. 2012. Cultural conflict and the impact on non-adults at Puruchuco-Huaquerones in Peru: the case for refinement of the methods used to analyze violence against children in the archeological record. Int J Paleopathol 2:69–77.

Gallos P.L. 1985. Cure cottages of Saranac Lake: architecture and history of a pioneer health resort. Historic Saranac Lake.

Galor O. 2022. The journey of humanity: the origins of wealth and inequality. Dutton.

Gaľová J. et al. 2022. Ankylosing spondylitis on unidentified individual from early modern times found in reformed church (Silická Brezová, Slovakia): a case-based review. Rheumatol Int 42(10): 1873–1881.

Gamage U.S.H. et al. 2021. The impact of errors in medical certification on the accuracy of the underlying cause of death. PLoS One 16(11): e0259667. https://doi.org/10.1371/journal.pone.0259667.

Gandhi D., Shanbag P., and Vaidya M. 2003. Lead lines. Lancet 362(9379): 197.

Gancz A.S. et al. 2023. Ancient dental calculus reveals oral microbiome shifts associated with lifestyle and disease in Great Britain. Nat Microbiol 8(12): 2315–2325.

Gao G. et al. 2023. The largest headhunting event in prehistoric Asia: evidence of mass decapitation at the 4100-year-old Neolithic Age Honghe site, Heilongjiang, China. Archaeol Anthropol Sci 15:144. https://doi.org/10.1007/s12520-023-01845-x.

Gardner W., Kassebaum N., and McHugh T. 2023. Anemia afflicts nearly 1 in 4 people worldwide, but there are practical strategies for reducing it. Commentary. Institute for Health Metrics and Evaluation. September 8. https://www.healthdata.org/news-events/insights-blog/commentary/anemia-afflicts-nearly-1-4-people-worldwide-there-are.

Garne E. et al. 2011. EUROCAT Working Group. Paper 5: Surveillance of multiple congenital anomalies: implementation of a computer algorithm in European registers for classification of cases. Birth Defects Res A Clin Mol Teratol 91(Suppl 1): S44–S50. https://doi.org/10.1002/bdra.20777.

Garnett E. and Lewis M. 2022. The potential for over diagnosis of Paget's disease of bone using macroscopic analysis. Int J Paleopathol 38:55–63.

Garot E. et al. 2023. Insights into molar-incisor hypomineralisation in past populations: a call to anthropologists. Int J Paleopathol 42:18–26.

Garralda M.D., Maureille B., and Vandermeersch B. 2014. Hyperostosis frontalis interna in a Neandertal from Marillac (Charente, France). J Hum Evol 67:76–84.

Garrett R.D. et al. 2021. Forests and sustainable development in the Brazilian Amazon: history, trends, and future prospects. Annu Rev Environ Resour 46:625–652.

Geber J. 2016. 'Children in a ragged state': seeking a biocultural narrative of a workhouse childhood in Ireland during the Great Famine (1845–1852). Child Past 9(2):120–138. https://doi.org/ 10.1080/17585716.2016.1205344.

Geber J. and Murphy E. 2018. Dental markers of poverty: biocultural deliberations on oral health of the poor in mid-nineteenth-century Ireland. Am J Phys Anthropol 167:840–855.

Geber J. and Murphy E. 2012. Scurvy in the Great Irish Famine: evidence of vitamin C deficiency from a mid-19th century skeletal population. Am J Phys Anthropol 148(4): 512–524.

Gejvall N.G. 1960. Westerhus, medieval population and church in light of their skeletal remains. Hakak Ohlssons Boktryckeri.

Genetics and Rare Diseases Information Centre (GARD). https://rarediseases.info.nih.gov/. Accessed 13 March 2024.

Gennari L., Rendina D., Falchetti A., and Merlotti D. 2019. Paget's disease of bone. Calcif Tissue Int 104(5): 483–500.

Gennari L. et al. 2022. Update on the pathogenesis and genetics of Paget's disease of bone. Front Cell Dev Biol 10:932065. https://doi.org/10.3389/fcell.2022.932065.

Gerbault P. et al. 2011. Evolution of lactase persistence: an example of human niche construction. Philos Trans R Soc Lond B Biol Sci. 366(1566): 863–877. https://doi.org/10.1098/rstb.2010.0268.

Gerosa M., De Angelis V., Riboldi P., and Meroni P.L. 2008. Rheumatoid arthritis: a female challenge. Womens Health 4(2): 195–201. https://doi.org/10.2217/17455057.4.2.195.

Gerszten P.C. and Gerszten E. 1995. Intentional cranial deformation: a disappearing form of self-mutilation. Neurosurgery 37(3): 374–382.

Getz F.M. 1991. The Black Death and the silver lining: meaning, continuity and revolutionary change in histories of medieval plague. J Hist Biol 24(2): 265–289.

Ghosh S.K. and Kumar A. 2019. The rich heritage of anatomical texts during Renaissance and thereafter: a lead up to Henry Gray's masterpiece. Anat Cell Biol 52(4): 357–368. https://doi.org/10.5115/acb.19.102.

Giacaman R.A. 2018. Sugars and beyond: the role of sugars and the other nutrients and their potential impact on caries. Oral Dis 24(7): 1185–1197. https://doi.org/10.1111/odi.12778.

Giacani L. and Lukehart S.A. 2014. The endemic treponematoses. Clin Microbiol Rev 27(1): 89–115. https://doi.org/10.1128/CMR.00070-13.

Giardine B.M. et al. 2021. Clinically relevant updates of the HbVar database of human hemoglobin variants and thalassemia mutations. Nucleic Acids Res 49(1): 1192–1196.

Gibbon V.E. 2020. African ancient DNA research requires robust ethics and permission protocols. Nat Rev Genet 21:645–647. https://doi.org/10.1038/s41576-020-00285-w.

Giesen M., ed. 2013. Curating human remains: caring for the dead in the UK. Boydell Press.

Giffin K. et al. 2020. A treponemal genome from an historic plague victim supports a recent emergence of yaws and its presence in 15th century Europe. Sci Rep 10:9499. https://doi.org/10.1038/s41598-020-66012-x.

Gilchrist R. and Sloane B. 2005. Requiem: the medieval monastic cemetery in Britain. Museum of London Archaeology Service.

Giles M. 2020. Bog bodies: face to face with the past. Manchester University Press.

Gilio M. et al. 2019. Diffuse idiopathic skeletal hyperostosis [DISH] in an HLA-B27-positive subject. J Clin Rheumatol 25(6): e94–e98. https://doi.org/10.1097/RHU.0000000000000865, 10.1097/RHU.0000000000000865.

Gilmore J.K. 2008. Leprosy at the lazaretto on St Eustatius, Netherlands Antilles. Int J Osteoarchaeol 18:72–84.

Gilmour R. et al. 2015. Gendered differences in accidental trauma to upper and lower limb bones at Aquincum, Roman Hungary. Int J Paleopathol 11:75–91.

Gilmour R.J., Brickley M.B., Jurriaans E., and Prowse T.L. 2019. Maintaining mobility after fracture: a biomechanical analysis of fracture consequences at the Roman Sites of Ancaster (UK) and Vagnari (Italy). Int J Paleopathol 24:119–129. https://doi.org/10.1016/j.ijpp.

Gindhart S.P. 1969. The frequency of appearance of transverse lines in the tibia in relation to childhood illnesses. Am J Phys Anthropol 31(1): 17–22.

Giuffra V. and Fornaciari G. 2015. Pulverized human skull in pharmacological preparations: possible evidence from the 'martyrs of Otranto' (southern Italy, 1480). J Ethnopharmacol 160:133–139. https://doi.org/10.1016/j.jep.2014.11.042.

Giuffra V. et al. 2013. Rickets in a high social class of Renaissance Italy: the Medici children. Int J Osteoarchaeol 25(5): 608–624.

Gjestland T. 1955. The Oslo study of untreated syphilis: an epidemiological investigation of the natural course of the syphilitic infection based upon a re-study of the Boeck-Bruusgaard material. Acat Dermato-Venerologica 35(Suppl. 34).

Gladykowska-Rzeczycka J. 1980. Remains of achondroplastic dwarf from Legnica of XI–XIIth century. Ossa 7:71–74.

Gladykowska-Rzeczycka J.J. 1999. Tuberculosis in the past and present in Poland. In: Tuberculosis: past and present, ed. G. Pálfi, O. Dutour, J. Deák, and I. Hutás, 561–573. Golden Book Publishers and Tuberculosis Foundation.

Gladykowska-Rzeczycka J.J., and Urbanowicz M. 1970. Multiple osseous exostoses of the skeleton from a prehistoric cemetery of a former population of Pruszcz Gdanski. Folia Morphol 29(3): 284–296.

Glass G.B. 1991. Continuous eruption and periodontal status in pre-industrial dentitions. Int J Osteoarchaeol 1:265–271. https://doi.org/10.1002/oa.1390010322.
Glencross B. 2011. Skeletal injury across the life course: towards understanding social agency. In: Social bioarchaeology, ed. S. Agarwal and B. Glencross, 390–409. Wiley-Blackwell.
Glencross B. and Stuart-Macadam P. 2000. Childhood trauma in the archaeological record. Int J Osteoarchaeol 10:198–209.
Global Burden of Disease 2019 Fracture Collaborators. 2021. Global, regional, and national burden of bone fractures in 204 countries and territories, 1990–2019: a systematic analysis from the Global Burden of Disease Study 2019. Lancet Healthy Longev 2:e580–92. https://doi.org/10.1016/S2666-7568(21)00172-0.
Global History of Health Project. 2024. European module. https://economics.osu.edu/european-module. Accessed 1 June 2024.
Glorieux F.H. et al. 2002. Osteogenesis imperfecta type VI: a form of brittle bone disease with a mineralization defect. J Bone Miner Res 17(1):30–38.
Gluckman P. and Hanson M. 2006. Mismatch: the lifestyle diseases timebomb. University Press.
Godde K., Pasillas V., and Sanchez A. 2020. Survival analysis of the Black Death: social inequality of women and the perils of life and death in medieval London. Am J Phys Anthropol 173:168–178. https://doi.org/10.1002/ajpa.24081.
Goldberger J., Waring C.H., and Willets D.G. 1914. The treatment and prevention of pellagra. Public Health Rep 29(43): 2821–2825.
Goldmeier D. and Guallar C. 2003. Syphilis: an update. Clin Med 3(3): 209–211. https://dx.doi.org/10.7861/clinmedicine.3-3-209.
Gomes R.A.M.P., Petit J, Dutour O., and Santos A.L. 2022. Frequency and co-occurrence of porous skeletal lesions in identified non-adults from Portugal (19th to 20th centuries) and its association with respiratory infections as cause of death. Int J Osteoarchaeol 32(5): 1061–1072. https://doi.org/10.1002/oa.3132.
Gomes R.A.M.P., Santos A.L., and Catarino L. 2024. Using portable X-ray fluorescence elemental analysis to explore porous skeletal lesions: interplay of sex, age at death, and cause of death. Am J Biol Anthropol 184(4): e24954. https://doi.org/10.1002/ajpa.24954.
Gooderham E., Matias A., Liberato M., Santos H., Walshaw S., Albanese J., and Cardoso H.F. 2019. Linear and appositional growth in children as indicators of social and economic change during the medieval Islamic to Christian transition in Santarém, Portugal. Int J Osteoarchaeol 29(5): 736–746.
Goodman A.H., Lallo J., Armelagos G.J., and Rose J.C. 1984. Health changes at Dickson Mounds, Illinois (AD 950–1300). In: Paleopathology at the origins of agriculture, ed. M.N. Cohen and G.J. Armelagos, 271–306. Academic Press.
Gordon I., Shapiro H., and Berson S. 1988. Forensic medicine: a guide to principles. Churchill Livingstone.
Goude G., Dori I., Sparacello V.S., Starnini E., and Varalli A. 2020. Multi-proxy stable isotope analyses of dentine microsections reveal diachronic changes in life history adaptations, mobility, and tuberculosis-induced wasting in prehistoric Liguria (Finale Ligure, Italy, northwestern Mediterranean). Int J Paleopathol 28:99–111. https://doi.org/10.1016/j.ijpp.2019.12.007.
Gowland R.L. 2006. Ageing the past: examining age identity from funerary evidence. In: The social archaeology of funerary remains, ed. R.L. Gowland and C.J. Knüsel, 143–154. Oxbow Books.
Gowland R.L. 2015. Entangled lives: implications of the developmental origins of health and disease hypothesis for bioarchaeology and the life course. Am J Phys Anthropol 158(4): 530–540.
Gowland R.L. 2016. Elder abuse: evaluating the potentials and problems of diagnosis in the archaeological record. Int J Osteoarchaeol 26:514–523. https://doi.org/ 10.1002/oa.2442.
Gowland R., and Chamberlain A.T. 2005. Detecting plague: palaeodemographic characterisation of a catastrophic death assemblage. Antiquity 79:146–157.
Gowland R.L. and Western A.G. 2012. Morbidity in the marshes: using spatial epidemiology to investigate skeletal evidence for malaria in Anglo-Saxon England (AD 410–1050). Am J Phys Anthropol 147(2): 301–311.
Grauer A.L., ed. 2012. A companion to paleopathology. Cambridge University Press.
Grauer A.L. 2018. A century of paleopathology. Am J Phys Anthropol 165(4): 904–914.

Grauer A.L. 2019. Circulatory, reticuloendothelial, and hematopoietic disorders. In: Ortner's identification of pathological conditions in human skeletal remains, ed J.E. Buikstra, 491–529. Academic Press.

Grauer A.L. 2023. The Routledge handbook of paleopathology, ed. A.L. Grauer, 1–16. Routledge.

Grauer A.L. and Buikstra J.E. 2019a. Themes in paleopathology. In: Ortner's identification of pathological conditions in human skeletal remains, ed. J.E. Buikstra, 21–31. Academic Press.

Grauer A.L. and Roberts C.A. 1996. Paleoepidemiology, healing and possible treatment of trauma in the medieval cemetery population of St Helen-on-the-Walls, York, England. Am J Phys Anthropol 100:531–544.

Grauer A.L. and Roberts C.A. 2019b. Infectious diseases 4: Fungal, viral, multicelled parasitic and protozoan infections, and malaria. In Ortner's identification of pathological conditions in human skeletal remains, edited by J.E. Buikstra, 441–478. Elsevier.

Gray P.H. 1969. A case of osteogenesis imperfecta associated with dentinogenesis imperfecta, dating from antiquity. Clin Radiol 21:106–108.

Green M. 2020. The four Black Deaths. Am Hist Rev 125(5): 1601–1631. https://doi.org/10.1093/ahr/rhaa511.

Gregg J.B. and Gregg P.S. 1987. Dry bones: Dakota Territory reflected. Sioux Printing.

Gregoricka L.A. 2021. Moving forward: the bioarchaeology of mobility and migration. J Archaeol Res 29:581–635.

Gresky J., Dorn J., Teßmann B., and Petiti E. 2021. How rare is rare? A literature survey of the last 45 years of paleopathological research on ancient rare diseases. Int J Paleopathol 33:94–102. https://doi.org/10.1016/j.ijpp.2021.03.003.

Grimer R.J., Hogendoorn P.C.W., and Vanel D. 2013. Tumours of bone: introduction. In: WHO classification of tumours of soft tissue and bone, 4th ed., vol. 5, 244–247. IARC.

Grmek M. 1991. Diseases in the ancient Greek world. Translated by M. Muellner and L. Muellner. Johns Hopkins University Press.

Grmek M.D. and Gourevitch D. 1998. Les maladies dans l'art antique. Fayard.

Gron K. 1973. Leprosy in literature and art. Int J Lepr 41(2): 249–283.

Groumpos P.P. 2021. A critical historical and scientific overview of all industrial revolutions. IFAC-PapersOnLine 54(13): 464–471. https://doi.org/10.1016/j.ifacol.2021.10.492.

Gross C.G. 2009. A hole in the head: more tales in the history of neuroscience. MIT Press.

Groves S.E., Roberts C.A., Johnstone C., Hall R., and Dobney K. 2003. A high-status burial from Ripon Cathedral, north Yorkshire: differential diagnosis of a chest deformity. Int J Osteoarchaeol 13:358–368.

Grzybowski A. and Nita M. 2016. Leprosy in the Bible. Clin Dermatol 34:3–7. https://doi.org/10.1016/j.clindermatol.2015.10.003.

Gubbels Bupp M.R., Potluri T., Fink A.L., and Klein S.L. 2018. The confluence of sex hormones and aging on immunity. Front Immunol 9:1269. https://doi.org/10.3389/fimmu.2018.01269.

Guichón R.A. et al. 2015. Pre-Columbian tuberculosis in Tierra del Fuego? Discussion of the paleopathological and molecular evidence. Int J Paleopathol 11:92–101. https://doi.org/10.1016/j.ijpp.2015.09.003.

Guimarey Duarte R., Rubio Salvador Á., Alemán Aguilera I., and Botella López M.C. 2023. Two cases of pelvic trauma with survival in the necropolis of Qubbet el-Hawa (Egypt). Int J Paleopathol 40:56–62. https://doi.org/10.1016/j.ijpp.

Gulati N. and Allen C.E. 2021. Langerhans cell histiocytosis: Version 2021. Hematol Oncol 39:15–23.

Gump W. 2010. Modern induced skull deformity in adults. Neurosurg Focus 29(6): e4. https://doi.org/10.3171/2010.10.FOCUS10203.

Guo B. et al. 2020. Inequality in the health services utilization in rural and urban China: a horizontal inequality analysis. Medicine (Baltimore) 99(2): e18625. https://doi.org/10.1097/MD.0000000000018625.

Gurdjian E.S. 1973. Prevention and mitigation of head injury from antiquity to the present. J Trauma 13(11): 931–945.

Gurdjian E.S., Webster J. E., and Lissner H.R. 1950. The mechanism of skull fracture. J Neurosurg 7:106–114.

Guy de Chauliac. 1683. La grande chirurgie . . . tome premier. Paris.
Guyomarc'h P., Campagna-Vaillancourt M., Kremer C., and Sauvageau A. 2010. Discrimination of falls and blows in blunt head trauma: a multi-criteria approach. J Forensic Sci 55(2): 423–427.
Guzmán-Solís A.A. et al. 2021. Ancient viral genomes reveal introduction of human pathogenic viruses into Mexico during the transatlantic slave trade. eLife 10:e68612. https://doi.org/10.7554/eLife.68612.
Haas C.J. et al. 2000. Molecular evidence for different stages of tuberculosis in ancient bone samples from Hungary. Am J Phys Anthrop 113:2933–3304.
Hackett C. 1963. On the origin of the human treponematoses. Bull World Health Organ 29:7–41.
Hackett C. 1967. The human treponematoses. In: Diseases in antiquity, ed. D.R. Brothwell and A.T. Sandison, 152–170. Charles C. Thomas.
Hackett C. 1976. Diagnostic criteria of syphilis, yaws and treponarid (treponematoses) and of some other diseases in dry bones. Sitzungsberichte der Heidelberger Akademie der Wissenschaften Mathematisch- naturwissenschaftliche Klasse, Abhandlung 4. Springer-Verlag.
Hackett C. 1981. Development of caries sicca in a dry calvaria. Virchows Arch (Pathol Anat) 391:53–79.
Hagelberg E., Sykes B., and Hedges R. 1989. Ancient bone DNA amplified. Nature 342:485. https://doi.org/10.1038/342485a0.
Hagen E.H., Blackwell A.D., Lightner A.D., and Sullivan R.J. 2023. Homo medicus: the transition to meat eating increased pathogen pressure and the use of pharmacological plants in Homo. Am J Biol Anthropol 180(4): 589–617. https://doi.org/10.1002/ajpa.24718.
Hajishengallis G. 2022. Interconnection of periodontal disease and comorbidities: evidence, mechanisms, and implications. Periodontology 2000 89(1):9–18. https://doi.org/10.1111/prd.12430.
Halcrow S.E. and Gowland R., eds. 2019. The mother-infant nexus in anthropology: small beginnings, significant outcomes. Springer.
Halcrow S.E., Harris N.J., Tayles N., Ikehara-Quebral R., and Pietrusewsky M. 2013. From the mouths of babes: dental caries in infants and children and the intensification of agriculture in mainland Southeast Asia. Am J Phys Anthropol 150(3): 409–420. https://doi.org/10.1002/ajpa.22215.
Halcrow S.E., Miller M.J., Snoddy A.M.E., Fan W., and Pechenkina K. 2020. Growing up different in Neolithic China: a contextualised case study and differential diagnosis of a young adult with skeletal dysplasia. Int J Paleopathol 28:6–19.
Halcrow S.E. and Schug G.R. 2022. Structural violence as a holistic interpretive tool in paleopathology. In: The Routledge handbook of paleopathology, ed. A.L. Grauer, 417–432. Routledge.
Hall E.G. et al. 2020. SPECC1L regulates palate development downstream of IRF6. Hum Mol Genet 29(5): 845–858. https://doi.org/10.1093/hmg/ddaa002.
Hall W., McDonnell A., and O'Neill J. 2018. Superbugs: an arms race against bacteria. Harvard University Press.
Hallbäck D.A. 1976. A medieval (?) bone with a copper plate support indicating an open surgical treatment. Ossa 3/4:63–82.
Ham A.W. and Harris W.R. 1956. Repair and transplantation of bone. In: The biochemistry and physiology of bone, ed. G.H. Bourne, chap. 16. Academic Press.
Hamblen D.H. and Simpson H. 2007. Adams's outline of fractures: including joint injuries, 12th ed. Elsevier Health Sciences.
Hamperl H. 1967. The osteological consequences of scalping. In: Diseases in antiquity, ed. D. Brothwell and A. Sandison, 630–634. Charles C. Thomas.
Hancock S., Zinn C., and Schofield G. 2020. The consumption of processed sugar- and starch-containing foods, and dental caries: a systematic review. Eur J Oral Sci. 128(6): 467–475. https://doi.org/10.1111/eos.12743.
Haneveld G.T. and Perizonius W.R.K. 1980. Trepanning practice in the Netherlands. In: Proceedings of the 3rd Paleopathology Association European Meeting, Caen, France. Paris, Paleopathology Association.
Hao J.J. and Mittelman M. 2014. Acupuncture: past, present, and future. Glob Adv Health Med. 3(4): 6–8. https://doi.org/10.7453/gahmj.2014.042.

Harbeck M. and Seifert L. et al. 2013. *Yersinia pestis* DNA from skeletal remains from the 6th century AD reveals insights into Justinianic plague. PLoS Pathog 9(5): e1003349. https://doi.org/10.1371/journal.ppat.1003349.

Hardy A. 1992. Rickets and the rest: child-care, diet and the infectious children's diseases, 1850–1914. Soc Hist Med 5(3): 389–412.

Hardy K. et al. 2012. Neanderthal medics? Evidence for food, cooking, and medicinal plants entrapped in dental calculus. Naturwissenschaften 99(8): 617–626. https://doi.org/10.1007/s00114-012-0942-0.

Hardy K. et al. 2016. Dental calculus reveals potential respiratory irritants and ingestion of essential plant-based nutrients at Lower Palaeolithic Qesem Cave Israel. Quat Int 398:129–135.

Harper K. 2021. Plagues upon the earth: disease and the course of human history. Princeton University Press.

Harper K.N., Zuckerman M.K., Harper M.L., Kingston J.D., and Armelagos G.J. 2011. The origin and antiquity of syphilis revisited: an appraisal of Old World pre-Columbian evidence for treponemal infection. Am J Phys Anthropol 146(Suppl 53): 99–133. https://doi.org/10.1002/ajpa.21613.

Harper K.N., Zuckerman M.K., Turner B.L., and Armelagos G.J. 2013. Primates, pathogens, and evolution: a context for understanding emerging disease. Primates, Pathogens, and Evolution 3:389–409. https://doi.org/10.1007/978-1-4614-7181-3_13.

Harper K.N. et al. 2008. On the origin of the treponematoses: a phylogenetic approach. PLoS Negl Trop Dis 2(1): e148. https://doi.org/10.1371/journal.pntd.0000148.

Harper K.N. et al. 2012. *Treponema pallidum* infection in the wild baboons of East Africa: distribution and genetic characterization of the strains responsible. PLoS One. 7(12): e50882. https://doi.org/10.1371/journal.pone.0050882.

Harris H.A. 1931. Lines of arrested growth in the long bones in childhood: the correlation of histological and radiographic appearances in clinical and experimental conditions. Br J Radiol 18:622–640.

Harrod R. and Martin D. 2014. Bioarchaeology, climate change and violence: ethical considerations. Springer.

Harrod R., Martin D., and Perez V., eds. 2012. The bioarchaeology of violence. University of Florida Press. https://doi.org/10.5744/florida/9780813041506.001.0001.

Hart G.D. 1980. Ancient diseases of the blood. In: Blood pure and eloquent: a story of discovery, of people, and of ideas, ed. M.M. Wintrobe, 33–56. McGraw-Hil.

Hart N.H. et al. 2017. Mechanical basis of bone strength: influence of bone material, bone structure and muscle action. J Musculoskelet Neuronal Interact 17(3):114–39.

Haschka D., Hoffmann A., and Weiss G. 2021. Iron in immune cell function and host defense. Semin Cell Dev Biol 115(July): 27–36.

Hassan N.A.M., Brown K.A., Eyers J., Brown T.A., and Mays S. 2014. Ancient DNA study of the remains of putative infanticide victims from the Yewden Roman villa site at Hambleden, England. J Archaeol Sci 43:192–197.

Hassett B.R. 2014. Missing defects? A comparison of microscopic and macroscopic approaches to identifying linear enamel hypoplasia. Am J Phys Anthropol 153:463–472. https://doi.org/10.1002/ajpa.22445.

Hatch-McChesney A. and Lieberman H.R. 2022. Iodine and iodine deficiency: a comprehensive review of a re-emerging issue. Nutrients 14(17): 3474. https://doi.org/10.3390/nu14173474.

Hawkey D. 1998. Disability, compassion and the skeletal record: using musculoskeletal stress markers (MsM) to construct an osteobiography from early New Mexico. Int J Osteoarchaeol 8:326–340.

Hazer L. and Gredebäck G. 2023. The effects of war, displacement, and trauma on child development. Humanit Soc Sci Commun 10:909. https://doi.org/10.1057/s41599-023-02438-8.

He X.S. and Shi W.Y. 2009. Oral microbiology: past, present and future. Int J Oral Sci. 1(2): 47–58. https://doi.org/10.4248/ijos.09029.

Hedenstierna-Jonson C. et al. 2017. A female Viking warrior confirmed by genomics. Am J Phys Anthropol 164:853–860.

Heinrich S. 2001. Fractures of the shaft of the tibia and fibula. In: Rockwood and Wilkins' fractures in children. 5th edition, ed. J. Beaty and J. Kasser, 1077–1120. Lippincott Williams and Wilkins.
Hejna P., Šafr M., and Zátopková L. 2012. Suicidal decapitation by guillotine: case report and review of the literature. J Forensic Sci 57:1643–1645. https://doi.org/10.1111/j.1556-4029.2012.02153.x.
Helliwell T. 2010. Inflammatory diseases of the nasal cavities and paranasal sinuses. Diagn Histopathol (Oxf) 16(6): 255–264. https://doi.org/10.1016/j.mpdhp.2010.03.008.
Henderson C.Y. and Cardoso F.A. 2018. Identified skeletal collections: the testing ground of anthropology. Archaeopress.
Henderson C.Y., Mariotti V., Pany-Kucera D., Perréard-Lopreno G., Villotte S., and Wilczak C. 2012. The effect of age on entheseal changes at some fibrocartilaginous entheses. Am J Phys Anthropol 147(S54): 163.
Henderson C.Y., Mariotti V., Pany-Kucera D., Villotte S., and Wilczak C. 2013. Recording specific entheseal changes of fibrocartilaginous entheses: initial tests using the Coimbra method. Int J Osteoarchaeol 23(2): 152–162.
Henderson C.Y., Mariotti V., Pany-Kucera D., Villotte S., and Wilczak C. 2016. The new 'Coimbra method': a biologically appropriate method for recording specific features of fibrocartilaginous entheseal changes. Int J Osteoarchaeol 26(5): 925–932.
Henderson M., Miles A., and Walker D. 2013. He being dead yet speaketh: excavations at three post-medieval burial grounds in Tower Hamlets, East London, 2004–10. MOLA Monograph Series.
Hendy J. 2021. Ancient protein analysis in archaeology. Sci Adv 7(3): eabb9314. https://doi.org/10.1126/sciadv.abb9314.
Hendy J. 2023. Archaeological proteomics. In: Handbook of archaeological sciences, vol. 1., 2nd edition, ed. M. Pollard, R.A. Armitage, and C. Makarewicz, 501–510. Wiley.
Hendy J. et al. 2018. Proteomic evidence of dietary sources in ancient dental calculus. Proc Biol Sci 285(1883): 20180977. https://doi.org/10.1098/rspb.2018.0977.
Henneberg M., Holloway-Kew K., and Lucas T. 2021. Human major infections: tuberculosis, treponematoses, leprosy—a paleopathological perspective of their evolution. PLoS One 16(2): e0243687.
Henrichsen J.L., Wilhem S.K., Siljander M.P., Kalma J.J., and Karadsheh M.S. 2018. Treatment of patella fractures. Orthopedics 41(6): e747–e755. https://doi.org/10.3928/01477447-20181010-08.
Hernigou P. 2014. Crutch art painting in the Middle Ages as orthopaedic heritage. Pt I and Pt II. Int Orthop 38(6): 1329–1335, and 38(7): 1535–1542. https://dx.doi.org/10.1007/s00264-014-2278-1.
Hernigou P. 2015. Medieval orthopaedic history in Germany: Hieronymus Brunschwig and Hans von Gersdorff. Int Orthop 39:2081–2086.
Hershkovitz I. et al. 1997. Recognition of sickle cell anemia in skeletal remains of children. Am J Phys Anthropol 104:213–226.
Hershkovitz I. et al. 1999. Hyperostosis frontalis interna: an anthropological perspective. Am J Phys Anthropol 109:303–325.
Hershkovitz I. et al. 2002. Serpens endocrania symmetrica (SES): a new term and possible clue for identifying intrathoracic disease in skeletal populations. Am J Phys Anthrop 118:201–216.
Hershkovitz I. et al. 2008. Detection and molecular characterization of 9,000-year-old *Mycobacterium tuberculosis* from a Neolithic settlement in the eastern Mediterranean. PLoS One 3(10): e3426. https://doi.org/10.1371/journal.pone.
Hewison M., Bouillon R., Giovannucci E., Goltzman D., Meyer M., and Welsh J. 2023. Feldman and Pike's vitamin D. Academic Press.
Higgs D.R., Engel J.D., and Stamatoyannopoulos G. 2012. Thalassaemia. Lancet 379(9813): 373–383.
Higham C., Johannsson G., and Shalet M. 2016. Hypopituitarism. Lancet 388:2403–2415.
Hillson S. 1986. Teeth. Cambridge University Press.
Hillson S. 2001. Recording dental caries in archaeological human remains. Int J Osteoarchaeol 11:249–289.
Hillson S. 2023. Dental anthropology, 2nd ed. Cambridge University Press.

Hillson S. 2019. Dental pathology. In: Biological anthropology of the human skeleton, 3rd edition, ed. M.A. Katzenberg and A.L. Grauer, 295–333. Wiley-Blackwell.
Hillson S. and Bond S. 1997. Relationship of enamel hypoplasia to the pattern of tooth crown growth: a discussion. Am J Phys Anthropol 104(1): 89–103.
Hillson S., Grigson C., and Bond S. 1998. Dental defects of congenital syphilis. Am J Phys Anthropol 107:25–40.
Hinshaw W. and Quin L. 2015. Recognition of the causative agent of 'phossy jaw' and 'fragile femur' in fumes arising from white phosphorus. Phosphorus Sulfur Silicon Relat Elem 190(12): 2082–2093.
Hinson J., Raven P., and Chew S. 2010. The endocrine system: basic science and clinical conditions, 2nd ed. Churchill Livingstone Elsevier.
Hippocrates. 1999 (5th C BC). On head wounds. In: Corpus Medicorum Graecorum, vol. I.4.1, translated by M. Hanson. Akademie.
Hippocrates. 2022 (5th C BC). Airs, waters, places. In: Hippocrates, vol. 1, translated by P. Potter. Loeb Classical Library, Harvard University Press.
Hirata K., Oku C., and Morimoto I. 2000. A case of leprosy in a medieval Japanese. Anthropol Sci 108:114.
Hirst C.S., Gilmour R.J., Cardoso F.A. and Plomp K.A., eds. 2023. Behaviour in our bones: how human behaviour influences skeletal morphology. Elsevier.
Hockings K.J. et al. 2021. Leprosy in wild chimpanzees. Nature 598(7882): 652–656. https://doi.org/10.1038/s41586-021-03968-4.
Hodges D.C. 1987. Health and agricultural intensification in the prehistoric valley of Oaxaca, Mexico. Am J Phys Anthropol 73:323–332. https://doi.org/10.1002/ajpa.1330730305.
Hodges D.C. 1991. Temporomandibular joint osteoarthritis in a British skeletal population. Am J Phys Anthropol 85:367–377.
Hodson C.M. 2021. New prospects for investigating early life-course experiences and health in archaeological fetal, perinatal and infant individuals. Child Past 14(1): 3–12.
Holcomb R.C. 1940. The antiquity of congenital syphilis. Bull Hist Med 10(2): 148–177.
Holick M.F. and Adams J.S. 1998. Vitamin D metabolism and biological function. In: Metabolic bone disease and clinically related disorders, 3rd edition, ed. L.V. Avioli and S.M. Krane, 123–164. Academic Press.
Hollander E. 1913. Die Medizin in der Klassischen Malerie. Stuttgart.
Hollowell J. and Hannon W. 1997. Teratogen update: iodine deficiency, a community teratogen. Teratology 55:389–405.
Holmes B. 1999. Grains of gold. New Scientist (14 August): 12.
Hook E.W. 2017. Syphilis. Lancet 389(10078): 1550–1557.
Hoppa R. and Saunders S. 1998. The MAD legacy: how meaningful is mean age-at-death in skeletal samples. Hum Evol 13:1–14.
Horden P. 2000. The Millennium Bug: health and medicine around the year 1000. Soc Hist Med 13(2): 201–219.
Hosek L. and Robb J. 2019. Osteobiography: a platform for bioarchaeological research. Bioarchaeol Int 3(1): 1–15.
Huang J. et al. 2022. Distribution, risk factors, and temporal trends for lung cancer incidence and mortality: a global analysis. Chest 161(4): 1101–1111.
Huang S.H. et al. 2021. Inequality in health: the correlation between poverty and injury: a comprehensive analysis based on income level in Taiwan; a cross-sectional study. Healthcare (Basel) 9(3): 349. https://doi.org/10.3390/healthcare9030349.
Hudson E.H. 1946. Treponematosis. Oxford University Press.
Hudson E.H. 1965. Treponematosis and man's social evolution. Am Anthrop 67:885–901.
Hudson E.H. 1968. Christopher Columbus and the history of syphilis. Acta Tropica 25:1–16.
Hukeľová Z., Nováček J., Daňová K., and Ruttkay M. 2021. First reported archaeological case of leprosy in Slovakia. Int J Osteoarchaeol 31(5): 881–890. https://doi.org/10.1002/oa.3005.
Hull N.C. and Schumaker B.A. 2018. Comparisons of brucellosis between human and veterinary medicine. Infect Ecol Epidemiol 8(1): 1 sss500846. https://doi.org/10.1080/20008686.
Humphrey J.H. and Hutchinson D.L. 2001. Macroscopic characteristics of hacking trauma. J Forensic Sci 46(2): 228–233.

Hunt D.R. and Albanese J. 2005. History and demographic composition of the Robert J Terry anatomical collection. Am J Phys Anthropol 127:406–417.
Hunt D.R., and Bullen L. 2007. The frequency of os acromiale in the Robert J. Terry Collection. Int J Osteoarchaeol 17:309–317. https://doi.org/10.1002/oa.877.
Hunt K., Kirkpatrick C., Campbell R., and Willoughby J. 2024. Cancer research in ancient bodies: (CRAB) Database. https://www.cancerantiquity.org/crabdatabase. Accessed 8 June 2024.
Hunt K., Roberts C., and Kirkpatrick C. 2018. Taking stock: a systematic review of archaeological evidence of cancers in human and early hominin remains. Int J Paleopathol 21:12–26.
Hurst S.A., Gregory T.M., and Reilly P. 2019. Os acromiale: a review of its incidence, pathophysiology, and clinical management. EFORT Open Rev 4(8): 525–532.
Huss-Ashmore R., Goodman A.H., and Armelagos G.J. 1982. Nutritional inference from paleopathology. In: Advances in archaeological method and theory, ed. M.B. Schiffer, vol. 5: 395–474. Academic Press.
Hutchinson D.L. 1996. Brief encounters: Tatham Mound and the evidence for Spanish and native American confrontation. Int J Osteoarchaeol 6:51–65.
Hwang M.C., Ridley L., and Reveille J.D. 2021. Ankylosing spondylitis risk factors: a systematic literature review. Clin Rheumatol 40:3079–3093.
Hymes R. and Green M.H. 2022. New evidence for the dating and impact of the Black Death in Asia. Edited by C. Symes. Arc Humanities Press. https://doi.org/10.2307/j.ctv33f0zwr.
Idris O.A., Wintola, O.A., and Afolayan A.J. 2019. Evaluation of the bioactivities of *Rumex crispus* L. leaves and root extracts using toxicity, antimicrobial, and antiparasitic assays. Evid Based Complement Alternat Med 2019(1): 6825297. https://doi.org/10.1155/2019/6825297.
Imani D., Rezaei R., Razi B., Alizadeh S., and Mahmoudi M. 2017. Association between IL6-174 G/C polymorphism and Graves' disease: a systematic review and meta-analysis. Acta Medica Iranica 55(11): 665–671.
Indra L.I., Alterauge A., and Lösch S. 2020. A probable case of diffuse idiopathic skeletal hyperostosis from an early modern crypt in eastern Germany. Int J Osteoarchaeol 30(6): 903–908.
Inhorn M.C. and Brown P.J. 1997. The anthropology of infectious disease. In: The anthropology of infectious disease: international health perspectives, ed. M.C. Inhorn and P.J. Brown, 31–67. Gordon and Breach.
Inskip S., Taylor G.M., Anderson S., and Stewart G. 2017. Leprosy in pre-Norman Suffolk, UK: biomolecular and geochemical analysis of the woman from Hoxne. J Med Microbiol 66(11): 1640–1649.
Inskip S.A. et al. 2015. Osteological, biomolecular and geochemical examination of an early Anglo-Saxon case of lepromatous leprosy. PLoS One 10(5): e0124282. https://doi.org/10.1371/journal.pone.0124282.
Ioannou S. and Henneberg M. 2017. Dental signs attributed to congenital syphilis and its treatments in the Hamann-Todd skeletal collection. Anthropol Rev 80:449–465. https://doi.org/10.1515/anre-2017-0032.
Ioannou S., Sassani S., Henneberg M., and Henneberg R.J. 2015. Diagnosing congenital syphilis using Hutchinson's method: differentiating between syphilitic, mercurial, and syphilitic-mercurial dental defects. Am J Phys Anthropol 159:617–629. https://doi.org/10.1002/ajpa.22924.
Irurita J., Alemán I., Viciano J., López-Lázaro S., and Botella M. C. 2015. Alterations of skull bones found in anencephalic skeletons from an identified osteological collection. Two case reports. Int J Legal Med 129:903–912.
Isler M. and Turcotte R. 2003. Bone tumors in children. In: Pediatric bone: biology and diseases, ed. F. Glorieux, J. Pettifor, and M. Jüppner, 703–743. Academic Press.
Itan Y., Jones B.L., Ingram C.J., Swallow D.M., and Thomas M.G. 2010. A worldwide correlation of lactase persistence phenotype and genotypes. BMC Evol Biol 10:36. https://doi.org/10.1186/1471-2148-10-36.
Ives R. and Brickley M.B. 2004. A procedural guide to metacarpal radiogrammetry in archaeology. Int J Osteoarchaeol 14:7–17.
Ives R. and Brickley M. 2014. New findings in the identification of adult vitamin D deficiency osteomalacia: results from a large-scale study. Int J Paleopathol 7:45–56.
Ives R., Mant M., de la Cova C., and Brickley M.B. 2017. A large-scale palaeopathological study of hip fractures from post-medieval urban England. Int J Osteoarchaeol 27:261–275.

Jackson C. et al. 2023. Barriers and drivers of positive COVID-19 vaccination behaviours among healthcare workers in Europe and central Asia: a qualitative cross-country synthesis. Humanit Soc Sci Commun 10:926. https://doi.org/10.1057/s41599-023-02443-x.

Jackson I., Mattiangeli V., Cassidy L.M., Murphy E., and Bradley D.G. 2022. Millennium-old pathogenic Mendelian mutation discovery for multiple osteochondromas from a Gaelic medieval graveyard. Eur J Hum Genet 31(2): 248–251.

Jacob J.T. and Franco-Paredes C. 2008. The stigmatization of leprosy in India and its impact on future approaches to elimination and control. PLoS Negl Trop Dis 2(1): e113. https://doi.org/10.1371/journal.pntd.0000113.

Jacobsen S.E., Sørensen M., Pedersen S.M., and Weiner J. 2013. Feeding the world: genetically modified crops versus agricultural biodiversity. Agron Sustainable Dev 33:651–662.

Jaffe H.L. 1958. Tumors and tumorous conditions of bones and joints. Lea and Febiger.

Jaffe H.L. 1972. Metabolic, degenerative and inflammatory disease of bones and joints. Lea and Febiger.

Jagadesh S., Combe M., and Gozlan R.E. 2022. Human-altered landscapes and climate to predict human infectious disease hotspots. Trop Med Infect Dis. 7(7): 124. https://doi.org/10.3390/tropicalmed7070124.

Jain M., Parija D., Nayak M., and Ajay S.C. 2021. Garre's sclerosing chronic osteomyelitis of femur in an adolescent. J Orthop Case Rep 11(12): 15–18. https://doi.org/10.13107/jocr.2021.v11.i12.2546.

Jain N. 2020. The early life education of the immune system: moms, microbes and (missed) opportunities. Gut Microbes 12(1): 1824564. https://doi.org/10.1080/19490976.2020.1824564.

James R. and Nasmyth-Jones R. 1992. The occurrence of cervical fractures in victims of judicial hanging. Forensic Sci Int 54:81–91.

Janakiram C. and Dye B.A. 2020. A public health approach for prevention of periodontal disease. Periodontol 2000 84(1): 202–214. https://doi.org/10.1111/prd.12337.

Jankauskas R. 2003. The incidence of diffuse idiopathic skeletal hyperostosis and social status correlations in Lithuanian skeletal materials. Int J Osteoarchaeol 13:289–293.

Janssens P. 1970. Palaeopathology. John Baker.

Janssens P. 1987. A copper plate on the upper arm in a burial at the church in Vrasene (Belgium). J Paleopatholo 1(1): 15–18.

Jarman P. and Vivekananda U. 2021. Neurology. In: Kumar and Clark's clinical medicine, 10th edition, ed. A. Feather, D. Randall, and M. Waterhouse, 801–897. Elsevier.

Jeong Y.J. et al. 2023. Global burden of gout in 1990–2019: a systematic analysis of the Global Burden of Disease study 2019. Eur J Clin Invest 53(4): e13937. https://dx.doi.org/10.1111/eci.13937.

Jersie-Christensen R.R. et al. 2018. Quantitative metaproteomics of medieval dental calculus reveals individual oral health status. Nat Commun 9:4744. https://doi.org/10.1038/s41467-018-07148-3.

Jheon A.H., Seidel K., Biehs B., and Klein O.D. 2013. From molecules to mastication: the development and evolution of teeth. Wiley Interdiscip Rev Dev Biol 2(2): 165–182. https://doi.org/10.1002/wdev.63.

Jiménez-Brobeil S.A., Al Oumaoui I., Fernández de la Gala J.V., Laffranchi Z., and Roca M.G. 2011. An example of a severe neck injury with survival seen in a Bronze Age burial. Int J Osteoarchaeol 21:247–252.

Jing S.S. 2020. Hand dominance: nature, nurture, and relevance for hand surgeons. J Hand Microsurg 14(1): 111–112. https://doi.org/10.1055/s-0040-1713557.

Johanson C., Duncan J. III, Klinge P., Brinker T., Stopa E., and Silverberg G. 2008. Multiplicity of cerebrospinal fluid functions: new challenges in health and disease. Cerebrospinal Fluid Res 5(10): 1–32.

Johnson A. et al. 2021. Agricultural injuries among farmers and ranchers in the central United States during 2011–2015. J Agromed 26(1):62–72. https://doi.org/10.1080/1059924X.2020.1845268.

Johnston F.E. 1963. Some observations on the roles of achondroplastic dwarfs through history. Clin Pediatr (Phila) 2:703–708.

Johnson R.C et al. 1980. Reported lactose tolerance of members of various racial/ethnic groups in Hawaii and Asia. Behav Gen 10: 377–385.

Jolly S. and Kurin D. 2017. Surviving trepanation: approaching the relationship of violence and the care of 'war wounds' through a case study from prehistoric Peru. In: New developments in the bioarchaeology of care: bioarchaeology and social theory, ed. L. Tilley and A. Schrenk, 175–195. Springer. https://doi.org/10.1007/978-3-319-39901-0_9.
Jones A.K.G. 1985. Trichurid ova in archaeological deposits: their value as indicators of ancient faeces. In: Palaeobiological investigations: research design, methods and data analysis, ed. N.J. Feiller, D.D. Gilbertson, and N.G.A. Ralph, 105–119. British Archaeological Reports International Series 266. BAR.
Jones C. 2014. The smile revolution in eighteenth-century Paris. Oxford University Press.
Jones L. 2022. Patterns of plague: changing ideas about plague in England and France. McGill-Queen's University Press.
Jones L. and Varlick N. 2022. Death and disease in the medieval and early modern world: perspectives from across the Mediterranean and beyond. University of York, York Medieval Press.
Jones M.W. 1990. A study of trauma in an Amish community. J Trauma 30(7): 899–902.
Jónsdóttir B., Ortner D.J., and Frohlich B. 2003. Probable destructive meningioma in an archaeological adult male skull from Alaska. Am J Phys Anthropol 122:232–239.
Jónsson B., Gardsell P., Johnell O., Redlund-Johnell I., and Sernbo I. 1992. Differences in fracture pattern between an urban and a rural population: a comparative population-based study in southern Sweden. Osteoporosis Int 2:269–273.
Jónsson B., Gardsell P., Johnell O., Sernbo I., and Gullberg B. 1993. Life-style and different fracture prevalence: a cross sectional comparative population-based study. Calcif Tissue Int 52:425–433.
Jordana X. et al. 2009. The warriors of the steppes: osteological evidence of warfare and violence from Pazyryk tumuli in the Mongolian Altai. J Archaeol Sci 36:1319–1327. https://doi.org/10.1016/j.jas.2009.01.008.
Jordana X., Galtés I., Busquets F., Isidro A., and Malgosa A. 2006. Clay-shoveler's fracture: an uncommon diagnosis in palaeopathology. Int J Osteoarchaeol 16:366–372. https://doi.org/10.1002/oa.829.
Judd M. 2000. Trauma and interpersonal violence in ancient Nubia during the Kerma period (ca. 2500–1500 BC). Ph.D. dissertation, University of Alberta, Edmonton, Canada.
Judd M. 2002. Comparison of long bone trauma recording methods. J Archaeol Sci 29:1255–1265.
Judd M. 2004. Trauma in the city of Kerma: ancient versus modern injury patterns. Int J Osteoarchaeol 14:34–51.
Judd M. and Roberts C.A. 1998. Fracture patterns at the medieval leper hospital in Chichester. Am J Phys Anthropol 105:43–55.
Judd M. and Roberts C.A. 1999. Fracture trauma in a medieval British farming village. Am J Phys Anthropol 109:229–243.
Judd M.A. 2006. Continuity of interpersonal violence between Nubian communities. Am J Phys Anthropol 131(3): 324–333. https://doi.org/10.1002/ajpa.20401.
Judd M.A. 2008. The parry problem. J Archaeol Sci 35:1658–1666. https://doi.org/10.1016/j.
Judd M.A. 2023. Living with lower limb traumas and below-knee amputation in a Jordanian Late Ottoman nomadic community. Int J Paleopathol 41:110–116. https://doi.org/10.1016/j.ijpp.2023.04.002.
Juengst S.L., Chávez S.J., Hutchinson D.L., and Mohr Chávez K.L. 2017. Trauma in the Titicaca Basin, Bolivia (AD 1000–1450). Int J Osteoarchaeol 27:67–75. https://doi.org/ 10.1002/oa.2469.
Jung B.K. and Yun I.S. 2020. Diagnosis and treatment of positional plagiocephaly. Arch Craniofac Surg 21(2): 80–86. https://doi.org/10.7181/acfs.2020.00059.
Jurmain R.D. 1999. Stories from the skeleton: behavioral reconstruction in human osteology. Gordon and Breach Publishers.
Jurmain R., Alves Cardoso F., Henderson C. and Villotte S., 2012. Bioarchaeology's holy grail: the reconstruction of activity. In: A companion to paleopathology, ed. A.L. Grauer, 531–552. Wiley-Blackwell.
Kacki S. 2013. Erosive polyarthropathy in a Late Roman skeleton from northern France: a new case of rheumatoid arthritis from the pre-Columbian Old Word. Int J Paleopathol 3(1): 59–63.

Kacki S., Rahalison L., Rajerison M., Ferroglio E., and Bianucci R. 2011. Black Death in the rural cemetery of Saint-Laurent-de-la-Cabrerisse Aude-Languedoc, southern France, 14th century: immunological evidence. J Archaeol Sci 38:581–587. https://doi.org/10.1016/j.jas.2010.10.012.
Kalter H. 2003. Teratology in the 20th century: environmental causes of congenital malformations in humans and how they were established. Neurotoxicol Teratol 25(2): 131–282.
Kappelman J. et al. 2008. First *Homo erectus* from Turkey and implications for migrations into temperate Eurasia. Am J Phys Anthropol 135:110–116. https://doi.org/10.1002/ajpa.20739.
Karaguzel G. and Holick M.F. 2010. Diagnosis and treatment of osteopenia. Rev Endocr Metab Disord 11 (4): 237–251.
Karapanou O. and Papadimitriou A. 2010. Determinants of menarche. Reprod BiolEndocrinol 8(1): 115. https://doi.org/10.1186/1477-7827-8-115.
Karenberg A. 2009. Retrospective diagnosis: use and abuse in medical historiography. Prague Med Rep 110(2): 140–145.
Karn K.W., Shockett H.D., Moffitt W.C., and Gray J.L. 1984. Topographic classification of deformities of the alveolar process. J Periodontol 55:336–340.
Karsh R.S. and McCarthy J.D. 1960. Archaeology and arthritis. Intern Med 105:640–644.
Karsten J., Heins S., Madden G., and Sokhatskyi M. 2015. Dental health and the transition to agriculture in prehistoric Ukraine: a study of dental caries. Eur J Archaeol 18:562–579. https://doi.org/10.1179/1461957115Y.0000000004.
Kattamis A., Forni G.L., Aydinok Y., and Viprakasit V. 2020. Changing patterns in the epidemiology of β-thalassemia. Eur J Haematol 105(6): 692–703.
Kattamis A., Kwiatkowski J.L., and Aydinok Y. 2022. Thalassaemia. Lancet 399(10343): 2310–2324.
Katzenberg A. 2012. The ecological approach: understanding past diet and the relationship between diet and disease. In: A companion to paleopathology, ed. A.L. Grauer, 97–113. Wiley-Blackwell.
Katzenberg M.A. and Lovell N.C. 1999. Stable isotope variation in pathological bone. Int J Osteoarchaeol 9:316–324.
Katzenberg M.A., Schwarcz H.P., Knyf M., and Melbye F.J. 1995. Stable isotope evidence for maize horticulture and paleodiet in southern Ontario, Canada. Am Antiq 60:335–350.
Katzenberg M.A. and Waters-Rist A.L. 2018. Stable isotope analysis: a tool for studying past diet, demography, and life history. In: Biological anthropology of the human skeleton, ed. M.A. Katzenberg and A. Grauer, 467–504. Wiley and Sons.
Kaufman M.H., Whitaker D., and McTavish J. 1997. Differential diagnosis of holes in the calvarium: application of modern clinical data to palaeopathology. J Archaeol Sci 24:193–218.
Kaufman M.R., Eschliman E.L., and Karver T.S. 2023. Differentiating sex and gender in health research to achieve gender equity. Bull World Health Organ 101(10): 666–671. https://doi.org/10.2471/BLT.22.289310.
Kaupová S.D., Limburský P., and Vélová L. 2023. Isotopic reconstruction of the early life experience of individuals from the early Bronze Age Vliněves site (Czech Republic). J Archaeol Sci: Rep 50:104085. https://doi.org/10.1016/j.jasrep.2023.104085.
Kaushik R. and Sougat R. 2018. War and epidemics: a chronicle of infectious diseases. J Marine Med Soc 20(1): 50–54. https://doi.org/10.4103/jmms.jmms_34_18.
Keene M.R., Heslop I.M., Sabesan S.S., and Glass B.D. 2019. Complementary and alternative medicine use in cancer: a systematic review. Complement Ther Clin Pract 35:33–47. https://doi.org/10.1016/j.ctcp.2019.01.004.
Keller M. et al. 2019. Ancient *Yersinia pestis* genomes from across Western Europe reveal early diversification during the First Pandemic (541–750). Proc Natl Acad Sci USA 116(25): 12363–12372. https://doi.org/10.1073/pnas.1820447116.
Kelley M. and Micozzi M. 1984. Rib lesions in chronic pulmonary tuberculosis. Am J Phys Anthropol 65:381–387.
Kelley M., Murphy S., Levesque D., and Sledzik P. 1994. Respiratory disease among protohistoric and early historic Plains Indians. In: Skeletal biology in the Great Plains: migration, warfare, health, and subsistence, ed. D.W. Owsley and R.L. Jantz, 123–130. Smithsonian Institution Press.
Kelley M.A. 1979. Skeletal changes produced by aortic aneurysms. Am J Phys Anthropol 51(1): 35–38. https://doi.org/10.1002/ajpa.1330510104.

Kendall E.J., Montgomery J., Evans J.A., Stantis C., and Mueller V. 2013. Mobility, mortality, and the Middle Ages: identification of migrant individuals in a 14th century Black Death cemetery population. Am J Phys Anthropol 150:210–222.

Kennedy G.E. 1986. The relationship between auditory exostoses and cold water: a latitudinal analysis. Am J Phys Anthropol 71:401–415.

Kępa M. et al. 2013. A case of the execution of Swedish soldiers at the market square in Cracow (17th c.). Int J Osteoarchaeol 23:730–736. https://doi.org/10.1002/oa.1291.

Kerner G. et al. 2023. Genetic adaptation to pathogens and increased risk of inflammatory disorders in post-Neolithic Europe. Cell Genom 3(2): 100248. https://doi.org/10.1016/j.xgen.2022.100248.

Kerr N.W. 1988. A method of assessing periodontal status in archaeologically derived skeletal material. J Paleopathol 2:67–78.

Kesling E. 2020. Medical texts in Anglo-Saxon literary culture. D.S. Brewer.

Kessel A. 2006. Air, the environment and public health. Cambridge University Press.

Khan F.Q., Deshmukh P.T., and Gaurkar S.S. 2022. Pneumatization pattern and status of the mastoid antrum in chronic otitis media: a review. Cureus 14(7): e27068. https://doi.org/10.7759/cureus.27068.

Khanna P., Thapa M., and Prasad S. 2011. Pictorial essay: the many faces of craniosynostosis. Indian J Radiol Imaging 21(1): 49–56.

Khoriati A.A., Rajakulasingam R., and Shah R. 2013. Sternal fractures and their management. J Emerg Trauma Shock 6(2): 113–116. https://doi.org/10.4103/0974-2700.110763.

Khoshnood S. et al. 2022. Prevalence, diagnosis, and manifestations of brucellosis: a systematic review and meta-analysis. Front Vet Sci 9:976215. https://doi.org/10.3389/fvets.2022.976215.

Khudaverdyan A. 2011. Trepanation and artificial cranial deformations in ancient Armenia. Anthropol Rev 74:39–55. https://doi.org/10.2478/v10044-010-0004-1.

Khudaverdyan A.Y., Devejyan S.H., Davtyan R.H., Yengibaryan A.A., Hovhanesyan A.A., and Vardanyan S.A. 2021. Female with ankylosing spondylitis from the 7th–6th century BCE Lori Berd burial (Armenia). Anthropol Rev 84(1): 85–100.

Khurana J., and Unni K. 2003. Pathological diagnosis of common tumours of bone and cartilage. In: Handbook of histology methods for bone and cartilage, ed. H. Yuehuei and K. Martin, 447–494. Humana Press.

Kickbusch I. and Alakija A. 2023. The Sustainable Development Goals should be reset to prioritize poverty, health and climate. Nat Med 29:2399–2401. https://doi.org/10.1038/s41591-023-02546-7.

Kilgore L., Jurmain R.D., and VanGerven D. 1997. Palaeoepidemiological patterns of trauma in a medieval Nubian skeletal population. Int J Osteoarchaeol 7:1103–1114.

King M., Speck P., and Thomas A. 1999. The effect of spiritual beliefs on outcome from illness. Soc Sci Med 48:1291–1299.

King S. 1994. The human skeletal remains from Glasgow Cathedral excavations 1992–3. Unpublished skeletal report.

King's Fund. 2024. https://www.kingsfund.org.uk/. Accessed 7 July 2024.

Kinkopf K.M. et al. 2023. Contextualizing bilateral asymmetry and gender: a multivariate approach to femoral cross-sectional geometry at rural medieval Pieve di Pava, Italy. Am J Biol Anthropol 180(1): 173–195.

Kinsman S.L. and Johnston M.V. 2016. Hydrocephalus. In: Nelson textbook of pediatrics, 20th edition, ed. R.M. Kliegman, B.F. Stanton, J. St. Geme, and N.F. Schor, 2814–2817. Elsevier.

Kintigh K.W. et al. 2014. Grand challenges for archaeology. Proc Natl Acad Sci USA 111(3): 879–880. https://doi.org/10.1073/pnas.1324000111.

Kishimoto M. et al. 2021. Clinical features of psoriatic arthritis. Best Pract Res Clin Rheumatol 35(2): 101670. https://doi.org/10.1016/j.berh.2021.101670.

Kjellström A. 2012. Possible cases of leprosy and tuberculosis in medieval Sigtuna, Sweden. Int J Osteoarchaeol 22:261–283.

Klaassen M. and Wille M. 2023. The plight and role of wild birds in the current bird flu panzootic. Nat Ecol Evol 7:1541–1542. https://doi.org/10.1038/s41559-023-02182-x.

Klaus H. 2010. Oral health and the postcontact adaptive transition: a contextual reconstruction of diet in Morrope, Peru. Am J Phys Anthropol 141:594–604.

Klaus H. 2014a. A probable case of acute childhood leukemia: skeletal involvement, differential diagnosis, and the bioarchaeology of cancer in South America. Int J Osteoarchaeol 26(2): 348–358.

Klaus H.D. 2014b. Frontiers in the bioarchaeology of stress and disease: cross-disciplinary perspectives from pathophysiology, human biology, and epidemiology. Am J Phys Anthropol 155(2): 294–308. https://doi.org/10.1002/ajpa.22574.

Klaus H.D. 2018. Possible prostate cancer in northern Peru: differential diagnosis, vascular anatomy, and molecular signaling in the paleopathology of metastatic bone disease. Int J Paleopathol 21:147–157.

Klaus H.D. and Lynnerup N. 2019. Abnormal bone: considerations for documentation, disease process identification, and differential diagnosis. In: Ortner's identification of pathological conditions in human skeletal remains, ed. J. E. Buikstra, 59–89. Academic Press.

Kleinman P.K. and Walters M.M. 2015. Dating fractures. In: Diagnostic imaging of child abuse, ed. P.K. Kleinman, 208–216. Cambridge University Press. https://doi.org/10.1017/CBO978051186 2366.014.

Knauf S., Liu H., and Harper K.N. 2013. Treponemal infection in nonhuman primates as possible reservoir for human yaws. Emerg Infect Dis 19(12): 2058–2060. https://doi.org/10.3201/eid1912.130863.

Knight B. 1991. Forensic pathology. Edward Arnold.

Knorr D.A. et al. 2019. Intestinal parasites in six Islamic medieval period latrines from 10th–11th century Córdoba (Spain) and 12th–13th century Mértola (Portugal). Int J Paleopathol 26:75–83. https://doi.org/10.1016/j.ijpp.2019.06.004.

Knudson K.J. and Stojanowski C.M., eds. 2020. Bioarchaeology and identity revisited. University Press of Florida.

Knüsel C. 2001. Activity-related skeletal change. In: Blood red roses: the archaeology of a mass grave from the Battle of Towton AD 1461, ed. V. Fiorato, A. Boylston, and C. Knüsel, 103–118. Oxbow Books.

Knüsel C. and Smith M., eds. 2014. The Routledge handbook of the bioarchaeology of human conflict. Routledge.

Knüsel C.J., Chundun Z.C., and Cardwell P. 1992. Slipped proximal femoral epiphysis in a priest from the medieval period. Int J Osteoarchaeol 2:109–119. https://doi.org/10.1002/oa.1390020203.

Knüsel C.J., Göggel S., and Lucy D. 1997. Comparative degenerative joint disease of the vertebral column in the medieval monastic cemetery of the Gilbertine Priory of St Andrew, Fishergate, England. Am J Phys Anthropol 103:481–495.

Knüsel C.J., Kemp R.L., and Budd P. 1995. Evidence for remedial treatment of a severe knee injury from the Fishergate Gilbertine Monastery in the City of York. J Archaeol Sci 22: 369–384.

Knüsel C.J., Roberts C.A., and Boylston A. 1996. Brief communication: when Adam delved . . . an activity-related lesion in three human skeletal populations. Am J Phys Anthropol 100:427–434.

Ko A. et al. 2013. ALPK1 genetic regulation and risk in relation to gout. Int J Epidemiol 42(2): 466–474.

Kobayashi D. et al. 2005. Musculoskeletal conditions of acute leukemia and malignant lymphoma in children. J Pediatr Orthop B 14(3): 156–161.

Koch V.H., Lopes M.T., Furusawa E., Vaz K., and Barroso U. 2024. Multidisciplinary management of people with spina bifida across the lifespan. Pediatr Nephrol 39(3): 681–697.

Köhler K. et al. 2017. Possible cases of leprosy from the late Copper Age (3780–3650 cal BC) in Hungary. PLoS One 12(10): e0185966.

Konrad G.G., Kundel K., Kreuz P.C., Oberst M., and Sudkamp N.P. 2007. Monteggia fractures in adults. J Bone Joint Surg Br 89(3): 354–360. https://doi.org/10.1302/0301-620X.89B3.18199.

Koukli M., Siegmund F., and Papageorgopoulou C. 2023. Stature estimation in Ancient Greece: population-specific equations and secular trends from 9000 BC to 900 AD. Archaeol Anthropol Sci 15:53. https://doi.org/10.1007/s12520-023-01744-1.

Kowal E. et al. 2023. Community partnerships are fundamental to ethical ancient DNA research. Hum Genet Genom Adv 4(2):100161. https://doi.org/10.1016/j.xhgg.2022.100161.

Kowal W.A., Krahn P.M., and Beattie O. 1989. Lead levels in human tissues from the Franklin Forensic Project. Int J Environ Anal Chem 35:119–126.

Kozakaitė J. et al. 2018. A rare case of child abuse from early modern Lithuania. Int J Paleopathol 22:189–197. https://doi.org/10.1016/j.ijpp.

Kozłowski T. 2012. Stan Biologiczny i Warunki Życia Ludności in Culmine na Pomorzu Nadwiślańskim (X–XIII wiek): Studium Antropologiczne [Biological state and life conditions of the population living in Culmine, Pomerania Vistula (10th–13th century: an anthropological study]. Mons Sancti Laurentii vol. 7. Toruń: Wydawnictwo Naukowe Uniwersytetu Mikołaja Kopernika. (In Polish with English abstract.)

Kremer C., Racette S., Dionne C.-A., and Sauvageau A. 2008. Discrimination of falls and blows in blunt head trauma: systematic study of the hat brim line rule in relation to skull fractures. J Forensic Sci 53:716–719. https://doi.org/10.1111/j.1556-4029.2008.00725.x.

Kremer C. and Sauvageau A. 2009. Discrimination of falls and blows in blunt head trauma: assessment of predictability through combined criteria. J Forensic Sci 54:923–926.

Krenz-Niedbała M. and Łukasik S. 2016a. Prevalence of chronic maxillary sinusitis in children from rural and urban skeletal populations in Poland. Int J Paleopathol 15:103–112. https://doi.org/10.1016/j.ijpp.2016.10.003.

Krenz-Niedbała M. and Łukasik S. 2016b. Skeletal evidence for otitis media in medieval and post-medieval children from Poland, Central Europe. Int J Osteoarchaeol 27(3): 375–386. https://doi.org/10.1002/oa.2545.

Krenz-Niedbała M. and Łukasik S. 2020. Urban-rural differences in respiratory tract infections in medieval and early modern Polish subadult samples. In: The bioarchaeology of urbanization: the biological, demographic, and social consequences of living in cities, ed. T.K. Betsinger and S. DeWitte, 245–272. Springer Nature.

Kroman A., Kress T., and Porta D. 2011. Fracture propagation in the human cranium: a re-testing of popular theories. Clin Anat 24(3): 309–318. https://dx.doi.org/10.1002/ca.21129.

Krugman J. and Chorba T. 2022. When a touch of gold was used to heal the King's Evil. Emerg Infect Dis 28(3): 765–767. https://doi.org/10.3201/eid2803.AC2803.

Kulus M.J. and Dąbrowski P. 2019. How to calculate the age at formation of Harris lines? A step-by-step review of current methods and a proposal for modifications to Byers' formulas. ArchaeolAnthropol Sci 11(4): 1169–1185.

Kumar D.V., Chaitanya D.K., Singh V., Sridhar Reddy D. 2018. A morphometric study of human middle ear ossicles in cadaveric temporal bones of Indian population and a comparative analysis. Journal of the Anatomical Society of India 67(1): 12–17. https://doi.org/10.1016/j.jasi.2018.01.001.

Kuo C.F., Grainge M.J., Zhang W., and Doherty M. 2015. Global epidemiology of gout: prevalence, incidence and risk factors. Nat Rev Rheumatol 11(11): 649–662.

Kuperus J.S. et al. 2018. Simultaneous occurrence of ankylosing spondylitis and diffuse idiopathic skeletal hyperostosis: a systematic review. Rheumatology 57(12): 2120–2128. https://dx.doi.org/10.1093/rheumatology/key211.

Kuperus J.S., Hoesein F.A.M., de Jong P.A., and Verlaan J.J. 2020. Diffuse idiopathic skeletal hyperostosis: etiology and clinical relevance. Best PractRes Clin Rheumatol 34(3): 101527. https://doi.org/10.1016/j.berh.2020.101527.

Kyei-Baafour E. et al. 2020. Impact of an irrigation dam on the transmission and diversity of *Plasmodium falciparum* in a seasonal malaria transmission area of northern Ghana. J Trop Med. 2020 (Mar 19). https://doi.org/10.1155/2020/1386587.

Kyere K.A. et al. 2012. Schmorl's nodes. Eur Spine J 21:2115–2121.

L'Abbé E.N. and Steyn M. 2007. Health status of the Venda, a post-antibiotic community in rural South Africa. Int J Osteoarchaeol 17:492–503.

Laes C. 2008. Learning from silence: disabled children in Roman antiquity. Arctos 42:85–122.

Laes C., Goodey C., and Rose M., eds. 2013. Disabilities in Roman antiquity: disparate bodies a capite ad calcem. Vol. 356. Brill.

Lagia A., Eliopoulos C., and Manolis S. 2006. Thalassemia: macroscopic and radiological study of a case. Int J Osteoarchaeol 17(3): 269–285.

Lagia A., Petroutsa I., Dretaki O., and Manolis S.K. 2006. Demographic and paleopathologic analysis of an early Christian era population from the Kos Island (Aegean Archipelago, Greece). Paper presented at the 16th European meeting of the Paleopathology Association, Santorini, Greece, August 28–September 1.

Laine C.G., Johnson V.E., Scott H.M., and Arenas-Gamboa A.M. 2023. Global estimate of human brucellosis incidence. Emerg Infect Dis 29(9): 1789–1797. https://doi.org/10.3201/eid2909.230052.

Lambert P.M. 2002. Rib lesions in a prehistoric Puebloan sample from southwestern Colorado. Am J Phys Anthropol 117:281–292.

Lambert P.M. 2012. Ethics and issues in the use of human skeletal remains in paleopathology. In: Companion to paleopathology, ed. A.L. Grauer, 17–33. Wiley-Blackwell.

Lambert P.M. and Walker P.L. 2018. Bioarchaeological ethics: perspectives on the use and value of human remains in scientific research. In: Biological anthropology of the human skeleton, 3rd edition, ed. A. Katzenberg and A. Grauer, 3–42. Wiley-Blackwell.

Lambert P.M., and Welker M.H. 2017. Traumatic injury risk and agricultural transitions: a view from the American Southeast and beyond. Am J Phys Anthropol 162:120–142. https://doi.org/10.1002/ajpa.23103.

Lampert F. 1998. Langerhans cell histiocytosis: historical perspectives. Hematol Oncol Clin 12(2): 213–219.

Lampl M., Kuzawa C., Jeanty P. 2003. Prenatal smoke exposure alters growth in limb proportions and head shape in the midgestation human fetus. Am J Human Biol 15:533–546.

Lancet. 2017. Editorial. Syndemics: health in context. Lancet 389:881.

Langgut D. 2022. Mid-7th century BC human parasite remains from Jerusalem, Int J Paleopathol 36:1–6. https://doi.org/10.1016/j.ijpp.2021.10.005.

Langley-Evans S. 2015. Nutrition in early life and the programming of adult disease: a review. J Hum Nutr Diet 28(Suppl. 1): 1–14.

Larentis O., Tonina E., Iorio S., Tesi C., Fusco R., and Licata M. 2023. A possible case of 'kissing' osteochondroma and multiple enchondromas in a medieval skeleton from the church of Sant'Agostino in Caravate (Northern Italy). Anthropologischer Anzeiger 80(2): 191–203.

Larsen C.S. 1984. Health and disease in prehistoric Georgia: the transition to agriculture. In: Paleopathology at the origins of agriculture, ed. M.N. Cohen and G.J. Armelagos, 367–392. Academic Press.

Larsen C.S. 2015. Bioarchaeology: interpreting behavior from the human skeleton. Cambridge University Press.

Larsen P. et al. 2015. Incidence and epidemiology of tibial shaft fractures. Injury 46(4): 746–750. https://doi.org/10.1016/j.injury.2014.12.027.

Larson H.J., Lin L., and Goble R. 2022. Vaccines and the social amplification of risk. Risk Analysis 42:1409–1422. https://doi.org/10.1111/risa.13942.

Lascaratos J. and Assimakopoulos D. 1999. From the roots of otology: diseases of the ear and their treatment in Byzantine times (AD 324–1453). Am J Otol 20(3): 397–402.

Laurence K.M. 1958. The natural history of hydrocephalus. Lancet 29:1152–1154.

Law A.S. 2012. Kalaupapa: a collective memory. University of Hawaii Press.

Lawler D.F. 2017. Differential diagnosis in archaeology. Int J Paleopathol 10:119–123.

Lawler D.F., Tangredi B.P., and Widga C.C. 2020. Organism migration in soils: should we be so comfortable with diagnosing ancient infectious diseases? Int J Osteoarchaeol 30:297–306. https://doi.org/10.1002/oa.2855.

Lazenby R. and Pfeiffer S. 1993. Effects of a 19th century below-knee amputation and prosthesis on femoral morphology. Int J Osteoarchaeol 3:19–28.

Le Page M. 2002. Gene battle goes south. New Scientist (21–28 December): 25.

Leden I., Forslind K., Svensson B., and BARFOT Study Group. 2012. Ankylosis of wrist and small joints of the hand occurs in rheumatoid arthritis: diagnostic implication in paleopathology. Int J Paleopathol 2(4): 249–251.

Ledger M.L. and Mitchell P.D. 2022. Evolutionary perspectives on human parasitic infection: from ancient parasites to modern medicine. In: Palaeopathology and evolutionary medicine: an integrated approach, ed. K. Plomp, C.A. Roberts, S. Elton, and G. Bentley, 204–221. Oxford University Press.

Lee C. 2019. A bioarchaeological and biocultural investigation of Chinese footbinding at the Xuecun archaeological site, Henan Province, China. Int J Paleopathol 25:9–19. doi.org/10.1016/j.

Lee M.J., Siek T.J., and Hirst C.S. 2024. Chronic maxillary sinusitis in palaeopathology: a review of methods. Int J Paleopathol 44:51–64. https://doi.org/10.1016/j.ijpp.2023.11.005.

Lee Y.H. et al. 2020. Patients with rheumatoid arthritis increased risk of developing osteoarthritis: a nationwide population-based cohort study in Taiwan. Front Med 7:392. https://doi.org/10.3389/fmed.2020.00392.

Leestma J.E. and Kirkpatrick J.B. 1988. Forensic neuropathology. Raven Press.

Legge S.S. 2010. Brief communication: transportation and trauma: dog-sledding and vertebral compression in Alaskan Eskimos. Am J Phys Anthropol 141(4): 632–637. https://doi.org/10.1002/ajpa.21220.

Leisen J.C.C., Duncan H., and Riddle J.M. 1991. Rheumatoid erosive arthropathy as seen in macerated (dry) bone specimens. In: Human paleopathology: current syntheses and future options, ed. D.J. Ortner and A. Aufderheide, 211–215. Smithsonian Institution Press.

Leitman T., Porco T., and Blower S. 1997. Leprosy and tuberculosis: the epidemiological consequences of cross-immunity. Am J. Public Health 87(12): 1923–1927.

Leone A., Cianfoni A., Cerase A., Magarelli N., and Bonomo L. 2011. Lumbar spondylolysis: a review. Skeletal Radiol 40(6): 683–700. https://doi.org/10.1007/s00256-010-0942-0.

Leowattana W., Leowattana P., and Leowattana T. 2023. Tuberculosis of the spine. World J Orthop 14(5): 275–293. https://doi.org/10.5312/wjo.v14.i5.275.

Lessa A. 2011. Daily risks: a biocultural approach to acute trauma in pre-colonial coastal populations from Brazil. Int J Osteoarchaeol 21:159–72. https://doi.org/10.1002/oa.1118.

Levene M. 1991. Metabolic disorders. In: Jolly's diseases of children, 6th edition, ed. M. Levene, 370–381. Blackwell Scientific Publications.

Levers R.G.H. and Darling A.I. 1983. Continuing eruption of some adult human teeth of ancient populations. Arch Oral Biol 28(5): 401–408.

Lewis B.A. 1998. Prehistoric juvenile rheumatoid arthritis in a precontact Louisiana native population reconsidered. Am J Phys Anthropol 106:229–248.

Lewis C.M., Akinyi M.Y., DeWitte S.N., and Stone A.C. 2023. Ancient pathogens provide a window into health and well-being. Proc Natl Acad Sci USA 120(4): e2209476119.

Lewis M. 2000. Non-adult palaeopathology: current status and future potential. In: Human osteology in archaeology and forensic science, ed. M. Cox and S. Mays, 39–57. Greenwich Medical Media.

Lewis M. 2002. Impact of industrialisation: comparative study of child health in four sites from medieval and post-medieval England (AD 850–1859). Am J Phys Anthropol 119(3): 211–223.

Lewis M. 2007. The bioarchaeology of children: current perspectives in biological and forensic anthropology. Cambridge University Press.

Lewis M. 2008. A traitor's death? The identity of a drawn, hanged and quartered man from Hulton Abbey, Staffordshire. Antiquity 82(315): 113–124.

Lewis M. 2010. Life and death in a Civitas Capital: metabolic disease and trauma in the children from late Roman Dorchester, Dorset. Am J Phys Anthropol 142: 405–416.

Lewis M. 2011. Thalassaemia: its diagnosis and interpretation in past skeletal populations. Int J Osteoarchaeol 21(2): 685–693.

Lewis M. 2016. Work and the adolescent in medieval England (AD 900–1050): the osteological evidence. Mediev Archaeol 60(1): 138–171.

Lewis M. 2018. Palaeopathology of children: identification of pathological conditions in the human skeletal remains of non-adults. Academic Press.

Lewis M. 2019a. Children in bioarchaeology: methods and interpretations. In: Biological anthropology of the human skeleton, 3rd edition, ed. A. Katzenberg and A.L. Grauer, 119–143. Wiley and Sons.

Lewis M. 2019b. Endocrine disturbances. In: Ortner's identification of pathological conditions in human skeletal remains, ed J.E. Buikstra, 567–584. Elsevier.

Lewis M. 2022. Exploring adolescence as a key life history stage in bioarchaeology. Am J Biol Anthropol 179(4): 519–534.

Lewis M. and Montgomery J. 2023. Youth mobility, migration, and health before and after the Black Death. Bioarchaeol Int 7(2): 111–129.

Lewis M. and Roberts C.A. 1997. Growing pains: the interpretation of stress indicators. Int J Osteoarchaeol 7:581–586.

Lewis M., Roberts C.A., and Manchester K. 1995a. A comparative study of the prevalence of maxillary sinusitis in medieval urban and rural populations in northern England. Am J Phys Anthropol 98(4): 497–506.

Lewis M., Roberts C.A., and Manchester K. 1995b. Inflammatory bone changes in leprous skeletons from the medieval hospital of St. James and St. Mary Magdalene. Int J Lepr 63(1): 77–85.

Lewis M.J., Owen-Crocker G.R., and Terkla D. 2011. The Bayeux tapestry: new approaches. In: Proceedings of a conference at the British Museum, 81–85. Oxbow Books.

Lewis M., Shapland F., and Watts R. 2016. The influence of chronic conditions and the environment on pubertal development: an example from medieval England. Int J Paleopathol 12:1–10.

Li H., He L., Gibbon V.E., Xiao X., and Wang B. 2021. Individual centred social-care approach: using computer tomography to assess a traumatic brain injury in an Iron Age individual from China. Int J Osteoarchaeol 31:99–107. https://doi.org/10.1002/oa.2928.

Li M., Chen L., Zhao D., and Roberts C.A. 2019. A male adult skeleton from the Han Dynasty in Shaanxi, China (202 BC–220 AD) with bone changes that possibly represent spinal tuberculosis. Int J Paleopathol 27:9–16.

Li N. et al. 2022. Spondylolysis. Orthop Rev (Pavia) 14(3): 37470. https://doi.org/10.52965/001c.37470.

Li Y. et al. 2023. Dynamics of oral microbiome acquisition in healthy infants: a pilot study. Front Oral Health 4:1152601. https://doi.org/10.3389/froh.2023.1152601.

Liebe-Harkort C. 2012. Cribra orbitalia, sinusitis and linear enamel hypoplasia in Swedish Roman Iron Age adults and subadults. Int J Osteoarchaeol 22(4): 387–397. https://doi.org/10.1002/oa.1209.

Lieverse A.R. 1999. Diet and the aetiology of dental calculus. Int J Osteoarchaeol 9:219–232.

Lieverse A.R., Cooper D.M.L., and Bazaliiskii V.I. 2017. Penetrating spinal injury: an extraordinary case of survival in early Neolithic Siberia. Int J Osteoarchaeol 27:508–514. https://doi.org/10.1002/oa.2568.

Lieverse A.R., Temple D.H., and Bazaliiskii V.I. 2014. Paleopathological description and diagnosis of metastatic carcinoma in an Early Bronze Age (4588+ 34 Cal. BP) forager from the Cis-Baikal region of eastern Siberia. PLoS One 9(12): e113919. https://doi.org/10.1371/journal.pone.0113919.

Lima M.F. et al. 2022. The presence of *Mycobacterium leprae* in wild rodents. Microorganisms 10(6): 1114. https://doi.org/10.3390/microorganisms10061114.

Lin H. and Gong Y.Z. 2017. Association of HLA-B27 with ankylosing spondylitis and clinical features of the HLA-B27-associated ankylosing spondylitis: a meta-analysis. Rheumatol Int 37:1267–1280.

Lind J. 1772. A treatise on scurvy, 3rd ed. S. Crowder.

Ling N.Y., Halcrow S.E., and Buckley H.R. 2023. Gout in paleopathology: a review with some etiological considerations. Gout Urate Cryst Depos Dis 1(4): 217–233.

Linhuan Q. and Fajun L. 2021. Morphological analysis of bones on the foot-binding female deformity of Taohuayuan Cemetery of Ming and Qing Dynasties in Ji County, Tianjin. Acta Anthropologica Sinica 40:787–800.

Lipton J.F. and Vigorita V.J. 2016. Metastatic bone disease. In: Orthopaedic pathology, 594–619. Wolter Kluwers.

Liston M. and Rotroff S. 2013. Babies in the well: archaeological evidence for newborn disposal in Hellenistic Greece. In: The Oxford handbook of childhood and education in the Classical world, ed. J. Evans Grubbs, T. Parkin, and R. Bell, 62–83. Oxford University Press.

Little R.E., Long C.M., Loehrl T.A., and Poetker D.M. 2018. Odontogenic sinusitis: a review of the current literature. Laryngoscope Investig Otolaryngol 3(2): 110–114. https://doi.org/10.1002/lio2.147.

Littlejohn G. 2022. Historical bioarcheological aspects of diffuse idiopathic skeletal hyperostosis in humans. Semin Arthritis Rheum 52:151942. https://doi.org/10.1016/j.semarthrit.2021.12.010.

Littleton J. 1998. A Middle Eastern paradox: rickets in skeletons from Bahrain. J Palaeopathol 10(1): 13–30.

Liu T. and Liu S. 2020. The impacts of coal dust on miners' health: a review. Environ Res 190:109849: https://doi.org/10.1016/j.envres.2020.109849.

Lockau L. et al. 2016. 'Buck and ball': identification and interpretation of buckshot injuries to the pelvis from the War of 1812. J Archaeol Sci: Rep 6:424–33. https://doi.org/10.1016/j.

Lockau L., et al. 2019. Vitamin D deficiency and the ancient city: skeletal evidence across the life course from the Roman period site of Isola Sacra, Italy, Journal of Anthropological Archaeology 55. https://doi.org/10.1016/j.jaa.2019.101069.

Loe L., Boyle A., Webb H., and Score D. 2014. 'Given to the ground': a Viking age mass grave on Ridgeway Hill, Weymouth. Dorset Natural History and Archaeology Society and Oxford Archaeology.

Loeser R.F., Goldring S.R., Scanzello C.R., and Goldring M.B. 2012. Osteoarthritis: a disease of the joint as an organ. Arthritis Rheum 64(6): 1697–1707.

Lombard J.E. et al. 2021. Human-to-cattle *Mycobacterium tuberculosis* complex transmission in the United States. Front Vet Sci. 8 (12 Jul). https://doi.org/10.3389/fvets.2021.

Longo U.G. et al. 2023. Colles' fracture: an epidemiological nationwide study in Italy from 2001 to 2016. Int J Environ Res Public Health 20(5): 3956. https://doi.org/10.3390/ijerph20053956.

Lopez A., Cacoub P., Macdougall I.C., and Peyrin-Biroulet L. 2016. Iron deficiency anaemia. Lancet 387(10021): 907–916.

López-Durán L. 1995. Traumatología Y Ortopedia. Madrid.

Lopopolo M. et al. 2025. Pre-European contact leprosy in the Americas and its current persistence. Science 389(6758). https://doi.org/10.1126/science.adu7144.

Lorentz K.O. and Casa B. 2020. First metacarpal fractures from Chalcolithic Cyprus: a fall or a fist? Int J Osteoarchaeol 30:712–735. https://doi.org/10.1002/oa.2905.

Lorkiewicz W. et al. 2019. Osteoporotic bone fractures and age-related bone loss in males inhabiting the Kujawy region in north-central Poland from the Neolithic to early modern times. J Archaeol Sci 103(March): 16–25.

Lorrio A.J. 2010. Enterramientos infantiles en el oppidum en El Mólón (Camporrobles, Valencia) [Children's burials at the oppidum at El Mólón]. Cuadernos de Arqueología de la Universidad de Navarra 18:201–262.

Loveland C.J., Gregg J.B., and Bass W.M. 1984. Osteochondritis dissecans from the Great Plains of north America. Plains Anthrop 105:239–246.

Lovell N.C. 1997. Trauma analysis in paleopathology. Yearbook of Physical Anthropology 40:139–70.

Lovell N.C. and Grauer A.L. 2019. Analysis and interpretation of trauma in skeletal remains. In: Biological anthropology of the human skeleton. 3rd edition, ed. M.A. Katzenberg and A.L. Grauer, 335–383. Wiley-Blackwell.

Lucero-Prisno D.E. et al. 2023. Top 10 public health challenges to track in 2023: shifting focus beyond a global pandemic. Public Health Chall 2:e86. https://doi.org/10.1002/puh2.86.

Lugli F. et al. 2019. Strontium and stable isotope evidence of human mobility strategies across the Last Glacial Maximum in southern Italy. Nat Ecol Evol 3:905–911. https://doi.org/10.1038/s41559-019-0900-8.

Lukacs J.R. 1989. Dental paleopathology: methods for reconstructing dietary patterns. In: Reconstruction of life from the skeleton, ed. M.Y. Iscan and K.A.R. Kennedy, 261–286. Alan Liss.

Lukacs J.R. 1995. The 'caries correction factor': a new method of calibrating dental caries rates to compensate for antemortem loss of teeth. Int J Osteoarchaeol 5:151–156.

Lukacs J.R. 2007. Dental trauma and antemortem tooth loss in prehistoric Canary Islanders: prevalence and contributing factors. Int J Osteoarchaeol 17:157–173. https://doi.org/10.1002/oa.864.

Lukacs J.R. 2011. Sex differences in dental caries experience: clinical evidence, complex etiology. Clin Oral Investig 15(5): 649–656. https://doi.org/10.1007/s00784-010-0445-3.

Lukacs J.R. and Largaespada LL. 2011. Explaining sex differences in dental caries prevalence: saliva, hormones, and 'life-history' etiologies. Am J Hum Biol 18:540–555.

Lukacs J.R. and Walimbe S.R. 1998. Physiological stress in prehistoric India: new data on localized hypoplasia of primary canines linked to climate and subsistence change. J Archaeol Sci 25:571–585.

Luna L.H. et al. 2020. Oldest evidence of tuberculosis in Argentina: a multidisciplinary investigation in an adult male skeleton from Saujil, Tinogasta, Catamarca (905–1030 CE). Tuberculosis 125:101995. https://doi.org/10.1016/j.tube.2020.101995.

Lundin N. et al. 2021. Epidemiology and mortality of pelvic and femur fractures—a nationwide register study of 417,840 fractures in Sweden across 16 years: diverging trends for potentially lethal fractures. Acta Orthop 92(3): 323–328. https://doi.org/10.1080/17453674.2021.1878329.

Lurie M.B. 1955. A pathogenetic relationship between tuberculosis and leprosy: the common denominators in the tissue response to mycobacteria. In: CIBA Foundation symposium on experimental tuberculosis, 340–343. Little, Brown.

Lurie S. and Glezerman M. 2003. The history of Cesarean technique. Am J Obstet Gynecol 189(6): 1803–1806.

Lux M.K. 2016. Separate beds: a history of Indian hospitals in Canada, 1920s–1980s. University of Toronto Press.

Lyall H. and Mann G. 1993. Diaphyseal aclasis in citizens of ancient Jerico. Int J Osteoarchaeol 3:233–240.

Lynnerup N. 2019. Mummies and palaeopathology. In: Ortner's identification of pathological conditions in human skeletal remains, ed. J.E. Buikstra, 799–807. Academic Press.

Lynnerup N. and Klaus H.D. 2019. Fundamentals of human bone, and dental biology: structure, function, and development. In: Ortner's identification of pathological conditions in human skeletal remains, ed. J.E. Buikstra, 35–58. Academic Press.

Ma K.-W. 2000. Hare-lip surgery in the history of traditional Chinese medicine. Med Hist 44:489–512.

Ma Y. et al. 2023. Racial/ethnic disparities in $PM_{2.5}$-attributable cardiovascular mortality burden in the United States. Nat Hum Behav 7:2074–2083. https://doi.org/10.1038/s41562-023-01694-7.

Maas A.I.R. et al. 2022. Traumatic brain injury: progress and challenges in prevention, clinical care, and research. Lancet Neurol 21(11): 1004–1060. https://doi.org/10.1016/S1474-4422(22)00309-X.

Maat G.J.R. 1982. Scurvy in Dutch whalers buried at Spitsbergen. In: Proceedings of the 4th European Meeting of the Paleopathology Association, Middelberg/Antwerpen, 82–93.

Maat G.J.R. 2004. Scurvy in adults and youngsters: the Dutch experience; a review of the history and pathology of a disregarded disease. Int J Osteoarchaeol 14:77–81.

Maat G.J.R. and Baig M. 1991. Scanning electron microscopy of fossilised sickle cells. Int J Anthrop 5(3): 271–276.

Maat G.J.R. and Uytterschaut H.T. 1984. Microscopic observations on scurvy in Dutch whalers buried at Spitsbergen. In: Proceedings of the Paleopathology Association 5th European Meeting, 1984, Siena, 211–216.

Machado M.P. et al. 2016. A wormian bone, mimicking an entry gunshot wound of the skull, in an anthropological specimen. J Forensic Sci 61(3): 855–857. https://doi.org/10.1111/1556-4029.13043.

Mackay I.R. 2010. Travels and travails of autoimmunity: a historical journey from discovery to rediscovery. Autoimmun Rev 9(5): A251–A258. https://doi.org/10.1016/j.autrev.2009.10.007.

Mackenzie J.S. and Jeggo M. 2019. The One Health approach: why is it so important? Trop Med Infect Dis 4(2): 88. https://doi.org/10.3390/tropicalmed4020088.

Mackenzie L., Radini A., and Speller C. 2018. Dental tartar. In: Lost lives, new voices: unlocking the stories of the Scottish soldiers from the Battle of Dunbar, ed. C.M. Gerrard, P. Graves, A. Millard, R. Annis, and A. Caffell, 98–99. Oxbow Books.

Mackenzie L., Speller C.F., Holst M., Keefe K., and Radini A. 2023. Dental calculus in the industrial age: human dental calculus in the post-medieval period, a case study from industrial Manchester. Quat Int 653–654:114–126. https://doi.org/10.1016/j.quaint.2021.09.020.

MacKinnon M. 2016. Diagnosing a possible case of juvenile idiopathic arthritis: a palaeopathology study from the Ishkeenickh River Cave Site. Int J Paleopathol 15:69–75.

Mader R. et al. 2017. Diffuse idiopathic skeletal hyperostosis (DISH): where we are now and where to go next. RMD Open 3(1). https://doi.org/10.1136%2Frmdopen-2017-000472.

Madhok R., Melton L.J. III, Atkinson E.J., O'Fallon W.M., and Lewallen D.G. 1993. Urban vs rural increase in hip fracture incidence: age and sex of 901 cases 1980–89 in Olmsted County, USA. Acta Orthop Scand 64(5): 543–548.

Magalhães B.M. 2018. When breathing is a burden: sinonasal variations and diseases affecting the human skull in three Portuguese identified osteological collections (19th–20th centuries). PhD dissertation, University of Coimbra, Portugal.

Magalhães B.M., Lopes C., and Santos A.L. 2017. Differentiating between rhinosinusitis and mastoiditis surgery from postmortem medical training: a study of two identified skulls and hospital records from early 20th century Coimbra, Portugal. Int J Paleopathol 17:10–17. https://doi.org/10.1016/j.ijpp.2017.03.002.

Magalhães B.M., Mays S., Stark S., and Santos A.L. 2023. A biocultural study of nasal fracture, violence, and gender using 19th–20th century skeletal remains from Portugal. Int J Osteoarchaeol 33(5): 858–867. https://doi.org/10.1002/oa.3233.

Magennis A.L.1990. Growth velocity as a factor influencing the formation of transverse lines. Am J Phys Anthropol 81(2): 262.

Magilton J.R., Lee F., and Boylston A., eds. 2008. 'Lepers outside the gate': excavations at the cemetery of the Hospital of St James and St Mary Magdalene, Chichester, 1986'87 and 1993. Council for British Archaeology Research Report 158 and Chichester Excavations vol. 10; Council for British Archaeology.

Magnússon, Þ. 1970. Skýrsla um Þjóðminjasafnið 1969 [Report from the Icelandic national museum 1969]. Árbók Hins Íslenzka Fornleifafélags 1969:127–146.

Mahone S. 2014. 'Hat on—hat off': Trauma and trepanation in Kisii, Western Kenya. J Eastern Afr Stud 8(3): 331–345. http://dx.doi.org/10.1080/17531055.2014.900959.

Mahoney P. 2006. Microwear and morphology: functional relationships between human dental microwear and the mandible. J Hum Evol 50:452–459. https://doi.org/10.1016/j.jhevol.2005.11.003.

Maixner F. et al. 2018. The Iceman's last meal consisted of fat, wild meat, and cereals. Curr Biol 28(14): 2348–2355.

Maixner F., Gresky J., and Zink A. 2021. Ancient DNA analysis of rare genetic bone disorders. Int J Paleopathol 33:182–187.

Majander K. et al. 2024. Redefining the treponemal history through pre-Columbian genomes from Brazil. Nature 627:182–188. https://doi.org/10.1038/s41586-023-06965-x.

Majno G. 1975. The healing hand: man and wound in the ancient world. Harvard University Press.

Manabe Y. et al. 2011. Nonmetric dental characteristics of the early modern population of Okinawa Island in Nansei Islands, Japan. Int J Osteoarchaeol 21:679–693.

Manchester K. 1978. Palaeopathology of a royalist garrison. Ossa 5:25–33.

Manchester K. 1980. Hydrocephalus in an Anglo-Saxon child. Arch Cantiana 96:77–82.

Manchester K. 1982. Spondylolysis and spondylolisthesis in two Anglo-Saxon skeletons. Paleopathol Newsl 37: 9–12.

Manchester K. 1984. Tuberculosis and leprosy in antiquity: an interpretation. Med Hist 28(2): 162–173. https://doi.org/10.1017/S0025727300035705.

Manchester K. 1991. Tuberculosis and leprosy: evidence for interaction of disease. In: Human paleopathology: current syntheses and future options, ed. D. Ortner and A. Aufderheide, 23–35. Smithsonian Institution Press.

Manchester K. 1994. Rhinomaxillary lesions in syphilis: differential diagnosis. In: L'origine de la syphilis en Europe: avant ou après 1493?, ed. O. Dutour, G. Pálfi, J. Bérato and J.-P. Brun, 79–80. Centre Archéologique du Var, Éditions Errance.

Manchester K. 2002. Infective bone changes of leprosy. In: The past and present of leprosy: archaeological, historical, palaeopathological and clinical approaches, ed. C.A. Roberts, M.E. Lewis, and K. Manchester, 69–72. British Archaeological Reports International Series 1054. Archaeopress.

Manchester K. and Elmhirst O.E.C. 1980. Forensic aspects of an Anglo-Saxon injury. Ossa 7:179–188.

Manchester K. and Knüsel C. 1994. A medieval sculpture of leprosy in the Cistercian Abbaye de Cadouin. Med Hist 38(2): 204–206.

Manchester K., Ogden A., and Storm R. 2016. Nomenclature in palaeopathology. https://paleopathology-association.wildapricot.org/resources/Documents/PPA%20Monographs/Nomenclature%20in%20Palaeopathology%20Web%20Document.pdf.

Manes C. 2013. Out of the shadow of leprosy: the Carville letters and stories of the Landry family. University Press of Mississippi.

Mank E., de Boer H.H., Versluis J.M., Oostra R.J., and van der Merwe A.E. 2023. Microcephaly as observed in the late 19th century cemetery of the Meerenberg psychiatric hospital: diagnostic issues and the value of population-specific data. Int J Osteoarchaeol 3 (1): 128–135.

Mann R.W. and Owsley D.W. 1989. Anatomy of uncorrected talipes equinovarus in a fifteenth century American Indian. J Am Podiatric Med Assoc 79(9): 436–440.

Mann R.W., Sledzik P.S., Owsley D.W., and Droulette M.R. 1990. Radiographic examination of Chinese foot binding. J Am Podiatric Med Assoc 80(8): 405–409.

Mansilla J. and Pijoan C.M. 1995. Brief communication: a case of congenital syphilis during the colonial period in Mexico City. Am J Phys Anthropol 97:187–195.

Mansukoski L. and Sparacello V.S. 2018. Smaller long bone cross-sectional size in people who died of tuberculosis: insights on frailty factors from a 19th and early 20th century Finnish population. Int J Paleopathol 20:38–44. https://doi.org/10.1016/j.ijpp.2017.12.005.

Mant M. 2019. Time after time: individuals with multiple fractures and injury recidivists in long eighteenth-century (c. 1666–1837) London. Int J Paleopathol 24:7–18. https://doi.org/10.1016/j.ijpp.2018.08.003.

Mant M., de la Cova C., and Brickley M.B. 2021. Intersectionality and trauma analysis in bioarchaeology. Am J Phys Anthropol 174 (4): 583–594.

Mant M., Pitre M., Dancer S., and Gatto M. 2024. A case of rheumatoid arthritis in a Nubian woman from the site of Sheikh Mohamed, near Aswan, Egypt. Int J Paleopathol 44:8–84.

Mant M. and Roberts C.A. 2014. Diet, sex and status in post-medieval London. Int J Hist Archaeol 19:188–207.

Manzi G., Sperduit A., and Passarello P. 1991. Behavior-induced auditory exostoses in Imperial Roman society: evidence from coeval urban and rural communities near Rome. Am J Phys Anthropol 85:253–260.

Mao J.J. et al. 2021. Integrative oncology: addressing the global challenges of cancer prevention and treatment. CA: A Cancer Journal for Clinicians 72(2):144–164.

Marchetti A., Pelligrini S., Bevilacqua G., and Fornaciari G. 1996. K-ras mutation of the tumour of Ferrante I of Aragon, King of Naples. Lancet 347:1272.

Marcombe D. and Manchester K. 1990. The Melton Mowbray 'leper head': an historical and medical investigation. Med Hist 34:86–91.

Marden K. and Ortner D.J. 2011. A case of treponematosis from pre-Columbian Chaco Canyon, New Mexico. Int J Osteoarchaeol 21:19–31.

Margerison B. and Knüsel C. 2002. Paleodemographic comparison of a catastrophic and attritional death assemblage. Am J Phys Anthrop 119:134–143.

Marine M.B. and Forbes-Amrhein M.M. 2021. Fractures of child abuse. Pediatr Radiol 51:1003–1013. https://doi.org/10.1007/s00247-020-04945-1.

Mariotti V. et al. 2015. Skeletal evidence of tuberculosis in a modern identified human skeletal collection (Certosa cemetery, Bologna, Italy). Am J Phys Anthropol 157:389–401.

Mark S.E. 2002. Alexander the Great, seafaring, and the spread of leprosy. J Hist Med Allied Sci 57 (3): 285–311. https://www.muse.jhu.edu/article/15345.

Marklein K.E., and Crews D.E. 2022. Highs and lows of frailty: skeletal frailty differentials among socioeconomic groups in post-medieval London. Archaeol Anthropol Sci 14(3): 43.

Marklein K.E., Leahy R.E., and Crews D.E. 2016. In sickness and in death: assessing frailty in human skeletal remains. Am J Phys Anthropol 161(2): 208–225.

Marks M. and Mabey D. 2020. Syphilis and the endemic treponematoses. In: Hunter's tropical medicine and emerging infectious diseases, 10th edition, ed. E.T. Ryan, D.R. Hill, T. Solomon, N.E. Aronson, and T.P. Endy, 534–540. Elsevier. https://doi.org/10.1016/B978-0-323-55512-8.00057-0.

Marks M., Mitjà O., Solomon A.W., Asiedu K.B., and Mabey D.C. 2015. Yaws. *Br Med Bull* 113: 91–100.

Marks M., Solomon A.W., and Mabey D.C. 2014. Endemic treponemal diseases. Trans R Soc Trop Med Hyg 108(10): 601–607. https://doi.org/10.1093/trstmh/tru128.

Marmot M. 2015. The health gap: the challenge of an unequal world. Bloomsbury.

Marques C. 2019. Tumors of bone. In: Ortner's identification of pathological conditions in human skeletal remains, ed. J.E Buikstra, 639–717. Academic Press.

Marques C., Compton Z., and Boddy A.M. 2022. Connecting palaeopathology and evolutionary medicine to cancer research: past and present. In: Palaeopathology and evolutionary medicine: an integrated approach, ed. K.A. Plomp, C.A. Roberts, S. Elton, and G.R. Bentley, 239–260. Oxford University Press.

Marques C., Matos V., Costa T., Zink A., and Cunha E. 2018. Absence of evidence or evidence of absence? A discussion on paleoepidemiology of neoplasms with contributions from two Portuguese human skeletal reference collections (19th–20th century). Int J Paleopathol 21:83–95.

Marques C., Matos V., and Meinzer N.J. 2019. Proliferative periosteal reactions: assessment of trends in Europe over the past two millennia. In: The backbone of Europe: health, diet, work and violence over two millennia, ed. R.H. Steckel, C.S. Larsen, C.A. Roberts, and J. Baten, 137–174. Cambridge University Press.

Marques C., Roberts C., Matos V.M., and Buikstra J.E. 2021. Cancers as rare diseases: terminological, theoretical, and methodological biases. Int J Paleopathol 32:111–122.

Márquez-Grant N. and Fibiger L., eds. 2011. The Routledge handbook of archaeological human remains and legislation. Routledge.

Márquez-Grant N. et al. 2022. How do drugs affect the skeleton? Implications for forensic anthropology. Biology (Basel) 11(4): 524. https://doi.org/10.3390/biology11040524.

Marshall J.S., Warrington R., Watson W., and Kim H.L. 2018. An introduction to immunology and immunopathology. Allergy Asthma Clin Immunol 14(Suppl 2): 49. https://doi.org/10.1186/s13223-018-0278-1.

Martensen R.L. 2004. The brain takes shape: an early history. Oxford University Press.

Martin C. 2023. Histories of medieval plague in Renaissance Italy. J Hist Med Allied Sci 78(2): 131–148. http://dx.doi.org/10.1093/jhmas/jrad001.

Martin D.L. and Frayer D.W., eds. 1997. Troubled times: violence and warfare in the past. Routledge.

Martin D.L. and Harrod R.P. 2015. Bioarchaeological contributions to the study of violence. Am J Phys Anthropol 156:116–145. https://doi.org/10.1002/ajpa.22662.

Martin D.L., Harrod R.P., and Fields M. 2010. Beaten down and worked to the bone: bioarchaeological investigations of women and violence in the ancient southwest. Landscapes of Violence 1(1): 3. https://scholarworks.umass.edu/lov/vol1/iss1/3.

Martin D.L., Harrod R.P., and Pérez V.R. 2013. Bioarchaeology: an integrated approach to working with human remains. Springer.

Martinez L. et al. 2019. Detection, survival and infectious potential of *Mycobacterium tuberculosis* in the environment: a review of the evidence and epidemiological implications. Eur Respir J 53(6): 1802302. https://doi.org/10.1183/13993003.02302-2018.

Martini E. 2002. Jacques Cartier witnesses a treatment for scurvy. Vesalius 8(1): 2–6.

Martini M., Bifulco M., Orsini D. 2022. Smallpox vaccination and vaccine hesitancy in the Kingdom of the Two Sicilies (1801) and the great modernity of Ferdinand IV of Bourbon: a glimpse of the past in the era of the SARS-COV-2 (COVID-19) pandemic. Public Health 213:47–53. doi: 10.1016/j.puhe.2022.09.012.

Martini M., Gazzaniga V., Behzadifar M., Bragazzi N.L., and Barberis I. 2018. The history of tuberculosis: the social role of sanatoria for the treatment of tuberculosis in Italy between the end of the 19th century and the middle of the 20th. J Prev Med Hyg 59(4): E323–E327. https://doi.org/10.15167/2421-4248/jpmh2018.59.4.1103.

Masiu R., Pedersen D.D., Hill L., and Steyn M. 2023. The association between skeletal lesions and tuberculosis in a pre-antibiotic South African sample. Int J Paleopathol 40:20–32. https://doi.org/10.1016/j.ijpp.2022.11.001.

Massler M., Schour J., and Poncher H. 1941. Development pattern of the child as reflected in the calcification pattern of the teeth. Am J Dis Child 62:33–67.

Masnicová S. and Beňus R. 2003. Developmental anomalies in skeletal remains from the Great Moravia and Middle Ages cemeteries at Devin (Slovakia). Int J Osteoarchaeol 13:266–274.

Masson M. et al. 2013. Osteological and biomolecular evidence of a 7000-year-old case of hypertrophic pulmonary osteopathy secondary to tuberculosis from Neolithic Hungary. PLoS One. https://doi.org/10.1371/journal.pone.0078252.

Masters E.A. et al. 2022. Skeletal infections: microbial pathogenesis, immunity and clinical management. Nat Rev Microbiol 20:385–400. https://doi.org/10.1038/s41579-022-00686-0.

Mastroiacovo P. et al.1999. Congenital malformations in twins: an international study. Am J Med Genet 83(2): 117–124.

Mathews C.J., Weston V.C., Jones A., Field M., and Coakley G. 2010. Bacterial septic arthritis in adults. Lancet 375(9717): 846–855.

Matić U. and Jensen B., eds. 2017. Archaeologies of gender and violence. Oxbow Books. https://doi.org/10.2307/j.ctvh1dp2p.

Matos V. 2009a. Broken ribs: paleopathological analysis of costal fractures in the human identified skeletal collection from the Museu Bocage, Lisbon, Portugal (late 19th to middle 20th centuries). Am J Phys Anthropol 140(1): 25–38. https://doi.org/10.1002/ajpa.21032.

Matos V.M.J. 2009b. Odiagnóstico retrospective da lepra: Complimentaridade clínica e paleopatológica no arquivo médico do Hospital-Colónia Rovisco Pais (Século X. X., Tocha, Portugal) e na Colecção de Esqueletos da Leprosaria Medieval de St Jørgen's (Odense, Dinamarca) [The retrospective diagnosis of leprosy: clinical and paleopathological complementarities in the medical files from the Rovisco Pais Hospital-Colony (20th Century, Tocha, Portugal) and in the skeletal collection from the medieval leprosarium of St. Jørgen's (Odense, Denmark)]. PhD dissertation, Universidade de Coimbra, Faculdade de Ciências e Technologia, Coimbra.

Matos V. and Santos A.L. 2006. On the trail of pulmonary tuberculosis based on rib lesions: results from the human identified skeletal collection from the Museu Bocage (Lisbon, Portugal). Am J Phys Anthropol 130:190–200. https://doi.org/10.1002/ajpa.20309.

Matos V.M.J. and Santos A.L. 2013. Leprogenic odontodysplasia: new evidence from the Jørgen's medieval leprosarium cemetery (Odense, Denmark). Anthropol Sci 121:43–47.

Mattei T. and Rehman A. 2014. Schmorl's nodes: current pathophysiological, diagnostic and therapeutic paradigms. Neurosurg Rev 37:39–46.

Mattingly D. and Foster S. 2023. This is archaeology: impacting heritage, landscapes and lives. Br Archaeol 188(Jan–Feb): 44–51.

Maurer A.F. et al. 2019. Testing LA-ICP-MS analysis of archaeological bones with different diagenetic histories for paleodiet prospect. Palaeogeogr Palaeoclimatol Palaeoecol 534:109287. https://doi.org/10.1016/j.palaeo.2019.109287.

Mavroforou A., Malizos K., Karachalios T., Chatzitheofilou K., and Giannoukas A.D. 2014. Punitive limb amputation. Clin Orthop Related Res 472(10): 3102–3106. https://dx.doi.org/10.1007/s11999-014-3480-6.

May H., Peled N., Dar G., Abbas J., and Hershkovitz I. 2011. Hyperostosis frontalis interna: what does it tell us about our health? Am J Hum Biol 23(3): 392–397.

May W.P. 1897. Rheumatoid arthritis (osteitis deformans) affecting bones 5500 years old. Br Med J 2:1631–1632.

Maymone M.B.C. et al. 2020. Leprosy: clinical aspects and diagnostic techniques, J Am Acad Dermatol 83:1–14. https://doi.org/10.1016/j.jaad.2019.12.080.

Mays S. 1993. Infanticide in Roman Britain. Antiquity 67:883–888.

Mays S. 1996a. Healed limb amputations in human osteoarchaeology and their causes: a case study from Ipswich. Int J Osteoarchaeol 6:101–113.

Mays S. 1996b. Age-dependent cortical bone loss in a medieval population. Int J Osteoarchaeol 6:144–154.

Mays S. 2006. A palaeopathological study of Colles' fracture. Int J Osteoarchaeol 16(5): 415–428.

Mays S. 2007a. Spondylolysis in non-adult skeletons excavated from a medieval rural archaeological site in England. Int J Osteoarchaeol 17(5): 504–513.

Mays S. 2007b. Lysis at the anterior vertebral body margin: evidence for brucellar spondylitis? Int J Osteoarchaeol 17(2): 107–118. https://doi.org/10.1002/oa.903.

Mays S. 2010. The archaeology of human bones. Routledge.

Mays S. 2012. Nasal septal deviation in a mediaeval population. Am J Phys Anthropol 148:319–326. https://doi.org/10.1002/ajpa.22046.

Mays S. 2015. Age-associated reduction in cortical bone in males, trends from the third century AD to the present day. Calcif Tissue Int 96:370–371.

Mays S. 2016. Bone-formers and bone-losers in an archaeological population. Am J Phys Anthropol 159(4): 577–584.

Mays S. 2018. How should we diagnose disease in palaeopathology? Some epistemological considerations. Int J Paleopathol 20:12–19.

Mays S. 2023. The macroscopic study of human skeletal pathology. In: The Routledge handbook of paleopathology, ed. A.L. Grauer, 19–42. Routledge.

Mays S. and Beattie O. 2015. Evidence for end-stage cannibalism on Sir John Franklin's last expedition to the Arctic, 1845. Int J Osteoarchaeol 26(5): 778–786. https://doi.org/10.1002/oa.2479.

Mays S., Brickley M., and Ives R. 2009a. Growth and vitamin D deficiency in a population from 19th century Birmingham, England. Int J Osteoarchaeol 19 (3): 406–415.

Mays S., Crane-Kramer G, and Bayliss A. 2003. Two probable cases of treponemal disease of medieval date from England. Am J Phys Anthropol 120:133–143.

Mays S. and Eyers J. 2011. Perinatal infant death at the Roman villa site at Hambleden, Buckinghamshire, England. J Archaeol Sci 38:1931–1938.
Mays S. and Faerman M. 2001. Sex identification in some putative infanticide victims from Roman Britain using ancient DNA. J Archaeol Sci 28:555–559.
Mays S., Harding C., and Heighway C. 2007. The churchyard. Wharram. A study of settlement on the Yorkshire Wolds XI. York University Publications 13. English Heritage.
Mays S. and Holst M. 2006. Palaeo-otology of cholesteatoma. Int J Osteoarchaeol 16:1–15. https://doi.org/10.1002/oa.801.
Mays S., Ives R., and Brickley M. 2009b. The effects of socioeconomic status on endochondral and appositional bone growth, and acquisition of cortical bone in children from 19th century Birmingham, England. Am J Phys Anthropol 140(3): 410–416.
Mays S., Lees B., and Stevenson J.C. 1998. Age-dependent bone loss in the femur in a medieval population. Int J Osteoarchaeol 8:97–106.
Mays S., Zakrzewski S., and Field S. 2022. The relationship between dental wear and age at death in British archaeological human skeletal remains: a re-evaluation of the 'Brothwell chart.' J Archaeol Sci: Rep 46:103707. https://doi.org/10.1016/j.jasrep.2022.103707.
Mbouaka A.L. et al. 2021. The elusive parasite: comparing macroscopic, immunological, and genomic approaches to identifying malaria in human skeletal remains from Sayala, Egypt (third to sixth centuries AD). Archaeol Anthropol Sci 13:115. https://doi.org/10.1007/s12520-021-01350-z.
McAllister J.P II. 2012. Pathophysiology of congenital and neonatal hydrocephalus. SeminFetal Neonat Med 17(5): 285–294.
McFadden C. 2021. The past, present and future of skeletal analysis in palaeodemography. Philos Trans R Soc Lond B Biol Sci 376:20190709. https://doi.org/10.1098/rstb.2019.0709.
McGivern L., Shulman L., Carney J.K., Shapiro S., and Bundock E. 2017. Death certification errors and the effect on mortality statistics. Public Health Rep 132(6): 669–675. https://doi.org/10.1177/0033354917736514.
McKeown T. 1988. The origins of human disease. Oxford University Press.
McKinley J.I. 1994. Spong Hill Part VIII: the cremations. East Dereham, East Anglian Archaeology 69.
McKinley J.I. 2000. The analysis of cremated bone. In: Human osteology, ed. M. Cox and S. Mays, 403–421. Greenwich Medical Media.
McNeill W.H. 1976. Plagues and peoples. Anchor Books.
Meinzer N.J., Steckel, R.H., and Baten J. 2019. Agricultural specialization, urbanization, workload, and stature. In: The backbone of Europe: health, diet, work and violence over two millennia, ed. R.H. Steckel, C.S. Larsen, C.A. Roberts, and J. Baten, 231–252. Cambridge University Press.
Mendes M.M., Charlton K., Thakur S., Ribeiro H., and Lanham-New S.A. 2020. Future perspectives in addressing the global issue of vitamin D deficiency. Proc Nutr Soc 79(2): 246–251.
Menéndez-Bueyes L.R. and Soler Fernández M.D. 2017. Paget's disease of bone: approach to its historical origins. Reumatol Clin 13(2): 66–72. https://doi.org/10.1016/j.reuma.2016.02.008.
Merbs C.F. 1983. Patterns of activity induced pathology in a Canadian Inuit population. Archaeological Survey of Canada Paper no. 119. National Museums of Canada.
Merbs C.F. 1989. Trauma. In: Reconstruction of life from the skeleton, ed. M.Y. Iscan and K.A.R. Kennedy, 161–189. Alan Liss.
Merbs C. 2004. Sagittal clefting of the body and other vertebral developmental errors in Canadian Inuit skeletons. Am J Phys Anthropol 123:236–249.
Merbs C.F. 2002. Asymmetrical spondylolysis. Am. J. Phys. Anthrop. 119: 156–174.
Merrett D.C. et al. 2016. Enamel hypoplasia in northeast China: evidence from Houtaomuga. Quat Int 405(B): 11–21. https://doi.org/10.1016/j.quaint.2015.06.004.
Merrett D. and Pfeiffer S. 2000. Maxillary sinusitis as an indicator of respiratory health in past populations. Am J Phys Anthrop 111:301–318.
Messina C. et al. 2022. Evidence of possible lower limb amputation in a tomb in an ancient Egyptian necropolis: the case report of an on-site radiographic analysis. BJR Case Rep 8 (6): 20220090. https://doi.org/10.1259/bjrcr.20220090.
Metzler I. 2006. Disability in medieval Europe: thinking about physical impairment during the High Middle Ages c. 1100–1400. Routledge.

Meyer A., and Steyn M. 2016. Chinese indentured mine labour and the dangers associated with early 20th-century deep-level mining on the Witwatersrand Gold Mines, South Africa. Int J Osteoarchaeol 26:648–660. https://doi.org/ 10.1002/oa.2455.

Meyer C. et al. 2018. Early Neolithic executions indicated by clustered cranial trauma in the mass grave of Halberstadt. Nat Commun 9:2472. https://doi.org/10.1038/s41467-018-04773-w.

Meyer-Rochow V.B. 2009. Food taboos: their origins and purposes. J Ethnobiol Ethnomed 5:18: https://doi.org/10.1186/1746-4269-5-18.

Michel M. et al. 2024. Ancient Plasmodium genomes shed light on the history of human malaria. Nature 631:125–133. https://doi.org/10.1038/s41586-024-07546-2.

Michou L. and Orcel P. 2019. Has Paget's bone disease become rare? Joint Bone Spine 86(5): 538–541.

Milella M., Belcastro M.G., Zollikofer C.P.E., Mariotti V. 2012. The effect of age, sex and physical activity on entheseal morphology in a contemporary Italian skeletal collection. Am J Phys Anthropol 148:379–388.

Milella M. et al. 2021 Troubles in Tuva: patterns of perimortem trauma in a nomadic community from Southern Siberia (second to fourth c. CE). Am J Phys Anthropol 174:3–19. https://doi.org/10.1002/ajpa.24142.

Miles A.E.W. 1994. Non-union of the epiphysis of the acromion in the skeletal remains of a Scottish population of ca. 1700. Int J Osteoarcheol 4:149–163.

Miliauskienė Ž. and Jankauskas R. 2015. Social differences in oral health: dental status of individuals buried in and around Trakai Church in Lithuania (16th–17th C). Anthropologischer Anzeiger 72(1): 89–106. https://doi.org/10.1127/anthranz/2014/0407.

Millard A.R. et al. 2020. Scottish soldiers from the Battle of Dunbar 1650: a prosopographical approach to a skeletal assemblage. PLoS One 15(12): e0243369. https://doi.org/10.1371/journal.pone.0243369.

Miller E., Ragsdale B.D., and Ortner D.J. 1996. Accuracy in dry bone diagnosis: a comment on palaeopathological methods. Int J Osteoarchaeol 6:221–229.

Millett M. and Gowland R. 2015. Infant and child burial rites in Roman Britain: a study from East Yorkshire. Britannia 46:171–189.

Milner G.R., Boldsen J.L., Weise S., Lauritsen J.M., and Freund U.H. 2015. Sex-related risks of trauma in medieval to early modern Denmark, and its relationship to change in interpersonal violence over time. Int J Paleopathol 9:59–68.

Milstein M.S. et al. 2020. An ethnographic approach to characterizing potential pathways of zoonotic disease transmission from wild meat in Guyana. EcoHealth 17:424–436. https://doi.org/10.1007/s10393-021-01513-3.

Min K.B. and Min J.Y. 2017. Increased risk for hyperuricemia in adults sensitized to cow milk allergen. Clin Rheumatol 36:1407–1412. Missios S. 2007. Hippocrates, Galen, and the uses of trepanation in the ancient classical world. Neurosurg Focus 23(1): E11. https://doi.org/10.3171/foc.2007.23.1.11.

Miszkiewicz J.J. 2015. Histology of a Harris line in a human distal tibia. J Bone Miner Metab 33:462–466.

Miszkiewicz J.J. et al. 2021. Bone loss markers in the earliest Pacific Islanders. Sci Rep 11(1): 3981. https://doi.org/10.1038/s41598-021-83264-3.

Mitchell P.D. 2017. Improving the use of historical written sources in paleopathology. Int J Paleopathol 18:88–95.

Mitchell P. and Brickley M., eds. 2017. Updated guidelines to the standards for recording human remains. Reading, BABAO and CIfA, 44–47; and a longer, expanded document at https://durham-repository.worktribe.com/output/1653844.

Mitchell P. and Redfern R. 2008. Diagnostic criteria for developmental dislocation of the hip in human skeletal remains. Int J Osteoarchaeol 18:61–71.

Mitchell P.D. 2013. The origins of human parasites: exploring the evidence for endoparasitism throughout human evolution. Int J Paleopathol 3(3): 191–198. https://doi.org/10.1016/j.ijpp.2013.08.003.

Mitchell P.D. et al. 2021. The prevalence of cancer in Britain before industrialization. Cancer 127(17): 3054–3059.

Mittal M., Gupta P., Kalra S. Bantwal G., and Mahendra K. 2021. Short stature: understanding the stature of ethnicity in height determination. Indian J Endocrinol Metab 25(5): 381–388. https://doi.org/10.4103/ijem.ijem_197_21.

Modell B. et al. 2018. Congenital disorders: epidemiological methods for answering calls for action. J Community Genet 9(4): 335–340.

Moghaddam N. et al. 2015. Survival after trepanation; early cranial surgery from late Iron Age Switzerland. Int J Paleopathol 11:56–65. https://doi.org/10.1016/j.ijpp.

Mogle P. and Zias J. 1995. Trephination as a possible treatment for scurvy in a Middle Bronze Age (ca. 2200 BC) skeleton. Int J Osteoarchaeol 5:77–81.

Møller P. and Møller-Christensen V. 1952. A mediaeval female skull showing evidence of metastases from a malignant growth. Acta Path Microbiol Scand 30:336–342.

Møller-Christensen V. 1953. Ten lepers from Naestved. Danish Science Press.

Møller-Christensen V. 1961. Bone changes in leprosy. Munksgaard.

Møller-Christensen V. 1969a. A rosary bead as tooth filling in a human mandibular canine tooth: a unique case from the Danish Middle Ages. Presented at the 21st International Congress of the History of Medicine, Siena. Atti del Congresso Internazionale di Storia Dela Medicina, Siena (Italia) Settembre 22–28, 1968, pp. 800–811.

Møller-Christensen V. 1969b. Provisional results of the examination of the whole Naestved Leprosy Hospital Churchyard—ab. 1250–1550 A.D. Nordisk Medicinhistorik Årsbok Part 4: 29–36.

Møller-Christensen V. 1978. Leprosy changes of the skull. Odense University Press.

Møller-Christensen V. and Inkster RG. 1965. Cases of leprosy and syphilis in the osteological collection of the Department of Anatomy, University of Edinburgh, with a note on the skull of Robert the Bruce. Danish Med Bull 12:11–18.

Molleson T. 1989. Seed preparation in the Mesolithic: the osteological evidence. Antiquity 63:356–362.

Molnar P. 2008. Dental wear and oral pathology: possible evidence and consequences of habitual use of teeth in a Swedish Neolithic sample. Am J Phys Anthropol 136:423–431. https://doi.org/10.1002/ajpa.20824.

Molto J. E. 1990. Differential diagnosis of rib lesions: a case study from Middle Woodland, southern Ontario. Am J Phys Anthropol 83:439–447.

Molto J.E. 2002. Leprosy in Roman period skeletons from Kellis 2, Dahkleh, Egypt. In: The past and present of leprosy: archaeological, historical, palaeopathological and clinical approaches, ed. C.A. Roberts, M.E. Lewis, and K. Manchester, 179–192. British Archaeological Reports International Series 1054. Archaeopress.

Molto J.E. and Kirkpatrick C.L. 2018. How short is short, and why? A probable case of proportionate dwarfism from Egypt's third intermediate period in the Dakhleh Oasis, Egypt. Int J Osteoarchaeol 28(1): 3–17.

Monot M. et al. 2005. On the origin of leprosy. Science 308(5724): 1040–1042.

Monot M. et al. 2009. Comparative genomic and phylogeographic analysis of *Mycobacterium leprae*. Nat Genet **41**:1282–1289.

Montgomery J., Evans J.A., Chenery S.R., Pashley V., and Killgrove K. 2010. 'Gleaming, white and deadly': using lead to track human exposure and geographic origins in the Roman period in Britain. Journal of Roman Archaeology Suppl 78:199–226.

Montiel R. et al. 2012. Neonate human remains: a window of opportunity to the molecular study of ancient syphilis. PLoS One 7(5): e36371. https://doi.org/10.1371/journal.pone.0036371.

Moodie R.L. 1923a. Paleopathology: an introduction to the study of ancient evidences of disease. University of Illinois Press.

Moodie R.L. 1923b. The antiquity of disease. Chicago University Press.

Moodie R.L. 1927. Injuries to the head among the pre-Columbian Peruvians. Ann Mediev Hist 9(3): 277–307.

Moodley K. et al. 2022. Ethics and governance challenges related to genomic data sharing in southern Africa: the case of SARS-Cov-2. Lancet Glob Health 10(12): e1855–e1859. https://doi.org/10.1016/S2214-109X(22)00417-X.

Moore J. and Buckberry J. 2016. The use of corsetry to treat Pott's disease of the spine from 19th century Wolverhampton, England. Int J Paleopathol 14:74–80. doi.org/10.1016/j.

Moore J. et al. 2020. A multi-isotope (C, N, O, Sr, Pb) study of Iron Age and Roman period skeletons from east Edinburgh, Scotland exploring the relationship between decapitation burials and geographical origins. J Archaeol Sci: Rep 29:102075. https://doi.org/10.1016/j.jasrep.2019.102075.

Moore K. and Persaud T. 2007. The developing human: clinically orientated embryology. Saunders.
Moore K., Persaud T., and Torcia M. 2019. The developing human: clinically orientated embryology, 11th ed. Saunders.
Moore W.J. and Corbett E. 1975. Distribution of dental caries in ancient British populations III: the 17th century. Caries Res 9:163–175.
Mora C. et al. 2022. Over half of known human pathogenic diseases can be aggravated by climate change. Nat Clim Chang 12:869–875. https://doi.org/10.1038/s41558-022-01426-1.
Moreno E. 2014. Retrospective and prospective perspectives on zoonotic brucellosis. Front Microbiol 5:213. https://doi.org/10.3389/fmicb.2014.00213.
Morgan B., Prakash K., Mayberry J.C., and Brickley M.B. 2022. Thoracic trauma: clinical and paleopathological perspectives. Int J Paleopathol 39:50–63. https://doi.org/10.1016/j.ijpp.
Morgan Jones M., Abrams D., and Lahiri A. 2020. Shape the future: how the social sciences, humanities and the arts can SHAPE a positive, post-pandemic future for peoples, economies and environments. J Br Acad 8:167–266. https://doi.org/10.5871/jba/008.167.
Mörgeli C. and Schulz S., 1996. Repeat caesarean delivery by the Zurich city wound physician Johann Jakob Locher 1817/18. Gesnerus 53(3–4): 194–216.
Morrow J.J., Newby J., Piombino-Mascali D., and Reinhard K.J. 2016. Taphonomic considerations for the analysis of parasites in archaeological materials. Int J Paleopathol 13:56–64. https://doi.org/10.1016/j.ijpp.2016.01.005.
Morse D., Brothwell D., and Ucko P. 1964. Tuberculosis in ancient Egypt. Am Rev Resp Dis 90:524–541.
Morse J. 1900. The frequency of rickets in infancy in Boston and vicinity. J Am Med Assoc 34(12): 724–726.
Mosekilde L. 1990. Consequences of the remodelling process for vertebral bone structure: an SEM study (uncoupling of loaded structures). Bone Miner 10:13–35.
Mukherjee S. 2010. The emperor of all maladies: a biography of cancer. Scribner.
Müldner G. 2018. Investigating medieval diet and society by stable isotope analysis of human bone. In: Reflections: 50 years of medieval archaeology, 1957–2007: No. 30, ed. R. Gilchrist and A. Reynolds, 327–346. Routledge.
Müldner G. and Richards M.P. 2007. Stable isotope evidence for 1500 years of human diet at the city of York, UK. Am J Phys Anthrop 133(1): 682–697.
Müldner G., Chenery C., and Eckardt H. 2011. The 'Headless Romans': multi-isotope investigations of an unusual burial ground from Roman Britain. J Archaeol Sci 38:280–290.
Müldner G. et al. 2009. Isotopes and individuals: diet and mobility among the medieval bishops of Whithorn. Antiquity 83:1119–33.
Mulhern D. 2005. A probable case of gigantism in a fifth dynasty skeleton from the western cemetery at Giza, Egypt. Int J Osteoarchaeol 15(4): 261–275.
Müller R., Roberts C.A., and Brown T.A. 2014. Biomolecular identification of ancient *Mycobacterium tuberculosis* complex DNA in human remains from Britain and continental Europe. Am J Phys Anthropol 153(2): 178–189.
Müller R., Roberts C.A., and Brown T.A. 2016. Complications in the study of ancient tuberculosis: presence of environmental bacteria in human archaeological remains. J Archaeol Sci 68:5–11.
Mummolo S. et al. 2020. Oral microbiota in mouth-breathing patients. J Oral Hyg Health 8:259. https://doi.org/10.4172/2332-0702.1000259.
Munizaga J., Allison M.J., Gerszten E., and Klurfeld D.M. 1975. Pneumoconiosis in Chilean miners of the 16th century. Bull New York Acad Med 5(11): 1281–1293.
Muñoz-Garach A., García-Fontana B., and Muñoz-Torres M. 2020. Nutrients and dietary patterns related to osteoporosis. Nutrients 12(7): 1986. https://doi.org/10.3390/nu12071986.
Munteanu O. et al. 2020. The etiopathogenic and morphological spectrum of anencephaly: a comprehensive review of literature. Rom J Morphol Embryol 61(2): 335–343.
Murphy E.M. 1996. A possible case of hydrocephalus in a medieval child from Doonbought Fort, Co. Antrim, Northern Ireland. Int J Osteoarchaeol 6:435–442.
Murphy E.M. 2000. Developmental defects and disability: the evidence from the Iron Age semi-nomadic peoples of Aymyrlyg, south Siberia. In: Madness, disability and social exclusion: the archaeology and anthropology of 'difference,' ed. J. Hubert, 60–80. Routledge.

Murphy E.M., Chistov Y.K., Hopkins R., Rutland P., and Taylor G.M. 2009. Tuberculosis among Iron Age individuals from Tyva, South Siberia: palaeopathological and biomolecular findings. J Archaeol Sci 36:2029–2038.

Murphy E.M., Gokhman I., Christov Y., and Barkova, L. 2002. Prehistoric Old World scalping: new cases from the cemetery of Aymyrlyg. Am J Archaeol 106:1–10.

Murphy K. 1999. A prehistoric case of polydactyly from the Iron Age site of Simbusenga, Zambia. Am J Phys Anthropol 108:311–319.

Murphy M. and McKenzie C. 2010. Multiple osteochondromas in the archaeological record: a global review. J Archaeol Sci 37:2255–2264.

Murphy M.F., Wainscoat J., and Colvin B.T. 2002. Haematological disease. In: Clinical medicine, 5th edition, ed. P. Kumar and M. Clark, 405–471. W.B. Saunders.

Murphy M.S. and Juengst S.L. 2020. Patterns of trauma across Andean South America: new discoveries and advances in interpretation. Int J Paleopathol 29:35–44. https://doi.org/10.1016/j.ijpp.2019.09.004.

Musallam K.M. et al. 2021. Survival and causes of death in 2,033 patients with non-transfusion-dependent β-thalassemia. Haematologica 106(9): 2489–2492.

Museum of London. 2024. Wellcome Osteological Research Database. https://www.museumoflondon.org.uk/collections/other-collection-databases-and-libraries/centre-human-bioarchaeology/osteological-database. Accessed 30 May 2024.

Mushrif-Tripathy V. 2014. Maxillary sinusitis from India: a bio-cultural approach. Korean J Phys Anthropol 27(1): 11. https://doi.org/10.11637/kjpa.2014.27.1.11.

Myszka A., Popowska-Nowak E., and Tomczyk J. 2022. Osteoarthritis in past human populations from Radom (14th–17th and 18th–19th century). Anthropologischer Anzeiger 79(4): 467–474.

Nagaoka T. et al. 2019. A health crisis during the Japanese medieval period: a new paleodemographic perspective. Int J Paleopathol 26:145–156.

Nakayama N. 2016. The relationship between linear enamel hypoplasia and social status in 18th to 19th century Edo, Japan. Int J Osteoarchaeol 26:1034–1044. https://doi.org/10.1002/oa.2515.

Nase J.B., Kollmann D.D., Dikin D.A., and Montoya C. 2022. Therapeutic dentistry in prehistoric Maryland—new analyses from the Hughes (18MO1) archeological site. Int J Osteoarchaeol 32:1011–1019. https://doi.org/10.1002/oa.3127.

Naser Moghadasi A. 2015. First visual evidence of leprosy in the continental shelf of Iran. Iranian aJ Public Health 44(8): 1162–1163.

National Museum of the American Indian. 2024. Repatriation. https://americanindian.si.edu/explore/repatriation. Accessed 8 July 2024.

National Park Service. 2024. Facilitating respectful return. https://www.nps.gov/subjects/nagpra/index.htm. Accessed 8 July 2024.

Nature. 2023. The world's goals to save humanity are hugely ambitious—but they are still the best option. Nature 621(7978): 227–229. https://doi.org/10.1038/d41586-023-02844-7.

Neary P. 1998. Venereal disease and public health administration in Newfoundland in the 1930s and 1940s. Can Bull Med Hist 15: 129–151.

Needleman H.L., Tuncay O.C., and Shapiro I.M. 1972. Lead levels in deciduous teeth of urban and suburban American children. Nature 235(5333): 111–112.

Nelson E.A., Buikstra J.E., Herbig A., Tung T.A., and Bos K.A. 2020. Advances in the molecular detection of tuberculosis in pre-contact Andean South America. Int J Paleopathol 29:128–140. https://doi.org/10.1016/j.ijpp.2019.12.006.

Neri R. and Lancelloti L. 2004. Fractures of the lower limbs and their skeletal adaptations: a 20th century example of pre-modern healing. Int J Osteoarchaeol 14:60–66.

Nerlich A., Peschel O., Löhrs U., Parsche F., and Betz, P. 1991. Juvenile gigantism plus polyostotic fibrous dysplasia in the Tegernsee giant. Lancet 338(8771): 886–887.

Nerlich A. and Zink A. 1995. Evidence of Langerhans cell histiocytosis in an infant of a late Roman cemetery. J Paleopathol 7(2): 119.

Nerlich A., Zink A., Hagedorn H.G., Szeimies U., and Weyss C. 2000. Anthropological and palaeopathological analysis of the human remains from three 'Tombs of the Nobles' of the necropolis of Thebes-West, Upper Egypt. Anthropologischer Anzeiger 58 (4): 321–343.

Nerlich A.G. 2018. Molecular paleopathology and paleo-oncology—state of the art, potentials, limitations and perspectives. Int J Paleopathol 21:77–82.

Nerlich A.G., Zink A., Szeimies U., and Haagedorn H.G. 2000. Ancient Egyptian prosthesis of the big toe. Lancet 356:2176–2179.

Nesse R.M. and Williams G.C. 1994. Why we get sick: the new science of Darwinian medicine. Vintage Books.

Neves W.A., Barros A.M., and Costa M.A. 1999. Incidence and distribution of postcranial fractures in the prehistoric population of San Pedro de Atacama, northern Chile. Am J Phys Anthropol 109:253–258.

Newman L. et al. 2013. Global estimates of syphilis in pregnancy and associated adverse outcomes: analysis of multinational antenatal surveillance data. PLoS Med. 10(2):e1001396. https://doi.org/10.1371/journal.pmed.1001396.

Newman S.L. and Gowland R.L. 2015. The use of non-adult vertebral dimensions as indicators of growth disruption and non-specific health stress in skeletal populations. Am J Phys Anthropol 158(1): 155–164.

Ni X. et al. 2020. Earliest-known intentionally deformed human cranium from Asia. Archaeol Anthropol Sci 12:93. https://doi.org/10.1007/s12520-020-01045-x.

Nicklisch N. et al. 2012. Rib lesions in skeletons from early Neolithic sites in central Germany: on the trail of tuberculosis at the onset of agriculture. Am J Phys Anthropol 149:391–404.

Nield L., Stenger J., and Kamat D. 2008. Common pediatric dental dilemmas. Clin Pediatr 47:99–105.

Nikiforuk A. 1996. The fourth horseman: a short history of plagues, scourges and emerging viruses. Penguin.

Nizam S., Virk H.S., and Sen I.S. 2022. High levels of fluoride in groundwater from northern parts of Indo-Gangetic plains reveals detrimental fluorosis health risks. Environ Adv 8:100200. https://doi.org/10.1016/j.envadv.2022.100200.

Novak S. 2001. Battle-related trauma. In: Blood red roses: the archaeology of a mass grave from the Battle of Towton AD 1461, ed. V. Fiorato, A. Boylston, and C. Knüsel, 90–102. Oxbow Books.

Nuki G. and Simkin P.A. 2006. A concise history of gout and hyperuricemia and their treatment. Arthritis Res Therapy 8(Suppl 1): S1. https://doi.org/10.1186/ar1906.

Nunn N. and Qian N. 2010. The Columbian exchange: a history of disease, food, and ideas. J Econ Persp 24(2): 163–188.

Nutton V. 2004. Ancient medicine. Routledge.

Nystrom K., Piombino-Mascali D., Buikstra J.E., and Watson Jiménez L. 2023. Mummified remains. In: The Routledge handbook of paleopathology, ed. A.L. Grauer, 210–228. Routledge.

O'Brien T.G., Peters L.R., and Hines M.E. 2013. Artificial cranial deformation: potential implications for affected brain function. Anthropology 1:107. https://doi.org/10.4172/2332-0915.1000107.

O'Connell T.C. 2023. Palaeodiet through stable isotope analysis. In: Handbook of archaeological sciences, vol. 1., 2nd edition, ed. M. Pollard, R.A. Armitage, and C. Makarewicz, 437–452. Wiley.

O'Connor D.B., Thayer J.F, and Vedhara K. 2021. Stress and health: a review of psychobiological processes. Annu Rev Psychol 72:663–688.

O'Donnell L., Buikstra J.E., Hill E.C., Anderson A.S., and O'Donnell M.J. Jr. 2023. Skeletal manifestations of disease experience: length of illness and porous cranial lesion formation in a contemporary juvenile mortality sample. Am J Hum Biol 35(8): e23896. https://doi.org/10.1002/ajhb.23896.

O'Donnell L., Hill E.C., Anderson A.S.A., and Edgar H.J. 2020. Cribra orbitalia and porotic hyperostosis are associated with respiratory infections in a contemporary mortality sample from New Mexico. Am J Phys Anthropol 173(4): 721–733.

O'Riordan J.L. and Bijvoet O.L. 2014. Rickets before the discovery of vitamin D. Bonekey Rep 3:478. https://doi.org/10.1038/bonekey.2013.212.

Oakberg K., Levy T., and Smith P. 2000. A method for skeletal arsenic analysis applied to the Chalcolithic copper smelting site of Shiqmim, Israel. J Archaeol Sci 27:895–901.

Oakley K.P., Brooke W.M.A., Akester A.R., and Brothwell D.R. 1959. Contributions on trepanning or trephination in ancient and modern times. Man 59:93–96.

Oehler R.L. and Vega V.R. 2022. Worldwide vaccine inequality threatens to unleash the next COVID-19 variant. Int J Infect Dis 123:133–135. https://doi.org/10.1016/j.ijid.2022.08.010.

Ogden A. 2008. Advances in the palaeopathology of teeth and jaws. In: Advances in human palaeopathology, ed. R. Pinhasi and S. Mays, 283–307. Wiley.

Ogden A., Pinhasi R., and White W. 2007. Gross enamel hypoplasia in molars from subadults in a 16th–18th century London graveyard. Am J Phys Anthropol 133(3): 957–966.

Okazaki K. et al. 2019. A paleopathological approach to early human adaptation for wet-rice agriculture: the first case of Neolithic spinal tuberculosis at the Yangtze River delta of China. Int J Paleopathol 24:236–244. https://doi.org/10.1016/j.ijpp.2019.01.002.

Olivé-Busom J., López-Costas O., Quer-Agustí M., Márquez-Grant N., and Kirchner H. 2021. Evidence of otitis media and mastoiditis in a medieval Islamic skeleton from Spain and possible implications for ancient surgical treatment of the condition. Int J Paleopathol 32:17–22. https://doi.org/10.1016/j.ijpp.2020.10.009.

Oliveira I.V.P.M., Deps P.D., and Antunes J.M.A.P. 2019. Armadillos and leprosy: from infection to biological model. Rev Inst Med Trop Sao Paulo. 61:e44. https://doi.org/10.1590/S1678-9946201961044.

Oliveira R., Strauss A., Murrieta R., Castro, C., and Matioli A. 2023. An early holocene case of congenital syphilis in South America. Int J Osteoarchaeol 33(1): 164–169. https://doi.org/10.1002/oa.3180.

Oliver K. and Cairney P. 2019. The dos and donts of influencing policy: a systematic review of advice to academics. Palgrave Commun 5(1): 21. https://doi.org/10.1057/s41599-019-0232-y.

Olsen S. and Shipman P. 1994. Cutmarks and perimortem treatment of skeletal remains on the northern Plains. In: Skeletal biology of the Great Plains: migration, warfare, health and subsistence, ed. D.W. Owsley and R.L. Jantz, 377–387. Smithsonian Institution Press.

One Health. 2024. One health. https://www.onehealth.co.uk/. Accessed 1 June 2024.

Oner D.A. and Tastan H. 2020. Cleft lip and palate: epidemiology and etiology. Otorhinolaryngol Head Neck Surg 5(4): 1–5. https://doi.org/10.15761/OHNS.1000246.

Oostra R.-J., van der Wolk S., Maas M., and Hennekam R. 2005. Malformations of the axial skeleton in the Museum Vrolik II: craniostenosis and suture related conditions. Am J Med Genet 136A: 327–342.

Ordonez-Ponce E. 2023. Exploring the impact of the Sustainable Development Goals on sustainability trends. Sustainability 15(24): 16647.

Orhan C.C. and Guajardo M. 2021. Analytics in developing countries: methods, applications, and the impact on the UN Sustainable Development Goals. Int Trans Oper Res 29(4): 2041–2081.

Orkar K., Ugwu B., and Momoh J. 2002. Cleft lip and palate: the Jos experience. East Afr Med J 79(10): 510–513.

Orr J. et al. 2021. Regional differences in short stature in England between 2006 and 2019: a cross-sectional analysis from the National Child Measurement Programme. PLoS Med 18(9): e1003760. https://doi.org/10.1371/journal.pmed.1003760.

Ortner D. 1979. Disease and mortality in early Bronze Age people of Bab edh-Dhra, Jordan. Am J Phys Anthropol 51:589–598.

Ortner D.J. 2003. Identification of pathological conditions in human skeletal remains. 2nd ed. Academic Press.

Ortner D.J., Butler W., Cafarella J., and Milligan L. 2001. Evidence of probable scurvy in non-adults from archeological sites in North America. Am J Phys Anthropol 114:343–351.

Ortner D.J. and Ericksen M.F. 1997. Bone changes in the human skull probably resulting from scurvy in infancy and childhood. Int J Osteoarchaeol 7:212–220.

Ortner D.J., Kimmerle E., and Diez M. 1999. Probable evidence of scurvy in non-adults from archeological sites in Peru. Am J Phys Anthropol 108:321–331.

Ortner D.J. and Mays S.A. 1998. Dry bone manifestations of rickets in infancy and childhood. Int J Osteoarchaeol 8(1): 45–55.

Ortner D. and Putschar W.J. 1981. Identification of pathological conditions in human skeletal remains. Smithsonian Institution Press.

Ortner D.J. and Ribas C. 1997. Bone changes in a human skull from the early Bronze site of Bab edh-Dhra', Jordan, probably resulting from scalping. J Paleopathol 9(3): 37–42.
Oskarsson V. et al. 2022. Influence of geographical latitude on vitamin D status: cross-sectional results from the BiomarCaRE consortium. Br J Nutr 128(11): 2208–2218. https://doi.org/10.1017/S0007114521005080.
Osterholtz A.J. 2012. The social role of hobbling and torture: violence in the prehistoric Southwest. Int J Paleopathol 2(2–3): 148–155. https://doi.org/10.1016/j.ijpp.2012.09.011.
Owen R.K. et al. 2023. Effect on life expectancy of temporal sequence in a multimorbidity cluster of psychosis, diabetes, and congestive heart failure among 1.7 million individuals in Wales with 20-year follow-up: a retrospective cohort study using linked data. *Lancet Public Health* 8(7): e535–e545. https://doi.org/10.1016/S2468-2667(23)00098-1.
Owsley D.W. 1994. Warfare in coalescent traditional populations of the Northern Plains. In: Skeletal biology of the Great Plains: migration, warfare, health and subsistence, ed. D.W. Owsley and R.L. Jantz, 333–343. Smithsonian Institution Press.
Owsley D.W., and Mann R.W. 1990. An American Indian skeleton with clubfoot from the Cabin burial site (A1184), Hemphill County, Texas. Plains Anthropol 35(128): 93–101.
Oxenham M. and Cavill I. 2010. Porotic hyperostosis and cribra orbitalia: the erythropoietic response to iron-deficiency anaemia. Anthropol Sci 118(3): 199–200.
Oyebola D.D.O. 1980. Yoruba traditional bonesetters: the practice of orthopaedics in a primitive setting in Nigeria. J Trauma 20(4): 312–322.
Özbek M. 2001. Cranial deformation in a subadult sample from Değirmentepe (Chalcolithic, Turkey). Am J Phys Anthropol 115:238–244.
Ozga A.T. et al. 2016. Successful enrichment and recovery of whole mitochondrial genomes from ancient human dental calculus. Am J Phys Anthropol 160:220–228. https://doi.org/10.1002/ajpa.22960.
Pääbo S. 1985. Molecular cloning of Ancient Egyptian mummy DNA. Nature 314:644–645. https://doi.org/10.1038/314644a0.
Pabst M.A. and Hofer F. 1998. Deposits of different origin in the lungs of the 5,300 year old Tyrolean Iceman. Am J Phys Anthropol 107:1–12.
Padala S.A. et al. 2021. Epidemiology, staging, and management of multiple myeloma. Med Sci 9(1): 3. https://doi.org/10.3390/medsci9010003.
Padyukov L. 2022. Genetics of rheumatoid arthritis. Semin Immunopathol 44:47–62.
Paine R.R. and Harpending H.C. 1998. Effect of sample bias on paleodemographic fertility estimates. Am J Phys Anthropol 105:231–240.
Paleopathology Association. 2023. Statement of ethical principles. https://paleopathology-association.wildapricot.org/Directors. Accessed 8 July 2024.
Palmeira P. and Carneiro-Sampaio M. 2016. Immunology of breast milk. Rev Assoc Med Bras 62:584–593.
Pankowská A., Galeta P., Spěváčková P.U., and Nováček K. 2019. Violence in European medieval monasteries: skeletal trauma in Teplá monastery (Czech Republic). Int J Osteoarchaeol 29:908–921. https://doi.org/10.1002/oa.2804.
Pantazis I. et al. 2020. A Ptolemaic mummy reveals evidence of invasive dentistry in ancient Egypt. Anat Rec (Hoboken) 303(12): 3129–3135. https://doi.org/10.1002/ar.24487.
Panter-Brick C. 2002. Sexual division of labor: energetic and evolutionary scenarios. Am J Hum Biol 14:627–640.
Panzer S., Grillhösl A., Zesch S., Haubenreisser H., and Rosendahl W. 2019. Evidence of pituitary tumor and acromegaly in an Ancient Egyptian mummy head. RöFo 191(8): 756–758.
Papageorgopoulou C., Suter S.K., Rühli F.J., and Siegmund F. 2011. Harris lines revisited: prevalence, comorbidities, and possible etiologies. Am J Hum Biol 23(3): 381–391.
Papas R.S. and Kutteh W.H. 2020. A new algorithm for the evaluation of recurrent pregnancy loss redefining unexplained miscarriage: review of current guidelines. Curr Opin Obstet Gynec 32(5): 371–379.
Papathanasiou A. 2003. Stable isotope analysis in neolithic Greece and possible implications on human health. Int J Osteoarchaeol 13:314–324.
Papathanasiou A., Meinzer N.J., Williams K.D., and Larsen C.S. 2019. In: The backbone of Europe: health, diet, work and violence over two millennia, ed. R.H. Steckel, C.S. Larsen, C.A. Roberts, and J. Baten, 198–230. Cambridge University Press.

Parascandola J. 2009. Quarantining women: venereal disease rapid treatment centers in World War II America. Bull Hist Med 83(3): 431–459. https://dx.doi.org/10.1353/bhm.0.0267.
Park E.A. and Richter C.P. 1953. Transverse lines in bone: the mechanism of their development. Bull Johns Hopkins Hosp 93:234–248.
Parker S., Roberts C.A., and Manchester K. 1986. A review of British trepanations with reports on two new cases. Ossa 12:141–157.
Parkhill J., Wren B.W., Thomson N.R., Titball R.W., Holden M.T.G. et al. 2001. Genome sequence of *Yersinia pestis*, the causative agent of plague. Nature 413:523–527.
Partiot C. et al. 2020. Cranial trepanation and healing process in modern patients: bioarchaeological and anthropological implications. J Anat 237(6): 1049–1061. https://doi.org/10.1111/joa.13266.
Pasero G. and Marson P. 2004. Hippocrates and rheumatology. Clin ExperRheumatol 22(6): 687–689.
Paterson D.E. and Rad M. 1961. Bone changes of leprosy: their incidence, progress, prevention and arrest. Int J Leprosy Other Mycobact Dis 29:393–422.
Patil K., Patil M., and Khemka A. 2012. Osteochondromatosis: a rare clinical condition. Journal of the Scientific Society 39(1): 40–41.
Patrick P. and Waldron T. 2003. Congenital absence of the patella in an Anglo-Saxon skeleton. Int J Osteoarchaeol 13:147–149.
Patton M. 2008. Genetics. In: Forfar and Arneil's textbook of pediatrics, ed. N. McIntosh, P. Helms, R. Smyth, and S. Logan, 379–409. Elsevier.
Payne L. 2017. The best surgeon in England: Percivall Pott, 1713–88. Peter Lang Inc., International Academic Publishers.
Pearce D. and Goldblatt P., eds. 2001. United Kingdom Health Statistics. 2001 edition. Her Majesty's Stationery Office.
Pechenkina E.A. and Benfer R.A. 2002. The role of occlusal stress and gingival infection in the formation of exostoses on mandible and maxilla from Neolithic China. Homo 53:112–130. https://doi.org/10.1078/0018-442X-00040.
Pedersen D.D., Milner G.R., Kolmos H.J., and Boldsen J.L. 2019. The association between skeletal lesions and tuberculosis diagnosis using a probabilistic approach. Int J Paleopathol 27:88–100. https://doi.org/10.1016/j.ijpp.2019.01.001.
Pedersen S. and Anton S. 1998. Bicoronal synostosis in a child from historic Omaha cemetery 25DK10. Am J Phys Anthropol 105:369–376.
Perry M. and Gowland R. 2022. Compounding vulnerabilities: syndemics and the social determinants of disease in the past. Int J Paleopathol 39:35–49.
Perry M.A., Coleman D.S., Dettman D.L., Grattan J.P., and al-Shiyab A.H. 2011. Condemned to metallum? The origin and role of 4th–6th century AD Phaeno mining camp residents using multiple chemical techniques. J Archaeol Sci 38(3): 558–569.
Persson E.K., Hagberg G., and Uvebrant P. 2005. Hydrocephalus prevalence and outcome in a population-based cohort of children born in 1989–1998. Acta Paediatr 94(6): 726–732.
Peterson C., Miller G.F., Barnett S.B.L., and Florence C. 2021. Economic cost of injury—United States, 2019. MMWR Morb Mortal Wkly Rep 70(48): 1655–1659. https://doi.org/10.15585/mmwr.mm7048a1.
Petersone-Gordina E. et al. 2020. Investigating dietary life histories and mobility of children buried in St Gertrude Church cemetery Riga, Latvia, 15th–17th centuries AD. Archaeometry 62(Suppl. 1): 3–18.
Pēterstone-Gordina E., Gerhards G., and Jakob T. 2013. Nutrition-related health problems in a wealthy 17–18th century German community in Jelgava, Latvia. Int J Paleopathol 3:30–38.
Pettifor J. 2003. Nutritional rickets. In: Pediatric bone: biology and diseases, ed. F. Glorieux J. Pettifor and M. Jüppner, 541–565. Academic Press.
Pettifor J. and Daniels E. 1997. Vitamin D deficiency and nutritional rickets in children. In: Vitamin D, ed. D. Feldman, F. Glorieux, and J. Pike, 663–678. Academic Press.
Pfeiffer S. 1991. Rib lesions and New World tuberculosis. Int J Osteoarchaeol 1:191–198.
Pfeiffer S. 2016. An exploration of interpersonal violence among Holocene foragers of southern Africa. Int J Paleopathol 13:27–38. https://doi.org/10.1016/j.ijpp.2016.01.001.
Pfeiffer S. and Crowder C. 2004. An ill child among mid-Holocene foragers of southern Africa. Am J Phys Anthropol 123:23–29.

Pfrengle S. et al. 2021. *Mycobacterium leprae* diversity and population dynamics in medieval Europe from novel ancient genomes. BMC Biol 19:220. https://doi.org/10.1186/s12915-021-01120-2.
Phillips M. et al. 2021. Two (missing) left feet: caring for foot amputees in late pre-Hispanic Túcume, Lambayeque Peru. Bioarchaeol Int 5:1–20.
Piel F.B. et al. 2010. Global distribution of the sickle cell gene and geographical confirmation of the malaria hypothesis. Nat Commun 1:104.
Pietrobelli A. et al. 2020. Syphilis in an Italian medieval Jewish community: a bioarchaeological and cultural perspective. Int J Paleopathol 30:85–97. https://doi.org/10.1016/j.ijpp.2020.06.001.
Pietrusewsky M. and Douglas M.T. 2002. Ban Chiang, a prehistoric village site in northeast Thailand 1: the human skeletal remains. University of Pennsylvania, University Museum Monograph 11.
Pietrusewsky M. and Douglas M.T. 1994. An osteological assessment of health and disease in precontact and historic (1778) Hawai'i. In: In the wake of contact: biological responses to conquest, ed. C.S. Larsen and G.R. Milner, 179–196. Wiley-Liss.
Piggott S. 1940. A trepanned skull of the Beaker period from Dorset and the practice of trepanning in prehistoric Europe. Proc Prehist Soc 6:112–133.
Pisarenko S.V. et al. 2018. Global evolution and phylogeography of *Brucella melitensis* strains. BMC Genom 19:353. https://doi.org/10.1186/s12864-018-4762-2.
Plomp K.A., Been E., and Collard M. 2022a. Acquired spinal conditions in humans: the roles of spinal curvature, the shape of the lumbar vertebrae, and evolutionary history. In: Palaeopathology and evolutionary medicine: an integrated approach, ed. K.A. Plomp, C.A. Roberts, S. Elton, and G.R. Bentley, 42–61. Oxford University Press.
Plomp K.A., Dobney K., and Collard M. 2020a. Spondylolysis and spinal adaptations for bipedalism: The overshoot hypothesis. Evol Med Public Health 2020 (1): 35–44. https://doi.org/10.1093/emph/eoaa003.
Plomp K.A., Roberts C.A., Elton S., and Bentley G., eds. 2022b. Palaeopathology and evolutionary medicine: an integrated approach. Oxford University Press.
Plomp K.A., Roberts C.A., and Strand Viðarsdóttir U. 2012. Vertebral morphology influences the development of Schmorl's nodes in the lower thoracic vertebrae. Am J Phys Anthropol 149(4): 572–582.
Plomp K.A., Roberts C.A., and Strand Vidarsdottir U. 2015. Does the correlation between Schmorl's nodes and vertebral morphology extend into the lumbar spine? Am J Phys Anthropol 157(3): 526–534.
Plomp E. et al. 2020b. Strontium, oxygen, and carbon isotope variation in modern human dental enamel. Am J Phys Anthropol 172:586–604. https://doi.org/10.1002/ajpa.24059.
Pobiner B., Pante M., and Keevil T. 2023. Early Pleistocene cut marked hominin fossil from Koobi Fora, Kenya. Sci Rep 13:9896. https://doi.org/10.1038/s41598-023-35702-7.
Polak A., Pawlikowska-Łagód K., Zagaja A., and Grzybowski A. 2023. The history of louse-borne typhus and geomedizine. Clin Dermatol 41:767–771. https://doi.org/10.1016/j.clindermatol.2023.09.009.
Polson C.J., Gee D.J., and Knight B. 1985. Essentials of forensic medicine. Pergamon Press.
Porter R. 1997. The greatest benefit to mankind: a medical history of humanity from antiquity to the present. Harper Collins.
Powell M.L. and Cook D.C., eds. 2005. The myth of syphilis: the natural history of treponematosis in North America. University Press of Florida.
Pradhan S. et al. 2022. Overall effects and moderators of rehabilitation in patients with wrist fracture: a systematic review. Phys Ther 102(6): pzac032. https://doi.org/10.1093/ptj/pzac032.
Price N. et al. 2019. Viking warrior women? Reassessing Birka chamber grave Bj.581. Antiquity 93(367): 181–198. https://doi.org/10.15184/aqy.2018.258.
Price S.D.R., Keenleyside A., and Schwarcz H.P. 2018. Testing the validity of stable isotope analyses of dental calculus as a proxy in paleodietary studies. J Archaeol Sci 91:92–103. https://doi.org/10.1016/j.jas.2018.01.008.
Primeau C., Jakobsen L.S., and Lynnerup N. 2016. CT imaging vs. traditional radiographic imaging for evaluating Harris Lines in tibiae. Anthropologischer Anzeiger 73:99–108.
Propst K.B., Danforth M.E., and Jacobi, K. 1994. Replicability in scoring enamel hypoplasias: a preliminary report. Paleopathol Assoc Newsl 87:11–12.

Prowse T.L. et al. 2008. Isotopic and dental evidence for infant and young child feeding practices in an imperial Roman skeletal sample. Am J Phys Anthropol 137:294–308. https://doi.org/10.1002/ajpa.20870.

Purchase S.L., Bazaliiskii V.I., and Lieverse A.R. 2019. An innovative method to visualise mastoiditis using a hand-held X-ray system. Int J Paleopathol 26:22–26. https://doi.org/10.1016/j.ijpp.2019.05.006.

Purnell T.S. et al. 2016. Achieving health equity: closing the gaps in health care disparities, interventions, and research. Health Aff (Millwood) 35(8): 1410–1415. https://doi.org/10.1377/hlthaff.

Püschel T.A., Friess M., and Manríquez G. 2020. Morphological consequences of artificial cranial deformation: modularity and integration. PLoS One 15(1): e0227362. https://doi.org/10.1371/journal.pone.0227362.

Pyatt F.B. and Grattan J.P. 2001. Some consequences of ancient mining activities on the health of ancient and modern human populations. J Public Health Med 23(3): 235–236.

Quade L. and Binder M. 2018. Life on a Napoleonic battlefield: a bioarchaeological analysis of soldiers from the Battle of Aspern, Austria. Int J Paleopathol 22:23–38.

Quatrehomme G. and Iscan M.Y. 1997. Post-mortem skeletal lesions. Forensic Sci Int 89:155–165.

Quiñonez C., Ieraci L., and Guttmann A. 2011. Potentially preventable hospital use for dental conditions: implications for expanding dental coverage for low-income populations. J Health Care Poor Underserved 22(3): 1048–1058. https://doi.org/10.1353/hpu.2011.0097.

Quintelier K. et al. 2014. Isotopic examination of links between diet, social differentiation, and DISH at the post-medieval Carmelite Friary of Aalst, Belgium. Am J Phys Anthropol 153:203–213.

Radini A. and Nikita E. 2023. Beyond dirty teeth: integrating dental calculus studies with osteoarchaeological parameters. Quat Int 653–654:3–18. https://doi.org/10.1016/j.quaint.2022.03.003.

Radini A., Nikita E., Buckley S., Copeland L., and Hardy K. 2017. Beyond food: the multiple pathways for inclusion of materials into ancient dental calculus. Am J Phys Anthropol 162:71–83. https://doi.org/10.1002/ajpa.23147.

Radu C., Andreica L., Constantinescu M., and Soficaru A. 2016. Multiple cases with probable treponemal infection from 16th to 19th centuries Romania. *Int J Osteoarchaeol* 26:563–573. https://doi.org/10.1002/oa.2444.

Ragan K.L. 2011. Fatal child maltreatment: the challenges of identifying the cause and incidence of deaths from abuse and neglect. In: The juvenile skeleton in forensic abuse investigations, ed. A.M. Ross and S.M. Abel, 7–18. Humana Press, Springer.

Ragsdale B.D. 1993. Morphologic analysis of skeletal lesions: correlation of imaging studies and pathologic findings. Adv Pathol Lab Med 6:445–490.

Ragsdale B.D., Campbell R.A., and Kirkpatrick C.L. 2018. Neoplasm or not? General principles of morphologic analysis of dry bone specimens. Int J Paleopathol 21:27–40.

Rajakumar K. 2001. Infantile scurvy: a historical perspective. Pediatrics 108(4): e76. https://doi.org/10.1542/peds.108.4.e76.

Rajkumar S.V. et al. 2014. International Myeloma Working Group updated criteria for the diagnosis of multiple myeloma. Lancet Oncol 15(12): e538–e548. https://doi.org/10.1016/S1470-2045(14)70442-5.

Ramirez D.A. et al. 2025. 4,000-year-old Mycobacterium lepromatosis genomes from Chile reveal long establishment of Hansen's disease in the Americas. Nat Ecol Evol. 9(9):1685–1693. https://doi.org/10.1038/s41559-025-02771-y.

Ramos Van Raap M.A. and Scabuzzo C. 2018. A case of nonvenereal treponematosis in a pre-Hispanic adult from north-eastern Argentina. Int J Osteoarchaeol 28:757–765. https://doi.org/10.1002/oa.2701.

Rando C. and Waldron T. 2012. TMJ osteoarthritis: a new approach to diagnosis. Am J Phys Anthropol 148(1): 45–53.

Rank M.G. and Heroux E.F.J. 2018. Military women and veterans. Mil Behav Health 6(1): 1–2. https://doi.org/ 10.1080/21635781.2017.1374222.

Rao P.N. and Suneetha S. 2021. Leprosy—the name and the stigma. Indian J Lepr 93:405–413.

Raoult D. et al. 2006. Evidence for louse-transmitted diseases in soldiers of Napoleon's Grand Army in Vilnius. J Infect Dis 193(1):112–120. https://doi.org/10.1086/498534.

Rasmussen K.L. et al. 2020. Trace element distribution in human cortical bone microstructure: the potential for unravelling diet and social status in archaeological bones. Heritage Sci 8(1): 1–23.

Rasmussen S. et al. 2015. Early divergent strains of *Yersinia pestis* in Eurasia 5,000 years ago. Cell 163(3): 571–582. https://doi.org/10.1016/j.cell.2015.10.009.

Rasool A. et al. 2018. A review of global outlook on fluoride contamination in groundwater with prominence on the Pakistan current situation. Environ Geochem Health 40(4): 1265–1281. https://doi.org/10.1007/s10653-017-0054-z.

Rather L.J. 1978. The genesis of cancer: a study in the history of ideas. Johns Hopkins University Press.

Ravelli A. and Martini A. 2007. Juvenile idiopathic arthritis. Lancet 369(9563): 767–778.

Rawcliffe C. 1997. Medicine and society in later medieval England. Sutton.

Rawcliffe C. 2006. Leprosy in medieval England. Boydell Press.

Rawcliffe C. 2013. Urban bodies. Communal health in late medieval English towns and cities. Boydell Press.

Razai M.S., Majeed A., and Esmail A. 2021. Structural racism is a fundamental cause and driver of ethnic disparities in health. BMJ 373:n938.

Redfern R.C. 2017a. Injury and trauma in bioarchaeology. Cambridge University Press.

Redfern R.C. 2017b. Identifying and interpreting domestic violence in archaeological human remains: a critical review of the evidence. Int J Osteoarchaeol 27:13–34. https://doi.org/10.1002/oa.2461.

Redfern R.C., Judd M.A., and DeWitte S.N. 2017. Multiple injury and health in past societies: an analysis of concepts and approaches, and insights from a multi-period study. Int J Osteoarchaeol 27:418–429. https://doi.org/ 10.1002/oa.2565.

Redfern R.C. and Roberts C.A. 2019. Trauma. In: Ortner's identification of pathological conditions in human skeletal remains, ed. J.E. Buikstra, 211–284. Elsevier.

Reed S.G. et al. 2017. Prenatal vitamin D and enamel hypoplasia in human primary maxillary central incisors: a pilot study. Pediatr Dent J 27(1): 21–28.

Reichart P., Ananatasan T., and Reznik G.1976. Gingiva and periodontium in leprosy: a clinical, radiological and microscopical study. J Periodontol 47:455–460.

Reid D.J. and Dean M.C. 2000. Brief communication: the timing of linear hypoplasias on human anterior teeth. Am J Phys Anthropol 113(1): 135–139. https://doi.org/10.1002/1096-8644(200009)113:1<135:AID-AJPA13>3.0.CO;2-A.

Reid D.J. and Dean M.C. 2006. Variation in modern human enamel formation times. J Hum Evol 50(3): 329–346. https://doi.org/10.1016/j.jhevol.2005.09.003.

Reid R. and Harrison D.J. 2008. Applications of pathology. In: Muir's textbook of pathology, 14th edition, ed. D.A. Levison, R. Reid, A.D. Burt, D.J. Harrison, and S. Fleming, 4–10. Hodder Arnold.

Reinhard K.J. 2017. Reestablishing rigor in archaeological parasitology. Int J Paleopathol 19:124–134. https://doi.org/10.1016/j.ijpp.2017.06.002.

Reinhard K.J. and Araújo A. 2012. Synthesizing parasitology with archaeology in paleopathology. In: The global history of paleopathology: pioneers and prospects, ed. J.E. Buikstra and C.A. Roberts, 751–764. Oxford University Press.

Reinhard K.J. and Camacho M. 2019. Parasitology. In: Ortner's identification of pathological conditions in human skeletal remains, ed. J.E. Buikstra, 479–489. Elsevier.

Reinhard K.J. et al. 2013. Food, parasites, and epidemiological transitions: a broad perspective. Int J Paleopathol 3:150–157. https://doi.org/10.1016/j.ijpp.2013.05.003.

Reitsema L.J. 2013. Beyond diet reconstruction: stable isotope applications to human physiology, health, and nutrition. Am J Hum Biol 25:445–456.

Reitsema L.J. and Holder S. 2018. Stable isotope analysis and the study of human stress, disease, and nutrition. Bioarchaeol Int 2(2): 63–74.

Reitz E.J. and Shackley M. 2012. Environmental archaeology. Springer.

Rembis M., Kudlick C., and Nielsen K., eds. 2018. The Oxford handbook of disability history. Oxford University Press.

Research Excellence Framework. 2022. Overview report by main panel c and sub-panels 13 to 24. https://2021.ref.ac.uk/media/1912/mp-c-overview-report-final-updated-september-2022.pdf.

Resnick D., Jacobson J.A., Chung C.B., Kransdorf M.J., and Pathria M., eds. 2024. Resnick's bone and joint imaging, 4th ed. Elsevier.
Retief F.P. and Cilliers L. 2011. Breast cancer in antiquity. South Afr Med J 101(8): 513–515.
Reuland-Bosma W. and van Dijk J. 1986. Periodontal disease in Down's syndrome: a review. J Clin Periodontol 13:64–73.
Reverby S.M. 2009. Examining Tuskegee: the infamous syphilis study and its legacy. University of North Carolina Press.
Reverby S.M. 2016. Restorative justice and restorative history for the sexually transmitted disease inoculation experiments in Guatemala. Am J Public Health 106(7): 1163–1164. https://doi.org/10.2105/AJPH.2016.303205.
Ricci F. et al. 2008. Evidence of artificial cranial deformation from the later prehistory of the Acacus Mts. (southwestern Libya, central Sahara). Int J Osteoarchaeol 18:372–391. https://doi.org/10.1002/oa.946.
Ricci S. et al. 2016. Toothpick use among Epigravettian humans from Grotta Paglicci (Italy). Int J Osteoarchaeol 26:281–289. https://doi.org/10.1002/oa.2420.
Riccomi G., Aringhieri G., Serritella A., and Giuffra V. 2023. Solitary osteochondromas in paleo-oncology: a case report from 4th-century BCE Pontecagnano (southern Italy).Int J Paleopathol 41:101–109.
Riccomi G., Fornaciari G., and Giuffra V. 2019. Multiple myeloma in paleopathology: a critical review. Int J Paleopathol 24:201–212.
Riccomi G., Minozzi S., Aringhieri G., and Giuffra V. 2021. A possible case of juvenile idiopathic arthritis from Renaissance Lucca (Tuscany, central Italy). Int J Paleopathol 33:72–83.
Riccomi G. et al. 2017. Trepanation to treat a head wound: a case of neurosurgery from 13th-century Tuscany. World Neurosurg 104:9–13. https://doi.org/10.1016/j.wneu.2017.04.160.
Richards G.D. and Anton S.C. 1991. Craniofacial configuration and postcranial development of a hydrocephalic child (ca. 2500 BC–AD 500): with a review of cases and comment on diagnostic criteria. Am J Phys Anthropol 85:185–200.
Richards M. and Montgomery J. 2012. Isotope analysis and paleopathology: a short review and future developments. In: The global history of paleopathology: pioneers and prospects, ed. J. Buikstra and C. Roberts, 718–731. Oxford University Press. https://doi.org/10.1093/acprof:osobl/9780195389807.003.0072.
Richards M.P., Mays S., and Fuller B.T. 2002. Stable carbon and nitrogen isotope values of bone and teeth reflect weaning age at the medieval Wharram Percy site, Yorkshire, UK. Am J Phys Anthropol 118:205–210.
Ridley D.S. and Jopling W.H. 1966. Classification of leprosy according to immunity: a five group system. Int J Lepr 34:255–273.
Riggs E. et al. 2019. Interventions with pregnant women, new mothers and other primary caregivers for preventing early childhood caries. Cochrane Database Syst Rev 2019(11): CD012155. https://doi.org/10.1002/14651858.CD012155.pub2.
Rinaldo N., Pasini A., Donati R., Belcastro M.G., and Gualdi-Russo E. 2018. Quantitative ultrasonometry for the diagnosis of osteoporosis in human skeletal remains: new methods and standards. J Archaeol Sci 99:153–161.
Ríos J.L., Francini F., and Schinella G.R., 2015. Natural products for the treatment of type 2 diabetes mellitus. Planta Medica 81: 975–994.
Rissech C. et al. 2023. Skeletal remains of human perinatal individuals from the fortified Iberian Period settlement of Ca n'Oliver (6th century to 50 years BCE). Archaeol Anthropol Sci 15. https://doi.org/10.1007/s12520-023-01863-9.
Rivollat M., Castex D., Hauret L., and Tillier A. 2014. Ancient Down syndrome: an osteological case from Saint-Jean-des-Vigne, from the 5–6th century AD. Int J Palaeopathol 7:8–14.
Robb R., Cessford C., Dittmar J., Inskip S.A., and Mitchell P.D. 2021. The greatest health problem of the Middle Ages? Estimating the burden of disease in medieval England. Int J Paleopathol 34:101–112. https://doi.org/10.1016/j.ijpp.2021.06.011.
Roberts C.A. 1986. Leprosy and leprosaria in medieval Britain. MASCA J 4(1): 15–21.
Roberts C.A. 1987. Possible pituitary dwarfism from the Roman period. British Medical J. 295:1659–1660.

Roberts C.A. 1988. Trauma and treatment in British antiquity: an osteoarchaeological study of macroscopic and radiological features of long bone fractures from the Historic period with a comparative study of clinical radiographs, supplemented by contemporary documentary, iconographical and archaeological evidence. Ph.D. dissertation, University of Bradford, Bradford, West Yorkshire, UK.
Roberts C.A. 1989. Trauma and treatment in British antiquity: a radiographic study. In: Proceedings of the Science and Archaeology Conference, Glasgow, September 1987, ed. J. Tate and E. Slater, 339–359. British Archaeological Reports British series 196. BAR.
Roberts C.A. 1991. Trauma and treatment in the British Historic period: a design for multidisciplinary research. In: Human paleopathology: current syntheses and future options, ed. D. Ortner and A. Aufderheide, 225–240. Smithsonian Institution Press.
Roberts C.A. 1999. Rib lesions and tuberculosis: the current state of play. In: Tuberculosis: past and present, ed. G. Pálfi, O. Dutour, J. Deák, and I. Hutás, 311–316. Golden Book Publishers and Tuberculosis Foundation.
Roberts C.A. 2000. Did they take sugar? The use of skeletal evidence in the study of disability in past populations. In: Madness, disability and social exclusion: the archaeology and anthropology of exclusion, ed. J. Hebert, 46–59. Routledge.
Roberts C.A. 2007. A bioarcheological study of maxillary sinusitis. Am J Phys Anthropol 133(2): 792–807.
Roberts C.A. 2017. Applying the 'index of care' to a person who experienced leprosy in late medieval Chichester, England. In: New developments in the bioarchaeology of care, ed. L. Tilley and A.A. Schrenk, 101–124. Springer.
Roberts C.A. 2018. Human remains in archaeology: a handbook, 2nd ed. Council for British Archeology.
Roberts C.A. 2019a. Ethical challenges of working with archaeological human remains, with a focus on the UK. In: Ethical challenges in the analysis of human remains, ed. K. Squires, D. Errickson, and N. Márquez-Grant, 133–155. Elsevier.
Roberts C.A. 2019b. Infectious disease: introduction, periostosis, periostitis, osteomyelitis, and septic arthritis. In: Ortner's identification of pathological conditions in human skeletal remains, ed. J.E. Buikstra, 285–319. Academic Press.
Roberts C.A. 2020a. Words, stigma and the coronavirus: implications of COVID-19 for holistic approaches to infectious diseases. J Br Acad 8:240–244. https://doi.org/10.5871/jba/008.167.
Roberts C.A. 2020b. Mortui vivos docent: let the dead teach the living in a postpandemic landscape. In: What makes a community more vulnerable to COVID-19?, ed. D. Abrams et al., 41–46. British Academy.
Roberts C.A. 2020c. Fashionable but debilitating diseases: tuberculosis past and present. In: Purposeful pain: the bioarchaeology of intentional suffering, ed. S. Sheridan and L. Gregoricka, 21–38. Springer.
Roberts C.A. 2020d. Leprosy: past and present. University of Florida Press.
Roberts C.A. 2022. Conceptual approaches to the bioarchaeology of 'community' care using knowledge from personal experiences of care giving. In: A community of care: expanding bioarchaeology of care to population level analyses, ed. L. Tremblay and A. Schrenk, 15–36. University of Florida Press.
Roberts C.A. 2023a. Evolution to revolution: human bioarchaeology is riding high. In: Handbook of archaeological sciences, vol. 1., 2nd edition, ed. M. Pollard, R.A. Armitage, and C. Makarewicz, 339-357. Wiley.
Roberts C.A. 2023b. Exploring the sources of indirect evidence for cardiovascular disease in bioarchaeology: potential impact on understanding its evolution. In: The bioarchaeology of cardiovascular disease, ed. M. Binder, C.A. Roberts, and D. Antoine, 8–38. Cambridge University Press.
Roberts C.A. 2024. Expertise for a new world: is bioarchaeology fit for purpose? In: Philosophy, expertise, and the myth of neutrality, ed. M. Farina and A. Lavazzo, 278–300. Routledge.
Roberts C.A., Blevins K., Filipek K.L., and Pacheco A. 2023. Here and now, there and then: two mycobacterial diseases still with us today. In: The Routledge handbook of paleopathology, ed. A.L. Grauer, chap. 17. Routledge.
Roberts C.A., Lewis M., and Boocock P. 1998a. Infectious disease, sex and gender: the complexity of it all! In: Sex and gender in palaeopathological perspective. ed. A. Grauer and P. Stuart-Macadam, 93–113. Cambridge, University Press.

Roberts C.A., Boylston A., Buckley L., Chamberlain A., and Murphy E. 1998b. Rib lesions and tuberculosis: the palaeopathological evidence. Tubercle Lung Dis 79(1):55–60.

Roberts C.A. and Buikstra J. E. 2003. The bioarchaeology of tuberculosis: a global view on a reemerging disease. University Press of Florida.

Roberts C.A. and Buikstra J.E. 2019. Bacterial infections. In: Ortner's identification of pathological conditions in human skeletal remains, ed. J.E. Buikstra, 321–439. Elsevier.

Roberts C.A., Caffell A., Filipek-Ogden K.L., Gowland R., and Jakob T. 2016. 'Til poison phosphorous brought them death': a potentially occupationally-related disease in a post-medieval skeleton from north-east England. Int J Paleopathol 13:39–48.

Roberts C.A. and Cox M. 2003. Health and disease in Britain: prehistory to the present day. Sutton.

Roberts C.A., Davies P.D.O., Stone A.C., and Blevins K. 2022a. Preventable and curable, but still a global problem: tuberculosis from an evolutionary perspective. In: Palaeopathology and evolutionary medicine: an integrated approach, ed. K. Plomp, C.A. Roberts, S. Elton, and G. Bentley, 179–203. Oxford University Press.

Roberts C.A. and Ingham S. 2008. Using ancient DNA analysis in palaeopathology: a critical analysis of published papers, with recommendations for future work. Int J Osteoarchaeol 18:600–613. https://doi.org/10.1002/oa.966.

Roberts C.A., Knüsel C., and Race L. 2004. A foot deformity from a Romano-British cemetery at Gloucester, England and the current evidence for Talipes in palaeopathology. Int J Osteoarchaeol 14(5): 389–403.

Roberts C.A., Lewis M.E., and Boocock P. 1998b. Infectious disease, sex and gender: the complexity of it all. In: Sex and gender in paleopathological perspective, ed. A. Grauer and P. Stuart-Macadam, 93–113. Cambridge University Press.

Roberts C.A., Lucy D., and Manchester K. 1994. Inflammatory lesions of ribs: an analysis of the Terry Collection. Am J Phys Anthropol 95(2): 169–182.

Roberts C.A., and Manchester K. 2005. The Archaeology of Disease, 3rd edition. Cornell University Press.

Roberts C.A. and Mays S. 2011. Study and restudy of curated skeletal collections in bioarchaeology: a perspective on the UK and its implications for future curation of human remains. Int J Osteoarchaeol 21:626–630.

Roberts C.A. and McKinley J. 2003. Review of trepanations in British antiquity focusing on funerary context to explain their occurrence. In: Trepanation: history, discovery, theory, ed. R. Arnott, S. Finger, and C.U.M. Smith, 56–78. Swets and Zeitlinger.

Roberts C.A., Millard A., Pearson G. et al. 2013. The origin and mobility of people with venereal syphilis buried in Hull, England in the late medieval period. Am J Phys Anthropol 150:273–285.

Roberts C.A., Pfister L., and Mays S. 2009. Letter to the editor: was tuberculosis present in Homo erectus in Turkey? Am J Phys Anthropol 139:442–444.

Roberts C.A. and Redfern R. 2019. The history of treponematosis continues to be one of the most contentious issues in science' (Ortner 2003:273)—some perspectives from bioarchaeology. In: The hidden affliction: sexually transmitted infections in history and infertility, ed. S. Sretzer, 93–123. Rochester University Press and Boydell and Brewer.

Roberts C.A., Scollard D.M., and Fava V.M. 2022b. Leprosy is down but not yet out: new insights shed light on its origin and evolution. In: Palaeopathology and evolutionary medicine: an integrated approach, ed. K. Plomp, C.A. Roberts, S. Elton, and G. Bentley, 155–178. Oxford University Press.

Roberts C.A. and Steckel R.H. 2019. The developmental origins hypothesis and the history of health project. In: The backbone of Europe: health, diet, work and violence over two millennia, ed. R.H. Steckel, C.S. Larsen, C.A. Roberts, and J. Baten, 325–351. Cambridge University Press.

Roberts C.A. and Wakely J. 1992. Microscopical findings associated with the diagnosis of osteoporosis in palaeopathology. Int J Osteoarchaeol 2:23–30.

Robinson P.C. et al. 2022. Consensus statement regarding the efficacy and safety of long-term low-dose colchicine in gout and cardiovascular disease. Am J Med 135(1): 32–38.

Roffey S. et al. 2017. Investigation of a medieval pilgrim burial excavated from the leprosarium of St Mary Magdalen Winchester, UK. PLoS Negl Trop Dis 11(1): e0005186. https://doi.org/10.1371/journal.pntd.0005186.

Rogers J. 2000. The palaeopathology of joint disease. In: Human osteology in archaeology and forensic science, ed. M. Cox and S. Mays, 163–182. Greenwich Medical Media.
Rogers J. and Waldron T. 1995. A field guide to joint disease in archaeology. Wiley.
Rogers J. and Waldron T. 2001. DISH and the monastic way of life. Int J Osteoarchaeol 11:357–365.
Rogers J., Shepstone L., and Dieppe P. 1997. Bone formers: osteophyte and enthesophyte formation are positively associated. Ann Rheum Dis 56(2): 85–90.
Rogers J., Waldron T., Dieppe P., and Watt I. 1987. Arthropathies in palaeopathology: the basis of classification according to most probable cause. J Archaeol Sci 14:179–193.
Rogers J., Watt I., and Dieppe P. 1990. Comparison of visual and radiographic defects of bony changes at the knee joint. Br Med J 300:367–368.
Rohnbogner A. 2016. Differential diagnosis of a probable case of non-adult thalassaemia from 4th century AD Romano-British Colchester, UK. Int J Paleopathol 15:39–49.
Rohrlach A.B. et al. 2024. Cases of trisomy 21 and trisomy 18 among historic and prehistoric individuals discovered from ancient DNA. Nat Commun 15(1): 1294. https://doi.org/10.1038/s41467-024-45438-1.
Rome K. et al. 2011. Functional and biomechanical characteristics of foot disease in chronic gout: a case-control study. Clin Biomech 26(1): 90–94.
Rose F.C. 1997. The history of head injuries: an overview. J Hist Neurosci 6(2): 154–180.
Rosen G. 2015. A history of public health, rev. ed. Johns Hopkins University Press.
Rostomyan L. et al. 2015. Clinical and genetic characterization of pituitary gigantism: an international collaborative study in 208 patients. Endocr Relat Cancer 22(5): 745–757.
Rothschild B.M. 2022. Recognizing and distinguishing the phenomenon referred to as meningioma. Anatomia 1(1): 107–118.
Rothschild B.M., Hershkovitz I., and Dutour O. 1998. Clues potentially distinguishing lytic lesions of multiple myeloma from those of metastatic carcinoma. Am J Phys Anthropol 105:241–250.
Rothschild B.M. and Rothschild C. 1995. Comparison of radiologic and gross examination for detection of cancer in defleshed skeletons. Am J Phys Anthropol 96:357–363.
Rothschild B.M. and Woods R.J. 1990. Symmetrical erosive disease in Archaic Indians: the origin of rheumatoid arthritis in the New World? Semin Arthritis Rheum 19 (5): 278–284.
Rothschild B.M., Woods R.J., and Ortel W. 1990. Rheumatoid arthritis 'in the buff': erosive arthritis in defleshed bones. Am J Phys Anthropol 82:441–449.
Rothschild B.M. et al. 1997. Recognition of leukemia in skeletal remains: report and comparison of two cases. Am J Phys Anthropol 102:481–496.
Rubini M., Zaio P., and Roberts C.A. 2014. Tuberculosis and leprosy in Italy: new skeletal evidence. Homo 65:13–32.
Rubini M. et al. 2022. Metastatic cancer and endentulism: exploring comorbidity to assist with differential diagnosis in a case from Vico nel Lazio (Fr, Italy), 13th–15th century CE. Int J Paleopathol 38:1–12. https://doi.org/10.1016/j.ijpp.2022.05.005.
Ruff C. 2019. Biomechanical analyses of archaeological human skeletons. In: Biological anthropology of the human skeleton, ed. A. Katzenberg and A.L. Grauer, 189–224. Wiley.
Ruff C.B., Holt B., and Trinkaus E. 2006. Who's afraid of the big bad Wolff? 'Wolff's law' and bone functional adaptation. Am J Phys Anthropol 129:484–498.
Ruffer M.A. 1910. Remarks on the histology and pathological anatomy of Egyptian mummies. Cairo 4:1–5.
Ruffer M.A. and Willmore J.G. 1914. Note on a tumour of the pelvis dating from Roman times (AD 250) and found in Egypt. J Path Bact 18:480–484.
Rufino R.I., Ferreira M.T., and Wasterlain S.N. 2017. Periapical lesions in intentionally modified teeth in a skeletal sample of enslaved Africans (Lagos, Portugal). Int J Osteoarchaeol 27:288–297.
Ruis G.J., Serrano S.C., and Guilliem A.S. 2020. Sociedad Novohispana y enfermedad. Un caso de lepra en el complejo funerario colonial de Tlatelolco, México [New Hispanic society and infirmity: a case of leprosy in the colonial funerary complex of Tlatelolco, Mexico]. Revista Española de Antropología Física 41:28–42. https://www.seaf.es/images/seaf/papers/vol41/4_Ruiz_Vol_41.pdf.
Ryan A.S. 1997. Iron-deficiency anaemia in infant development: implications for growth, cognitive development, resistance to infection, and iron supplementation. Yearbook of Physical Anthropology 40:25–62.

Ryan T.M. and Milner G.R. 2006. Osteological applications of high-resolution computed tomography: a prehistoric arrow injury. J Archaeol Sci 33:879. https://doi.org/10.1016/j.jas.2005.10.020.

Ryhl-Svendsen M., Clausen G., Chowdhury Z., and Smith K.R. 2010. Fine particles and carbon monoxide from wood burning in 17th–19th century Danish kitchens: measurements at two reconstructed farm houses at the Lejre Historical–Archaeological Experimental Center. Atmos Environ 44:735–744. https://doi.org/10.1016/j.atmosenv.

Sabbatani S. and Fiorino S. 2008–2009. Apporti della paleopatologia alla definizione della patocenosi delle malattie infettive [Contribution of paleopathology to defining the pathocoenosis of infectious diseases (two parts)] Infezioni in Medicina 16(4): 236–250 and 7(1): 47–63.

Sabin S. and Atone A.C. 2023. Genetics and genomics. In: The Routledge handbook of paleopathology, ed. A.L. Grauer, 136–157. Routledge.

Sabin S. et al. 2020. A seventeenth-century *Mycobacterium tuberculosis* genome supports a Neolithic emergence of the *Mycobacterium tuberculosis* complex. Genome Biol 21:201. https://doi.org/10.1186/s13059-020-02112-1.

Sables A. 2010. Rare example of an early medieval dwarf infant from Brownslade, Wales. Int J Osteoarchaeol 20(1): 47–53.

Sager P. 1969. Spondylosis cervicalis: a pathological and osteoarchaeological study of osteochondrosis intervertebralis cervicalis, arthrosis uncovertebralis, and spondylarthrosis cervicalis. Munksgaard.

Salari N. et al. 2021. The global prevalence of osteoporosis in the world: a comprehensive systematic review and meta-analysis. J Orthop Surg Res 16(1): 1–20.

Salari N. et al. 2022a. Global prevalence of congenital anencephaly: a comprehensive systematic review and meta-analysis. Reprod Health 19(1): 201. https://doi.org/10.1186/s12978-022-01509-4.

Salari N. et al. 2022b. Global prevalence of cleft palate, cleft lip and cleft palate and lip: a comprehensive systematic review and meta-analysis. J Stomatol Oral Maxillofac Surg 123(2): 110–120.

Salazar-García D.C., Warinner C., Eerkens J.W.E., and Henry A.G. 2023. The potential of dental calculus as a novel source of biological isotopic data. In: Exploring human behavior through isotope analysis: applications in archaeological research, ed. M.M. Beasley and A.D. Somerville, 125–152. Springer Nature.

Salazar-Gómez A. and Alonso-Castro A.J. 2022. Medicinal plants from Latin America with wound healing activity: ethnomedicine, phytochemistry, preclinical and clinical studies: a review. Pharmaceuticals 15(9): 1095. https://doi.org/10.3390/ph15091095.

Saleem S.N. and Hawass Z. 2014. Brief report: ankylosing spondylitis or diffuse idiopathic skeletal hyperostosis in royal Egyptian mummies of the 18th–20th dynasties? CT [computed tomography] and archaeology studies. Arthritis Rheum 66(12): 3311–3316. https://doi.org/10.1002/art.38864.

Saleem S.N. and Hawass Z. 2017. Computed tomography study of the feet of mummy of Ramesses III: new insights on the harem conspiracy. J Comput Assist Tomogr 41(1): 15–17. https://dx.doi.org/10.1097/RCT.0000000000000489.

Salesse K., Kaupová S., Brůžek J., Kuželka V., and Velemínský P. 2013. An isotopic case study of individuals with syphilis from the pathological-anatomical reference collection of the national museum in Prague (Czech Republic, 19th century A.D.). Int J Paleopathol 25:46–55. https://doi.org/10.1016/j.ijpp.2019.04.001.

Sallares R. 2019. Malaria and Rome: a history of malaria in ancient Italy. Oxford University Press.

Salo W.L., Aufderheide A., Buikstra J., and Holcomb T.A. 1994. Identification of *Mycobacterium tuberculosis* DNA in a pre-Columbian mummy. Proc Nat Acad Sci USA 91:2091–2094.

Sampson P. et al. 1997. Incidence of fetal alcohol syndrome and prevalence of alcohol related neurodevelopment disorder. Teratology 56:317–326.

Sanderson K. 2023. How to convince a politician: a science advisor's lessons from the pandemic. Nature 616(7955): 20. https://doi.org/10.1038/d41586-023-00938-w.

Sankaran D., Partridge E., and Lakshminrusimha S. 2023. Congenital syphilis—an illustrative review. Children 10(8): 1310. https://doi.org/10.3390/children10081310.

Sankaye P. and Ostlere S. 2015. Arthritis at the shoulder joint. Semin Musculoskelet Radiol 19(30): 307–318.

Santana J., Rodríguez-Santos F.J., Camalich-Massieu M.D., Martín-Socas D., and Fregel R. 2019. Aggressive or funerary cannibalism? Skull-cup and human bone manipulation in Cueva

de El Toro (Early Neolithic, southern Iberia). Am J Phys Anthropol 169:31–54. https://doi.org/10.1002/ajpa.23805.
Santos A.L. 2020. A particular heritage: the importance of osteological collections. Metode Sci Stud J 10:91–97.
Santos A.L. and Roberts C.A. 2001. A picture of tuberculosis in young Portuguese people in the early 20th century: a multidisciplinary study of the skeletal and historical evidence. Am J Phys Anthropol 115:38–49.
Santos A.L. and Roberts C.A. 2006. Anatomy of a serial killer: differential diagnosis of tuberculosis based on rib lesions of adult individuals from the Coimbra Identified Skeletal Collection, Portugal. Am J Phys Anthropol 130:38–49.
Santos A.L. and Suby J.A. 2015. Skeletal and surgical evidence for acute osteomyelitis in non-adult individuals. Int J Osteoarchaeol 25:110–118, https://doi.org/10.1002/oa.2276.
Sarnat B.G. and Schour I. 1942. Enamel hypoplasia (chronologic enamel aplasia) in relation to systemic disease: a chronologic, morphologic and etiologic classification. J Am Dent Assoc 29(1): 67–75. ISSN 0002-8177. https://doi.org/10.14219/jada.archive.1942.0381.
Sarris P. 2022. Viewpoint: new approaches to the 'Plague of Justinian': *past and present*. 254(1): 315–346. https://doi.org/10.1093/pastj/gtab024.
Sasse T. and Haddon C. 2019. How academia can work with government. Institute for Government.
Satam H. et al. 2023. Next-generation sequencing technology: current trends and advancements. Biology 12(7): 997. https://doi.org/10.3390/biology12070997.
Saunders S.R. 1989. Non-metric skeletal variation. In: Reconstruction of life from the skeleton, ed. M.Y. Iscan and K.A.R. Kennedy, 95–108. Alan Liss.
Saunders S.R. and Hoppa R.D. 1993. Growth deficit in survivors and non-survivors: biological mortality bias in subadult skeletal samples. Yearbook of Physical Anthropology 36:127–151.
Saunders S.R. and Rainey D.L. 2008. Nonmetric trait variation in the skeleton: abnormalities, anomalies and atavisms. In: Biological anthropology of the human skeleton, 2nd edition, ed. M.A. Katzenberg and S.R. Saunders, 533–559. Wiley.
Scaffidi B.K. and Tung T.A. 2020. Endemic violence in a pre-Hispanic Andean community: a bioarchaeological study of cranial trauma from the Majes Valley, Peru. Am J Phys Anthropol 172:246–269. https://doi.org/10.1002/ajpa.24005.
Schats R. 2021. Cribriotic lesions in archaeological human skeletal remains: prevalence, co-occurrence, and association in medieval and early modern Netherlands. Int J Paleopathol 35:81–89.
Schell L.M. 1997. Culture as stressor: a revised model of biocultural interaction. Am J Phys Anthropol 102:67–77.
Scherer A.K. 2021. Recent research on the archaeology of war and violence. Annual Review of Anthropology 50:403–421.
Scheuer L. and Black S. 2004. The juvenile skeleton. Elsevier.
Schilder A.G. et al. 2016. Otitis media. Nat Rev Dis Primers 2(1): 16063. https://doi.org/10.1038/nrdp.2016.63.
Schlott T., Eiffert H., Schmidt-Schultz T., Gebhardt M., Parzinger H., and Schultz M. 2007. Detection and analysis of cancer genes amplified from bone material of a Scythian royal burial in Arzhan near Tuva, Siberia. Anticancer Research 27:4117–4119.
Schilling A.K. et al. 2019. British red squirrels remain the only known wild rodent host for leprosy bacilli. Front Vet Sci 6:8. https://doi.org/10.3389/fvets.2019.00008.
Schmit C.W. and Symes S.A., eds. 2008. The analysis of burnt human remains. Academic Press.
Schmitz-Cliever E. 1971. Zur Osteo-archaologie der Mittel-alterlichen Lepra: Ergebnis einer Probegrabung im Melaten bei Aachen. Medizinhist J 6: 249–263.
Schneider M.A. and Gilmour R.J. 2022. Exploring radiogrammetry beyond the second metacarpal: using the third, fourth, and fifth metacarpals to quantify cortical bone. Am J Hum Biol 35(3): e23831. https://doi.org/10.1002/ajhb.23831.
Schoenaker D.C.A., Jackson J.V., and Rowlands G.D. 2014. Mishra socioeconomic position, lifestyle factors and age at natural menopause: a systematic review and meta-analyses of studies across six continents. Int J Epidemiol 43(5): 1542–1562.
Schofield J.S. 2024. Wicked problems for archaeologists: heritage as transformative practice. Oxford University Press.

Schroeder H., Haviser J.B., Price T.D. 2014. The Zoutsteeg three: three new cases of African types of fental modification from Saint Martin, Dutch Caribbean. Int J Osteoarchaeol 2:688–696. https://doi.org/10.1002/oa.2253.

Schuenemann V.J. et al. 2013. Genome-wide comparison of medieval and modern *Mycobacterium leprae*. Science 341:179–183.

Schuenemann V.J. et al. 2018a. Ancient genomes reveal a high diversity of *Mycobacterium leprae* in medieval Europe. PLoS Pathog 14(5): e1006997. https://doi.org/10.1371/journal.ppat.1006997.

Schuenemann V.J. et al. 2018b. Historic *Treponema pallidum* genomes from colonial Mexico retrieved from archaeological remains. PLoS Negl Trop Dis 12(6): e0006447. https://doi.org/10.1371/journal.pntd.0006447.

Schug G.R., ed. 2021. The Routledge handbook of the bioarchaeology of environmental change. Routledge.

Schug G.R., Blevins K.E., Cox B., Gray K., and Mushrif-Tripathy V. 2013. Infection, disease, and biosocial processes at the end of the Indus civilization. PLoS One 8(12): e84814. https://journals.plos.org/plosone/article?id=10.1371/journal.pone.0084814.

Schug G.R and Halcrow S. 2022. Building a bioarchaeology of pandemic, epidemic, and syndemic diseases: lessons for understanding COVID-19. Bioarchaeol Int 6(1–2): 1–22. https://doi.org/10.5744/bi.2022.6000.

Schug G.R. et al. 2009. Ancient skeletal evidence for leprosy in India (2000 BC). PLoS One 4(5): 1–8.

Schug G.R. et al. 2023. Perspective: climate change, human health, and challenges to resilience in the Holocene. Proc Natl Acad Sci USA 120(4): e2209472120.

Schulting R.K. and Fibiger L. 2012. Sticks, stones, and broken bones: Neolithic violence in a European perspective. Oxford University Press.

Schultz M. 1979. Diseases of the ear region in early and prehistoric populations. J Hum Evol 8(6): 575–580.

Schultz M. 2001. Paleohistology of bone: a new approach to the study of ancient diseases. Yearbook of Physical Anthropology 44:106–147.

Schultz M. 2003. Light microscopic analysis in skeletal paleopathology. In: Identification of pathological conditions in human skeletal remains, ed. D.J. Ortner, 73–107. Academic Press.

Schultz M., Parzinger H., Posdnjakov D.V., Chikisheva T.A., and Schmidt-Schultz T. 2007. Oldest known case of metastasizing prostate carcinoma diagnosed in the skeleton of a 2,700-year-old Scythian king from Arzhan (Siberia, Russia). Int J Cancer 121:2591–2595.

Schulz D.C. et al. 2021. The many faces of ocular syphilis: case-based update on recognition, diagnosis, and treatment. Can J Ophthalmol 56(5): 283–293. https://dx.doi.org/10.1016/j.jcjo.2021.01.006.

Schwab T.R., Stillhard P.F., Schibli S., Furrer M., and Sommer C. 2018. Radial nerve palsy in humeral shaft fractures with internal fixation: analysis of management and outcome. Eur J Trauma Emerg Surg 44(2): 235–243. https://doi.org/10.1007/s00068-017-0775-9.

Schwartz J.H., Brauer J., and Gordon-Larsen P. 1995. Brief communication: Tigaran (Point Hope, Alaska) tooth drilling. Am J Phys Anthropol 97:77–82.

Scollard D.M. and Gillis T.P., eds. 2016. International textbook of leprosy. American Leprosy Missions. https://doi.org/10.1489/itl.11.1.

Scott G.R. and Pilloud M.A. 2019. Dental morphology. In: Biological anthropology of the human skeleton, 3rd edition, ed. M.A. Katzenberg and A.L. Grauer, 257–292. Wiley-Blackwell.

Scott G.R. and Turner C.G. 1997. The anthropology of modern human teeth. Cambridge University Press.

Scott R.M. et al. 2019. Domestication and large animal interactions: skeletal trauma in northern Vietnam during the hunter-gatherer Da But period. PLoS One 14(9): e0218777. https://doi.org/10.1371/journal.pone.0218777.

Scott-Clark C. and Levy A. 2003. Spectre orange. Guardian, 29 March: 20–27.

Scrimshaw N.S. 2000. Iron deficiency. In: Nutritional anthropology: biocultural perspectives on food and nutrition, ed. A.H. Goodman, D.L. Dufour, and G.H. Pelto, 252–258. Mayfield.

Scrimshaw S.C.M. 1984. Infanticide in human populations: societal and individual concerns. In: Infanticide: comparative and evolutionary perspectives, ed. G. Hausfater and S. Blaffer, 441–444. Aldine.

Scrivo R. et al. 2023. The conundrum of psoriatic arthritis: a pathogenetic and clinical pattern at the midpoint of autoinflammation and autoimmunity. Clin Rev Allergy Immunol 65(1): 72–85.

Seguin G., D'Incau E., Murail P., and Maureille B. 2014. The earliest dental prosthesis in Celtic Gaul? The case of an Iron Age burial at Le Chêne, France. Antiquity 88:488–500. https://doi.org/10.1017/S0003598X00101139.

Seiler R., Spigelman A.I., Zink A., and Rühli F. 2013. Oral pathologies of the Neolithic Iceman, c.3300BC. Eur J Oral Sci 121:137–141.

Sevitt S. 1981. Bone repair and fracture healing in man. Churchill Livingstone, Edinburgh.

Seyle H. 1950. The physiology and pathology of exposure to stress. Acta.

Shakespeare T. et al. 2022. Disabled people in Britain and the impact of the COVID-19 pandemic. Soc Policy Adm. 56(1): 103–117. https://doi.org/10.1111/spol.12758.

Shanko K., Kemal J, and Kenea D. 2015. A review on confronting zoonoses: the role of veterinarian and physician. J Veterinar Sci Technol 6:221.

Shao X. et al. 2018. Diagnosis and treatment of cerebral syphilitic gumma: a report of three cases. Front Neurosci. 12:100. https://doi.org/10.3389/fnins.2018.00100.

Shao Y.C., Harwood P., Grotz M.R.W., Limb D., and Giannoudis P.V. 2005. Radial nerve palsy associated with fractures of the shaft of the humerus. J Bone Joint Surg Br 87(12): 1647–1652. https://doi.org/10.1302/0301-620X.87B12.16132.

Shapiro F. and Yu J.Y. 2019. Woven bone overview: structural classification based on its integral role in development, repair and pathological bone formation throughout vertebrate groups. Eur Cell Mater 38:137–167.

Sharkia R., Khatib M., Sheikh-Muhammad A., Mahajnah M., and Zalan A. 2023. The prevailing trend of consanguinity in the Arab society of Israel: is it still a challenge? J Biosoc Sci 55(1): 169–173.

Sharma N., Bhatia S., Sodhi A.S., and Batra N. 2018. Oral microbiome and health. AIMS Microbiol 4(1): 42–66. https://doi.org/10.3934/microbiol.2018.1.42.

Shaw B. et al. 2019. Molecular insights into an ancient form of Paget's disease of bone. Proc Natl Acad Sci USA 116(21): 10463–10472.

Sheikh H. 2020. CAEP dental care statement. Can J Emerg Med 22(1): 36–39. https://doi.org/10.1017/cem.2019.437.

Shen Y., Liu J., Han Z., Jiang W., Cui H., and Xun Y. 2022. Risk prediction models for hepatocellular carcinoma in chronic hepatitis B patients on antiviral therapy: a meta-analysis. Clin Res Hepatol Gastroenterol 46(6): 101930. https://doi.org/10.1016/j.clinre.2022.101930.

Sheridan A. et al. 2018. A summary round-up list of Scottish archaeological human remains that have been sampled/analyzed for DNA as of January 2019. Discovery and Excavation in Scotland, New Series 19:228–250.

Sherwood J. 2010. Infection of the innocents: wet nurses, infants and syphilis in France 1780–1900. McGill-Queen's University Press.

Shillito L.M., Namdeo A., Bapat A.V., Mackay H., and Haddow S.D. 2022. Analysis of fine particulates from fuel burning in a reconstructed building at Çatalhöyük World Heritage Site, Turkey: assessing air pollution in prehistoric settled communities. Environ Geochem Health 44(3):1033–1048. https://doi.org/10.1007/s10653-021-01000-2.

Shin D.H. et al. 2013. The pattern of ancient parasite egg contamination in the private residence, alley, ditch and streambed soils of Old Seoul City, the capital of Joseon Dynasty. Int J Paleopathol 3:208–213. https://doi.org/10.1016/j.ijpp.2013.04.002.

Shriner D. and Rotimi C.N. 2018. Whole-genome-sequence-based haplotypes reveal single origin of the sickle allele during the Holocene wet phase. Am J Hum Genet 102(4): 547–556.

Siek T. 2013. The osteological paradox and issues of interpretation in paleopathology. vis-à-vis: Explorations in Anthropology 12 (1): 92–101.

Siek T. 2020. In defence of the osteoma: the relevance of benign tumours in bioarchaeology and palaeo-oncology. Int J Osteoarchaeol 30(2): 281–283.

Siek T., Rando C., Cieślik A., Spinek A., and Waldron T. 2021. A palaeoepidemiological investigation of osteomata, with reference to medieval Poland. Int J Osteoarchaeol 31(2): 154–161.

Silva F.J., Santos-Garcia D., Zheng X., Zhang L., and Han X.Y. 2022. Construction and analysis of the complete genome sequence of leprosy agent *Mycobacterium lepromatosis*. Microbiol Spectr 10(3): e0169221. https://doi.org/10.1128/spectrum.01692-21.

Silva M. et al. 2021. Biomolecular insights into North African-related ancestry, mobility and diet in eleventh-century Al-Andalus. Sci Rep 11:18121. https://doi.org/10.1038/s41598-021-95996-3.

Singh J.A. and Gaffo A. 2020. Gout epidemiology and comorbidities, Semin Arthritis Rheum 50:S11–S16. https://doi.org/10.1016/j.semarthrit.2020.04.008.

Singh J.A. and Strand V. 2008. Gout is associated with more comorbidities, poorer health related quality of life and higher healthcare utilisation in US veterans. Ann Rheum Dis 67(9): 1310–1316.

Sinigaglia R. et al. 2008. Musculoskeletal manifestations in pediatric acute leukemia. J Pediatr Orthop 28:20–28.

Sirak K. et al. 2020. Human auditory ossicles as an alternative optimal source of ancient DNA. Genome Res 30(3): 427–436. https://doi.org/10.1101/gr.260141.119.

Sirota M. et al. 2024. We must harness the power of social and behavioural science against the growing pandemic of antimicrobial resistance. Nat Hum Behav 8:11–13. https://doi.org/10.1038/s41562-023-01762-y.

Sjøvold T., Swedborg I., and Diener I. 1974. A pregnant woman from the Middle Ages with exostosis multiplex. Ossa 1:3–22.

Sketchfab. 2024. https://sketchfab.com/. Accessed 11 June 2024.

Skinsnes O.K. 1980. Leprosy in archaeologically recovered bamboo book in China. Int J Lepr 48:333.

Skinsnes O.K. and Chang P.H.C. 1985. Understanding of leprosy in ancient China. Int J Lepr 53(2): 289–307.

Slavin R.G. et al. 2005. The diagnosis and management of sinusitis: a practice parameter update. J Allergy Clin Immunol 116(6 Suppl): S13–47. https://doi.org/10.1016/j.jaci.2005.

Sledzik P. and Bellantoni N. 1994. Brief communication: bioarcheological and biocultural evidence for the New England vampire folk belief. Am J Phys Anthropol 94:269–274.

Slepchenko S. and Reinhard K. 2018. Paleoparasitology and pathoecology in Russia: investigations and perspectives. Int J Paleopathol 22:39–44. https://doi.org/10.1016/j.ijpp.2018.03.005.

Smelyansky E. 2020. The intolerant Middle Ages: a reader. University of Toronto Press.

Smith F.B. 1988. The retreat of tuberculosis, 1850–1950. Croom Helm.

Smith G.E. 1908. Anatomical report. Archaeological Survey of Nubia Bulletin 1:25–35.

Smith L. 2023. Air quality: policies, proposals, and concerns. House of Commons Library.

Smith M.E., Feinman G.M., Drennan R.D., Earle T., and Morris I. 2012. Archaeology as a social science. Proc Natl Acad Sci USA 109(20): 7617–7621. https://dx.doi.org/10.1073/pnas.1201714109.

Smith M.O. 1996. 'Parry' fractures and female-directed interpersonal violence: implications from the Late Archaic Period of west Tennessee. Int J Osteoarchaeol 6:84–91. https://doi.org/10.1002/(SICI)1099-1212(199601)6:1<84::AID-OA262>3.0.CO;2-G.

Smith M.O. 2003. Beyond palisades: the nature and frequency of late Prehistoric deliberate violent trauma in the Chickamauga Reservoir of east Tennessee. Am J Phys Anthropol 121:303–318.

Smith M.O., Dorsz J.R., and Betsinger T.K. 2013. Diffuse idiopathic skeletal hyperostosis (DISH) in pre-Columbian North America: evidence from the eastern Tennessee River Valley. Int J Paleopathol 3(1): 11–18.

Smith N.E. 2015. The paleoepidemiology of malaria in the ancient Near East. PhD dissertation, University of Arkansas. https://scholarworks.uark.edu/etd/28.

Smith P. and Kahila G. 1992. Identification of infanticide in archaeological sites: a case study from the late Roman–early Byzantine periods at Ashkelon, Israel. J Archaeol Sci 19:667–675.

Smith S.E. and Hirst C.S. 2019. 3D data in human remains disciplines: ethical challenges. In: Ethical challenges in the analysis of human remains, ed. K. Squires, D. Errickson, and N. Márquez-Grant, 315–346. Elsevier.

Smith T.M. and Warinner C. 2022. Developmental, evolutionary and behavioural perspectives on oral health. In: Palaeopathology and evolutionary medicine: an integrated approach, ed. K.A. Plomp, C.A. Roberts, S. Elton, and G.R. Bentley, 95–119. Oxford University Press.

Smith-Guzmán N.E. 2015. The skeletal manifestation of malaria: an epidemiological approach using documented skeletal collections. American Journal of Physical Anthropology 158(4):624–635.

Smith-Guzmán N.E., Rivera-Sandoval J., Knipper C., and Sánchez Arias G.A. 2020. Intentional dental modification in Panamá: new support for a late introduction of African origin. J Anthropol Archaeol 60(4): 101226. doi.org/10.1016/j.jaa.2020.101226.

Smith W.D., ed. and trans. 1994. Hippocrates. Epidemics 2, 4-7. Loeb Classical Library 477. Harvard University Press.

Smrčka V., Kuqelka V., and Melková J. 2003. Meningioma probable reason for trephination. Int J Osteoarchaeol 13:325–330.

Snoddy A.M.E. et al. 2019. 'Captain of all these men of death': an integrated case study of tuberculosis in nineteenth-century Otago, New Zealand. Bioarchaeol Int 3(4): 219–239.

Snow C.E. 1943. Two prehistoric Indian dwarf skeletons from Moundville. Alabama Museum of Natural History Museum Papers 21:1–90.

Sołtysiak A. 2017. Antemortem cranial trauma in ancient Mesopotamia. Int J Osteoarchaeol 27:119–128. https://doi.org/10.1002/oa.2478.

Somar P., Waltz M.M., and van Brakel W.H. 2020. The impact of leprosy on the mental wellbeing of leprosy-affected persons and their family members—a systematic review. Glob Ment Health (Camb) 7:e15. https://doi.org/10.1017/gmh.2020.3.

Souza G.C. et al. 2024. Experiences of social stigma of people living with Hansen's disease in Brazil: silencing, secrets and exclusion. Int Health 16(Suppl 1): i60–i67. https://doi.org/10.1093/inthealth/ihae005.

Spake L. and Cardoso H.F. 2019. Indirect evidence for biological mortality bias in growth from two temporo-spatially distant samples of children. Anthropologischer Anzeiger 76:379–390.

Spake L. and Cardoso H.F. 2021. Interpolation of the Maresh diaphyseal length data for use in quantitative analyses of growth. Int J Osteoarchaeol 31(2): 232–242.

Spake L., Hoppa R.D., Blau S., and Cardoso H.F. 2021. Lack of biological mortality bias in the timing of dental formation in contemporary children: implications for the study of past populations. Am J Phys Anthropol 174(4): 646–660.

Sparacello V.S., Roberts C.A., Canci A., Moggi-Cecchi J., and Marchi D. 2016. Insights on the paleoepidemiology of ancient tuberculosis from the structural analysis of postcranial remains from the Ligurian Neolithic (northwestern Italy). Int J Paleopathol 15:50–64. https://doi.org/10.1016/j.ijpp.2016.08.003.

Sparacello V.S., Roberts C.A., Kerudin A., and Müller R. 2017. A 6,500-year-old Middle Neolithic child from Pollera Cave (Liguria, Italy) with probable multifocal osteoarticular tuberculosis. Int J Paleopathol 17:67–74.

Spector L.G. et al. 2021. Comparative international incidence of Ewing sarcoma 1988 to 2012.Int J Cancer 149(5): 1054–1066.

Spekker O. et al. 2018. Rare manifestations of spinal tuberculosis in the Robert J. Terry Anatomical Skeletal Collection (National Museum of Natural History, Smithsonian Institution, Washington, DC, USA). Int J Osteoarchaeol 28:343–353. https://doi.org/10.1002/oa.2658.

Spekker O. et al. 2020a. Tracking down the white plague: the skeletal evidence of tuberculous meningitis in the Robert J. Terry Anatomical Skeletal Collection. PLoS One 15(3): e0230418. https://doi.org/10.1371/journal.pone.0230418.

Spekker O. et al. 2020b. Tracking down the white plague. Chapter two: the role of endocranial abnormal bloods vessel impressions and periosteal appositions in the paleopathological diagnosis of tuberculous meningitis. PLoS One 15(9): e0238444. https://doi.org/10.1371/journal.pone.0238444.

Sperduti A. et al. 2018. Tooth grooves, occlusal striations, dental calculus, and evidence for fiber processing in an Italian eneolithic/Bronze Age cemetery. Am J Phys Anthropol 167:234–243. https://doi.org/10.1002/ajpa.23619.

Spinek A.E., Kurek M., Kozakiewicz M., Głąb H., and Drążkowska A. 2023. A case of bilateral cleft palate with obturator prosthesis from XVIII century Cracow (Poland). J Archaeol Sci: Rep 51:104211. https://doi.org/10.1016/j.jasrep.2023.104211.

Spinks J. 2015. Monstrous births and visual culture in sixteenth-century Germany. Routledge.

Spyrou M.A. et al. 2022. The source of the Black Death in fourteenth-century central Eurasia. Nature 606:718–724 https://doi.org/10.1038/s41586-022-04800-3.

Squires K., Booth T., and Roberts C.A. 2019a. The ethics of sampling human skeletal remains for destructive analyses: a UK Perspective. In: Ethical challenges in the analysis of human remains, ed. K. Squires, D. Errickson, and N. Márquez-Grant, 265–297. Elsevier.

Squires K., Errickson D., and Márquez-Grant N., eds. 2019b. Ethical challenges in the analysis of human remains. Elsevier.
Squires K., Roberts C.A., Marquez-Grant N. 2022. Commentary: ethical considerations and publishing within biological anthropology. Am J Biol Anthropol 177:615–619. https://doi.org/10.1002/ajpa.24467.
Stamm L.V. 2015. Pinta: Latin America's forgotten disease? Am J Trop Med Hyg 93(5): 901–903. https://doi.org/10.4269/ajtmh.15-0329.
Standaert C.J. and Herring S.A. 2000. Spondylolysis: a critical review. Br J Sports Med 34:415–422.
Standen V.G. et al. 2020. Violence in hunters, fishermen, and gatherers of the Chinchorro culture: archaic societies of the Atacama Desert (10,000–4,000 cal yr BP). Am J Phys Anthropol 172:227–245. https://doi.org/10.1002/ajpa.24009.
Standen V.G., and Arriaza B. 2000. Trauma in the preceramic coastal populations of northern Chile: violence or occupational hazards. Am J Phys Anthropol 112:239–249.
Stantis C. and Kendall E.J. 2023. Isotopes in paleopathology. In: The Routledge handbook of paleopathology, ed. A.L. Grauer, 118–135. Routledge.
Stanton E., Urata M., Chen J.F., and Chai Y. 2022. The clinical manifestations, molecular mechanisms and treatment of craniosynostosis. Dis Model Mech 15(4): dmm.04390. https://doi.org/10.1242/dmm.049390.
Starbuck J. 2011. On the antiquity of Trisomy 21: moving towards a quantitative diagnosis of Down syndrome in historic material culture. Journal of Contemporary Anthropology 2(1): 61–89.
Steckel R., Sciulli P.W., and Rose J., eds. 2002. The backbone of history: health and nutrition in the Western Hemisphere. Cambridge University Press.
Steckel R.H. 1995. Stature and the standard of living. J Econ Lit 33:1903–1940.
Steckel R.H., Larsen C.S., Roberts C.A., and Baten J, eds. 2019. The backbone of Europe: health, diet, work and violence over two millennia. Cambridge University Press.
Steckel R.H., Larsen C.S., Sciulli P.W., and Walker P.L. 2005. The global history of health project: data collection codebook. https://www.uv.es/paleolab/Codebook-08-25-051%5B1%5D.pdf.
Steckel R.H., Sciulli P.W., and Rose J.C. 2002. A health index from skeletal remains. In: The backbone of history: health and nutrition in the Western Hemisphere, ed. R.H. Steckel, P.W. Sciulli, and J.C. Rose, 61–93. Cambridge University Press.
Steele J. 2000. Skeletal indicators of handedness. In: Human osteology in archaeology and forensic science, ed. M. Cox and S. Mays, 307–323. Greenwich Medical Media.
Steinbock R.T. 1976. Paleopathological diagnosis and interpretation: bone diseases in ancient human populations. Charles C. Thomas.
Steinbock R.T. 1993. Rickets and osteomalacia. In: The Cambridge world history of human disease, ed. K. Kiple, 978–980. Cambridge University Press.
Steinmann C. et al. 2011. Pectus excavatum and pectus carinatum patients suffer from lower quality of life and impaired body image: a control group comparison of psychological characteristics prior to surgical correction. Eur J Cardiothorac Surg 40:1138–1145. https://doi.org/10.1016/j.ejcts.2011.02.019.
Stephen J. et al. 2015. Mutations in patients with osteogenesis imperfecta from consanguineous Indian families. Eur J Med Genet 58(1): 21–27.
Stephenson L. and Byard R.W. 2020. An atlas overview of characteristic features of tuberculosis that may be encountered at autopsy. Forensic Sci Med Pathol 16(1): 143–151. https://doi.org/10.1007/s12024-019-00161-y.
Stern C. et al. 2020. Distal femoral cortical irregularity at knee MRI: increased prevalence in youth competitive alpine skiers. Radiology 296(2): 411–419.
Stevens G.C. and Wakely J. 1993. Diagnostic criteria for identification of seashell as a trephination implement. Int J Osteoarchaeol 3:167–176.
Stewart N.A., Gerlach R.F., Gowland R.L., Gron K.J., and Montgomery J. 2017. Sex determination of human remains from peptides in tooth enamel. Proc Natl Acad Sci USA 114(52): 13649–13654. https://doi.org/10.1073/pnas.1714926115.
Stewart T.D. 1958. Stone age skull surgery: a general review with emphasis on the New World. Smithsonian Inst Ann Rep 1957:461–491.
Steyn M., Scholtz Y., Botha D., and Pretorius S. 2013. The changing face of tuberculosis: trends in tuberculosis-associated skeletal changes. Tuberculosis 93:467–474. https://doi.org/10.1016/j.

Stini W.A. 1990. 'Osteoporosis': etiologies, prevention and treatment. Yearbook of Physical Anthropology 33:151–194.
Stirland A. 2000. Raising the dead: the skeleton crew of Henry VIII's great ship, the Mary Rose. Wiley.
Stirland A. and Waldron T. 1997. Evidence for activity-related markers in the vertebrae of the crew of the Mary Rose. J Archaeol Sci 24:329–335.
Stodder A.L.W. 2018. Taphonomy and the nature of archaeological assemblages. In: Biological anthropology of the human skeleton. 3rd edition, ed. A. Katzenberg and A. Grauer, 73–116. Wiley-Blackwell.
Stone A.C. and Ozaga A.T. 2019. Ancient DNA and the study of ancient disease. In: Ortner's identification of pathological conditions in human skeletal remains, ed. J.E. Buikstra, 183–210. Academic Press.
Stone J.H., Nelson G.C., and Fitzpatrick S.M. 2020. Temporomandibular joint osteoarthritis at Chelechol ra Orrak, Palau. Int J Paleopathol 28:20–31.
Stone P.K. 2012. Binding women: ethnology, skeletal deformations, and violence against women. Int J Paleopathol 2:53–60.
Storey G.O. and Scott D.L. 1998. Arthritis associated with venereal disease in nineteenth-century London. Clin Rheumatol 17:500–504. https://doi.org/10.1007/BF01451287.
Storey J.E. 2020. Risk factors for elder abuse and neglect: a review of the literature. Aggression and Violent Behavior 50:101339. https://doi.org/10.1016/j.avb.2019.101339.
Stout S.D., Cole M.E., and Agnew A.M. 2019. Histomorphology: deciphering the metabolic record. In: Ortner's identification of pathological conditions in human skeletal remains, ed. J.E. Buikstra, 91–167. Academic Press.
Strak M. et al. 2021. Long term exposure to low level air pollution and mortality in eight European cohorts within the ELAPSE project: pooled analysis. Br Med J 374:n1904. https://doi.org/10.1136/bmj.n1904.
Stroud G. and Kemp R. 1993. Cemeteries of St Andrew, Fishergate: the archaeology of York; the medieval cemeteries 12/2. Council for British Archaeology for York Archaeological Trust.
Strouhal E. and Němečková A. 2009. History and palaeopathology of malignant tumours. Anthropologie 47(3): 289–294.
Strouhal E., Horáčkova L., Likovsky J., Vargová L., and Daneš J. 2002. Traces of leprosy from the Czech Kingdom. In: The past and present of leprosy: archaeological, historical, palaeopathological and clinical approaches, ed. C.A. Roberts, M.E. Lewis, and K. Manchester, 223–232. British Archaeological Reports International Series 1054. Archaeopress.
Stuart-Macadam P. 1989. Porotic hyperostosis: relationship between orbital and vault lesions. Am J Phys Anthropol 80:187–193.
Stuart-Macadam P. 1992. Anemia in past human populations. In: Diet, demography and disease: changing perspectives on anemia, ed. P. Stuart-Macadam and S.K. Kent, 151–170. Aldine De Gruyter.
Stuart-Macadam P. and Dettwyler K.A., eds. 1995. Breastfeeding: biocultural perspectives. Aldine De Gruyter.
Stuckert C.M. and Kricun M.E. 2011. A case of bilateral forefoot amputation from the Romano-British cemetery of Lankhills, Winchester, UK. Int J Paleopathol 1:111–116. https://doi.org/10.1016/j.ijpp.2011.04.001.
Sture J. 2002. Biocultural perspectives on birth defects in late medieval rural and urban populations in northern England. Unpublished Ph.D. dissertation, Department of Archaeology, Durham University, England.
Suby J.A. 2014. Porotic hyperostosis and cribra orbitalia in human remains from southern Patagonia. Anthropol Sci 122(2): 69–79.
Suby J.A. and Giberto D.A. 2019. Temporomandibular joint osteoarthritis in human ancient skeletal remains from Late Holocene in southern Patagonia. Int J Osteoarchaeol 29(1): 14–25.
Sullivan E. 2010. Why Florence Nightingale is still relevant to us today? In: Nurse past, present and future: the making of modern nursing, ed. K. Trant and S. Usher, 24–27. Black Dog.
Sun L., Pechenkina K., Cao Y., Zhang H., and Qi X. 2019. Cases of endocranial lesions on juvenile skeletons from Longshan cultural sites in Henan Province, China. Int J Paleopathol 26:61–74. https://doi.org/10.1016/j.ijpp.2019.06.001.

Sun X., You S., Wang J., Zhang Q., and Wang Q. 2023. A commoner with advanced surgery: a bioarcheological study of a trepanation case with special reference to the medical care system during the Western Zhou Dynasty of China (1045–771 BCE). J Archaeol Sci: Rep 47:103830. https://doi.org/10.1016/j.jasrep.2023.103830.

Sundman E.A. and Kjellström A. 2013. Signs of sinusitis in times of urbanization in Viking age-early medieval Sweden. J Archaeol Sci 40: 4457–465. https://doi.org/10.1016/j.jas.2013.06.010.

Suter S. et al. 2008. Technical note: standardized and semiautomated Harris lines detection. Am J Phys Anthropol 137(3): 362–366.

Suzuki T. and Inoue T. 2007. Earliest evidence of spinal tuberculosis from the aneolithic Yayoi period in Japan. Int J Ostearchaeol 17:392–402.

Suzuki T., Fujita H., and Choi J.G. 2008. Brief communication: new evidence of tuberculosis from prehistoric Korea—population movement and early evidence of tuberculosis in Far East Asia. Am J Phys Anthropol 136:357–360.

Swali P. et al. 2023. *Yersinia pestis* genomes reveal plague in Britain 4000 years ago. Nat Commun 14:2930. https://doi.org/10.1038/s41467-023-38393-w.

Swinson D., Snaith J., Buckberry J., and Brickley M. 2010. High performance liquid chromatography (HPLC) in the investigation of gout in palaeopathology. Int J Osteoarchaeol 20(2): 135–143.

Szeniczey T. et al. 2019. Hyperostosis frontalis interna in ancient populations from the Carpathian Basin—a possible relationship between lifestyle and risk of development. Int J Paleopathol 24:108–118.

Szostakowski B., Smitham P., and Khan W.S. 2017. Plaster of Paris—short history of casting and injured limb immobilization. Open Orthop J. 17(11): 291–296. https://doi.org/10.2174/1874325001711010291.

Tagaya A. 2014. Human remains from Tappeh Sang-e Chakhmaq. In: The first farming village in northeast Iran and Turan: Tappeh Sang-e Chakhmaq and beyond, ed. A. Tsuneki, 39–42. Research Center for West Asian Civilization, University of Tsukuba.

Taher A.T., Weatherall D.J., and Cappellini M.D. 2018. Thalassaemia. Lancet 391(10116): 155–167.

Takahashi T. et al. 2023. Comparison of radiological characteristics between diffuse idiopathic skeletal hyperostosis and ankylosing spondylitis: a multicenter study. Sci Rep 13(1): 1849. https://doi.org/10.1038/s41598-023-28946-w.

Takashima K. et al. 2018. Ethical concerns on sharing genomic data including patients' family members. BMC Med Ethics 19:61. https://doi.org/10.1186/s12910-018-0310-5.

Tal L. and Jaramillo D. 2020. It's time to recognize the perichondrium. Pediatr Radiol 50(2): 153–160. https://doi.org/10.1007/s00247-019-04534-x.

Tancock D. 2014. Congenital defects in 18th and 19th century populations from rural and urban Northeast England. Unpublished PhD dissertation. Durham University, England.

Tang L. et al. 2023. Paleoproteomic evidence reveals dairying supported prehistoric occupation of the highland Tibetan Plateau. Sci Adv 9(15): eadf0345. https://doi.org/10.1126/sciadv.adf0345.

Tao Z. et al. 2023. Prevalence of developmental dysplasia of the hip (DDH) in infants: a systematic review and meta-analysis. BMJ Paediatr Open 7(1). https://doi.org/10.1136/bmjpo-2023-002080.

Tayles N. 1996. Anemia, genetic diseases, and malaria in prehistoric mainland southeast Asia. Am J Phys Anthrop 101:11–27.

Tayles N. and Buckley H.R. 2004. Leprosy and tuberculosis in Iron Age southeast Asia? Am J Phys Anthropol 125:239–256.

Taylor G.M. et al. 2024. Bioarchaeological investigation of individuals with suspected multibacillary leprosy from the mediaeval leprosarium of St Mary Magdalen, Winchester, Hampshire, UK. J Med Microbiol 73(2). https://dx.doi.org/10.1099/jmm.0.001806.

Taylor G.M., Murphy E., Hopkins R., Rutland P., and Chistov Y. 2007. First report of *Mycobacterium bovis* DNA in human remains from the Iron Age. Microbiology 153:1243–1249.

Taylor J.H. and Antoine D. 2014. Ancient lives, new discoveries: eight mummies, eight stories. British Museum.

Taylor M., Rutland P., and Molleson T. 1997. A sensitive polymerase chain reaction method for the detection of Plasmodium species in ancient human remains. Ancient Biomol 1:192–203.
Teerlink C.C. et al. 2021. A role for the MEGF6 gene in predisposition to osteoporosis. Ann Hum Genet 85(2): 58–72.
Temple D.H. and Edes A.N. 2022. Stress in bioarchaeology, epidemiology, and evolutionary medicine: an integrated conceptual model of shared history from the descriptive to the developmental. In: Palaeopathology and evolutionary medicine: an integrated approach, ed. K.A. Plomp, C.A. Roberts, S. Elton, and G.R. Bentley, 261–285. Oxford University Press.
Temple D.H. and Larsen C.S. 2007. Dental caries prevalence as evidence for agriculture and subsistence variation during the Yayoi period in prehistoric Japan: biocultural interpretations of an economy in transition. Am J Phys Anthropol 134:501–512.
Temple D.H. and Stojanowski C.M., eds. 2019. Hunter-gatherer adaptation and resilience: a bioarchaeological perspective. Cambridge University Press.
Theron G., Cohen T., and Dye C. 2021. Epidemiology. In: Clinical tuberculosis, 6th edition, ed. L. Friedman, M. Dedicoat, and P.D.O. Davies, 17–37. CRC Press.
Thomas R. 2012. Nonhuman paleopathology. In: The global history of paleopathology: pioneers and prospects, ed. J.E. Buikstra and C.A. Roberts, 652–664. Oxford University Press.
Thomas R. 2019. Non-human paleopathology—are we so different? In: Ortner's identification of pathological conditions in human skeletal remains, ed. J.E. Buikstra, 809–822. Academic Press.
Thompson T., ed. 2015. The archaeology of cremation. Oxbow Books.
Tiesler V. 2024. Ancient Maya teeth: dental modification, cosmology, and social identity in Mesoamerica. University of Texas Press.
Tiesler V., Coppa A., Zabala P. and Cucina A. 2016. Scurvy-related morbidity and death among Christopher Columbus' crew at La Isabela, the first European town in the New World (1494–1498): an assessment of the skeletal and historical information. Int J Osteoarchaeol 26(2): 191–202.
Tietze E., Berón M.A., Lucero E., and Beltrame M.O. 2023. Ancient parasite infections from the main Pampean-Patagonian cemetery of hunter-gatherer of prehistoric times: archaeological site Chenque I (Parque Nacional Lihué Calel, La Pampa Province, Argentina). J Archaeol Sci: Rep 49:104040. https://doi.org/10.1016/j.jasrep.2023.104040.
Tilley L. 2012. The bioarchaeology of care. SAA Archaeological Record 12(3): 39–41.
Tilley L. 2015. Theory and practice in the bioarchaeology of care. Springer.
Tilley L. and Cameron T. 2014. Introducing the Index of Care: a web-based application supporting archaeological research into health-related care. Int J Paleopathol 6:5–9.
Tilley L., and Oxenham M.F. 2011. Survival against the odds: modeling the social implications of care provision to seriously disabled individuals. Int J Paleopathology 1(1):35–42. https://doi.org/10.1016/j.ijpp.2011.02.003.
Tilley L. and Schrenk A.A. 2017. New developments in the bioarchaeology of care. Springer.
Tillier A.-M., Arensburg B., Duday H., and Vandermeersch B. 2001. Brief communication: an early case of hydrocephalus: the Middle Paleolithic Qafzeh child (Israel). Am J Phys Anthropol 114:166–170.
Timmins S., Seréville-Niel C., and Brickley M. 2017. Childhood cranial trauma from a Late Roman and Merovingian context from Michelet, Lisieux, France. Int J Osteoarchaeol 27: 715–722. https://doi.org/ 10.1002/oa.2581.
Tipper S., Wilson P., and Roberts C.A. 2023. Spondylolysis in ancient Nubian skeletal populations. Int J Osteoarchaeol 33(5): 876–885. https://doi.org/10.1002/oa.3241.
Titche L.L., Coulthard S.W., Wachter R.D., Thies A.C., and Harries L.L. 1981. Prevalence of mastoid infection in prehistoric Arizona Indians. Am J Phys Anthropol 56:269–273. https://doi.org/10.1002/ajpa.1330560306.
Titelbaum A.R. 2020. Developmental anomalies and South American paleopathology: a comparison of block vertebrae and co-occurring axial anomalies among three skeletal samples from the El Brujo archaeological complex of northern coastal Peru. Int J Paleopathol 29:76–93.
Titelbaum A.R., Burnett S.E., and Case D.T. 2022. Developmental conditions in paleopathology. In: The Routledge handbook of paleopathology, ed. A.L. Grauer, 250–270. Routledge.

Toikumo S. et al. 2024. A multi-ancestry genetic study of pain intensity in 598,339 veterans. Nat Med 30(4): 1075–1084. https://doi.org/10.1038/s41591-024-02839-5.
Tomczyk J. et al. 2014. The prevalence of pulp stones in historical populations from the middle Euphrates valley (Syria). Am J Phys Anthropol 153(1): 103–115. https://doi.org/10.1002/ajpa.22414.
Tomczyk J., Mankowska-Pliszka H., Palczewski P., and Olczak- Kowalczyk D. 2015a. Congenital syphilis in the skeleton of a child from Poland (Radom, 18th–19th century AD). Anthropol Rev 78:79–90.
Tomczyk J. et al. 2015b. Anaemia (thalassaemia) in the middle Euphrates valley of Syria in the second–fourth centuries AD? Antiquity 90(349): 157–171.
Torgerson P.R. et al. 2020. Source attribution of human echinococcosis: a systematic review and meta-analysis. PLoS Negl Trop Dis 14(6): e0008382. https://doi.org/10.1371/journal.pntd.0008382.
Tornberg A. and Jacobsson L. 2018. Care and consequences of traumatic brain injury in Neolithic Sweden: a case study of ante mortem skull trauma and brain injury addressed through the bioarchaeology of care. Int J Osteoarchaeol 28:188–198. https://doi.org/10.1002/oa.2646.
Torres-Rouff C. 2020. Cranial modification and the shapes of heads across the Andes. Int J Paleopathol 29:94–101. https://doi.org/10.1016/j.ijpp.2019.06.007.
Torres-Rouff C. and Costa Junqueira M.A. 2006. Interpersonal violence in prehistoric San Pedro de Atacama, Chile: behavioral implications of environmental stress. Am J Phys Anthropol 130(1): 60–70. https://doi.org/10.1002/ajpa.
Toyne J.M. 2011. Possible cases of scalping from pre-hispanic highland Peru. Int J Osteoarchaeol 21:229–42. https://doi.org/10.1002/oa.1127.
Toyne J.M. and Turner B.L. 2020. Linking isotope analysis and paleopathology: an Andean perspective. Int J Paleopathol 29:117–127.
Trembly D. 2002. Perspectives on the history of leprosy in the Pacific. In: The past and present of leprosy: archaeological, historical, palaeopathological and clinical approaches, ed. C.A. Roberts, M.E. Lewis, and K. Manchester, 233–238. British Archaeological Reports International Series 1054. Archaeopress.
Trevor J.C. 1950. Notes on the human remains of Romano-British date from Norton, Yorkshire. In: Roman pottery at Norton, East Yorkshire. Roman Malton and District Report 7, ed. P. Corder, 39–40. Roman Antiquities Committee of the Yorkshire Archaeological Society.
Trinkhaus E. 1983. Shanidar Neanderthals. Academic Press.
Trivellin G. et al. 2014. Gigantism and acromegaly due to Xq26 microduplications and GPR101 mutation. N Engl J Med 371(25): 2363–2374.
Tröhler U. 2005. Lind and scurvy: 1747 to 1795. J R Soc Med 98(11): 519–522.
Tromp M. et al. 2020. Exploitation and utilization of tropical rainforests indicated in dental calculus of ancient Oceanic Lapita culture colonists. Nat Hum Behav 4:489–495. https://doi.org/10.1038/s41562-019-0808-y.
Trumble B.C. and Finch CE. 2019. The exposome in human evolution: from dust to diesel. Q Rev Biol 94(4): 333–394.
Tucker B.K. et al. 2001. Microscopic characteristics of hacking trauma. J Forensic Sci 46(2): 234–240.
Tulumello G. et al. 2020. A possible case of palaeopathology of leukaemia from Late Antique southern Italy. Lancet Oncol 21(12): 1561–1562.
Tumler D., Paladin A., and Zink A.R. 2021. Trauma patterns and injury prevalence in early medieval Säben-Sabiona, Italy. Int J Osteoarchaeol 31(5): 820–832. https://doi.org/10.1002/oa.2993.
Tung T.A. 2012. Violence, ritual, and the Wari Empire: a social bioarchaeology of imperialism in the ancient Andes. University Press of Florida.
Tur S.S., Svyatko S.V., Beisenov A.Z., and Tishkin A.A. 2016. An exceptional case of healed vertebral wound with trapped bronze arrowhead: analysis of a 7th–6th c. BC individual from central Kazakhstan. Int J Osteoarchaeol 26:740–746. https://doi.org/ 10.1002/oa.2470.
Turankar R.P. et al. 2022. Existence of viable *Mycobacterium leprae* in natural environment and its genetic profiling in a leprosy endemic region. Front Trop Dis 3:972682. https://doi.org/10.3389/fitd.2022.972682.
Turner C. 1993. Cannibalism in Chaco Canyon: the charnel pit excavated in 1926 at Small House ruin by Frank H.H. Roberts, Jr. Am J Phys Anthropol 91:421–439.

Turner T.R., Wagner J.K., and Cabana G.S. 2018. Ethics in biological anthropology. Am J Phys Anthropol 165:939–951. https://doi.org/10.1002/ajpa.23367.

Turunen S. et al. 2020. Maternal hyperthyroidism and pregnancy outcomes: a population-based cohort study. Clin Endocrinol 93(6): 721–728.

Tyrrell A. 2000. Skeletal non-metric traits and the assessment of inter- and intra-population diversity: past problems and future potential. In: Human osteology in archaeology and forensic science, ed. M. Cox and S. Mays, 289–306. Greenwich Medical Media.

Ubelaker D. 1992. Hyoid fracture and strangulation. J Forensic Sci 37(5): 1216–1222.

Ubelaker D. and Adams B.J. 1995. Differentiation of perimortem and post-mortem trauma using taphonomic indicators. J Forensic Sci 40(3): 509–512.

Uhl E.W. and Thomas R. 2022. Uncovering tales of transmission: an integrated palaeopathological perspective on the evolution of shared human and animal pathogens. In: Palaeopathology and evolutionary medicine: an integrated approach, ed. K. Plomp, C.A. Roberts, S. Elton, and G. Bentley, 316–349. Oxford University Press.

Ullinger J. and Loewen T. 2023. Dental disease. In: The Routledge handbook of paleopathology, ed. A.L. Grauer, 360–378. Routledge.

Ulu-Kilic A. et al. 2014. Update on treatment options for spinal brucellosis. Clin Microbiol Infect 20:O75–O82.

Ungar P.S. and Crittenden A.N. 2017. Toddlers in transition: linear enamel hypoplasias in the Hadza of Tanzania: Hadza linear enamel hypoplasias. Int J Osteoarchaeol 27(4): 638–649. https://doi.org/10.1002/oa.2586.

United Nations. 2023. The Sustainable Development Goals report: towards a rescue plan for people and planet. Special edition. United Nations.

United Nations. 2024a. Department of economic and social affairs: sustainable development. https://sdgs.un.org/goals. Accessed 1 June 2024.

United Nations. 2024b. Universal health coverage. https://www.un.org/pga/73/event/universal-health-coverage/. Accessed 8 July 2024.

Urban C. et al. 2024. Ancient *Mycobacterium leprae* genome reveals medieval English red squirrels as animal leprosy host. Curr Biol 2024:S0960–9822(24)00446–9. https://doi.org/10.1016/j.cub.2024.04.006.

Ursin G. et al. 2005. Reproductive factors and subtypes of breast cancer defined by hormone receptor and histology. Br J Cancer 93(3): 364–371.

Urteaga O. and Pack G.T. 1966. On the antiquity of melanoma. Cancer 19:607–610.

Vågene Å.J. et al. 2022. Geographically dispersed zoonotic tuberculosis in pre-contact South American human populations. Nat Commun 13(1): 1195. https://doi.org/10.1038/s41467-022-28562-8.

Vairamuthu T. and Pfeiffer S. 2018. A juvenile with compromised osteogenesis provides insights into past hunter-gatherer lives. Int J Paleopathol 20:1–9.

Vaishya R., Vijay V., Nwagbara I.C., and Agarwal A.K. 2017. Diffuse idiopathic skeletal hyperostosis (DISH)—a common but less known cause of back pain. J Clin Orthop Trauma 8(2): 191–196. https://doi.org/10.1016/j.jcot.2016.11.006.

Valente de Souza L., Hoffmann A., and Weiss G. 2021. Impact of bacterial infections on erythropoiesis. Expert Rev Anti Infect Ther 19(5): 619–633.

Valoriani S., Eliopoulos C., Irish J.D. and Borrini M. 2019. Health and safety issues in the Victorian workplace: an example of mandibular phosphorus necrosis from Gloucester, UK. Int J Osteoarchaeol 30(1): 73–79.

Van Arsdall A. 2010. Medieval herbal remedies: the Old English herbarium and Anglo-Saxon medicine. Routledge.

Van der Merwe A.E., Steyn M., and L'Abbé E.N. 2010. Trauma and amputations in 19th century miners from Kimberley, South Africa. Int J Osteoarchaeol 20(3): 291–306. https://doi.org/10.1002/oa.1035.

Van Spelde A.M., Schroeder H., Kjellström A., and Lidén K. 2021. Approaches to osteoporosis in paleopathology: how did methodology shape bone loss research? Int J Paleopathol 33:245–257.

Van't Noordende A.T. et al. 2021. Leprosy perceptions and knowledge in endemic districts in India and Indonesia: differences and commonalities. PLoS Negl Trop Dis 15 (1): e0009031. https://doi.org/10.1371/journal.pntd.0009031.

Vanhoenacker F., Van Hul W., Wuyts W., Willems P., and De Schepper A. 2001. Hereditary multiple exostoses: from genetics to clinical syndrome and complications. Eur J Radiol 40:208–217.

Varkey B. 2021. Principles of clinical ethics and their application to practice. Med Princ Pract 30(1): 17–28. https://doi.org/10.1159/000509119.

Varlık N. 2017. Review essay: beyond Eurocentric histories of plague. Early Sci Med 22(4): 361–373. https://doi.org/10.1163/15733823-00224P04.

Vaz F., Mehta N., and Hamilton R.D. 2021. Ear, nose and throat and eye disease. In: Kumar and Clark's clinical medicine, 10th edition, ed. A. Feather, D. Randall, and M. Waterhouse, 899–925. Elsevier.

Velasco G.C., Artates A, M.V., Castañeda S.S., and Castillo R.M. 2020. Leprosy of the larynx and its clinical manifestations—a case report. Otolaryngol Case Rep 15:100176. https://doi.org/10.1016/j.xocr.2020.100176.

Velasco-Vázquez J., Delgado-Darias T., and Alberto-Barroso V. 2018. Violence targeting children or violent society? Craniofacial injuries among the pre-Hispanic subadult population of Gran Canaria (Canary Islands). Int J Osteoarchaeol 28:388–396. https://doi.org/10.1002/oa.2662.

Velmurugan H. and Thangaraju P. 2024. Nutritional status in leprosy patients: a systematic review and meta-analysis. Infect Disord Drug Targets 24(3): e211123223670. https://doi.org/10.2174/01 18715265263893231102114955.

Velsko I.M., Fellows Yates J.A., Aron F. et al. 2019. Microbial differences between dental plaque and historic dental calculus are related to oral biofilm maturation stage. Microbiome 7:102. https://doi.org/10.1186/s40168-019-0717-3.

Ventades N.G., Perez-Rubio C., Hervella M., and de-la-Rúa C. 2020. Rickets in a non-industrialised Iberian population: a case study in Vitoria-Gasteiz (Basque Country, Spain) between the 12th and 18th centuries. Quat Int 566:245–255.

Ventades N.G., Laza I.M., Hervella M., and de-la-Rúa C. 2018. A recording form for differential diagnosis of arthropathies. Int J Paleopathol 20:45–49.

Ventresca Miller A.R. et al. 2023. Permafrost preservation reveals proteomic evidence for yak milk consumption in the 13th century. Commun Biol 6:351. https://doi.org/10.1038/s42003-023-04723-3.

Ventura L. et al. 2021. Giant cell tumor of bone in an eighteenth-century Italian mummy. Virchows Archive 479(6): 1255–1261.

Verano J. 2016. Holes in the head: the art and archaeology of trepanation in ancient Peru. Studies in Pre-Columbian Art and Archaeology Series no. 38. Dumbarton Oaks Research Library Collection.

Verano J.W., Anderson L.S., and Franco R. 2000. Foot amputation by the Moche of ancient Peru: osteological evidence and archaeological context. Int J Osteoarchaeol 10:177–188.

Verhoeff M., van der Veen E., Rovers M., Sanders E., and Schilder A. 2006. Chronic suppurative otitis media: a review. Int J Otorhinolaryngol 70:1–12.

Verlinden P. and Lewis M.E. 2015. Childhood trauma: methods for the identification of physeal fractures in non-adult skeletal remains. Am J Phys Anthropol 157(3): 411–420. https://doi.org/10.1002/ajpa.22732.

Vernon-Roberts B. and Pirie C.J. 1973. Healing trabecular microfractures in the bodies of lumbar vertebrae. Ann Rheum Dis 32:406–412.

Veselka B., Hoogland M., and Waters-Rist A. 2015. Rural rickets: vitamin D deficiency in a post-medieval farming community from the Netherlands. Int J Osteoarchaeol 25(5): 666–675.

Vested A. et al. 2018. A nationwide follow-up study of occupational organic dust exposure and risk of chronic obstructive pulmonary disease (COPD). Occup Environ Med 76(2): 105–113. https://doi.org/10.1136/oemed-2018-105323.

Viciano J., De Luca S., López-Lázaro S., Botella D., and Diéguez-Ramírez J.P. 2015. A probable case of gigantism/acromegaly in skeletal remains from the Jewish necropolis of 'Ronda Sur' (Lucena, Córdoba, Spain; VIII–XII centuries CE). Anthropologischer Anzeiger 72(1): 67–87.

Vikatou I., Hoogland M.L.P., and Waters-Rist A.L. 2017. Osteochondritis dissecans of skeletal elements of the foot in a 19th century rural farming community from the Netherlands. Int J Paleopathol 19:53–63. https://doi.org/10.1016/j.ijpp.

Villa C. and *Jørkov M.L. 2023. Paleoradiology.* In: The Routledge handbook of paleopathology, ed. A.L. Grauer, 105–117. Routledge.

Villa P. et al. 1986. Cannibalism in the neolithic. Science 233:431–436.

Villotte S. and Knüsel C.J. 2013. Understanding entheseal changes: definition and life course changes. International Journal of Osteoarchaeology, 23(2): 135–146.
Villotte S. and Santos F. 2023. The effect of age on entheseal changes: a study of modifications at appendicular attachment sites in a large sample of identified human skeletons. Int J Osteoarchaeol 33(3): 389–401.
Villotte S. et al. 2016. In search of consensus: terminology for entheseal changes (EC). Int J Paleopathol 13:49–55.
Vilumets L., Aguraiuja-Lätti Ü., and Lewis M. 2024. Growing up in the suburbs: growth faltering and disease burden in the children from 16th to 18th century Tallinn, Estonia. Int J Osteoarchaeol 34(1): e3270. https://doi.org/10.1002/oa.3270.
Vincent M., Duval R.E., Hartemann P., and Engels-Deutsch M. 2018. Contact killing and antimicrobial properties of copper. J Appl Microbiol 124:1032–1046. https://doi.org/10.1111/jam.13681.
Visentin D., Gobin I., and Maglica Ž. 2023. Periodontal pathogens and their links to neuroinflammation and neurodegeneration. Microorganisms 11(7): 1832. https://doi.org/10.3390/microorganisms11071832.
Vlok M. 2023. Technical note: the use and misuse of threshold diagnostic criteria in paleopathology. Am J Biol Anthropol 181(2): 326–335.
Vlok M. and Buckley H.R. 2022. Palaeoepidemiological considerations of mobility and population interaction in the spread of infectious diseases in the prehistoric past. Bioarchaeol Int 6 (1–2): 77–107.
Vlok M. et al. 2021. Forager and farmer evolutionary adaptations to malaria evidenced by 7000 years of thalassemia in Southeast Asia. Sci Rep 11(1): 5677. https://doi.org/10.1038/s41598-021-83978-4.
Von Hunnius T., Roberts C.A., Saunders S., and Boylston A. 2006. Histological identification of syphilis in pre-Columbian England. Am J Phys Anthropol 129:559–566.
Von Hunnius T.E., Yang D., Eng B., Waye J.S., and Saunders S.R. 2007. Digging deeper into the limits of ancient DNA research on syphilis. J Arch Sci 34:2091–2100.
Vreeland J.M. and Cockburn A. 1980. Mummies of Peru. In: Mummies, disease and ancient cultures, ed. A. Cockburn and E. Cockburn, 135–174. Cambridge University Press.
Wagner J.K. et al. 2020. Fostering responsible research on ancient DNA. Am J Hum Genet 107:183–195. https://doi.org/10.1016/j.ajhg.2020.06.017.
Wakely J. and Young I. 1995. A medieval wrist injury fracture of the hook of the hamate bone. J Paleopathol 7(1): 51–56.
Wakely J., Manchester K., and Roberts C. 1991. Scanning electron microscopy of rib lesions. Int J Osteoarchaeol 1:185–189.
Waldron T. 1985. DISH at Merton Priory: evidence for a 'new' occupational disease. Br Med J 291:1762–1763.
Waldron T. 1993. The distribution of osteoarthritis of the hands in a skeletal population. Int J Osteoarchaeol 3:213–218.
Waldron T. 1994. Counting the dead: the epidemiology of skeletal populations. Wiley.
Waldron T. 1998. An unusual cluster of meningiomas? Int J Osteoarchaeol 8:213–217.
Waldron T. 2007. St Peter's, Barton-upon-Humber, Lincolnshire. Vol. 2: The human remains. Oxbow Books.
Waldron T. 2015. Roy Lee Moodie (1880–1934) and the beginnings of palaeopathology. J Med Biogr 23(1): 8–13.
Waldron T. 2019. Joint disease. In: Ortner's identification of pathological conditions in human skeletal remains, ed. J.E. Buikstra, 719–748. Academic Press.
Waldron T. 2021. Palaeopathology, 2nd ed. Cambridge University Press.
Waldron T. and Cox M. 1989. Occupational arthropathy: evidence from the past. Br J Industrial Med 46:420–422.
Waldron T. and Rogers J. 1991. Inter-observer variation in coding osteoarthritis in human skeletal remains. Int J Osteoarchaeol 1:49–56.
Walker D. 2012. Disease in London, 1st–19th centuries. Museum of London Archaeology Monograph 56.
Walker D., Powers N., Connell B., and Redfern R. 2015. Evidence of skeletal treponematosis from the medieval burial ground of St Mary Spital, London, and implications for the origins of the disease in Europe. Am J Phys Anthrop 156:90–101.

Walker E.G. 1983. Evidence for prehistoric cardiovascular disease of syphilitic origin on the Northern Plains. Am J Phys Anthropol 60:499–503.

Walker P., Bathurst R., Richman R., Gjerdrum T., and Andrushko V. 2009. The causes of porotic hyperostosis and cribra orbitalia: a reappraisal of the iron-deficiency anemia hypothesis. Am J Phys Anthropol 139:109–125.

Walker P.L. 1989. Cranial injuries as evidence of violence in prehistoric southern California. Am J Phys Anthropol 80:313–323.

Walker P.L. 1997. Wife beating, boxing and broken noses: skeletal evidence for the cultural patterning of violence. In: Troubled times: violence and warfare in the past, ed. D.L. Martin and D.W. Frayer, 145–179. Gordon and Breach.

Walker P.L., Cook D.C., and Lambert P.M. 1997. Skeletal evidence for child abuse: a physical anthropological perspective. J Forensic Sci 42(2): 196–207.

Walser J.W. III, Kristjánsdóttir S., Gowland R., and Desnica N. 2019. Volcanoes, medicine, and monasticism: investigating mercury exposure in medieval Iceland. Int J Osteoarchaeol 29:48–61. https://doi.org/10.1002/oa.2712.

Walter B.S., DeWitte S.N., and Redfern R.C. 2016. Sex differentials in caries frequencies in medieval London. Arch Oral Biol 63:32–39. https://doi.org/10.1016/j.archoralbio.2015.11.024.

Wan A.K.L. et al. 2003. A longitudinal study of *Streptococcus mutans* colonization in infants after tooth eruption. J Dent Res 82(7): 504–508. http://dx.doi.org/10.1177/15440591 0308200703.

Wang F. et al. 2021. Effects of water improvement and defluoridation on fluorosis-endemic areas in China: a meta-analysis. Environ Pollut 270:116227. https://doi.org/10.1016/j.envpol.2020. 116227.

Wang T. et al. 2022. Intestinal parasite infection in the Augustinian friars and general population of Cambridge, UK. Int J Paleopathol 39:115–121. https://doi.org/10.1016/j.ijpp.2022.06.001.

Wang T., Dittmar J.M., Inskip S.A., Cessford C., and Mitchell P.D. 2024. Investigating the association between intestinal parasite infection and cribra orbitalia in the population of Cambridge, UK. Int J Paleopathol 44:20–26. https://doi.org/10.1016/j.ijpp.2023.11.001.

Wani A.L., Ara A., and Usmani J.A. 2015. Lead toxicity: a review. Interdiscip Toxicol 8(2): 55–64. https://doi.org/10.1515/intox-2015-0009.

Ward E., DeSantis C., Robbins A., Kohler B., and Jemal A. 2014. Childhood and adolescent cancer statistics, 2014. CA: A Cancer Journal for Clinicians 64(2): 83–103.

Warinner C. 2016. Dental calculus and the evolution of the human oral microbiome. J Calif Dent Assoc. 44(7):411–20.

Warinner C. et al. 2014. Pathogens and host immunity in the ancient human oral cavity. Nat Genet 46:336–344. https://doi.org/10.1038/ng.2906.

Wasterlain S.N., Cunha E., and Hillson S. 2011. Periodontal disease in a Portuguese identified skeletal sample from the late nineteenth and early twentieth centuries. Am J Phys Anthropol 145:30–42. https://doi-org.ezphost.dur.ac.uk/10.1002/ajpa.21464.

Wasterlain S.N., Neves M.J., and Ferreira M.T. 2019. Dental modifications in a skeletal sample of enslaved Africans found at Lagos (Portugal). Int J Osteoarchaeol 26:621–632.

Waters-Rist A. and Hoogland M. 2013. Osteological evidence of short-limbed dwarfism in a nineteenth century Dutch family: achondroplasia or hypochondroplasia. Int J Paleopathol 3(4): 243–256.

Watson G.L. and Gilchrist R. 2021. Objects: the archaeology of healing. In: A cultural history of medicine in the Middle Ages (800–1450), ed. I. McCleery, 107–129. Bloomsbury Academic.

Watson J.T. 2008. Prehistoric dental disease and the dietary shift from cactus to cultigens in northwest Mexico. Int J Osteoarchaeol 18:202–212.

Watts R. 2013. Lumbar vertebral canal size in adults and children: observations from a skeletal sample in London, England. Homo 64:120–128.

Watts R. 2015. The long-term impact of developmental stress. Evidence from later medieval and post-medieval London (AD1117–1853). Am J Phys Anthropol 158(4): 569–580.

Webb E.A. and Dattani M.T. 2015. Understanding hypopituitarism. Paediatr Child Health 25(7): 295–301.

Webb S. 1988. Two possible cases of trephination from Australia. Am J Phys Anthropol 75:541–548.

Wechter J.F., Sikka R.S., Alwan M., Nelson B.J., and Tompkins M. 2014. Proximal tibial morphology and its correlation with osteochondritis dissecans of the knee. Knee Surg Sports Traumatol Arthrosc 23(12): 3717–3722.

Weiss D.L. and Møller-Christensen V. 1971. Leprosy, echinococcosis and amulets: a study of a mediaeval Danish inhumation. Med Hist 15 (3): 260–267.

Weiss P. 1958. Cultural osteology: cephalic practices. Part 1: Trophy heads, trephanation and cauterization. Universidad Nacional Mayor de San Marcos.

Wells C. 1962. Three cases of aural pathology of Anglo-Saxon date. J Laryng Otol 76: 931–933.

Wells C. 1963. Ancient Egyptian pathology. J Laryng Otol 77(3): 261–265.

Wells C. 1964a. Bones, bodies and disease. Thames and Hudson.

Wells C. 1964b. Chronic sinusitis with alveolar fistulae of mediaeval date. J Laryng Otol 78(3): 320–322.

Wells C. 1964c. The study of ancient disease. Surgo 32(1): 3–7.

Wells C. 1965. Osteogenesis imperfecta from an Anglo-Saxon burial ground at Burgh Castle, Suffolk. Med Hist 9:88–89.

Wells C. 1974a. Osteochondritis dissecans in ancient British skeletal material. Med Hist 18(4): 365–369.

Wells C. 1974b. The results of 'bone setting' in Anglo-Saxon times. Med Biol Ill 24:215–220.

Wells C. 1977. Disease of the maxillary sinus in antiquity. Med Biol Ill 27:173–178.

Wells C. 1982. The human remains. In: Romano-British cemeteries at Cirencester, ed. A. McWhirr, L. Viner, and C. Wells, 135–202. Excavations Committee.

Wells C. and Woodhouse N. 1975. Paget's disease in an Anglo-Saxon. Med Hist 19(4): 396–400.

Welsh H., Nelson A.J., van der Merwe A.E., de Boer H.H., and Brickley M.B. 2020. An investigation of micro-CT analysis of bone as a new diagnostic method for paleopathological cases of osteomalacia. Int J Paleopathol 31:23–33. https://doi.org/10.1016/j.ijpp.2020.08.004.

Wenham S. 1987. Anatomical interpretations of Anglo-Saxon weapon injuries. In: Weapons and warfare in Anglo-Saxon England, 123–139. Oxford University Committee for Archaeology Monograph 21.

Western A. and Bekvalac J. 2020. Manufactured bodies: the impact of industrialisation on London health. Oxbow Books.

Western A.G. and Bekvalac J.J. 2017. Hyperostosis frontalis interna in female historic skeletal populations: age, sex hormones and the impact of industrialization. Am J Phys Anthropol 162(3): 501–515.

Weston D.A. 2008. Investigating the specificity of periosteal reactions in pathology museum specimens. Am J Phys Anthropol 137:48–59.

Weston D.A. 2009. Brief communication: paleohistopathological analysis of pathology museum specimens: can periosteal reaction microstructure explain lesion etiology? Am J Phys Anthropol 140:186–93.

Weyrich L. et al. 2017. Neanderthal behaviour, diet, and disease inferred from ancient DNA in dental calculus. Nature 544:357–361. https://doi.org/10.1038/nature21674.

Wheeler S.M., Williams L., Beauchesne P., and Dupras T.L. 2013. Shattered lives and broken childhoods: evidence of physical child abuse in Ancient Egypt. Int J Paleopathol 3:71–82.

Whelton H.P., Spencer A.J., Do L.G., and Rugg-Gunn A.J. 2019. Fluoride revolution and dental caries: evolution of policies for global use. J Dent Res 98(8): 837–846. https://doi.org/10.1177/0022034519843495.

Whitaker D.K. 1993. Oral health. In: The Spitalfields project. Vol. 2: The anthropology: the middling sort, ed. T. Molleson and M. Cox, 49–65. Council for British Archaeology Research Report 86. Council for British Archaeology.

Whitaker D.K. and White D. 1989. A colour atlas of forensic dentistry. Wolfe.

Whitaker I.S. et al. 2007. Larval therapy from antiquity to the present day: mechanisms of action, clinical applications and future potential. Postgrad Med J 83(980): 409–413.

White C.D. 1996. Sutural effects of fronto-occipital cranial modification. Am J Phys Anthropol 100:397–410.

White C.D. and Armelagos G.J. 1997. Osteopenia and stable isotope ratios in bone collagen of Nubian female mummies. Am J Phys Anthropol 103:185–199.

White T., Black M., and Folkens P. 2012. Human osteology. Academic Press.

White T.D. 1992. Prehistoric cannibalism at Mancos 5MTUMR-2346. Princeton University Press.

White T.D., DeGusta D., Richards G.D., and Baker S.D. 1997. Brief communication: prehistoric dentistry in the American Southwest: a drilled canine from Sky Aerie, Colorado. Am J Phys Anthropol 103:409–414.

White V. and Ruparella P. 2021. Respiratory disease. In: Kumar and Clark's clinical medicine, 10th edition, ed. A. Feather, D. Randall, and M. Waterhouse, 927–999. Elsevier.

White W. 1988. The cemetery of St Nicholas Shambles. Museum of London and the London and Middlesex Archaeological Society.

Whiten A., Hinde R.A., Laland K.N., and Stringer C.B. 2011. Culture evolves. Philos Trans R Soc Lond B Biol Sci 366(1567): 938–948. https://doi.org/10.1098/rstb.2010.0372.

Whiting R.J., Antoine D., and Hillson S. 2019. Periodontal disease and 'oral health' in the past: new insights from ancient Sudan on a very modern problem. Dent Anthropol 32:30–50.

Whitney W. 1886. Notes on the anomalies, injuries and diseases of the bones of the native races of North America. Annual Reports of the Peabody Museum of American Archaeology and Ethnology 3:433–466. https://nativehealthdatabase.net/system/files/atoms/file/9900160.pdf.

Wilbur A.K., Buikstra J.E., and Stojanowski C. 2002. Mycobacterial disease in North America: an epidemiological test of Chaussinand's cross-immunity hypothesis. In: The past and present of leprosy: archaeological, historical, palaeopathological and clinical approaches, ed. C.A. Roberts, M.E. Lewis, and K. Manchester, 247–258. British Archaeological Reports International Series 1054. Archaeopress.

Wiggins R., Boylston A., and Roberts C.A. 1993. Report on the human skeletal remains from Blackfriars, Gloucester (19/91). Unpublished.

Wilczak C. and Mulhern D. 2012. Co-occurrence of DISH and HFI in the Terry Collection. Int J Osteoarchaeol 22:452–459.

Wilczak C.A. and Ortner D.J. 2013. A case of lepromatous leprosy from Kodiak Island, Alaska. Paper presented at the 40th annual meeting of the Paleopathology Association, Knoxville, Tennessee.

Wilczak C.A. and Ousley SD. 2009. Test of the relationship between sutural ossicles and cultural cranial deformation: results from Hawikuh, New Mexico. Am J Phys Anthropol 139(4): 483–493. https://doi.org/10.1002/ajpa.21005.

Wilkinson R. and Pickett K. 2009. The spirit level: why equality is better for everyone. Penguin.

Willey P. and Scott D.D. 1996. 'The bullets buzzed like bees': gunshot wounds in skeletons from the Battle of the Little Bighorn. Int J Osteoarchaeol 6:15–27.

Williams C.D. 1935. Kwashiorkor: a nutritional disease of children associated with a maize diet. Lancet (November 16): 1151–1152.

Williams K., Meinzer N., and Larsen C.S. 2018. History of degenerative joint disease in people across Europe: bioarchaeological inferences about lifestyle and activity from osteoarthritis and vertebral osteophytosis. In: The backbone of Europe: health, diet, work and violence over two millennia, ed. R.H. Steckel, C.S. Larsen, C.A. Roberts, and J. Baten, 253–299. Cambridge University Press.

Williams T.N. and Thein S.L. 2018. Sickle cell anemia and its phenotypes. Annu Rev Genom Hum Genet 19:113–147.

Williamson M.A., Johnston C.A., Symes S.A., and Schultz J.J. 2003. Interpersonal violence between 18th century Native Americans and Europeans in Ohio. Am J Phys Anthropol 122:113–122.

Willis R.A. 1948. Pathology of tumours. Butterworth.

Willson J.K. 1959. The bone lesions of leukemia: a survey of 140 cases. Radiology 72(5): 672–681.

Wilson A.S., Mulhall I., Cerdeira V., and Schotsman E.M.J. 2023. Preserved human bodies. In: Handbook of archaeological sciences, vol. 1, 2nd edition, ed. M. Pollard, R.A. Armitage, and C. Makarewicz, 453–475. Wiley.

Wilson B. and Pyatt F.B. 2007. Heavy metal dispersion, persistence, and bioaccumulation around an ancient copper mine situated in Anglesey, UK. Ecotoxicol Environ Saf 66:224–231. https://doi.org/10.1016/j.ecoenv.2006.02.015.

Wilson M. 1995. Ross and Wilson anatomy and physiology in health and illness, 7th ed. Churchill Livingstone.

Wißing C. et al. 2019. Stable isotopes reveal patterns of diet and mobility in the last Neandertals and first modern humans in Europe. Sci Rep 9(1): 4433. https://doi.org/10.1038/s41598-019-41033-3.

Wispelwey B., Tanous O., Asi Y., Hammoudeh W., and Mills D. 2023. Because its power remains naturalized: introducing the settler colonial determinants of health. Front Public Health 11:1137428. https://doi.org/10.3389/fpubh.2023.

Witkin A. 2011. The human skeletal remains. In: Infernal traffic: excavations of a liberated African graveyard in Rupert's Valley, St Helena. CBA Research Report 169, ed. A. Pearson, B. Jeffs, A. Witkin, and H. MacQuarrie, 57–98. Council for British Archaeology.

Witwer-Backofen U., and Engel F. 2019. The history of European dental health. In: The backbone of Europe: health, diet, work and violence over two millennia, ed. R.H. Steckel, C.S. Larsen, C.A. Roberts, and J. Baten, 84–136. Cambridge University Press.

Wolday D. et al. 2021. Effect of co-infection with intestinal parasites on COVID-19 severity: a prospective observational cohort study. EClinicalMedicine. 39:101054. https://doi.org/10.1016/j.eclinm.2021.101054.

Wolfe N., Dunavan C., and Diamond J. 2007. Origins of major human infectious diseases. Nature 447:279–283. https://doi.org/10.1038/nature05775.

Wolff J. 1989. The science of cancerous disease from earliest times to the present. Translated by Barbara Ayoub. Science History Publications.

Woo E.J., Kim J.-H., Lee W.-J., Cho H., and Pak S. 2019. Syphilitic infection in a pre-modern population from South Korea (19th century AD). Anthropol Sci 127:55–63.

Wood J.W., Ferrell R.J., and Dewitte-Aviña S.N. 2003. The temporal dynamics of the fourteenth-century Black Death: new evidence from English ecclesiastical records. Hum Biol 75(4): 427–448. https://doi.org/10.1353/hub.2003.0067.

Wood J.W., Milner G.R., Harpending H.C., and Weiss K.M. 1992. The osteological paradox: problems of inferring prehistoric health from skeletal samples. Curr Anthrop 33(4): 343–370.

Woods A., Bresalier M., Cassidy A., and Dentinger R.M. 2017. Animals and the shaping of modern medicine: One Health and its histories. Palgrave Macmillan.

World Archaeological Congress. 2024. https://worldarchaeologicalcongress.com/code-of-ethics/.

World Health Organization (WHO). 2011. Global status report on noncommunicable diseases 2010 description of the global burden of NCDs, their risk factors and determinants. World Health Organization.

World Health Organization (WHO). 2014. Global nutrition targets 2025: anaemia policy brief (No. WHO/NMH/NHD/14.4). World Health Organization.

World Health Organization (WHO). 2018. Working for better health for everyone, everywhere. World Health Organization. https://www.who.int/about/what-we-do/who-brochure.

World Health Organization (WHO). 2019a. Global leprosy update, 2018: moving towards a leprosy-free world. Wkly Epidemiol Rec 94:389–412.

World Health Organization (WHO). 2019b. Lead poisoning. https://www.who.int/news-room/fact-sheets/detail/lead-poisoning-and-health. Accessed July 2024.

World Health Organization (WHO). 2019c. Osteoarthritis. https://www.who.int/news-room/fact-sheets/detail/osteoarthritis. Accessed October 2023.

World Health Organization (WHO). 2020. Cancer. https://www.who.int/news-room/fact-sheets/detail/cancer. Accessed February 2024.

World Health Organization (WHO). 2022a. Global oral health status report. World Health Organization. https://www.who.int/team/noncommunicable-diseases/global-status-report-on-oral-health-2022. Accessed April 2024.

World Health Organization (WHO). 2022b. Global tuberculosis report 2022. World Health Organization. https://iris.who.int/handle/10665/363752. Accessed October 2023.

World Health Organization (WHO). 2022c. Plague. https://www.who.int/news-room/fact-sheets/detail/plague. Accessed April 2024.

World Health Organization (WHO). 2023a. Anaemia. https://www.who.int/health-topics/anaemia#tab=tab_1. Accessed April 2024.

World Health Organization (WHO). 2023b. Congenital disorders. https://www.who.int/news-room/factsheets/detail/birthdefects. Accessed July 2024.

World Health Organization (WHO). 2023c. Osteoarthritis. https://www.who.int/news-room/fact-sheets/detail/osteoarthritis#:~:text=Osteoarthritis%20affects%20the%20entire%20joint,older%20age%20and%20being%20overweight. Accessed October 2023.

World Health Organization (WHO). 2023d. The top 10 causes of death. https://www.who.int/news-room/fact-sheets/detail/the-top-10-causes-of-death. Accessed November 2023.

World Health Organization (WHO). 2024a. Abuse of older people. https://www.who.int/news-room/fact-sheets/detail/abuse-of-older-people. Accessed July 2024.

World Health Organization (WHO). 2024b. Air pollution. https://www.who.int/news-room/fact-sheets/detail/ambient-(outdoor)-air-quality-and-health. Accessed April 2024.

World Health Organization (WHO). 2024c. Brucellosis. https://www.who.int/news-room/fact-sheets/detail/brucellosis. Accessed April 2024.

World Health Organization (WHO). 2024d. Leprosy. https://www.who.int/news-room/fact-sheets/detail/leprosy. Accessed April 2024.

World Health Organization (WHO). 2024e. Malaria. https://www.who.int/news-room/fact-sheets/detail/malaria. Accessed April 2024.

World Health Organization (WHO). 2024f. Neglected tropical diseases. https://www.who.int/news-room/questions-and-answers/item/neglected-tropical-diseases. Accessed April 2024.

World Health Organization (WHO). 2024g. Primary health care. https://www.who.int/health-topics/primary-health-care#tab=tab_1. Accessed July 2024.

World Health Organization (WHO). 2024h. Rheumatoid arthritis. https://www.who.int/news-room/fact-sheets/detail/rheumatoid-arthritis. Accessed July 2024.

World Health Organization (WHO). 2024i. Syphilis. https://www.who.int/news-room/fact-sheets/detail/syphilis. Accessed April 2024.

World Health Organization (WHO). 2024j. Yaws (endemic treponematoses). https://www.who.int/health-topics/yaws#tab=tab_1. Accessed July 2024.

Wright L. 2011. Bilateral talipes equinovarus from Tikal, Guatemala. Int J Paleopathol 1(1): 55–62.

Wright L.E. and Schwarcz H.P. 1998. Stable carbon and oxygen isotopes in human tooth enamel: identifying breastfeeding and weaning in prehistory. Am J Phys Anthropol 106:1–18.

Wright S.L., Dobney K., and Weyrich L.S. 2021. Advancing and refining dental calculus research using multiomic frameworks. Sci Technol Archaeol Res 7:13–30.

Wrobel G.D., Biggs J.A., and Hair A.L. 2019. Digital modeling for bioarchaeologists. Adv Archaeol Pract 7(1): 47–54. https://doi.org/10.1017/aap.2018.47.

Wujastyk D. 1998. The roots of Ayurveda: selections from Sankskrit medical writings. Penguin.

Wysocka J. and Cieślik. 2023. The frequency and macromorphological classification of abnormal blood vessel impressions and periosteal appositions of the dura mater in an early modern osteological collection from Poland. Int J Paleopathol 41:78–87. https://doi.org/10.1016/j.ijpp.2023.04.001.

Xiong J.X. et al. 2021. A study of maxillary sinusitis infections of the Han Dynasty people from the Heishuiguo site [Chinese with English abstract]. Acta Anthropologica Sinica 40(5): 776–786. https://doi.org/10.16359/j.cnki.cn11-1963/q.2020.0031.

Yadav R., Verma A.K., Uppal A., Chahar H.S., Patel J. and Pal C.P., 2022. Prevalence of primary knee osteoarthritis in the urban and rural population in India. Indian J Rheumatol 17(3): 239–243.

Yamada R., Suzuki A., Chang X., and Yamamoto K. 2005. Citrullinated proteins in rheumatoid arthritis. Front Biosci 10:54–64.

Yang S. et al. 2023. Trepanation during the late Neolithic Age from the Mapai cemetery in the Gan-Qing region, northwestern China—a bioarcheological and experimental study. Int J Osteoarchaeol 33(1): 70–82.

Yapijakis C. et al. 2023. Molecular mechanisms involved in craniosynostosis. In Vivo 37(1): 36–46.

Yaussy S. 2022. Intersectionality and the interpretation of past pandemics. Bioarchaeol Int 6:58–76.

Yaussy S. 2023. Epidemiology and mathematical modelling. In: The Routledge handbook of paleopathology, ed. A.L. Grauer, 64–81. Routledge.

Yeap S.S. 2009. Rheumatoid arthritis in paintings: a tale of two origins. Int J Rheum Dis 12(4): 343–347. https://dx.doi.org/10.1111/j.1756-185X.2009.01434.x.

Yeh H.Y. and Mitchell P.D. 2016. Ancient human parasites in ethnic Chinese populations. Korean J Parasitol 54(5): 565–572. https://doi.org/10.3347/kjp.2016.54.5.565.

You S. et al. 2021. First case of juvenile primary bone malignant neoplasm in ancient China: a skeleton from the Northern Wei Dynasty (386–534 CE). Int J Osteoarchaeol 32(1): 182–191.

You T., Frostick S., Zhang W.T., and Yin Q. 2019. Os acromiale: reviews and current perspectives. Orthop Surg 11(5): 738–744. https://doi.org/10.1111/os.12518.

Young M.F., Luo H., and Suchdev P.S. 2023. The challenge of defining the global burden of iron deficiency anaemia. Lancet Haematol 10(9): e702–e704. https://doi.org/10.1016/S2352-3026(23)00168-0.

Yu D. et al. 2022. The gut microbiome and metabolites are altered and interrelated in patients with rheumatoid arthritis. Front Cell Infect Microbiol 11:763507. https://doi.org/10.3389/fcimb.2021.763507.

Zariņa G. et al. 2016. Cribra orbitalia as a potential indicator of childhood stress: evidence from paleopathology, stable C, N, and O isotopes, and trace element concentrations in children from a 17th–18th century cemetery in Jēkabpils, Latvia. J Trace Elem Med Biol 38:131–137.

Zäuner S.P., Wahl J., Boyadziev Y., and Aslanis I. 2013. A 6000-year-old hand amputation from Bulgaria: the oldest case from south-east Europe? Int J Osteoarchaeol 23:618–625. https://doi.org/10.1002/oa.1277.

Zedda N., Bramanti B., Gualdi-Russo E., Ceraico E., and Rinaldo N. 2021. The biological index of frailty: a new index for the assessment of frailty in human skeletal remains. Am J Phys Anthropol 176(3): 459–473.

Zhan X., Shao J., Zhu Y., and Yeh H.Y. 2023. A case of septic arthritis of the hip in Central Plains, China, during the Western Han Dynasty (3rd century BCE–1st century CE). Int J Paleopathol 40:87–92.

Zhang H., Liu M., Fan W., Sun S., and Fan X. 2022. The impact of *Mycobacterium tuberculosis* complex in the environment on One Health approach. Front Public Health 10:994745. https://doi.org/10.3389/fpubh.2022.994745.

Zhang H. et al. 2016. A comparative study of oral health in three Late Bronze Age populations with different subsistence practices in North China. Quat Int 405:44–57. https://doi.org/10.1016/j.quaint.2015.05.029.

Zhang J.S., Chu C.-H., and Yu O.Y. 2022. Oral microbiome and dental caries development. Dent J 10(10): 184. https://doi.org/10.3390/dj10100184.

Zhang W. et al. 2021. Violence in the first millennium BCE Eurasian steppe: cranial trauma in three Turpan Basin populations from Xinjiang, China. Am J Phys Anthropol 175:81–94. https://doi.org/10.1002/ajpa.24194.

Zhang X., Zhao Y., Niu Y., Wang Z., and Zeng W. 2020. Two probable cases of mastoiditis in a cemetery from the Warring States to Han Dynasty (475 BCE–220 CE) in Qufu, Shandong Province, China. Int J Paleopathol 30:77–84. https://doi.org/10.1016/j.ijpp.2020.03.001.

Zhang X. et al. 2021. A case of well-healed foot amputation in early China (8th–5th centuries BCE). Int J Osteoarchaeol 32:132–141.

Zhao D., He L., and Xing F. 2023. Skeletal evidence for two external auditory canal disorder cases from China. Int J Osteoarchaeol 33(1): 170–177. https://doi.org/10.1002/oa.3187.

Zhenbiao Z. 1994. The skeletal evidence of human leprosy and syphilis in ancient China. Acta Anthropologica Sinica 13:294–298.

Zhou Y. et al. 2022. Identifying treponemal disease in early East Asia. Am J Biol Anthropol 178(3): 530–543. https://doi.org/10.1002/ajpa.24526.

Zhou Y., Xi F., Zhao F., and Berger E. 2024. A probable case of multiple osteochondromas in a Qing period (1644–1911) individual from Shandong, China. Int J Osteoarchaeol https://doi.org/10.1002/oa.3323.

Zias J. and Mitchell P. 1996. Psoriatic arthritis in a fifth-century Judaean monastery. Am J Phys Anthropol 101:491–502.

Zias J. and Mumcuoglu K. 1991. Pre-pottery neolithic B headlice from Nahal Hemar Cave. Atiquot (Jerusalem) 20:167–168.

Zias J. and Numeroff K. 1987. Operative dentistry in the 2nd century BC. J Am Dental Assoc. 114:665–666.

Zias J. and Pomeranz S. 1992. Serial craniectomies for intracranial infection 5.5 millennia ago. Int J Osteoarchaeol 2:183–186.

Zimmermann M.B. 2009. Iodine deficiency. *Endocr Rev* 30:376–408. https://doi.org/10.1210/er.2009-0011.

Zink A. et al. 2007. Molecular history of tuberculosis from ancient mummies and skeletons. Int J Osteoarchaeol 17:380–391. https://doi.org/10.1002/oa.909.

Zink A. et al. 2014. Genomic correlates of atherosclerosis in ancient humans. Glob Heart 9:203–209. https://doi.org/10.1016/j.gheart.2014.03.2453.

Zink A. et al. 2023. The genetic background of atherosclerosis in ancient mummies. In: The bioarchaeology of cardiovascular disease, ed. M. Binder, C.A. Roberts, D. Antoine, 81–98. Cambridge University Press.

Zou J. et al. 2020. Association between rare variants in specific functional pathways and human neural tube defects multiple subphenotypes. Neural Dev 15:1–15. https://doi.org/10.1186/s13064-020-00145-7.

Zubir M.Z.M., Holloway S., and Mohd Noor N. 2020. Maggot therapy in wound healing: a systematic review. Int J Environ Res Public Health 17(17): 6103. https://doi.org/10.3390/ijerph17176103.

Zubova A., Moiseyev V., Ananyeva N., Stulov I., and Andreev E. 2022. Chronic maxillary sinusitis recorded in archaeological samples: geographical distribution and predisposing factors. Archaeol Ethnol Anthropol Eurasia 50(1): 147–157.

Zuckerman M.K. 2017. The 'poxed' and the 'pure': a bioarchaeological investigation of community and marginalization relative to infection with acquired syphilis in post-medieval London. Archeological Papers of the American Anthropological Association 28:91–103. https://doi.org/10.1111/apaa.12091.

Zuckerman M.K. et al. 2023. Sex, gender, and sexuality in paleopathology: select current developments and pathways forward. Int J Paleopathol 41:8–21.

Zuckerman M.K., Turner B.L., and Armelagos G.J. 2012. Evolutionary thought in paleopathology and the rise of the biocultural approach. In: A companion to paleopathology, ed. A.L. Grauer, 34–57. Wiley-Blackwell.

Zuckerman M.K., Harper K.N., and Armelagos G.J. 2016. Adapt or die: three case studies in which the failure to adopt advances from other fields has compromised paleopathology. Int J Osteoarchaeol 26:375–383. https://doi.org/10.1002/oa.2426.

Zwick E.D. and Pepperell C.S. 2020. Tuberculosis sanatorium treatment at the advent of the chemotherapy era. BMC Infect Dis 20(1): 831. https://doi.org/10.1186/s12879-020-05539-w.

Index

Pages with figures are in italics.